BSAVA Manual of Canine and Feline Dentistry and Oral Surgery
fourth edition

Editors:

Alexander M. Reiter
DipTzt DrMedVet DipAVDC DipEVDC
School of Veterinary Medicine,
University of Pennsylvania, Philadelphia, PA 19104–6010, USA

Margherita Gracis
DVM DipAVDC DipEVDC
Clinica Veterinaria San Siro,
Via Lampugnano 99, Milan, 20154, Italy

Published by:

British Small Animal Veterinary Association
Woodrow House, 1 Telford Way, Waterwells Business Park, Quedgeley, Gloucester GL2 2AB

A Company Limited by Guarantee in England
Registered Company No. 2837793 • Registered as a Charity

Published 2018
Reprinted 2019, 2021, 2023
Copyright © 2023 BSAVA

All rights reserved. No part of this publication may be reproduced, stored in a retrieval system, or transmitted, in form or by any means, electronic, mechanical, photocopying, recording or otherwise without prior written permission of the copyright holder.

Figures 2.9e and 2.9f and illustrations in Operative Technique 9.2 (part) were drawn by David Crossley and are printed with his permission.

Figures 2.1, 4.13a, 4.14a, 4.15a, 4.16a, 4.17a, 4.18a, 4.19a, 4.20a, 4,21a, 6.7, 10.37, 10.38 and 10.39 and illustrations in Operative Technique 9.2 (part) were drawn by S.J. Elmhurst BA Hons (www.livingart.org.uk) and are printed with her permission.

A catalogue record for this book is available from the British Library.

ISBN 978 1 905319 60 2

The publishers, editors and contributors cannot take responsibility for information provided on dosages and methods of application of drugs mentioned or referred to in this publication. Details of this kind must be verified in each case by individual users from up to date literature published by the manufacturers or suppliers of those drugs. Veterinary surgeons are reminded that in each case they must follow all appropriate national legislation and regulations (for example, in the United Kingdom, the prescribing cascade) from time to time in force.

Printed in the UK by Hobbs the Printers Ltd, Totton SO40 3WX
Printed on ECF paper made from sustainable forests

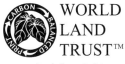

www.carbonbalancedprint.com
CBP2250

Carbon Balancing is delivered by World Land Trust, an international conservation charity, who protects the world's most biologically important and threatened habitats acre by acre. Their Carbon Balanced Programme offsets emissions through the purchase and preservation of high conservation value forests.

Save 15% off the digital version of this manual. By purchasing this print edition we are pleased to offer you a reduced price on online access at www.bsavalibrary.com Enter offer code 15DOS224 on checkout

Please note the discount only applies to a purchase of the full online version of the *BSAVA Manual of Canine and Feline Dentistry and Oral Surgery, 4th edition* via **www.bsavalibrary.com**. The discount will be taken off the BSAVA member price or full price, depending on your member status. The discount code is for a single purchase of the online version and is for your personal use only. If you do not already have a login for the BSAVA website you will need to register in order to make a purchase.

18379UBS23

Titles in the BSAVA Manuals series

For further information on these and all BSAVA publications, please visit our website: **www.bsava.com**

Contents

Contributors

Ana Castejon-Gonzalez
DVM PhD DipAVDC
School of Veterinary Medicine,
University of Pennsylvania,
Philadelphia, PA 19104-6010, USA

Margherita Gracis
DVM DipAVDC DipEVDC
Clinica Veterinaria San Siro,
Via Lampugnano 99,
Milan, 20154, Italy

Norman Johnston
BVM&S FAVD DipAVDC DipEVDC FRCVS
DentalVets Ltd,
29-31 Station Hill, North Berwick,
East Lothian EH39 4AS, UK

Simone Kirby
FHEA DipEVDC MRCVS
Chess Veterinary Clinic,
97 Uxbridge Road,
Rickmansworth,
Hertfordshire WD3 7DJ, UK

Helena Kuntsi
ELL DipEVDC DipAVDC
Veterinary Specialist for Small Animal Diseases,
Anident, Lamminpätie 41,
02880, Veikkola, Finland

M. Paula Larenza Menzies
DVM DrMedVet PhD DipECVAA
University of Veterinary Medicine – Vienna,
Veterinaerplatz 1, 1210, Vienna, Austria

Loic Legendre
DVM FAVD DipAVDC DipEVDC
West Coast Veterinary Dental Services,
1350 Kootenay Street, Vancouver,
BC, V5K 4R1, Canada

John R. Lewis
VMD FAVD DipACVD
NorthStar Vets,
315 Robbinsville-Allentown Road,
Robbinsville, NJ 08691, USA

Wilfried Mai
DrMedVet MSc PhD
School of Veterinary Medicine,
University of Pennsylvania,
Philadelphia, PA 19104-6010, USA

Bonnie Miller
BS RDH
School of Veterinary Medicine,
University of Pennsylvania,
Philadelphia, PA 19104-6010, USA

Laura Ordeix
LdaVet MSc DipECVD
Universitat Autònoma de Barcelona
08193 Bellaterra, Barcelona, Spain

Alexander M. Reiter
DipTzt DrMedVet DipAVDC DipEVDC
School of Veterinary Medicine,
University of Pennsylvania,
Philadelphia, PA 19104-6010, USA

Giorgio Romanelli
DipECVS MRCVS
Centro Specialistico Veterinario,
via dei Fontanili 11/a, Milan, 20134, Italy

Tobias Schwarz
DrMedVet MA DVR DipECVDI DipACVR FRCVS
Royal (Dick) School of Veterinary Studies,
Easter Bush Campus, Midlothian EH25 9RG, UK

Peter Southerden
BVSc MBA DipEVDC MRCVS
Eastcott Referrals,
Edison Park, Dorcan Way,
Swindon, Wiltshire SN3 3FR, UK

Jerrold Tannenbaum
MA JD
School of Veterinary Medicine,
University of California, Davis,
One Shields Avenue, Davis, CA 95616, USA

Frank J.M. Verstraete
DrMedVet BVSc(Hons) MMedVet DipAVDC DipECVS DipEVDC
School of Veterinary Medicine,
University of California, Davis,
One Shields Avenue, Davis, CA 95616, USA

Foreword

In 1987–88, I spent a sabbatical year as a Visiting Professor jointly at the Dental and Veterinary Schools of Liverpool University; this led to an invitation to edit the first *BSAVA Manual of Small Animal Dentistry*, which was published in 1990 as a modest volume of 158 pages, limited to black-and-white illustrations.

When the first edition was written, dental equipment and instruments in the typical UK small animal practice consisted of an ultrasonic scaler and a limited selection of tooth extraction instruments. The intervening 30 years have seen an explosion in awareness of small animal dentistry. Now, even in a non-specialist practice, a high-speed dental unit with hand-pieces, burs and an air-water spray, and a dental radiographic unit, preferably digital, are considered essential to practicing good quality general dentistry. This book fills a very useful purpose, because dentistry has yet to achieve the veterinary school 'curriculum time' appropriate for its clinical importance. Continued professional development and reading expert texts such as this book are critical means of closing the dental knowledge circle for veterinary practitioners.

To match the need for greatly expanded dental information, the Editors of this fourth edition have assembled a very strong group of contributors. The book is logical in its organization, thorough in its depth of coverage, well referenced, and very well illustrated with several excellent 'how-to' sequences. It tackles the controversial topics, such as 'anaesthesia-free dentistry' and 'use and abuse of antibiotics in association with dental treatment' in a fair and useful way.

While it remains unlikely that every small animal practice will ever have the expertise, experience, equipment, instruments and supplies to offer the full range of veterinary dental procedures, all small animal practices should be capable of two things:

1. Effective management of the common dental and oral conditions in cats and dogs.
2. Recognition of the full range of dental and oral conditions, so that informed referrals can be made to dental specialists who are able to offer equipment- and knowledge-intensive procedures.

This book provides the detailed, well-illustrated information required for the first of these critical items, and sufficient detail for the second to ensure that accurate information about treatment and prognosis can be provided to owners when a referral to a specialist is indicated.

One area in which significant progress has been made is in the understanding of the interactions between the oral cavity and the rest of the body. The association of distant organ pathology (cardiac, renal, hepatic) and systemic response to increasing severity of periodontal disease is now well documented in dogs, and provides a powerful stimulus to establish an effective periodontal disease preventive program in every practice. As is well described in this book, this consists of professional scaling when indicated, extractions when necessary, and an effective home-care oral hygiene program. The general health of our pets will benefit when early attention is paid to prevention as well as treatment of this, the most common disease occurring in dogs and cats.

Please take time to read through this book, and then be sure to 'lift-the-lip' every time you see any patient for any reason, so that you can recognize the oral-dental conditions that are so well described here.

I hope you will find, as I did, that dentistry offers a challenging, interesting and professionally satisfying use of your veterinary skills!

Colin Harvey BVSc DipACVS DipAVDC DipEVDC FRCVS
Emeritus Professor of Surgery and Dentistry, School of Veterinary Medicine,
University of Pennsylvania

Preface

It has been 6 years since we were first approached to edit the 4th edition of this book, thus continuing a series of BSAVA manuals on dentistry and oral surgery in dogs and cats. We found it important to add 'and oral surgery' to its title, as many procedures performed in and around the mouth involve surgical techniques beyond the treatment of teeth.

This book has been written to reach veterinarians, veterinary technicians and nurses, and veterinary students. It contains 13 chapters and is intended to educate the reader about the following topics:

Ethical aspects; anatomy and physiology; examination; diagnostic imaging; common pathology; anaesthesia and analgesia; management of periodontal disease, non-periodontal inflammatory, infectious and reactive conditions, dental and oral trauma, developmental disorders, and oral and maxillofacial neoplasia; tooth extraction; and perioperative considerations.

We come from both academia and private practice, and put great thought and effort into this project. The reader can hope to learn the basics of dentistry and oral surgery in dogs and cats by reading this manual, and we also included intermediate and advanced information for those that already have a special interest in the discipline. While no attempt was made to be all-inclusive, we wanted to deliver well-referenced knowledge that is supported by an abundance of image material.

We selected authors that are known leaders and experienced professionals in their field of expertise. They were instrumental in the writing of this manual, and we thank them for having made significant contributions to the veterinary literature. We are also grateful to our partners, families, friends and colleagues who supported us during this journey. Our special gratitude goes to our mentors Dr Colin Harvey, Dr Paul Orsini and Mrs Bonnie Miller, who were influential in making us become who we are today.

Respectfully,

Alexander M. Reiter and Margherita Gracis
June 2018

Chapter 1

Ethics in dentistry and oral surgery

Frank J.M. Verstraete and Jerrold Tannenbaum

Veterinary practice on companion animals raises unavoidable and sometimes challenging ethical issues. Veterinary surgeons (veterinarians) are committed to protect the health and welfare of patients. They also serve clients, who receive substantial benefits from the human–animal bond and who pay veterinary surgeons for agreed-upon services. What is in the best interest of a patient is not always what the client wants or needs, and what a client wants or needs is not always best for the patient. It is sometimes unclear how such conflicts ought to be resolved. Veterinary surgeons also have legitimate interests in furthering their knowledge and skills and in adequate and fair compensation for their services.

This chapter considers a number of ethical issues that are distinctive to small animal dentistry and oral surgery. The discussion presents several general principles of veterinary ethics. It is then suggested how these principles apply in various ways to branches or aspects of veterinary dentistry. The first two principles – which are arguably the most important core principles of veterinary ethics (Tannenbaum, 2013) – are quoted from the Royal College of Veterinary Surgeons (RCVS) Code of Professional Conduct for Veterinary Surgeons. In substance, all the principles stated here are explicitly included in or are implied by the official ethical codes or positions of veterinary associations worldwide. Therefore, these principles provide strong foundations for ethical approaches to veterinary dentistry. The chapter cannot consider all ethical principles that apply to dental and oral care of companion animals. It also must be recognized that generally accepted ethical principles do not always result in universal consensus. There can be disagreement about how strongly to weigh conflicting interests and considerations in a particular case. Some clinical situations may present unique or complex facts that can make it difficult for a veterinary surgeon to decide what is ethically permissible or required.

Principles of veterinary ethics

Principles of veterinary ethics relevant to small animal dentistry and oral surgery include:

- Veterinary surgeons must make animal health and welfare their first consideration when attending to animals (RCVS, 2013a)
- Veterinary surgeons must be open and honest with clients and respect their needs and requirements (RCVS, 2013b)

- The potential benefits of a procedure to a patient and client must justify the potential risks or costs to the patient and client, and the greater these risks or costs, the more important must be the benefits
- A veterinary procedure that is performed solely for cosmetic or aesthetic reasons does not justify subjecting the patient to pain, distress or discomfort, or to any significant medical risks associated with the procedure
- A veterinary surgeon should not offer as a service that promotes patients' health and welfare a procedure that does not benefit patients, or in fact presents risks to their health and welfare
- Veterinary surgeons should base diagnoses and treatments on the best available scientific knowledge, and should not employ techniques of which the efficacy and safety have not been established by sufficient scientific evidence
- The veterinary surgeon must obtain informed consent from the client for any proposed procedure or treatment
- The veterinary surgeon must have sufficient training and skill to perform a procedure. The veterinary surgeon should not delegate the procedure or aspects of the procedure to colleagues or staff who do not have sufficient training and skill. When appropriate, a case should be referred to a specialist or a practitioner with sufficient background and skill.

Principle 1: Veterinary surgeons must make animal health and welfare their first consideration when attending to animals

Although they serve humans as well as animals, veterinary surgeons are animal doctors – experts in prevention, diagnosis and treatment of animal disease and the promotion of animal health and welfare. There are vigorous and sometimes contentious debates about when, if ever, it is ethically appropriate to favour the interests of owners over those of their animals (Tannenbaum, 2013). There are also disagreements about how to define animal 'welfare' (Tannenbaum, 1995a). Nevertheless, there is general agreement among veterinary surgeons about certain core components of animal health and welfare that veterinary surgeons should make their primary considerations in dealing with patients and clients. As stated by the Principles of Veterinary Medical Ethics of the AVMA (American Veterinary Medical Association), at the very least, 'Veterinarians should first consider the needs of the patient: to prevent and relieve disease, suffering, or disability while minimizing pain or fear' (AVMA, 2015a).

Principle 2: Veterinary surgeons must be open and honest with clients and respect their needs and requirements

Clients have important needs, interests and expectations. Clients expect that their veterinary surgeon will accept and promote these interests in return for payment of their fees. For clients with companion animals, these interests typically include the desire to keep or make their animals healthy and happy – a desire motivated by sincere devotion and love that is part of a genuine human–companion animal bond. In order to serve these interests and expectations, veterinary surgeons must listen carefully and empathetically to clients and respond honestly to their questions and concerns. Veterinary surgeons must respect and attempt to fulfil the desires of clients once there has been an agreement about the patient's care. In a real sense, small animal veterinary surgeons are doctors not just to their animal patients, but to the human–companion animal bond, which of course includes the human as well as the animal component (Tannenbaum, 1995b).

Principle 3: The potential benefits of a procedure to a patient and client must justify the potential risks or costs to the patient and client, and the greater these risks or costs, the more important must be the benefits

This principle is easily stated but can be difficult to apply in particular circumstances because one must take into account, and sometimes prioritize, different and sometimes conflicting interests of the patient and client. Among potential benefits to veterinary patients are cure, palliation or prevention of disease, infirmity or pain; a continuing life; and a good quality of life. Among potential benefits to clients are the ability to continue enjoyment of a human–animal bond and knowing that their animals are healthy and happy. Among typical potential risks or harms to veterinary patients are the risk of death that might be associated with a procedure; pain, distress or discomfort that can be part of or result from the procedure; and a poor or unimproved quality of life. Among typical potential harms to veterinary clients are the significant financial cost of some procedures; and psychological or physical burdens caring for the animal during or after a procedure.

Principle 4: A veterinary procedure that is performed solely for cosmetic or aesthetic reasons does not justify subjecting the patient to pain, distress or discomfort, or to any significant medical risks associated with the procedure

This principle follows from principle 1; procedures performed solely for cosmetic or aesthetic considerations of the client do not protect the patient's health or welfare.

Principle 3 also counts against a procedure that subjects a patient to pain, distress, or discomfort, or medical risks for no benefit to it, to obtain what most people would regard as a relatively trivial 'benefit' to the client. Principle 4 is reflected in the long-standing prohibition of the RCVS (RCVS, 1987) and the more recent disapproval of the AVMA (AVMA, 2008; Nolen, 2008) of ear trimming and tail-docking of dogs when done for purely cosmetic reasons and not for the medical benefit of the animal.

Principle 5: A veterinary surgeon should not offer as a service that promotes patients' health and welfare a procedure that does not benefit to patients, or in fact presents risks to their health and welfare

This principle also follows from principles 1 and 2. Providing a useless or potentially harmful service does not promote – and indeed expresses great disregard of and disrespect for – the patient's health and welfare. It also reflects dishonesty to clients who are led to believe that a useless or harmful procedure will help their animals.

Principle 6: Veterinary surgeons should base diagnoses and treatments on the best available scientific knowledge, and should not employ techniques of which the efficacy and safety have not been established by sufficient scientific evidence

This is more than just an ethical principle that follows from a veterinary surgeon's ethical responsibilities to the patient and client. The principle is part of the very definition of veterinary medicine itself. Veterinary surgeons are not simply members of the profession that seeks to help animals and people by preventing, alleviating and curing animal injury, infirmity and disease. Veterinary medicine is the discipline that pursues these aims supported and guided by scientific knowledge.

Principle 7: The veterinary surgeon must obtain informed consent from the client for any proposed procedure or treatment

This principle follows from principle 2. Because patients are typically the property of clients and, in the case of companion animals, are likely to be of great personal and emotional importance to clients and their families, clients have an ethical (as well as a legal) right to decide what care their animals shall receive. Although precise legal requirements for informed consent vary among jurisdictions, in essence the ethical requirement of informed consent means that a client must voluntarily agree to a procedure after having been given, and understanding, information regarding the procedure that an ordinarily reasonable client would want to have. Such information typically includes potential risks of the procedure to the animal, likely outcomes if the procedure is performed, and likely outcomes of medically reasonable alternatives, including (sometimes) not performing any procedure or euthanasia.

Principle 8: The veterinary surgeon must have sufficient training and skill to perform a procedure. The veterinary surgeon should not delegate the procedure or aspects of the procedure to colleagues or staff who do not have sufficient training and skill. When appropriate, a case should be referred to a specialist or a practitioner with sufficient background and skill

This principle follows from a veterinary surgeon's ethical obligations to protect the health and welfare of the patient, and to respect the needs, requirements and expectations of clients.

Application of ethical principles to branches and aspects of small animal dentistry and oral surgery

Orthodontics

Orthodontics is the branch of dentistry dealing with malocclusions. Malocclusion is the abnormal spatial relationship between individual teeth, which can be caused by the abnormal position or orientation of teeth, or by discrepancies in jaw length. The clinical importance of malocclusion varies greatly. Some malocclusions are incidental findings with no clinical significance other than a visible abnormality, which may or may not affect the aesthetic appearance of the pet. On the other hand, some malocclusions cause pathological tooth attrition, due to an abnormal tooth-to-tooth contact. The most significant malocclusions are those that cause soft tissue trauma due to an abnormal contact between teeth and oral soft tissues, resulting in obvious pain and discomfort; linguoversion of the mandibular canine teeth, which causes trauma to the palatal mucosa, is a good example. Abnormal forces acting upon teeth can cause periodontal trauma, which in turn may contribute to a more rapid progression of periodontitis in the absence of oral hygiene.

In considering orthodontic treatment, the attending veterinary surgeon should, first and foremost, in accordance with the first ethical principle discussed above, determine whether there is a true medical problem that requires correction. If there is a medical problem, the potential advantages and disadvantages of orthodontic treatment versus other methods of treatment, such as selective extractions, must be evaluated. Among relevant considerations are the number of anaesthesias and the nature of the proposed procedures and associated discomfort, distress and risks (principles 3 and 4). If orthodontic treatment is deemed justified, the client should be counselled about the possible genetic background of the problem to be corrected, and neutering the animal should strongly be recommended. This is especially important regarding show and breeding animals. The rules of the American Kennel Club (AKC) as well as other kennel clubs and registries worldwide specifically state that altering the natural appearance of a dog for the purpose of correcting an abnormality is cause for disqualification (AKC, 2013).

The veterinary surgeon must be completely honest with the client regarding the need for orthodontic treatment and treatment planning, so that the client can exercise a truly informed consent (principles 2 and 7). Sometimes, there can be professional temptations and client and peer pressures, which may cloud the decision-making of the veterinary surgeon. Clients may insist on orthodontic treatment, even though there is no obvious medical need, for cosmetic or aesthetic reasons or because of their intention to use the patient as a show or breeding animal. Additionally, board-certified veterinary dentists and veterinary general practitioners with a professional interest in dentistry may be tempted to recommend orthodontic treatment in order to be seen as offering a state-of-the-art clinical service. Veterinary surgeons who are aspiring to submit their credentials to the European Veterinary Dental College (EVDC) or American Veterinary Dental College (AVDC), which have a minimum required case log quota system, may be tempted to perform orthodontic procedures on questionable cases for the sole purpose of meeting the quota requirement.

When a malocclusion is corrected, or indeed any alteration is made to an animal's appearance, privacy and confidentiality laws in the USA and most European countries prevent the veterinary surgeon from disclosing anything regarding the procedure, including the names of the client and patient, to anyone without the client's permission (AVMA, 2015b). However, in the UK, the Kennel Club makes it a condition of registration that the owner consents that a veterinary surgeon report any Caesarean operation or correction or alteration of a dog's appearance to the Kennel Club (Kennel Club, 2014). Moreover, the RCVS Code of Professional Conduct for Veterinary Surgeons specifically provides that 'registration of a dog with the Kennel Club permits a veterinary surgeon who carries out a Caesarean section on a bitch, or surgery to alter the natural conformation of a dog, to report this to the Kennel Club' without violating the duty of confidentiality (RCVS, 2015).

Periodontics

The standard of care in small animal periodontics includes periodontal probing and dental charting and the removal of supragingival and subgingival plaque and calculus (AVDC, 2013a). It is generally accepted within the veterinary community that this can be achieved safely and effectively only if the patient is placed under general anaesthesia (AVDC, 2013a). Anaesthesia-free dental cleaning is a relatively recent phenomenon. Several companies and individuals can be found on the Internet promoting this service, usually claiming a 'proprietary' method of restraining the animal. Many of the individuals performing this practice are not licensed veterinary surgeons, veterinary technicians or veterinary nurses. Some even use the term 'veterinary dental hygienist', which creates the perception that these individuals have received appropriate training. In many instances, anaesthesia-free cleaning is performed at grooming businesses. Some techniques used in such dental cleaning (such as the use of scalers) typically constitute the practice of veterinary medicine and can only be performed lawfully in the USA or UK by licensed veterinary surgeons.

Several medical and ethical issues are raised by anaesthesia-free dental cleaning. First, a full oral examination with periodontal probing and radiographs is not tolerated by animals without anaesthesia, and many lesions may go unnoticed without diagnostic charting and radiographs.

Secondly, without anaesthesia it is practically impossible to remove the subgingival plaque and calculus, which are the deposits that are most important, as they are in close proximity to the periodontal disease site. Removing only supragingival plaque and calculus is ineffective and does not improve the pet's health (AVDC, 2013a). Thirdly, anaesthesia-free dental cleaning is deceptive, as it gives the client a false sense of accomplishment. Fourthly, periodontal instruments are sharp and can cause injury to an awake and moving animal. Finally, scaling teeth without an endotracheal tube in place may result in accidental aspiration of dental calculus (AVDC, 2013a).

A recent worrisome development is the providing of anaesthesia-free dental cleaning by some veterinary practices under supervision of a licensed veterinary surgeon. Although this may make anaesthesia-free cleaning legal, it would still be at odds with principles 4 and 5 described above because such cleaning would not benefit the animal, would be done in essence for cosmetic reasons, and would be associated with distress and risk of injury. Anaesthesia-free dental cleaning also violates principle 6, which requires treatment based on the best available scientific knowledge, the efficacy and safety of which has been well established. Principle 8 also prohibits veterinary surgeons from delegating procedures to individuals with insufficient training and skill.

Another aspect of periodontics that has ethical implications is the plethora of available oral veterinary healthcare products, such as gels or creams, and additives to water that are supposed to prevent or remove dental plaque. Ideally, the safety and efficacy of such products should be documented in peer-reviewed publications in respectable scientific journals. Unfortunately this has not been the case. The Veterinary Oral Health Council (VOHC) grants a 'seal of acceptance' to products that meet certain requirements based on information provided by the manufacturer (VOHC, 2013). Unfortunately, the safety and efficacy of many of these products are often not documented, except for promotional documents provided by the manufacturer. If such products are sold or recommended in a veterinary practice, clients are likely to believe that the veterinary surgeon has evaluated the products and believes that they are effective and safe. It is a violation of principle 6 for a veterinary surgeon to sell or recommend a dental product that is represented as benefiting the patient, unless the clinician has in fact evaluated its efficacy and safety and has sound medical reasons for selling or recommending the product.

Endodontics

Endodontics is the branch of dentistry dealing with diseases of the pulp. Endodontic treatment is a commonly performed procedure to address pulp exposure or necrosis, often caused by a complicated crown fracture. The procedure is safe and effective, if properly performed, but technique-sensitive. It is not part of the regular veterinary curriculum. Therefore, endodontic treatment should only be performed by veterinary surgeons who have the necessary advanced training and skill (principle 8). If a veterinary surgeon lacks such training and skill, referral to a specialist is indicated.

Endodontic treatment requires follow-up radiographs obtained under sedation or general anaesthesia, as the documented success rate of the procedure is in the order of 94% (Kuntsi-Vaattovaara et al., 2002). Therefore, if the client will not consent to follow-up examination, or if the overall health status of the animal is such that prolonged chemical restraint is contraindicated, the affected tooth should simply be extracted. Again, this would be a recommendation by the veterinary surgeon based on the

animal's health and welfare (principle 1) and appropriate and complete informed consent (principle 7). The veterinary surgeon should not be tempted to opt for endodontic treatment based on professional temptations and client and peer pressures, as noted in the discussion of Orthodontics above.

Prosthodontics

A prosthetic crown is a restoration that covers all or most of the coronal part of a tooth. It is rarely medically necessary in the dog and cat (AVDC, 2013b). A prosthetic crown may be indicated to prevent further damage to the tooth, for example, if a crack is noted in the remaining crown or if abrasion has weakened the remaining crown. Fractures of the canine teeth in working dogs are commonly mentioned as an indication for crowning (AVDC, 2013b). It must be borne in mind, however, that a crowned tooth does not regain its original strength, force distribution on a crowned tooth is different from that on a normal tooth, and even a working dog can be fully functional with short canine teeth.

The routine use of prosthodontic crowns following endodontic treatment is controversial in veterinary dentistry. Non-vital dentine is 3.5% more brittle than vital dentine, which is probably clinically irrelevant (Sedgley and Messer, 1992). Endodontic treatment weakens the crown structure; however, subsequent fracture following endodontic treatment and simple restoration is uncommon, with a reported incidence of 3.7% in the dog (Kuntsi-Vaattovaara et al., 2002). The incidence of fracture of a prosthodontically treated tooth has recently been found to be 10.3% (Fink and Reiter, 2015).

Contraindications for crowning techniques include deep crown-root fractures, non-vital teeth without endodontics, questionable endodontic treatment, and abnormal chewing behaviour. Given the fact that the preparation and placement of a prosthetic crown requires additional anaesthesia, medically compromised patients are not considered good candidates. A prosthetic crown may be lost due to cement failure. It may also be lost as a result of a fracture of the remaining tooth substance; if this causes a deep crown-root fracture the tooth will need to be extracted.

The application of a prosthetic crown for the sole purpose of restoring a cosmetic appearance at the request of the client is ethically questionable. A crucial element in clinical decision-making regarding prosthetic crowns is the informed consent of the client. A client must be told about all available options, including their advantages and disadvantages (principle 7). Questions about functionality and medical need should be honestly answered. Thus, a client should not be told that a prosthetic crown is medically necessary after root canal therapy if in fact (as is often the case) the animal will do perfectly well without the crown. It is also important that veterinary surgeons in EVDC or AVDC training programmes always put the interests of the patient first, and not be tempted to place prosthetic crowns to meet the minimum case log quotas required for the purposes of demonstrating their credentials (principle 1).

Dental implants have until recently rarely been used in dogs and cats. However, they have recently been promoted as a 'cutting edge' development in veterinary dentistry, with several unsubstantiated claims, such as improved bone integrity (Tannenbaum et al., 2013). This raises several ethical concerns, the main one being principle 6, namely that efficacy and safety have not been established by sufficient scientific evidence. Furthermore, there is no evidence that implants are medically beneficial (principles 1 and 5).

Exodontics

Exodontics is the branch of dentistry dealing with tooth extractions. As with all dental procedures, extractions should not be performed without the client's informed consent (principle 7). Medical indications for extraction are well established (Lommer, 2012). The veterinary surgeon's responsibility is to recommend extraction if this is in the best interest of the animal (principle 1). Although the veterinary surgeon must respect the client's needs and requirements (principle 2), this should not take precedence over the animal's welfare. If a client refuses permission to extract unsalvageable teeth, a sound client–veterinary surgeon relationship is absent and the veterinary surgeon should not proceed with any treatment.

One should always obtain permission from a client before disposing of extracted teeth. In humans, extracted teeth may be returned to patients upon request and in the USA are not subject to the provisions of the Occupational Safety and Health Administration (OSHA) Bloodborne Pathogens Standard (Centers for Disease Control and Prevention (CDC), 2013). It is reasonable for clients to expect that their pet's teeth will be returned to them if they so wish. If extracted teeth are returned, it is good practice to properly decontaminate them (CDC, 2013).

The AVDC considers extraction of teeth to be included in the practice of veterinary dentistry (AVDC, 2013c): 'Decision-making is the responsibility of the veterinarian, with the consent of the pet owner, when electing to extract teeth. Only veterinarians shall determine which teeth are to be extracted and perform extraction procedures'. The RCVS (RCVS, 2013c) is in agreement and specifically precludes veterinary nurses from performing extractions, as 'the extraction of teeth using instruments may readily become complicated and should only be carried out by veterinary surgeons'. The legal situation in the USA is less clear and varies by state (AVMA, 2013a; Veterinary Medical Board, 2013). In most states, extraction by veterinary technicians, when allowed, can only be done under the direct supervision of a veterinary surgeon. Irrespective of legal requirements, the veterinary surgeon should ensure that, if the procedure or aspects of the procedure are delegated to staff, they should have sufficient training and skill (principle 8).

Removal and reduction of teeth

Uncontrollable aggression is not a valid indication for the extraction of teeth, canine teeth in particular. An animal cannot be converted into a manageable pet by means of dental extractions or by crown amputation followed by vital pulp therapy, occasionally referred to as 'disarming' (Shipp, 1991). The AVMA (AVMA, 2013b) recently issued a position statement condemning such practices: 'The AVMA is opposed to removal or reduction of healthy teeth in nonhuman primates and carnivores, except when required for medical treatment or approved scientific research. Animals may still cause severe injury with any remaining teeth and this approach does not address the cause of the behavior'. As alternatives, behaviour modification and improved husbandry techniques are recommended by the AVMA.

References and further reading

American Kennel Club (2013) *Rules, Policies and Guidelines for Conformation Dog Show Judges.* (http://images.akc.org/pdf/rulebooks/REJ999.pdf.)

American Veterinary Dental College (2013a) *Dental scaling without anesthesia.* (http://www.avdc.org/dentalscaling.html.)

American Veterinary Dental College (2013b) *Crowns in veterinary patients.* (http://www.avdc.org/crowns.html.)

American Veterinary Dental College (2013c) *AVDC Position Statements.* (http://www.avdc.org/statements.html.)

American Veterinary Medical Association (2008) *Ear cropping and tail docking of dogs.* (https://www.avma.org/KB/Policies/Pages/Ear-Cropping-and-Tail-Docking-of-Dogs.aspx.)

American Veterinary Medical Association (2013a) *Authority of veterinary technicians and other non-veterinarians to perform dental procedures.* (https://www.avma.org/Advocacy/StateAndLocal/Pages/sr-dental-procedures.aspx.)

American Veterinary Medical Association (2013b) *Removal or reduction of teeth in nonhuman primates and carnivores.* (https://www.avma.org/KB/Policies/Pages/Removal-or-Reduction-of-Teeth-in-Non-Human-Primates-and-Carnivores.aspx.)

American Veterinary Medical Association (2015a) *Principles of veterinary medical ethics of the AVMA: the principles with supporting annotations Ia.* (https://www.avma.org/KB/Policies/Pages/Principles-of-Veterinary-Medical-Ethics-of-the-AVMA.aspx)

American Veterinary Medical Association (2015b) *Principles of veterinary medical ethics of the AVMA: the principles with supporting annotations Va.* (https://www.avma.org/KB/Policies/Pages/Principles-of-Veterinary-Medical-Ethics-of-the-AVMA.aspx)

Centers for Disease Control and Prevention (2013) *Infection control in dental settings.* (http://www.cdc.gov/oralhealth/infectioncontrol/questions/extracted-teeth.htm.)

Fink L and Reiter AM (2015) Assessment of 68 prosthodontic crowns in 41 pet and working dogs (2000–2012). *Journal of Veterinary Dentistry* **32**, 148–152

Kennel Club (2014) *Caesarean operations and procedures which alter the natural conformation of a dog.* (http://www.thekennelclub.org.uk/vets-reseachers/caesarean-operations-and-procedures-which-alter-the-natural-conformation-of-a-dog)

Kuntsi-Vaattovaara H, Verstraete FJM and Kass PH (2002) Results of root canal treatment in dogs: 127 cases (1995–2000). *Journal of the American Veterinary Medical Association* **220**, 775–780

Lommer MJ (2012) Principles of exodontics. In: *Oral and Maxillofacial Surgery in Dogs and Cats*, ed. FJM Verstraete and MJ Lommer, pp.97–114. Saunders Elsevier, Edinburgh

Nolen RS (2008) AVMA opposes cosmetic ear cropping, tail docking of dogs. *Journal of the American Veterinary Medical Association* **233**, 1811

Royal College of Veterinary Surgeons (1987) *Report of the Royal College of Veterinary Surgeons Council to Consider the Mutilation of Animals.* RCVS, London

Royal College of Veterinary Surgeons (2013a) *Royal College of Veterinary Surgeons Code of Professional Conduct for Veterinary Surgeons, 1.1.* (http://www.rcvs.org.uk/advice-and-guidance/code-of-professional-conduct-for-veterinary-surgeons/#principles.)

Royal College of Veterinary Surgeons (2013b) *Royal College of Veterinary Surgeons Code of Professional Conduct for Veterinary Surgeons, 2.1.* (http://www.rcvs.org.uk/advice-and-guidance/code-of-professional-conduct-for-veterinary-surgeons/#principles.)

Royal College of Veterinary Surgeons (2013c) *Delegation to veterinary nurses.* (http://www.rcvs.org.uk/advice-and-guidance/code-of-professional-conduct-for-veterinary-surgeons/supporting-guidance/delegation-to-veterinary-nurses/.)

Royal College of Veterinary Surgeons (2015) *Royal College of Veterinary Surgeons Code of Professional Conduct for Veterinary Surgeons 14.4.* (http://www.rcvs.org.uk/advice-and-guidance/code-of-professional-conduct-for-veterinary-surgeons/supporting-guidance/client-confidentiality/.)

Sedgley CM and Messer HH (1992) Are endodontically treated teeth more brittle? *Journal of Endodontics* **18**, 332–335

Shipp AD (1991) Crown reduction – disarming of biting pets. *Journal of Veterinary Dentistry* **8**, 4–6

Tannenbaum J (1995a) What is animal welfare? In: *Veterinary Ethics, 2nd edn*, pp.150–175. Mosby, St. Louis

Tannenbaum J (1995b) The human–companion animal bond. In: *Veterinary Ethics, 2nd edn*, pp.184–192. Mosby, St. Louis

Tannenbaum J (2013) Veterinary ethics. In: *The International Encyclopedia of Ethics*, ed. H LaFollette, pp.5317–5329. Wiley-Blackwell, West Sussex

Tannenbaum J, Boaz A, Reiter AM *et al.* (2013) The case against the use of dental implants in dogs and cats. *Journal of the American Veterinary Medical Association* **243**, 1680–1685

Veterinary Medical Board (2013) *Registered Veterinary Technician Job Task Regulations.* (http://www.vmb.ca.gov/laws_regs/rvttasks.shtml.)

Veterinary Oral Health Council (2013) (http://www.vohc.org/.)

Chapter 2

Dental anatomy and physiology

Margherita Gracis

Teeth are very important components of the digestive system and perform a number of invaluable tasks. In dogs and cats they are used for hunting, cutting food into pieces to allow ingestion, prehending food, and mechanically reducing the size of ingested food particles. Chewing helps to increase the surface area of the food for chemical and microbiological degradation and allows mixing of food with saliva, which in turns facilitates swallowing the bolus. Furthermore, teeth are utilized as weapons for offence and defence and, together with the tongue, for grooming activities.

Dentition of dogs and cats

Dogs and cats belong taxonomically to the order Carnivora and the families Canidae and Felidae, respectively. The dentition of carnivores is:

- Diphyodont: deciduous and permanent sets of teeth
- Heterodont: morphologically different teeth
- Anelodont: limited period of growth
- Brachyodont: short crown and relatively long root(s).

Furthermore, their teeth may be:

- Secodont: with sharp cutting edges
- Bunodont: with prominent cusps.

Odontogenesis

Odontogenesis, or tooth development, is initiated in the early embryonic development stages and continues for some time after birth. Compared with humans, it is a rather rapid process in dogs and cats. Size, shape and location are genetically and independently determined for each tooth, and tooth size is independent of mandibular and maxillary dimensions.

Teeth form in a coronoapical direction, from the tip of the crown to the root. The biological principles and rules that regulate and influence tooth development and eruption are the same for deciduous and permanent teeth (Figure 2.1). However, it is believed that development of the permanent teeth is dependent on the normal odontogenesis of the deciduous predecessors. If a deciduous tooth is congenitally missing, the succeeding tooth usually will not form.

For the tooth to develop, embryonic mesenchyme and epithelium have to interact closely. Initially, mesenchymal cells migrate from the neural crest into the tooth-forming region of the jaws, inducing proliferation of odontogenic epithelial cells. The odontogenic epithelium forms a local thickening called the primary epithelial band, which gives rise to the dental lamina in the medial nasal (premaxillary), maxillary and mandibular processes.

During the initial stages of tooth development (bud and cap stages), proliferation and migration of cells of both epithelial and mesenchymal origin form a structure called the tooth germ or organ. In particular, the epithelium invaginates and gives rise to the dental organ (also known as the enamel organ). The ectomesenchyme condenses, partially in the dental papilla, which is surrounded by the dental organ, and partially in the dental follicle, encapsulating the dental organ and papilla.

During the succeeding stages of development, the processes of histodifferentiation and morphogenesis take place. The mesenchyme of the dental papilla gives rise to the odontoblasts in the pulp that produce dentine. After the first dentine (predentine) has formed, the epithelial cells of the tooth germ (enamel organ) differentiate into ameloblasts that secrete enamel matrix.

As enamel formation along the crown is completed, root formation commences, with differentiation of the cells of the dental follicle into cementoblasts, which produce cementum, and cells that give rise to the periodontal ligament and the alveolar lamina dura. Root formation is guided by a layer of epithelial cells (Hertwig's root sheath) originating from the dental organ. These cells do not differentiate but induce histodifferentiation of the odontoblasts.

When roots have developed about three-quarters of their length, tooth eruption occurs. As the crown penetrates through the gingival tissues, emerging into the oral cavity, the ameloblastic layer loses its nutritive supply and degenerates. For this reason, enamel cannot be repaired or replaced after tooth eruption. With completed tooth formation, the Hertwig's epithelial root sheath is stretched and fragmented to form a fenestrated network of cells called the epithelial cell rests of Malassez. These epithelial cells persist throughout life within the periodontal ligament, retaining their odontogenic potential and being able to give rise to cystic or neoplastic lesions when stimulated.

Alterations of any specific phase of the odontogenic process may induce specific developmental disturbances or structural defects (see Figure 2.1). Tooth number and size may be altered when the induction phase (bud and cap stages of development) is disturbed, while structural

Stage	Microscopic appearance	Main processes involved	Description	Possible developmental disturbances
Initiation stage		Induction	Ectoderm lining stomodeum gives rise to oral epithelium and then to dental lamina, adjacent to the deeper ectomesenchyme, which is influenced by the neural crest cells. Both tissues are separated by a basement membrane	Anodontia, supernumerary teeth
Bud stage		Proliferation	Dental lamina grows into a bud that penetrates the growing ectomesenchyme	Macrodontia, microdontia
Cap stage		Proliferation, differentiation, morphogenesis	Dental organ forms into a cap, surrounding the mass of dental papilla from the ectomesenchyme and surrounded by a mass of dental follicle also from the ectomesenchyme. The tooth germ forms	Dens in dente, germination, fusion, tubercles
Bell stage		Proliferation, differentiation, morphogenesis	Dental organ differentiates into a bell with four cell types, and the dental papilla into two cell types. Crown assumes its final shape	Dens in dente, germination, fusion, tubercles
Apposition stage		Induction, proliferation	Dental tissues secreted as a matrix in successive layers. Crown and root develop	Enamel or dentine dysplasia, with hypoplasia or hypocalcification (e.g. amelogenesis or dentinogenesis imperfecta), enamel pearls, concrescence, dilaceration, accessory roots
Maturation stage		Maturation	Dental tissues fully mineralize to their mature level. Root develops and tooth erupts	Enamel or dentine dysplasia, with hypoplasia or hypocalcification (e.g. amelogenesis or dentinogenesis imperfecta), enamel pearls, concrescence, dilaceration, accessory roots, included and embedded teeth (dentigerous cyst formation)

2.1 Stages of tooth development and possible consequences of any disturbance of the physiological processes.
(Modified from Bath-Balogh and Fehrenbach (2006) with permission from the publisher)

changes, such as enamel and dentinal hypoplasia or dysplasia, may develop if disturbances occur during apposition and maturation (bell and maturation stages). In the case of genetic anomalies, all the teeth of an individual may be affected, such as with amelogenesis imperfecta and dentinogenesis imperfecta (see Chapter 10). Environmental factors, such as trauma, metabolic, chemical or infectious agents, may affect one or more teeth.

Tooth eruption and exfoliation

Tooth eruption

Tooth eruption is defined as the process of migration of a tooth from its site of development within the bone to its functional position within the oral cavity. Although dental development begins at the fetal stage, dogs and cats are born without visible crowns and teeth begin to erupt a few weeks after birth (Figure 2.2).

Many theories have been developed about the possible mechanisms of eruption of deciduous and permanent teeth, but they remain poorly understood events. Eruption begins only after the dental crown has completely formed and the roots have begun to develop, showing strict chronological coordination and exhibiting precise timing in bilateral symmetry. The intraosseous phase of tooth eruption seems to depend on regulation by the embryonic dental follicle of bone metabolism on opposite sides of the tooth bud. Resorption of occlusal bone lying in the path of the erupting tooth and apical apposition seem to be essential for tooth eruption. Numerous studies, many performed in the dog and few in the cat, have shown that the tooth mainly plays a

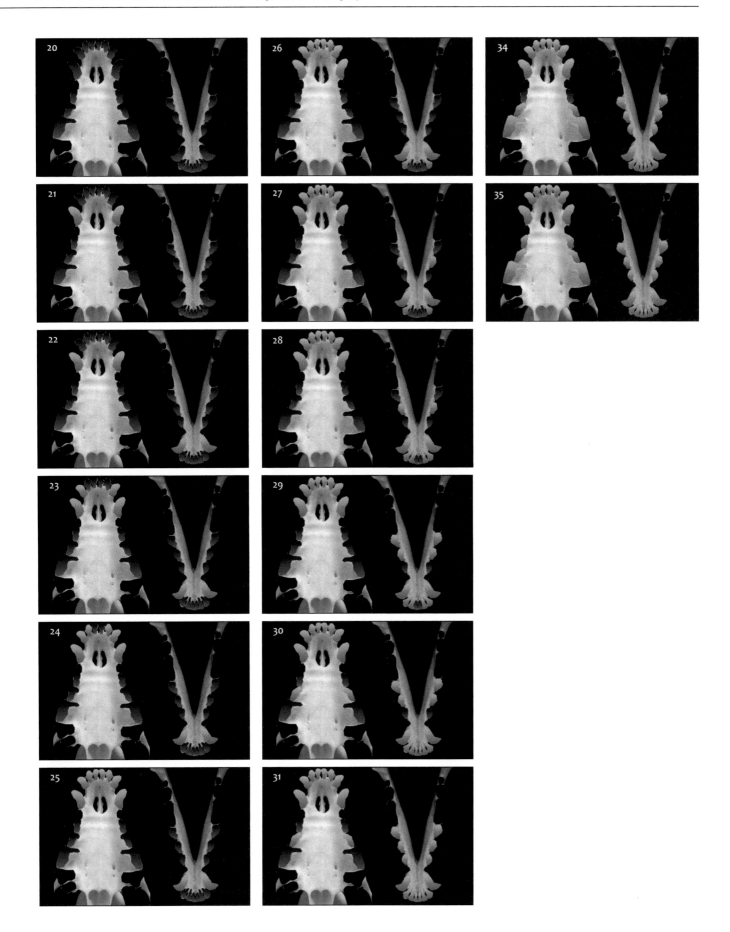

2.2 (a) Approximate eruption schedule and timing (age in days) of deciduous maxillary and mandibular teeth in dogs (black = missing teeth; orange = deciduous teeth). (continues)
(Modified from Gracis (2013) with permission from the publisher)

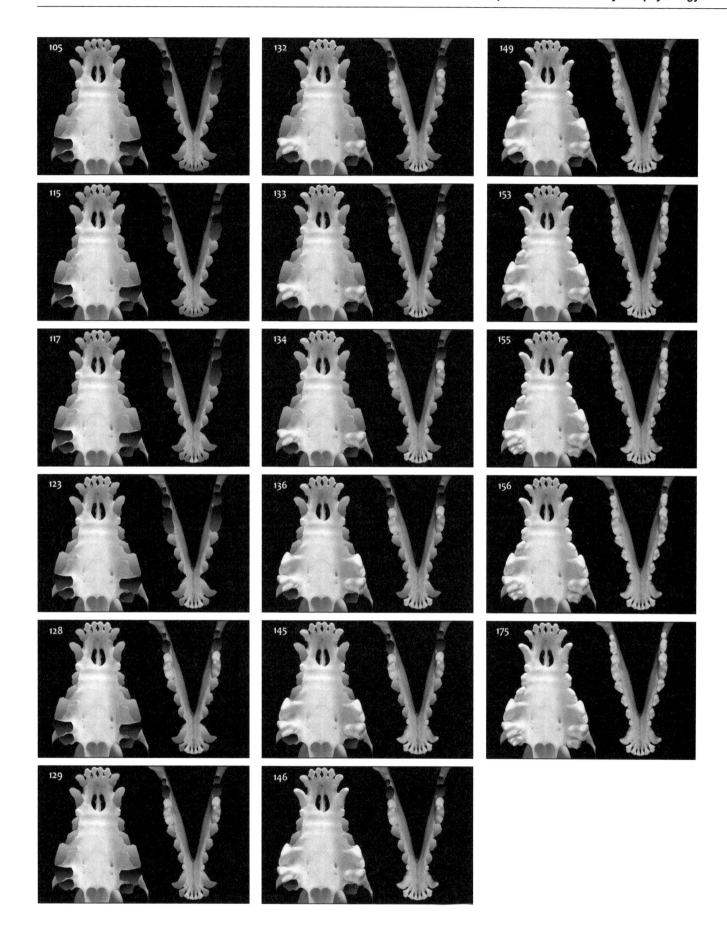

2.2 (continued) (b) Approximate eruption (gingival emergence) schedule and timing (age in days) of permanent maxillary and mandibular teeth in dogs (black = missing teeth; orange = deciduous teeth; white = permanent teeth). (continues)
(Modified from Gracis (2013) with permission from the publisher)

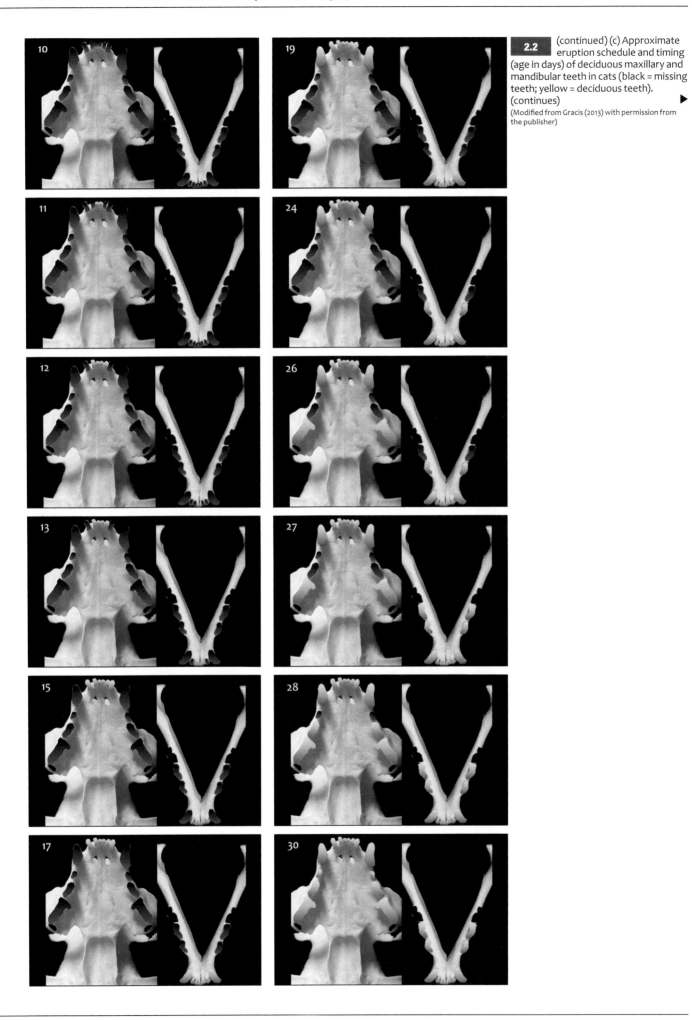

2.2 (continued) (c) Approximate eruption schedule and timing (age in days) of deciduous maxillary and mandibular teeth in cats (black = missing teeth; yellow = deciduous teeth). (continues) ▶

(Modified from Gracis (2013) with permission from the publisher)

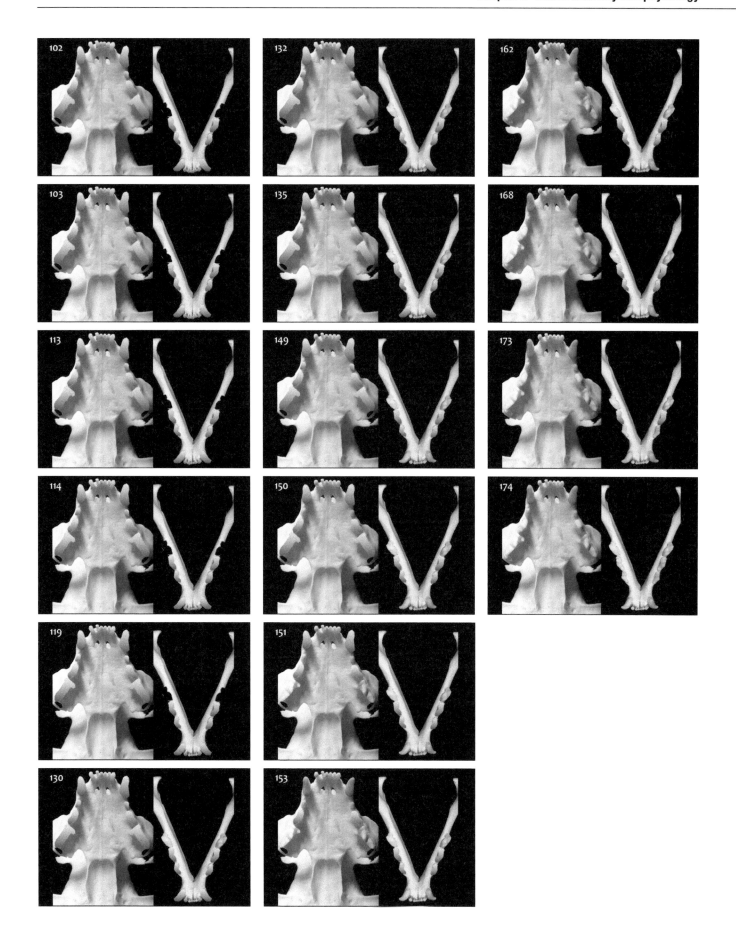

2.2 (continued) (d) Approximate eruption (gingival emergence) schedule and timing (age in days) of permanent maxillary and mandibular teeth in cats (black = missing teeth; yellow = deciduous teeth; white = permanent teeth).
(Modified from Gracis (2013) with permission from the publisher)

passive role. This theory has been supported by demonstrating that eruption is not affected by surgical destruction of the roots and periodontal ligament of developing mandibular premolars, or removal of the crown and substitution with sterile metal and silicone replicas.

Control of tooth eruption is possibly multifactorial and includes genetic, environmental, infectious and traumatic factors. Some of the recognized non-genetic causes of delayed or retarded eruption in dogs and cats are radiation therapy of the head, canine distemper virus infection, dwarfism, hypervitaminosis A, and physical impediment by trauma, supernumerary teeth, cysts or tumours.

The definitive spatial position of an erupted tooth does not always coincide with that of the corresponding dental germ. Due to the small size of the growing skull, dental germs may develop with their long axis oblique or perpendicular to the dental arch. As the skull grows, the space for the teeth increases, and during eruption the teeth rotate in either a lingual/palatal or a buccal/labial

direction to form, with the adjacent elements, an ordered arch. Typically, the type of rotation of the maxillary second and third premolars is such that the mesial portion of the tooth rotates buccally (B type of rotation). On the contrary, the mesial portion of the mandibular fourth premolar tooth normally rotates lingually (L rotation). However, if the mesiodistal dimension of the teeth is excessive compared with the total dental arch length, the dental germs fail to rotate, teeth erupt in the original position and tooth crowding develops, as often occurs in brachycephalic or small-breed animals.

Tooth exfoliation

Both dogs and cats have a diphyodont dentition, with deciduous and permanent sets of teeth (see Figures 2.2, 2.3 and 2.4). As in eruption, exfoliation of the deciduous dentition is a relatively enigmatic process, accomplished by root resorption. Normally, the deciduous teeth start

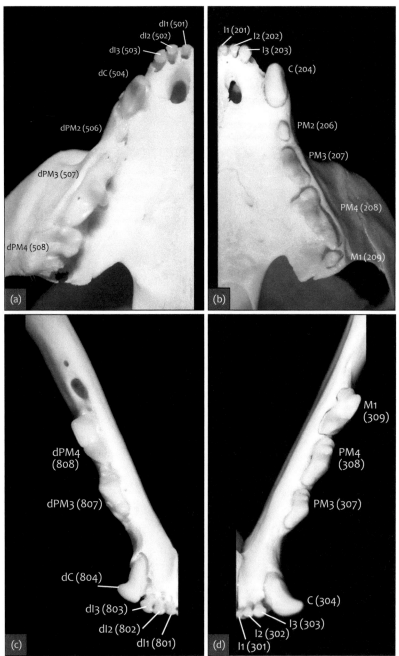

2.3 Occlusal view of feline deciduous and permanent dentition based on the Modified Triadan System. (a) Deciduous right maxillary teeth. (b) Permanent left maxillary teeth. (c) Deciduous right mandibular teeth. (d) Permanent left mandibular teeth. C = canine tooth; d = deciduous tooth; I = incisor tooth; M = molar tooth; PM = premolar tooth.
(© Dr Margherita Gracis)

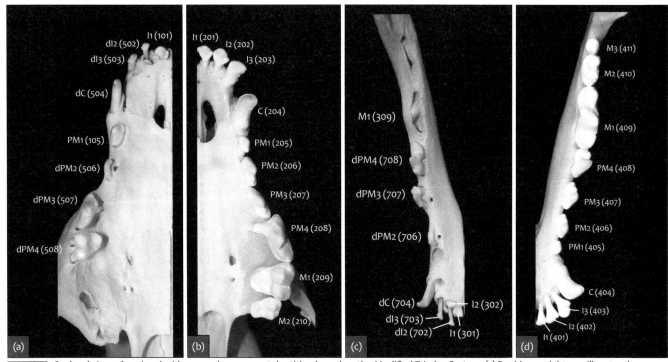

2.4 Occlusal view of canine deciduous and permanent dentition based on the Modified Triadan System. (a) Deciduous right maxillary teeth. (b) Permanent left maxillary teeth. (c) Deciduous right mandibular teeth. (d) Permanent left mandibular teeth. Some permanent teeth have already erupted and are visible on (a) and (c). C = canine tooth; d = deciduous tooth; I = incisor tooth; M = molar tooth; PM = premolar tooth.
(© Dr Margherita Gracis)

exfoliating and are lost before the succeeding permanent teeth begin to erupt into the oral cavity. A deciduous tooth still present in the mouth at the time of eruption of the succeeding permanent tooth is defined as 'persistent'. However, the emergence of the maxillary permanent canine teeth before exfoliation of the deciduous corresponding teeth is considered to be normal, and the deciduous canines can persist for several days or weeks after eruption of their permanent counterparts. Eruption and root growth of the permanent teeth are normally preceded by resorption of the deciduous tooth roots, but the root of a deciduous tooth may be resorbed even when the corresponding succeeding permanent tooth is missing. Furthermore, in the case of a missing permanent tooth it is possible that the deciduous tooth will be maintained in the oral cavity much longer than normally expected and may even be present for the entire life of the animal.

Differences between deciduous and permanent teeth

The deciduous and permanent dentitions differ in number of teeth present due to the fact that not every tooth in the mouth has a corresponding deciduous tooth (see Figures 2.3 and 2.4). The difference between a premolar and a molar tooth is the presence of deciduous predecessors for premolars but not for molar teeth. An exception is the first premolar tooth in dogs, which does not have a deciduous counterpart (see Figure 2.4).

Tooth shape is also somewhat different, with crowns of deciduous teeth being more simple and rounded (incisor and premolar teeth) or pointed (canine teeth). An interesting process is the so-called 'molarization' of deciduous premolar teeth (Figure 2.5). Crown morphology and number of roots of each deciduous premolar tooth are

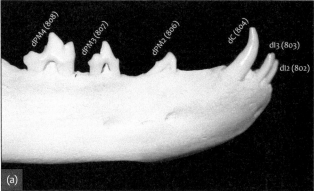

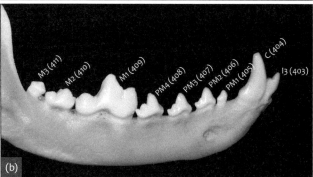

2.5 Lateral view of the right mandible in (a) a young dog with deciduous dentition and (b) an adult dog with permanent dentition. C = canine tooth; d = deciduous tooth; I = incisor tooth; M = molar tooth; PM = premolar tooth.
(© Dr Margherita Gracis)

typical of the permanent tooth positioned distal to it, rather than that of its true successor. For example, the deciduous maxillary third premolar tooth has three roots, like the three-rooted permanent fourth premolar and unlike the two-rooted permanent third premolar. Its crown shape resembles that of the permanent fourth premolar tooth, with a large mesial cusp, a shorter distal cusp and a small palatal cusp. An exception to the rule is the deciduous maxillary second premolar tooth in cats, which has a similar shape to its successor (see Figure 2.3).

Finally, the deciduous and permanent dentitions differ in colour (the crowns of deciduous teeth are usually whiter because their enamel is less mineralized than in permanent teeth) and size (deciduous teeth have smaller crowns and relatively longer, thinner roots) (Figures 2.5 and 2.6).

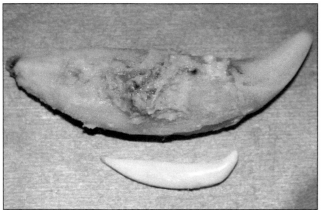

2.6 Permanent (top) and deciduous (bottom) mandibular canine teeth extracted from two related male Rhodesian Ridgebacks. The adult dog was 9 years old, and the tooth measured 6.2 cm in length. The immature dog was 4 months old, and the deciduous tooth measured 2.5 cm in length.
(© Dr Margherita Gracis)

Dental formula and eruption schedule

Based on palaeontological studies, primitive carnivore dentition used to comprise four premolar and three molar teeth in each jaw quadrant. The carnassial teeth (lacerating teeth, namely the mandibular first molar and the maxillary fourth premolar) are the largest teeth in all carnivores and can be used as a reference to name the remaining teeth. The following abbreviations are used below: I = incisors; C = canines; PM = premolars; and M = molars.

Dogs

Deciduous dentition

The first premolar and the molar teeth in dogs do not have deciduous predecessors (see Figure 2.4ac). Therefore, the total deciduous dental formula comprises 28 teeth and is depicted as follows:

$$2 \times \left\{ I\,\frac{3}{3} \quad C\,\frac{1}{1} \quad PM\,\frac{3}{3} \right\} = 28$$

The earliest embryological evidence of tooth development in the dog is around day 25 of gestation (Zontine, 1975). The deciduous teeth start erupting at about 3 weeks of age (see Figure 2.2a), when root formation is almost complete. Full eruption of the entire deciduous dentition is expected by about 40–50 days of age. Variations in eruption pattern and chronology are common and depend on the animal's health, breed, sex and other individual factors. There is possibly a tendency to earlier eruption in larger breeds compared with smaller

breeds. In addition, some teeth (i.e. deciduous maxillary second and fourth premolar teeth) seem to erupt earlier in males compared with females, while others (i.e. maxillary and mandibular deciduous canines, mandibular first incisors and second premolars) may erupt earlier in females. Furthermore, it should be noted that published studies often evaluate relatively small numbers of animals and few breeds. In some publications it is also unclear if the reported 'time of eruption' corresponds to the time of gingival emergence (defined as supragingival exposure of any portion of the tooth (Berman, 1974) or intraoral presence of at least 0.5 mm^2 of enamel surface (Kremenak, 1969)) or full eruption. The schedule and chronological order of tooth eruption shown in Figure 2.2a should therefore only be considered as approximate.

Mineralization of the deciduous crowns begins around day 50 of gestation and is complete 10–20 days after birth, representing a total of about 30 days for the mineralization process to occur. Partial mineralization of all deciduous teeth is visible radiographically at the time of birth. However, root formation and mineralization is complete at 40–50 days after birth (Zontine, 1975), and root apical closure occurs about 6–7 weeks after birth. Exfoliation generally occurs between 3.5 and 5 months of age during the eruption of the permanent teeth.

Permanent dentition

The permanent dentition of dogs comprises 10 teeth in each maxillary quadrant and 11 teeth in each mandibular quadrant (see Figure 2.4bd). It is depicted as:

$$2 \times \left\{ I\,\frac{3}{3} \quad C\,\frac{1}{1} \quad PM\,\frac{4}{4} \quad M\,\frac{2}{3} \right\} = 42$$

The relationship between deciduous and permanent teeth is as follows:

- The permanent maxillary and mandibular incisor teeth erupt palatally and lingually to their deciduous predecessors
- The permanent maxillary canine teeth erupt mesially to the deciduous canine teeth
- The permanent mandibular canine teeth erupt lingually to their deciduous counterparts
- The permanent maxillary second and third premolar teeth erupt palatally to the deciduous teeth
- The permanent maxillary fourth premolar tooth erupts mesiobuccally to its deciduous predecessor
- The permanent mandibular premolars usually erupt lingually to the deciduous teeth.

Variations in eruption schedule are common and depend on the animal's health, breed, sex and other individual factors, but the pattern and chronological order are approximately as indicated in Figure 2.2b.

Mineralization of the mandibular first molar tooth starts and is radiographically visible a few days before birth. Mineralization of all other permanent teeth, and therefore presence of a complete permanent dentition, cannot be demonstrated radiographically until 3–4 months of age. Roots reach their definitive length about 120 (first premolar teeth) to 180 days (canine teeth) after birth (Arnall, 1961). In dogs, on average, root apical closure occurs between 7 and 10 months of age, with the apices of the canine teeth closing last (Morgan and Miyabayashi, 1991; Wilson, 1996).

Cats

Deciduous dentition

The deciduous dental formula in cats includes seven teeth in each maxillary quadrant and six teeth in each mandibular quadrant (see Figure 2.3ac) and is depicted as:

$$2 \times \left\{ I\,\frac{3}{3} \quad C\,\frac{1}{1} \quad PM\,\frac{3}{2} \right\} = 26$$

Eruption of the deciduous dentition in cats begins 11–15 days after birth and is complete between 1 and 2 months of age. The approximate schedule and chronological order of tooth eruption is shown in Figure 2.2c.

Permanent dentition

The permanent dental formula in cats includes eight teeth in each maxillary quadrant and seven teeth in each mandibular quadrant (see Figure 2.3bd) and is depicted as follows:

$$2 \times \left\{ I\,\frac{3}{3} \quad C\,\frac{1}{1} \quad PM\,\frac{3}{2} \quad M\,\frac{1}{1} \right\} = 30$$

Eruption of deciduous and permanent rostral teeth follows a similar pattern, with the incisors erupting before the canine teeth (see Figure 2.2d). Permanent molar teeth usually start erupting just before the premolar teeth. Maxillary teeth may erupt slightly before the opposing mandibular teeth. Eruption of the permanent dentition is completed at about 6–7 months of age. The time of closure of the apices of the mandibular first molar, maxillary canine and mandibular premolar teeth occurs at about 7, 8 and 10 months of age, respectively, with some variations possible (Wilson, 1999).

Age estimation by dental methods

Estimating the age of an animal may be necessary in archaeological studies or for legal and medical reasons. Import and trade of underaged puppies and kittens are common problems in many countries, and veterinary surgeons (veterinarians) may be involved in determining their age in case of legal controversies or to decide the correct vaccination protocol.

Unfortunately, there is no single reliable method for making precise age estimates, either in humans or animals. Age estimation by dental methods is only approximate, especially when dealing with small temporal margins (e.g. is the dog 3 or 3.5 months old?). Age estimation by dental development and eruption is prone to a wide range of error due to the fact that sex, breed, individual and other factors may affect odontogenesis, eruption and even tooth growth. The fact that tooth development is so fast in dogs and cats (with the deciduous and permanent teeth completing their turnover on average by 6 months of age) may be advantageous in some cases but may represent a problem in others.

The evaluation of tooth mineralization and pulp cavity size may be used to determine an approximate age. At the time of tooth eruption in dogs, the size of the root canal corresponds to the width of the tooth root by a ratio of 66% (distal root of mandibular fourth premolar tooth) to 80% (canine teeth). Its size then decreases rapidly due to secondary dentine production, and by 2–3 years of age it becomes less than 10% of the width of the root (Morgan and Miyabayashi, 1991). Afterwards, changes are much slower and less evident, and therefore less reliable as an age indicator. Study results on the applicability of these methods are still controversial in humans, and specific studies are lacking in veterinary medicine. Furthermore, to obtain intraoral radiographs, sedation or general anaesthesia is required, which may be contraindicated in young and possibly unhealthy animals.

Tooth abrasion has also been suggested as a method to estimate the age of dogs and cats, based on that used in horses for centuries. However, the dentition of horses is clearly different (radicular hypsodont) to that of carnivores (anelodont). In dogs and cats, abrasion is influenced by external factors that have little to do with their age.

Combining dental methods with adjunctive information related to physical development (i.e. bodyweight, height, body mass) and skeletal maturity may reduce the margin of error when determining the age of young dogs and cats. It is still recommended that any clinical evaluation is worded with caution, indicating that the animal is probably, likely, possibly or unlikely to be of a certain age, and that the dentition is compatible or incompatible with a certain age.

Modified Triadan System

The Modified Triadan System is a numerical dental nomenclature system derived from the human New System by the International Dental Federation (Floyd, 1991). It consists of a three-digit number and provides a consistent method of numbering teeth across different animal species (Figure 2.7). The first digit of the number refers to the quadrant. For permanent teeth, the right maxillary quadrant is numbered 1, the left maxillary quadrant is numbered 2, the left mandibular quadrant is numbered 3, and the right mandibular quadrant is numbered 4. For deciduous teeth the quadrants are numbered from 5 to 8, following the same order.

The second and third digits of the number refer to the type and position of the tooth in the quadrant, beginning at the midline and proceeding caudally, from 01 (the first incisor tooth), to 10 (the second maxillary molar tooth) or 11 (the third mandibular molar tooth). The canine teeth are therefore teeth number 04 (the fourth tooth on the quadrant after the three incisor teeth), and the carnassial teeth 08 (maxillary fourth premolar tooth) and 09 (mandibular first molar tooth). These can be used to number the other premolar and molar teeth, especially in animals where teeth are missing compared with the ancestral carnivore. Therefore, in the cat, the maxillary fourth premolar tooth is tooth number 108 or 208; the premolar teeth rostral to it will be 107 and 106 or 207 and 206, respectively, and then a gap is left in the numbering sequence because in the cat, the first maxillary premolar teeth, 105 and 205, are missing.

Dental anatomy and tissues

Dental anatomical terminology is explained in Figure 2.8. Despite morphological differences between different groups of teeth, the basic structure and anatomy are identical for any tooth (Figure 2.9). Normal teeth are hollow structures consisting of enamel, dentine and cementum.

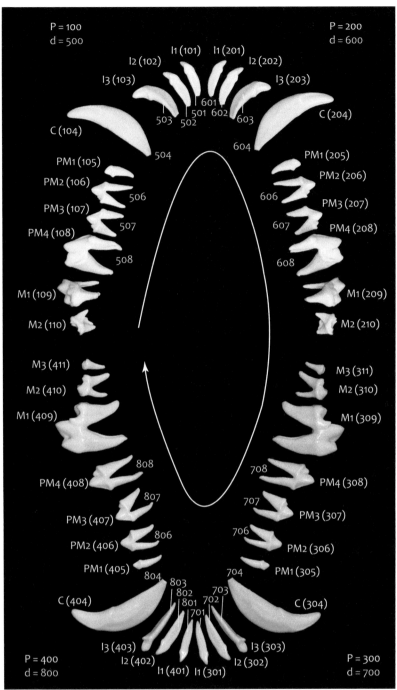

2.7 Modified Triadan System. Complete permanent canine dentition, showing the lingual side of the mandibular teeth and the palatal side of the maxillary teeth. The numbering for the deciduous dentition is shown in yellow. C = canine tooth; d = deciduous tooth; I = incisor tooth; M = molar tooth; P = permanent tooth; PM = premolar tooth.
(© Dr Margherita Gracis)

The bulk is composed of dentine. Enamel and cementum are the thin outer layers covering the anatomical crown and root, respectively. The clinical crown (the portion of the tooth visible above the gingival margin) and the clinical root (the portion of the tooth hidden below the gingival margin) do not always correspond to their anatomical counterparts, as in healthy teeth the free gingiva covers a small portion of the enamel and during disease the gingival margin may have migrated apically.

The inner space of the tooth, containing pulp tissues, is the pulp cavity. The portion of the pulp cavity contained in the crown is defined as the pulp chamber, and the portion contained in the roots as the root canal. The neck of the tooth or cervical region is the portion between the crown and root, where cementum and enamel meet (cemento-enamel junction, CEJ).

Dental hard tissues

Crown and enamel

The anatomical crown is the portion of the tooth covered by enamel. It can have one (canine teeth) or more tubercules or cusps, separated by developmental fissures or grooves. The portion of the crown just coronal to the neck of the tooth enlarges to form the so-called dental or tooth bulge (see Figure 2.9). The bulge has a protective function, deflecting food particles from the gingival margin during chewing. Its designation as the enamel bulge is inaccurate, as the bulk of the bulge is composed of dentine, and the thickness of enamel is the same as in adjacent areas (Crossley, 1995). Normally, enamel thickness is less than 0.3 mm in the cat and less than 0.6 mm in the dog. Thickness decreases from the crown tip to the mid-crown area and

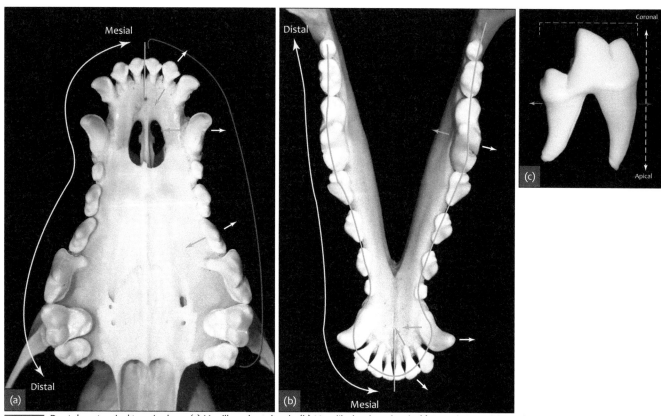

2.8 Dental anatomical terminology. (a) Maxillary dental arch. (b) Mandibular dental arch. (c) Buccal view of the right mandibular first molar tooth. Specific anatomical terms are used when describing dental structures. 'Cranial' and 'caudal', 'dorsal' and 'ventral' can be confusing terms and should not be used. The teeth on the lower jaw are the mandibular teeth, while those on the upper jaw are referred to as the maxillary teeth. Teeth are arranged in a larger maxillary and a narrower mandibular arch (green line indicates the mandibular arch). Each arch is divided into right and left quadrants (red line indicates the left maxillary quadrant). An area of a dental arch devoid of teeth is called a diastema. A large diastema exists between the maxillary third incisor tooth and the canine tooth in both dogs and cats. The surface of a tooth towards the tongue or the palate is defined as the lingual (for mandibular teeth) or palatal (for maxillary teeth) surface (light blue arrows). The portion facing the lips and cheeks is the labial or buccal surface, also defined as the vestibular surface (white arrows). The surfaces facing adjacent teeth are defined as interproximal and can be either mesial (light pink arrow) or distal (green arrow); the face of the tooth pointing towards the midline along the dental arch (the point between the right and left first incisor teeth, indicated by the light blue lines) is the mesial surface, and the opposite is the distal surface (yellow double arrows). The occlusal surface corresponds to the masticatory surface (blue interrupted line). The terms apical and coronal refer to directions towards the root apex or the crown of a tooth, respectively (interrupted double white arrow).
(© Dr Margherita Gracis)

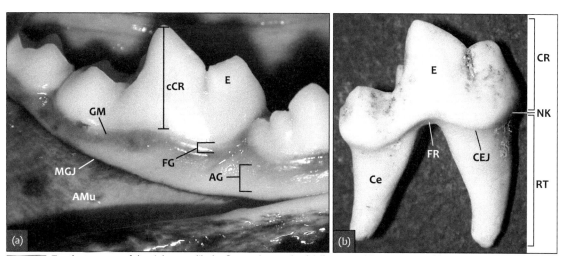

2.9 Tooth structure of the right mandibular first molar tooth of different middle-aged dogs. (a) Clinical aspect, buccal side. (b) Extracted tooth, buccal side. AG = attached gingiva; AMu = alveolar mucosa; cCR = clinical crown; Ce = cementum; CEJ = cementoenamel junction; CR = anatomical crown; E = enamel; FG = free gingiva; FR = furcation; GM = gingival margin; MGJ = mucogingival junction; NK = tooth neck; RT = anatomical root. (continues)
(a, b, © Dr Margherita Gracis)

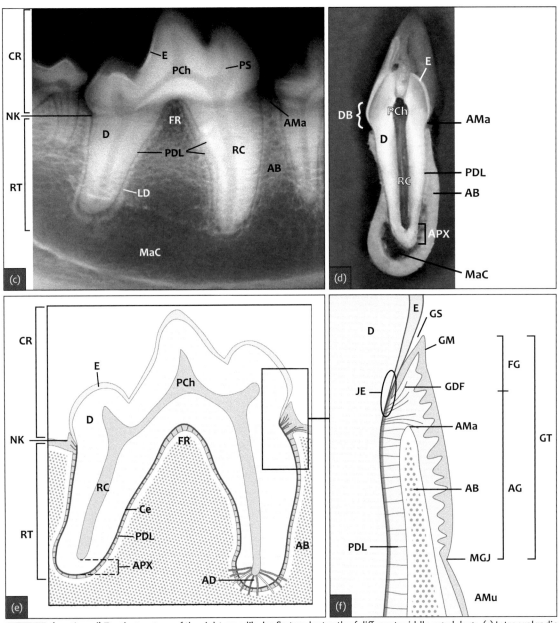

2.9 (continued) Tooth structure of the right mandibular first molar tooth of different middle-aged dogs. (c) Intraoral radiographic image. (d) Vertical section through the mesial root. (e) Schematic presentation. (f) Detail of (e), showing periodontal structures. AB = alveolar bone; AD = apical delta; AG = attached gingiva; AMa = alveolar margin; AMu = alveolar mucosa; APX = apex; Ce = cementum; CR = anatomical crown; D = dentine; DB = dental bulge; E = enamel; FG = free gingiva; FR = furcation; GDF = gingivodental fibres; GM = gingival margin; GS = gingival sulcus; GT = gingival tissue; JE = junctional epithelium; LD = lamina dura; MaC = mandibular canal; MGJ = mucogingival junction; NK = tooth neck; PCh = pulp chamber; PDL = periodontal ligament space; PS = pulp stone; RC = root canal; RT = anatomical root. (c, d, © Dr Margherita Gracis)

down to the CEJ (DeLauriel, 2006), reflecting the fact that tooth development and enamel production start from the tip of the crown and progress in an apical direction.

Enamel is the most highly mineralized and hardest tissue of the body, with about 96% inorganic material consisting mainly of hydroxyapatite crystals and less than 4% organic material (mainly proteins, and a few carbohydrates and lipid components) and water (Figure 2.10). Enamel mineralization decreases from the crown tip to the CEJ (DeLauriel et al., 2006). The microscopic, crystalline structural unit of enamel is defined as enamel rod or enamel prism, extending from the dentinoenamel junction to the outer enamel surface with an undulating course. One ameloblast produces one rod and its inter-rod enamel. The superficial layer of enamel is normally rodless, and therefore smooth. However, areas of

prismatic or 'cobbled' enamel, in which the prism-free surface otherwise covering the tooth is missing, may be present (DeLauriel et al., 2006).

Amelogenesis (or enamel formation) occurs during the apposition stage of tooth development and after dentinogenesis has started (see Figure 2.1). Ameloblasts are cells of ectodermal origin, deriving from oral epithelium, and responsible for enamel formation. They become functional after initial dentine production, lose their differentiation after enamel is completely formed, and disappear after tooth eruption. Therefore, enamel cannot be produced or regenerated after the initial stages of tooth development. Furthermore, enamel is avascular and has no nerve supply.

Tooth colour is mainly determined by enamel thickness and degree of mineralization. However, because of the enamel's semitranslucency the colour of the crown may

Parameter	Enamel	Dentine	Cementum	Alveolar bone
Embryological background	Enamel organ	Dental papilla	Dental papilla	Mesoderm
Type of tissue	Epithelial tissue	Connective tissue	Connective tissue	Connective tissue
Formative cells	Ameloblasts	Odontoblasts	Cementoblasts	Osteoblasts
Mature cells	None (lost with eruption)	Only dentinal tubules with odontoblastic processes	Cementocytes	Osteocytes
Resorptive cells	Odontoclasts	Odontoclasts	Odontoclasts	Osteoclasts
Mineral levels	96%	70%	65%	60%
Organic	1% organic	20% organic	23% organic	25% organic
Water levels	3% water	10% water	12% water	15% water
Tissue formation after eruption	None	Possible	Possible	Possible
Vascularity	None	None	None	Present
Innervation	None	Present	None	Present

2.10 Comparison of dental hard tissues and alveolar bone.
(Modified from Bath-Balogh and Fehrenbach (2006) with permission from the publisher)

change based on the colour of dentine or any material underneath the enamel. The whiter appearance of deciduous teeth compared with permanent teeth is due to a lower degree of mineralization of the enamel of deciduous teeth (see Figure 2.6).

Cementoenamel junction

The interface between enamel and cementum is called the CEJ (see Figure 2.9). It is located at the neck of the tooth where the gingiva attaches to the tooth surface and anatomically divides the anatomical crown from the anatomical root of the tooth.

Enamel and cementum do not always meet edge-to-edge, but there may be areas where cementum overlaps enamel for a short distance or where dentine is exposed because the enamel and cementum margins do not meet. Exposed dentine may be more susceptible to odontoclastic activity and resorption, possibly explaining why some tooth resorption commences at the neck of the tooth (DeLauriel et al., 2006).

Root and cementum

The tooth root is covered by a thin layer of cementum, which is a bone-like, mineralized connective tissue composed of inorganic material (about 50%) and an organic matrix rich in collagen (see Figure 2.10). Cementum is therefore less mineralized and softer than enamel and dentine, having a chemical composition similar to that of bone. Like enamel, cementum is avascular and has no nerve supply. It has a yellowish colour and shows some degree of permeability that decreases with age. Cementum is part of the periodontium, the anchoring system of the tooth within the alveolus. The collagen fibres (Sharpey's fibres) of the periodontal ligament are embedded in both cementum and bone.

Cementogenesis starts during tooth development, after dentine formation. Cementoblasts differentiate from mesenchymal cells and produce cementum continuously throughout the animal's life. Therefore, cementum slightly increases in thickness with time. Primary cementum is produced before tooth eruption, is highly mineralized and covers the coronal two-thirds of the root. Secondary cementum is formed less rapidly and is less mineralized, than primary cementum. It is mainly deposited around the apical third of the root after tooth eruption and throughout the animal's life. Cementum is normally resistant to

resorption, but a cellular type of reparative cementum may be produced in response to trauma and other external factors, causing hypercementosis.

The following root terminology is used (see Figure 2.9):

* The area between roots of multi-rooted teeth is called the furcation
* The tip of the root is called the apex
* The roots are seated into their bony sockets or alveoli (one alveolus per root)
* When the bone over the roots is particularly thin, such as in the maxilla, the alveolar wall may form a prominence or jugum that can be easily palpated through the alveolar mucosa.

Dentine

Dentine constitutes the bulk of the tooth. It supports enamel, which is very hard but also brittle because of its high mineral content. Dentine is a porous structure, slightly less mineralized than enamel, with an inorganic component of 70% (see Figure 2.10). Up to 50,000 dentinal tubules/mm^2 traverse the dentinal walls from the inner dentinal wall to the dentinoenamel and dentinocemental junctions. Each dentinal tubule is occupied by a single odontoblastic process and a small amount of gel with a rich organic component. Dentine mineralization varies at different levels and is lowest at the CEJ and cervical root (DeLauriel et al., 2006). In addition, the number of dentinal tubules is higher in the coronal dentine than in the radicular dentine, making the coronal portion of dentine more sensitive to external stimuli, when exposed.

The cells responsible for dentine production are the odontoblasts, which are situated on the outer surface of the pulp. Dentinogenesis begins at the late bell stage of development of the tooth and continues throughout the animal's life. Therefore, dentine thickens with time, which in turn causes a progressive reduction in size of the pulp cavity. Primary dentine is produced until root formation is completed. Secondary dentine is deposited after root formation is completed and, depending on the vitality of the pulp, continues throughout the animal's life.

Tertiary dentine may be quickly produced in response to a stimulus, such as caries, trauma and other external factors. It is defined as reparative if produced by odontoblast-like cells that differentiated from pulpal stem cells, or reactionary when produced by existing odontoblasts. The dentinal tubules of tertiary dentine may be absent or reduced in number and irregularly arranged and shaped. For this reason, tertiary dentine reflects light differently to normal dentine and is also more likely to absorb pigments and thus become discoloured. Its colour may therefore appear darker than the surrounding primary or secondary yellowish dentine. It may need to be differentiated from carious lesions, pulp exposure or other structural defects by gently exploring the surface with a fine dental explorer. The surface of tertiary dentine feels smooth.

The obliteration of the dentinal tubules by dentine is defined as dentinal sclerosis, which seems to be a defensive response to several physiological (i.e. ageing) and pathological stimuli. Sclerosis causes a reduction of dentine permeability. The sclerotic tooth often looks glossy and translucent. Unusual structures such as vasodentine (vascular inclusions) and osteodentine (intermediate cementum) have been described in the permanent teeth of cats.

Pulp cavity and pulp tissue

The pulp cavity is enclosed by dentine, and comprises the pulp chamber within the crown and the root canal within the root (see Figure 2.9). The pulp cavity is rather simple in dogs and cats, with one main canal for each root. The shape grossly follows the external shape of the tooth. In multi-rooted teeth, the pulp chamber communicates with each root canal. If endodontic disease develops in teeth with more than one root, the whole endodontic system will inevitably be affected.

The root canal communicates with the external environment (the periodontal space) almost exclusively at the root apex. The apex is open, with one large canal, until 7–11 months of age. Then it closes down, leaving behind the so-called apical delta, a group of 10–20 or more microscopic apical ramifications that allow passage of vessels and nerves to and from the root canal in a homogeneous (characterized by a large quantity of small canals of reduced size) or non-homogeneous (characterized by the division into smaller canals from a few larger canals) pattern (Lorenzo et al., 2001) (Figure 2.11).

Non-apical ramifications, canals that extend from the main root canal to the periodontal space anywhere along the root coronally to the apex, may be found with a relatively low prevalence in canine and feline teeth. Furcation canals may connect the pulp chamber with the periodontal space in multi-rooted teeth.

The pulp consists of blood vessels, sensory nerves, lymphatic capillaries and numerous cells immersed in a collagenous matrix, such as immunocompetent cells (lymphocytes, macrophages and dendritic cells), undifferentiated mesenchymal cells, fibroblasts and specialized odontoblasts. In addition to being responsible for dentine production, the pulp has nutritive, protective and sensory functions. Nutrition to the surrounding tissues is provided by the pulp's rich vascular supply.

Non-dental periodontal tissues

Together with cementum, the periodontal ligament, alveolar bone and gingiva form the supporting tissues of the tooth, called the periodontium (see Figure 2.9).

Gingiva

Teeth are the only structures in the body that perforate epithelium. The gingiva is that part of the oral mucosa that covers the alveolar process of the jaws and surrounds the neck of the teeth (see Figure 2.9). It is a resilient tissue, able and necessary to withstand continuous masticatory trauma.

The attached gingiva is tightly bound to the periosteum and separated from the alveolar mucosa by the mucogingival junction (MGJ), a line that is obviously demarcated in most dogs, but less visible in cats (see Figure 2.9). As the alveolar mucosa is somewhat loose, it can be stretched to visualize the MGJ. On the maxillary teeth, the attached gingiva blends palatally into the palatal mucosa without a clear demarcation. The width of the attached gingiva varies greatly among individuals and even in different areas of the same mouth. Typically, in dogs and cats the width is greatest at the maxillary canine teeth and diminishes in the incisor and premolar/molar regions.

The free gingiva is the unattached portion of the tissue, measured from the bottom of the gingival sulcus to the coronal border of the gingiva, the gingival margin (see Figure 2.9). It tapers to a knife edge at the gingival margin.

The gingival sulcus is a shallow space between the free gingiva and the tooth. Its depth is reported in the literature to be normally less than 1 mm in the cat and less than 3 mm in the dog, but variations are common, especially taking into account the great disparity in dog breeds and sizes. In addition, similarly to the attached gingiva, the sulcus depth may vary between different teeth in the same mouth.

The oral surface of the free gingiva is basically indistinguishable from the keratinized or parakeratinized

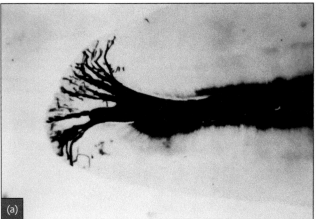
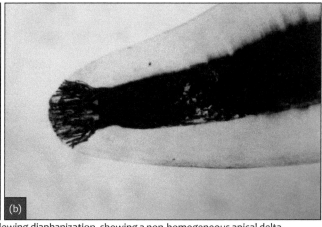

2.11 (a) Photomicrograph of the maxillary canine tooth of a dog following diaphanization, showing a non-homogeneous apical delta. (b) Photomicrograph of the maxillary canine tooth of a cat following diaphanization, showing a homogeneous apical delta.
(a, Reproduced from Lorenzo et al. (2001) with permission from InVet; b, Reproduced from Negro and Hernandez (2000) with permission from Veterinaria Argentina)

attached gingiva. Its internal lining, the sulcular epithelium, is a thin, non-keratinized stratified squamous epithelium. The apical portion of the sulcular epithelium, the junctional epithelium, consists of a band of stratified non-keratinized epithelium that connects to the tooth surface by means of hemidesmosomes.

The gingival tissue is rich in connective fibres, mainly collagen, that attach the gingiva to the underlying bone and cementum, encircling the tooth in a ring-like fashion and providing rigidity to the tissue, and are continuous with the periodontal ligament fibres (see Figure 2.9). Some of these gingival fibres, the transseptal group, extend between the cementum of approximating teeth and are considered responsible for orthodontic relapse or post-extraction tooth movement in human patients. In dogs and cats, however, the position of remaining teeth will not necessarily change following extraction of adjacent teeth. The reason is currently unknown, but it could be speculated that transseptal fibres are missing in domestic carnivores or have a different arrangement than in humans.

Alveolar bone

The portion of the jaw that accommodates the roots of the teeth is defined as the alveolar process and comprises cancellous or trabecular bone limited by a lingual and a labial external cortical plate covered by periosteum. The alveolar process is perforated by the alveolar sockets or alveoli. The alveolar walls are composed of a cribriform plate that provides attachment for the periodontal ligament fibres (Sharpey's fibres). The alveolar process forms and is maintained in relation to the teeth. If a tooth is congenitally missing, the alveolar process will not develop. If a tooth is lost or extracted, the alveolar process will gradually be resorbed. The alveolar margin is the coronal margin of the alveolar bone and normally located not more than 1 mm apical to the CEJ.

Periodontal ligament and space

The periodontal ligament, together with blood vessels, lymphatic vessels and nerves, occupies the narrow space between the tooth and the alveolar bone, the periodontal space. The terminal portions of its connective fibres (Sharpey's fibres) are embedded into cementum on one side and into alveolar bone on the other, holding the tooth in place and acting as a shock absorber in response to masticatory stimuli (see Figure 2.9). In fact, the fibres are not arranged in a 'mat' on the tooth surface, but in interwoven and interconnected bundles that can be classified based on their functional orientation into alveolar margin, horizontal, oblique, apical and interradicular fibres.

Tooth morphology

Tooth size and shape is determined genetically. Size does not seem to be strongly correlated with body or head size, but rather to the size of supporting structures. Small-breed dogs, however, show large teeth (in particular the mandibular first molar tooth) relative to bone height, which may predispose small dogs to pathological bony fractures (Gioso *et al.*, 2001).

Teeth can have one, two or three roots, with a relatively constant number for each tooth (Figure 2.12). However, variations resulting from fusion of two roots or from the presence of an extra or supernumerary root may occur.

Number of roots	Dogs		Cats	
	Deciduous	*Permanent*	*Deciduous*	*Permanent*
One	Max/man I, C	Max I, C, PM1 Man I, C, PM1, M3	Max I, C, PM2 Man I, C	Max I, C, PM2 Man I, C
Two	Max PM2 Man PM2, PM3, PM4	Max PM2, PM3 Man PM2, PM3, PM4, M1, M2	Man PM3, PM4 Max PM4	Max PM3, M1 Man PM3, PM4, M1
Three	Max PM3, PM4	Max PM4, M1, M2	Max PM3	Max PM4

2.12 Number of roots. C = canine tooth; I = incisor tooth; M = molar tooth; Man = mandibular; Max = maxillary; PM = premolar tooth.

Common examples are the permanent maxillary third premolar tooth of both dogs and cats that may have three rather than two roots, or the permanent maxillary second premolar tooth in the cat, which may have one or two roots. Roots of any multi-rooted tooth may differ in size and shape (see Figure 2.7).

Dental sexual dimorphism (size and shape differences between females and males) is minimal or absent in domestic dogs and cats. Dogs and cats have teeth that are morphologically different and serve distinct purposes (heterodont dentition) (see below).

Incisor teeth

Incisor teeth are relatively small compared with the rest of the dentition (see Figure 2.7). They are normally packed together either in a smooth arch (dogs) or in straight rows (cats). Especially in deciduous teeth, the sharp crown is normally much shorter than the single root (Figure 2.13). The crown of permanent teeth normally has a large middle cusp and one or two smaller mesial and distal cusps. In dogs, at the level of the normal gingival margin, there is a ridge called the cingulum on the lingual and palatal sides of the crown of mandibular and maxillary incisor teeth (Figure 2.14). In cats, a small tubercle (a secondary projection of the crown) is present instead. Incisor teeth are mainly used for cutting and for grooming activity.

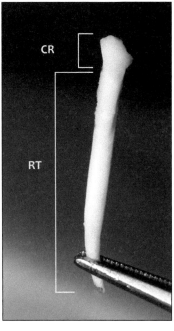

2.13 Extracted mandibular incisor tooth of a 4-month-old Rhodesian Ridgeback. The crown:root length ratio is about 1:6. CR = anatomical crown; RT = anatomical root.
(© Dr Margherita Gracis)

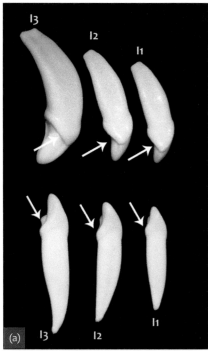

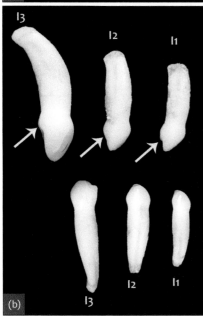

2.14 Left maxillary (top) and mandibular (bottom) incisor teeth of (a) a dog and (b) a cat. White arrows denote the cingulum. Yellow arrows denote the tubercle. I = incisor tooth.
(© Dr Margherita Gracis)

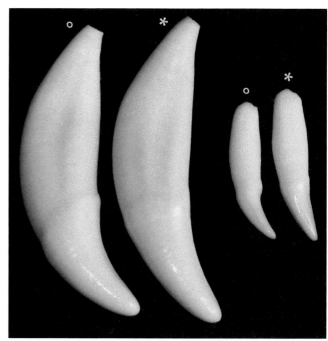

2.15 Mandibular (o) and maxillary (*) teeth from a dog (left) and a cat (right). The vestibular view is shown.
(© Dr Margherita Gracis)

curved than that of the mandibular canines. In cats, the roots are almost straight, the root of the maxillary tooth being slightly larger than that of the mandibular counterpart (see Figure 2.15). As in dogs, the crown of the mandibular canine is slightly shorter and more curved than that of the maxillary canine.

The oval pulp cavity follows the external shape of the tooth (Figure 2.16). In mature teeth (with a closed apex) the size of the pulp cavity also mimics the external morphology of the tooth, being narrower at the coronal and apical thirds and wider in the middle portion. This is an important consideration during endodontic treatment. As in all single-rooted teeth, the demarcation between the pulp chamber and the root canal is undefined.

Canine teeth

Canines are simple, single-rooted teeth with a strong, long, distally curved conical crown used to grasp and hold (Figure 2.15). They are characterized by the presence of coronal developmental grooves and shallow ridges that may allow drainage of blood while holding and killing prey. Canines are also used to lacerate flesh. They have an oval shape, being slightly flattened in a vestibulopalatal or vestibulolingual direction. The root is larger than the crown, with the maximum diameter at the middle third. Deciduous canine teeth are relatively small and pointed compared with their permanent counterparts (see Figure 2.6).

In dogs, the root of the maxillary and mandibular permanent canines is of almost identical size and shape, while the crown of maxillary canines is slightly longer and less

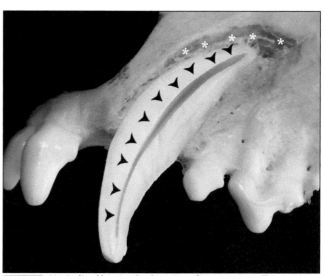

2.16 Mesiodistal longitudinal section of a mature maxillary canine tooth of a dog showing the pulp cavity (arrowheads) and dentinal thickness. A portion of the incisivomaxillary canal has been exposed (*).
(© Dr Margherita Gracis)

Premolar teeth

Premolar teeth presumably have a function in catching and holding prey. The shape, size and number of roots of permanent premolars vary significantly, ranging from the small single-rooted first premolar to the large three-rooted maxillary fourth premolar (Figure 2.17).

The two-rooted premolar teeth are grossly symmetrical, compressed buccolingually and have pointed cusps that do not necessarily meet when the jaws are closed. Carnassial teeth (permanent maxillary fourth premolar and mandibular first molar) have a blade-like shape and are used to cut skin and meat. The maxillary fourth premolar tooth has a similar shape in both dogs and cats, with a large distal root and two thinner mesial roots (buccal and palatal). The small mesiopalatal root is only connected to the mesiobuccal root (Figure 2.18), which is an important consideration for root separation during extractions.

Molar teeth

In dogs, molar teeth have a bunodont shape (Figure 2.19). Maxillary molars have two higher buccal (mesial and distal) cusps with long and relatively thin roots and a lower palatal cusp with a short and stubby root, connected to both vestibular roots (Figure 2.20). Often the distobuccal and palatal roots of the second molar tooth are fused together. Numerous fissures and pits are present on the crowns.

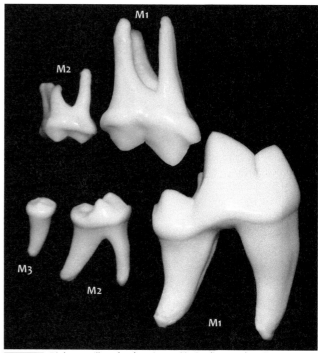

2.19 Right maxillary (top) and mandibular (bottom) molar teeth of a dog. The vestibular view is shown. M = molar tooth.
(© Dr Margherita Gracis)

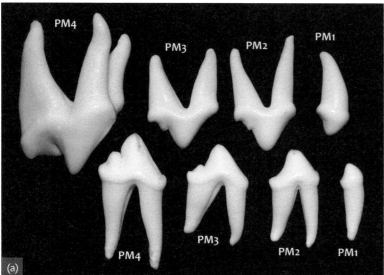

2.17 Right maxillary (top) and mandibular (bottom) premolar teeth of (a) a dog and (b) a cat. The vestibular view is shown. PM = premolar tooth.
(© Dr Margherita Gracis)

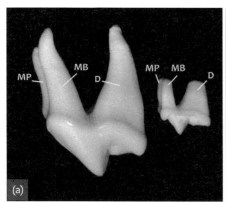
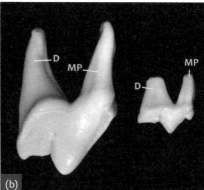
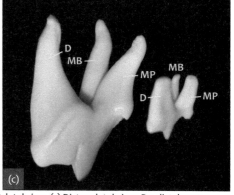

2.18 Left maxillary fourth premolar tooth of a dog (left) and a cat (right). (a) Buccal view. (b) Palatal view. (c) Distopalatal view. D = distal root; MB = mesiobuccal root; MP = mesiopalatal root.
(© Dr Margherita Gracis)

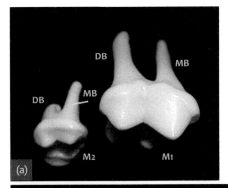

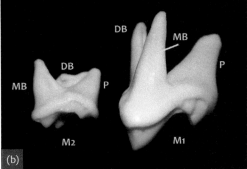

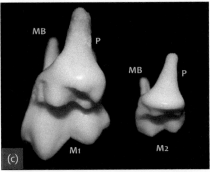

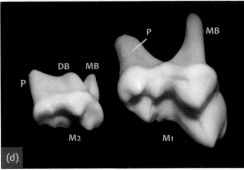

2.20 Right maxillary first and second molar teeth of a dog.
(a) Buccal view. (b) Mesial view. (c) Palatal view. (d) Distal view.
The distobuccal and palatal roots of the second molar tooth are fused in
this specimen. DB = distobuccal root; M = molar tooth; MB = mesiobuccal
root; P = palatal root.
(© Dr Margherita Gracis)

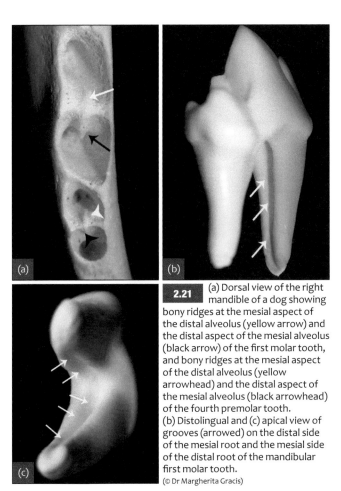

2.21 (a) Dorsal view of the right mandible of a dog showing bony ridges at the mesial aspect of the distal alveolus (yellow arrow) and the distal aspect of the mesial alveolus (black arrow) of the first molar tooth, and bony ridges at the mesial aspect of the distal alveolus (yellow arrowhead) and the distal aspect of the mesial alveolus (black arrowhead) of the fourth premolar tooth. (b) Distolingual and (c) apical view of grooves (arrowed) on the distal side of the mesial root and the mesial side of the distal root of the mandibular first molar tooth.
(© Dr Margherita Gracis)

The mandibular first molar tooth has two similarly elongated roots, slightly curved distally (see Figure 2.19). The crown has two tall mesial cusps and a lower distal cusp, which – with the occlusal surface of the other mandibular molars – creates an effective surface for crushing bones and hard materials against the maxillary molars.

The roots of multi-rooted premolar and molar teeth in dogs often present a longitudinal groove corresponding to a bony ridge in the alveolus (Figure 2.21). Normally the grooves are present on the mesial surface of the distal root and the distal surface of the mesial root. The interlock

between grooves and bony ridges improves root retention within the tooth socket.

Cats are true carnivores, and probably for this reason during evolution they have lost most bunodont molar teeth (Figure 2.22). Therefore, they have an almost exclusively secodont (cutting) post-canine dentition, with sharp dental cusps (see Figure 2.3). The mandibular molar has a large mesial root and a very thin, distally and slightly lingually angled, distal root. The crown has two equal cusps, separated by a deep developmental groove that is located more mesially than the root furcation. The maxillary first molar is a very small, two-rooted tooth with a bunodont crown. It is placed transversally in the dental arch (see Figure 2.3).

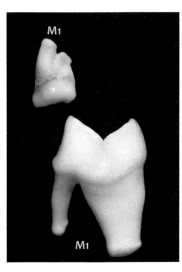

2.22 Right maxillary (top) and mandibular (bottom) molar teeth of a cat. The vestibular view is shown. M = molar tooth.
(© Dr Margherita Gracis)

Dental radiographic anatomy

Enamel, dentine and cementum

Enamel, dentine and cementum are highly mineralized tissues that appear radiographically opaque (see Figure 2.9). Their radiodensity is related to their mineral content (see Figure 2.10).

Enamel will appear more radiopaque than the other structures. However, enamel is not always detectable as it is normally very thin. Only when the radiographic beam passes tangential to a significant thickness of enamel will this show as a radiopaque line.

Due to their comparable mineral content, and to the fact that cementum is normally only a few microns thick, cementum and dentine are normally radiographically indistinguishable. In the case of a pathological increase in thickness (hypercementosis), cementum may become visible, showing as an external layer slightly more radiolucent layer than dentine.

Pulp cavity

The pulp cavity follows the external tooth shape and should always appear radiolucent. Even in the case of pulp death, the radiodensity of the pulp cavity will not change. However, radiopaque dystrophic pulp mineralization may rarely develop following trauma. Discrete calcifications (pulp stones) may also be seen within the pulp chamber or coronal third of the root canal as round or oval radiopaque structures. The aetiology of pulp stones is unknown, and in human patients they represent occasional findings with no clinical consequences. At times, pulp stones may be radiographically difficult to differentiate from a condition known as dens in dente, where the outer surface of the tooth folds inward. In young animals, the open apex is seen directly connected to the periodontal space, but the thin microscopic canals of the adult apical delta are not detectable radiographically.

Periodontal space

Healthy tooth roots are surrounded by a thin radiolucent line, the periodontal space (see Figure 2.9). The size of the space may vary slightly along a root, but should be consistently visible all around it. In cases of ankylosis, the periodontal space will be obliterated. Usually, the cross-section of canine and feline teeth is round or oval. Therefore, as the X-ray beam passes tangential to the root surface, a single radiolucent line is created on the radiograph. In dogs, however, some of the roots of the mandibular premolar and molar teeth may exhibit a cashew nut-like cross-section, with a concave area between two convex surfaces (see Figure 2.21bc). In this case the periodontal space may appear radiographically as a double radiolucent line.

Alveolar bone and lamina dura

The radiopaque alveolar bone is cancellous bone with a variable radiographic trabecular pattern, surrounding the roots and filling the furcation area of multi-rooted teeth. Its most coronal extension, the alveolar margin, should be not more than 1 mm apical to the cementoenamel junction. It appears as a radiopaque line continuous with the lamina dura, the wall of the alveolar socket (the cribriform plate), and is seen around the root as a line more radiopaque than the adjacent cancellous bone (see Figure 2.9). Despite its radiopacity, the lamina dura is not cortical bone. Its high radiopacity is due to a summatory effect of the X-ray beam passage through this thick layer of bone.

Dental occlusion

Dental occlusion is the spatial relationship between maxillary and mandibular dental arches when the jaws are closed and in the resting position (centric occlusion). Normal or eugnathic occlusion is termed **orthocclusion** and is described for the permanent dentition of dogs and cats as follows (Figures 2.23 and 2.24):

- Slight anisognathism (i.e. a lower dental arch that is shorter and narrower compared with the upper dental arch)
- Symmetrical right and left sides, with the midpoint of the upper and lower dental arches on the same plane as the median plane of the head
- The mandibular incisor teeth occlude on the palatal cingulum (dogs) or tubercle (cats) of the maxillary counterparts in the so-called 'scissors' bite. An edge-to-edge occlusion, with contact between the incisal

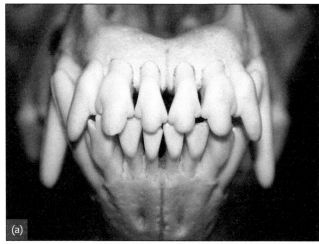

(a)

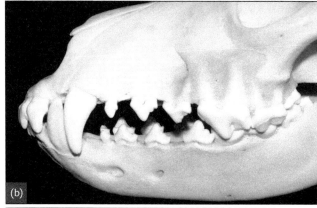

(b)

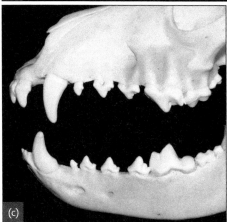

(c)

2.23 Skull of a mesocephalic dog showing dental occlusion.
(a) Rostral view.
(b) Left lateral view – closed mouth.
(c) Left lateral view – open mouth (separated mandible and maxilla).
(© Dr Margherita Gracis)

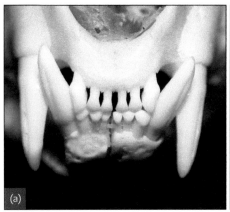
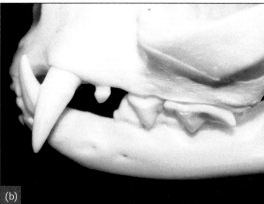
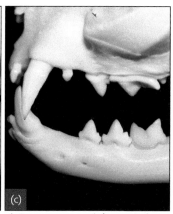

2.24 Skull of a cat showing dental occlusion. (a) Rostral view. (b) Left lateral view – closed mouth. (c) Left lateral view – open mouth (separated mandible and maxilla).
(© Dr Margherita Gracis)

margin of the mandibular and maxillary incisor teeth, is also acceptable for some canine and feline breeds, but may lead to attrition and traumatic dental fracture
- Due to the difference in size between maxillary and mandibular teeth, in dogs the maxillary first, second and third incisor teeth occlude in the interproximal spaces of the mandibular first and second incisor teeth, the second and third incisor teeth, and the third incisor teeth and canine teeth, respectively
- Each mandibular canine tooth occludes in the diastema mesial to the maxillary canine tooth, being equidistant from the ipsilateral maxillary third incisor and canine teeth
- The mandibular canine teeth are slightly labioversed (the tip of the crown is angled labially at an approximatively 110 degree angle to the occlusal plane) to compensate for anisognathism and avoid contact with the palatal mucosa
- The premolar teeth interdigitate, with the maxillary premolar teeth occluding distal to their mandibular counterparts (e.g. the maxillary first premolar tooth occludes between the mandibular first and second premolar teeth). The maxillary premolar teeth should be slightly labial to the mandibular premolar teeth, and there should not be any contact between them
- In dogs, the maxillary fourth premolar tooth occludes on the buccal side of the mesial cusp of the mandibular first molar tooth. In cats, the maxillary fourth premolar tooth completely overlaps the mandibular first molar

- In dogs, the occlusal surfaces of the maxillary and mandibular molar teeth (only the distal cusp of the mandibular first molar) come into contact. In cats, the small maxillary first molar is placed transversely as compared with the premolar teeth and occludes just distal to the mandibular first molar.

Chondrodystrophy of the chondrocranium, which causes an early interruption of growth at the base of the cranium in brachycephalic breeds, such as Bulldogs, Boxers and Pekingese, leads to the development of disharmony or malocclusion between upper and lower dental arches defined as relative mandibular mesiocclusion (Figure 2.25). This condition is due to a shorter upper jaw (maxillary brachygnathism) rather than a longer lower jaw and may result in extreme crowding and irregularity of the maxillary teeth. As the mandibles preserve their growth potential, an altered contact between the rostral portion of the mandibles and the rostral maxillary teeth often occurs, with resultant ventral bowing of the lower jaw and sympheseal soft tissue lesions secondary to occlusal trauma.

Even in brachycephalic breeds, an excessive difference in length between the mandibles and maxillae, where the mandibular incisor teeth are visible during closed-mouth examination, is considered a true defect, as it may cause a less efficacious bite. A short lower jaw (mandibular brachygnathism or distocclusion) is an unacceptable type of occlusion for any breed standard.

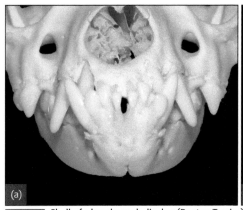
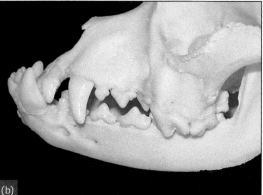
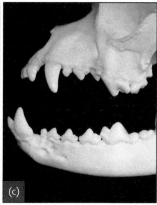

2.25 Skull of a brachycephalic dog (Boston Terrier) showing dental occlusion. (a) Rostral view. (b) Left lateral view – closed mouth. (c) Left lateral view – open mouth (separated mandible and maxilla).
(© Dr Margherita Gracis)

Surgical anatomy

Species, skull morphology, tooth type, size and position determine the relationship between teeth and the nearby anatomical structures (Figures 2.26 and 2.27). Knowing the regional surgical anatomy allows the veterinary surgeon to better understand and diagnose pathology and to correctly plan and perform treatment.

Maxillary teeth

Several important structures should be considered and recognized when working on the maxillary teeth (Figure 2.28).

Salivary ducts

In dogs and cats, the major parotid duct runs from the parotid gland lateral to the masseter muscle and opens in the upper cheek on the buccal mucosa opposite the

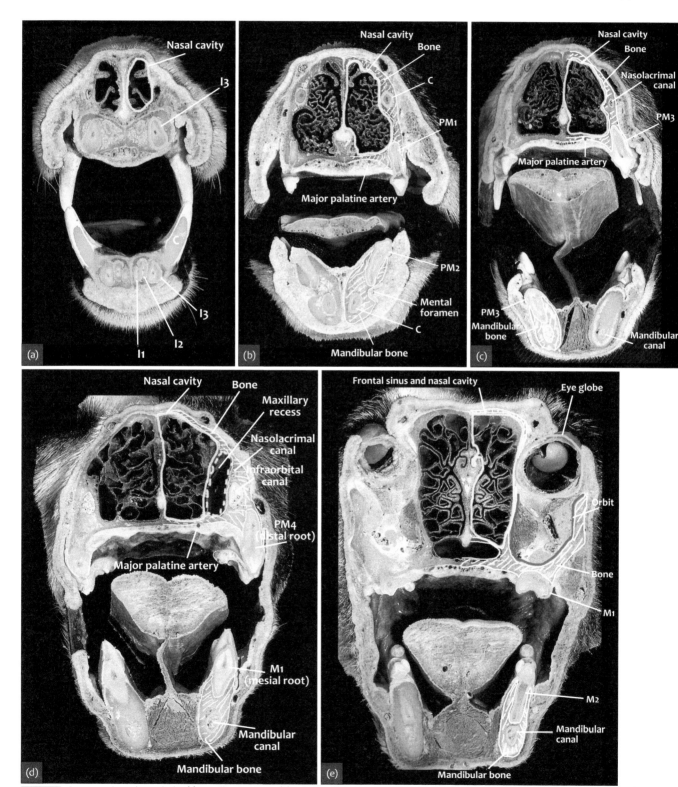

2.26 Cross-sections through the (a) maxillary incisors; (b) maxillary first premolar; (c) maxillary third premolar; (d) maxillary fourth premolar; (e) maxillary first molar in a dog. C = canine tooth; I = incisor tooth; M = molar tooth; PM = premolar tooth.
(Modified from Done *et al.* (1996) with permission from the publisher)

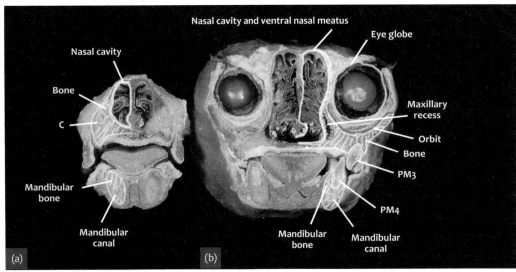

2.27 Cross-sections through the maxillary (a) canine and (b) third premolar tooth in a cat. C = canine tooth; PM = premolar tooth.
(Modified from Done et al. (1996) with permission from the publisher)

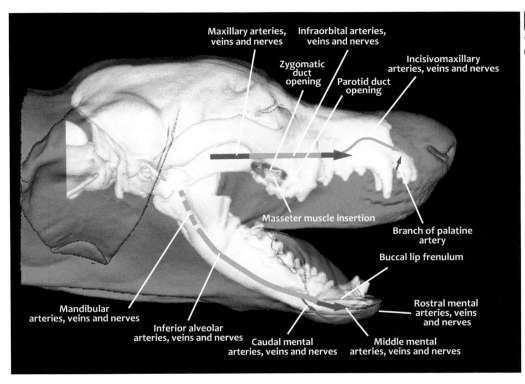

2.28 Important anatomical structures seen from the right side of a dog.
(Courtesy of Dr G Bertolini, modified)

maxillary fourth premolar tooth. The zygomatic glands lies in the pterygopalatine fossa, dorsal and lateral to the pterygoid muscles and ventral to the ventral orbital margin. The major zygomatic duct opens about 1 cm caudal to the parotid papilla, opposite the first molar teeth. Particular care should be taken when performing surgical procedures in this area, and soft tissue incisions should preferably be made rostral to the duct openings.

Masseter muscle

The masseter muscle arises from the zygomatic arch, covers the lateral surface of the ramus of the mandible, and inserts on the ventrolateral and ventromedial surface of the mandible. Some fibres may be found inserting on the caudal border of the maxilla, just ventral to the zygomatic process of the maxilla (Figure 2.29). After elevating mucogingival flaps in this area to reach the bone surface and perform partial alveolectomy for extraction of molar teeth, it may be necessary to elevate or incise some muscle fibres.

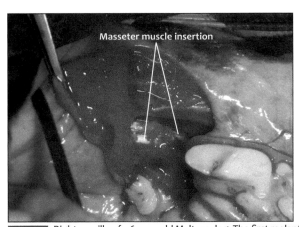

2.29 Right maxilla of a 6-year-old Maltese dog. The first molar tooth has been extracted. The masseter muscle insertion to the caudal maxilla is visible after elevation of a mucogingival flap created to close the defect. The incision on the mucosa was made rostral and dorsal to the zygomatic and parotid salivary gland duct openings.
(© Dr Margherita Gracis)

Orbit

The maxillary first (cat) and the second (dog) molar teeth are located just rostral to the caudal margin of the maxilla near the so-called maxillary tuberosity. The orbit and its contents (the zygomatic salivary gland in particular) are just caudodorsal to this area (see Figures 2.26e and 2.27b).

Nasolacrimal duct

The nasolacrimal duct conducts the lacrimal secretions from the eye to the nasal vestibule. Initially, the duct enters the lacrimal foramen and runs rostroventrally into the lacrimal canal of the lacrimal bone and maxilla (see Figure 2.26cd). It then makes a slight dorsomedial turn, thereafter running parallel to the hard palate and medial to the canine tooth root. Rostral to the nasal concha (at the level of the third premolar tooth) the duct is no longer covered by bone, but only by nasal mucosa, until it opens in the nasal vestibule.

The course of the nasolacrimal duct is strongly related to the shape of the skull (Breit *et al.*, 2003). In brachycephalic feline breeds the angle between the descending part and the rostral portion of the canal has been shown to become more acute, causing a sharp change in direction of the duct, which opens above the level of the lacrimal foramen. Independent of skull morphology, the nasolacrimal duct runs very close to the apex of the canine tooth, and dental pathology may lead to impaired nasolacrimal drainage.

Infraorbital artery, vein and nerve

In dogs, the infraorbital canal is in strict relation to the roots of the fourth premolar tooth, as it runs between the mesiobuccal and mesiopalatal roots and slightly dorsal and palatal to the distal root (see Figures 2.26d and 2.28). The infraorbital neurovascular bundle exits the infraorbital canal at the infraorbital foramen, dorsal to the apex of the distal root of the third premolar tooth. In cats and brachycephalic dogs, the infraorbital canal is no more than a few millimetres long and the foramen may be found just below the ventral margin of the orbit.

Other neurovascular structures

Two smaller vascular structures may be encountered during surgical procedures performed on the maxillary canine tooth (see Figure 2.28). One of the branches of the major palatine artery runs through the interproximal space between the canine and third incisor teeth and anastomoses with the lateral nasal artery in the width of the upper lip. A branch of the infraorbital artery runs in the incisivomaxillary canal, which borders the apex and the apical two-thirds of the mesial side of the canine root (see Figure 2.16). Brisk haemorrhage may therefore be expected when making an interproximal mucosal incision mesial to the canine tooth or when performing alveolectomy around its root.

Bone

The roots of all the maxillary teeth are deeply seated into the alveolar process of the incisive bones and maxillae (see Figures 2.26, 2.27, 2.30 and 2.31). Normally, the incisive bones carry the incisors, and the maxillae carry all remaining upper teeth. Both in dogs and cats the thickness of the vestibular alveolar walls of the maxillary teeth is rather thin (see Figures 2.26 and 2.27), which explains why fistulae of dental origin often open on the mucogingival tissues intraorally or on the skin extraorally.

The thickness of the alveolar wall on the palatal side of the teeth differs significantly between dogs and cats. In dogs, the palatal wall is often paper thin, and the alveoli are in close proximity to the nasal cavity, the maxillary recess and the orbit (see Figure 2.26). Pathological or iatrogenic communications may therefore easily develop. Oronasal fistulae may originate from the alveoli of the maxillary incisors, canines, and first, second and third premolar teeth. The relationship of the roots of the caudal teeth and the above structures varies based on skull morphology. In dolichocephalic and mesocephalic dogs the roots of the maxillary fourth premolar tooth are just lateral to the maxillary recess and the molars are located just ventral to the orbit (see Figures 2.26d and 2.30a).

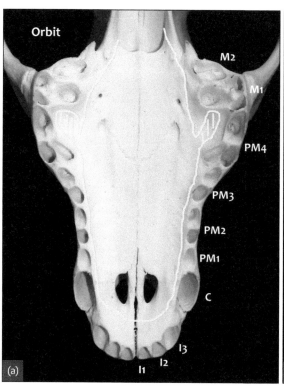

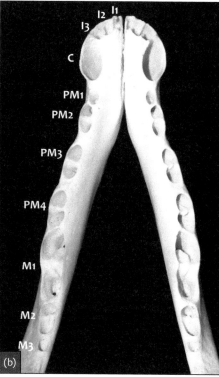

2.30 Skull of an adult dog. Empty alveoli of (a) the maxilla and (b) the mandible. In (a) the yellow line denotes the gross lateral margin of the nasal cavity and the striped area denotes the gross margins of the maxillary recess. C = canine tooth; I = incisor tooth; M = molar tooth; PM = premolar tooth. (continues) ▶

(a,b, © Dr Margherita Gracis)

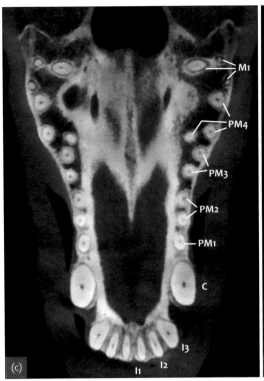

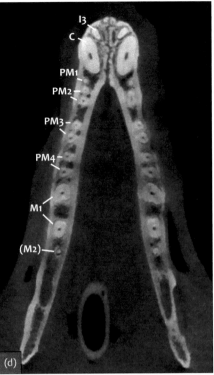

2.30 (continued) Skull of an adult dog. Dorsal plane cone beam computed tomography (CT) images through the roots of (c) the maxillary and (d) the mandibular teeth. The maxillary second molar tooth, the mandibular first and second incisor and third molar teeth are missing or not visible. Only the mesial root of the mandibular second molar tooth is visible. C = canine tooth; I = incisor tooth; M = molar tooth; PM = premolar tooth.
(c,d, Courtesy of Dr N. Girard)

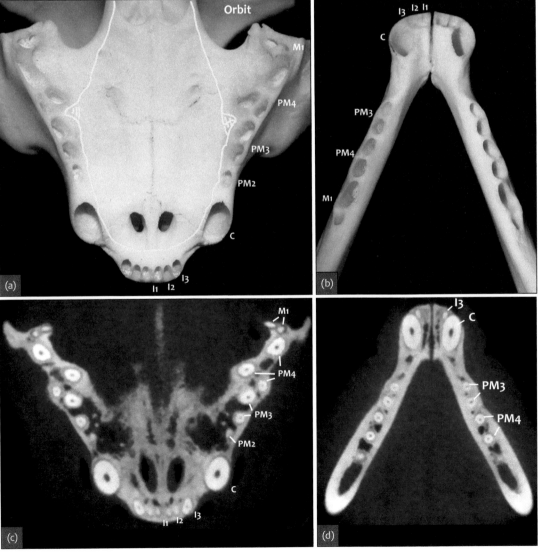

2.31 Skull of an adult cat. Empty alveoli of (a) the maxilla and (b) the mandible. In (a) the yellow line denotes the gross lateral margin of the nasal cavity and the striped area denotes the lateral margin of the maxillary recess. Dorsal plane cone beam computed tomography (CT) images through the roots of (c) the maxillary and (d) the mandibular teeth. The mandibular first and second incisor teeth are missing or not visible. C = canine tooth; I = incisor tooth; M = molar tooth; PM = premolar tooth.
(a,b, © Dr Margherita Gracis; c,d, Courtesy of Dr N. Girard)

Pathology affecting these teeth may therefore lead to oroantral or oro-orbital communications, respectively. In brachycephalic dogs the maxillary fourth premolar tooth is positioned relatively more caudally and laterally, at a certain distance from the nasal cavity and maxillary recess. Therefore, oronasal and oroantral communications originating from the alveoli of the fourth premolar tooth are less common in brachycephalic breeds. Similarly, in cats the bone palatal and apical to all maxillary teeth is relatively thick, and fistulae of dental origin are more likely to open on the cutaneous surface than in the nasal cavity, the small maxillary recess or the orbit (see Figures 2.27 and 2.31ac).

Mandibular teeth

A few important structures should be recognized when working on the mandibular teeth (see Figure 2.28).

Lower lip frenulum

On the rostrolateral side of each mandible, a mucosal fold connects the lower lip to the interproximal space between the canine and first premolar teeth (dog) or canine and third premolar teeth (cat). The *Nomina Anatomica Veterinaria* does not list or name it. This mucosal fold keeps the lip in position and should not be severed when mucogingival flaps are created. The mucosal fold also covers the middle mental foramen, and great care should be exercised when elevating tissue flaps in this area to avoid injuries to the associated neurovascular bundle.

Lingual molar salivary gland

In cats, there is a mucosal fold containing the lingual molar salivary gland distolingual to the mandibular first molar tooth.

Mental foramina

The three mental foramina located on the side of the rostral portion of each mandible represent openings of the mandibular canal. Rostral, middle and caudal mental foramina open apical to the mandibular first incisor and the second and third premolar teeth, respectively. The middle mental foramen is the largest one, and in dogs it can be palpated underneath the lower lip frenulum. This foramen is also lateral to the apex of the canine tooth (see Figure 2.26b). It should not be radiographically confused with periapical pathology affecting the rostral premolar teeth. It often represents the apical limit to bone removal during lateral alveolectomy of the canine alveolus.

Bone

Especially in dogs, bone thickness around the mandibular teeth varies greatly, as they are not placed in the middle of the mandible (see Figures 2.30d and 2.31d). The lower dental arch has a smooth sigmoid curvature, with the first and second molar teeth more laterally (see Figure 2.30). The alveolar bone over the roots of the caudal mandibular cheek teeth is particularly thick, making the access to the apices for apicoectomy very challenging. The thickness of the alveolar bone on the vestibular side of the mandibular canine tooth increases in the coronoapical direction, as the root is angled from a coronovestibular to an apicolingual direction. In small-breed dogs, the tooth size:mandibular bone height ratio is very high.

Therefore, the presence of advanced periodontal disease or improper application of forces during tooth extraction may lead to mandibular fracture.

Mandibular canal

The mandibular canal runs apically to the teeth (see Figures 2.26 and 2.27), extending from the medially located mandibular foramen to the laterally located mental foramina. It has been shown in brachycephalic dogs that the canal is slightly lingual to the molar teeth, then apical to the caudal premolar teeth, and finally it turns in a vestibular direction at the level of the second premolar tooth to open on the lateral side of the mandible. In mid-sized and small-sized dog breeds, the roots of some of the premolar and molar teeth can reach or even cross the mandibular canal, reaching into the ventral mandibular cortex. When extracting mandibular teeth, it is therefore important to consider the local anatomy, as improper placement of instruments can damage the inferior alveolar neurovascular bundle.

Incisor arrangement

Although the crowns of the mandibular incisor teeth are arranged in a smooth arch or line, the roots are not. The apices converge, and the root of the second incisor tooth is lingual to the roots of the first and third incisor teeth (see Figures 2.30d and 2.31d). This arrangement may help explain why the crowns of the second incisor teeth tend to deviate lingually, and those of the first and third incisor teeth displace in a labial direction, when dental malocclusion develops in this area.

Dental physiology

Tooth ageing

Following eruption, teeth do not change in size or shape, but dentine and pulp do have the ability to react to physiological and pathological stimuli. Newly erupted teeth usually have very thin dentinal walls (made up of so-called primary dentine), a wide pulp cavity with abundant pulp tissue, and incomplete roots with open apices (Figure 2.32). Apexogenesis (root development and apical closure) occurs within a few weeks (deciduous teeth) or months (permanent teeth) following eruption. This process occurs as a result of continuous activity of the epithelial cells of Hertwig's root sheath at the root apex. Apical closure of permanent teeth takes place in cats and dogs between 7 and 10 months of age, the roots of the mandibular first molar tooth being the first and the maxillary canine tooth root the last to form.

Following eruption/apexogenesis, the odontoblasts continue to produce dentine, known as secondary dentine. The odontoblastic layer lies on the periphery of the pulp, just below the dentine. As odontoblasts produce dentine, they move centripetally towards the centre of the canal. Therefore, the root canal becomes narrower with time, while the dentinal walls become thicker (see Figure 2.32).

Defence mechanisms

The ability to produce tertiary dentine is one of the most important defence mechanisms of the tooth pulp. External stimuli may also stimulate the thickening of the dentine around the tubules and obliteration of their lumina, which leads to dentinal sclerosis.

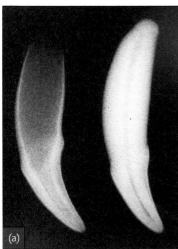

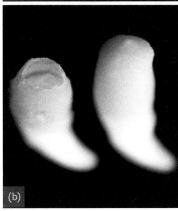

2.32 Extracted mandibular canine teeth from an immature 6-month-old cat (left) and an adult cat (right).
(a) Radiographic appearance.
(b) Apical view of the extracted specimens.
(© Dr Margherita Gracis)

Vascular supply

The vascular supply to the mandibular teeth comes from the inferior or mandibular alveolar artery, a branch of the maxillary artery. The inferior alveolar artery enters the mandibular canal through the mandibular foramen, on the medial side of each mandible. It is accompanied by a vein and nerve and during its course gives off small vessels that penetrate the bone, reaching the apices of the roots and periodontal structures, including the alveolar bone, periodontal ligament and gingiva. The artery exits through the mental foramina on the lateral and rostral surfaces of the mandible, branching into the caudal, middle and rostral mental arteries, supplying the rostrolateral part of the lower jaw and chin.

The maxillary teeth also receive their blood supply from different branches of the maxillary artery.

In the pterygopalatine fossa, just before it enters the maxillary foramen, the maxillary artery gives off the caudal dorsal alveolar artery. Small dental branches that leave the caudal dorsal alveolar artery supply the molar teeth. Within the infraorbital canal, the infraorbital artery, the main continuation of the maxillary artery, gives off the middle dorsal alveolar branches to the roots of the fourth premolar tooth.

Near the infraorbital foramen, the rostral opening of the infraorbital canal, the infraorbital artery gives off the rostral dorsal alveolar artery, which enters the incisivomaxillary canal. The incisivomaxillary canal and its neurovascular content run rostrally into the maxillary bone. They make a sharp turn dorsally, running towards the canine tooth root apex, then border the apical two-thirds of the mesial side of the canine root, and finally continue rostrally and medially into the incisive bone, supplying the first three premolar teeth, the canine tooth and incisor teeth (see Figure 2.16). The infraorbital artery exits the infraorbital foramen and divides into lateral and dorsal nasal arteries, supplying the muzzle.

Sensory system

Pulp tissue is rich in sensory nerve fibres entering the endodontic system through the apex in close association with arterioles, venules and lymphatic vessels. External stimuli (e.g. variation in tooth temperature or direct injury of pulp tissues) cause sensory nerve fibres to produce a sensation of pain. In human patients, dentine exposure associated with periodontitis or aggressive tooth brushing, caries and other pathological processes may also cause perception of pain. The currently accepted theory of dentine sensitivity is the hydrodynamic hypothesis of Brännström, whereby noxious stimuli cause fluid movement within the dentinal tubules, which is registered by the pulpal free endings of nerves located underneath the odontoblasts and possibly by the odontoblasts themselves. Dehydration of the exposed dentinal tubule results in tension on the odontoblastic process, causing pain.

References and further reading

Arnall L (1961) Some aspects of dental development in the dog – I. Calcification of crown and root of the deciduous dentition. *Journal of Small Animal Practice* **1**, 169–173

Bath-Balogh M and Fehrenbach MJ (2006) Tooth development and eruption. In: *Dental Embryology, Histology and Anatomy, 2nd edn*, ed. M Bath-Balogh and MJ Fehrenbach, pp. 61–91. Elsevier Saunders, St Louis

Berman E (1974) The time and pattern of eruption of the permanent teeth of the cat. *Laboratory Animal Science* **24**, 929–931

Breit S, Kunzel W and Oppel M (2003) The course of the nasolacrimal duct in brachycephalic cats. *Anatomia, Histologia, Embryologia* **32**, 224–227

Crossley DA (1995) Tooth enamel thickness in the mature dentition of domestic dogs and cats – Preliminary study. *Journal of Veterinary Dentistry* **12**, 111–113

DeLauriel A, Boyle A, Horton MA *et al.* (2006) Analysis of the surface characteristics and mineralization status of feline teeth using scanning electron microscopy. *Journal of Anatomy* **209**, 655–669

Done SH, Goody PC, Evans SA *et al.* (1996) *Color Atlas of Veterinary Anatomy. The Dog and Cat.* Mosby-Wolfe, London

Floyd MR (1991) The modified Triadan system: nomenclature for veterinary dentistry. *Journal of Veterinary Dentistry* **8**, 18–19

Gioso MA, Shofer F, Barros PSM *et al.* (2001) Mandible and mandibular first molar tooth measurements in dogs: relationship of radiographic height to body weight. *Journal of Veterinary Dentistry* **18**, 65–68

Gracis M (2013) *Odontostomatologia*. DVD multimediale, collana Med Tutor Veterinaria, UTET

Jayne H (1898) The teeth. In: *Mammalian anatomy. A preparation for human and comparative anatomy. Part I: The skeleton of the cat. Its muscular attachment, growth, and variations compared with the skeleton of man*, ed. H Jayne, pp. 402–457. Lippincott Co., London

Kremenak CR (1969) Dental eruption chronology in dogs: deciduous tooth gingival emergence. *Journal of Dental Research* **48**, 1177–1184

Lorenzo CE, Negro VB and Hernandez S (2001) Topografia de los conductos radiculares de los colmillos del perro. *InVet* **3**, 29–37

Morgan JP and Miyabayashi T (1991) Dental radiology: ageing changes in permanent teeth of beagle dogs. *Journal of Small Animal Practice* **32**, 11–18

Negro VB and Hernandez SZ (2000) Colmillos y muelas carniceras del gato domestico *(Felis catus)*: Caracteristicas anatomicas de importancia clinicoquirurgica. *Veterinaria Argentina* **17**, 62–77

Wilson GJ (1996) Implications of the time of apical closure in relation to tooth fracture in dogs. *Australian Veterinary Practitioner* **26**, 65–71

Wilson G (1999) Timing of apical closure of the maxillary canine and mandibular first molar teeth of cats. *Journal of Veterinary Dentistry* **16**, 19–21

Zontine WJ (1975) Canine dental radiology: radiographic technic, development, and anatomy of the teeth. *Journal of the American Veterinary Radiological Society* **16**, 75–82

Chapter 3

Dental and oral examination and recording

Simone Kirby and Bonnie Miller

A dental record is an essential part of the patient's medical record, as it helps the veterinary surgeon (veterinarian) to arrive at an accurate diagnosis and oral treatment plan. Dental charts are available to be purchased or downloaded or they may be included as part of an electronic medical record system (Figure 3.1). The record should be considered a legal permanent document, legibly written in ink and initialled by the clinician. Signalment information, essential medical and dental history, data collected during the oral assessment and periodontal evaluation, and a record of any treatment that is performed will become part of the dental record. It will serve as a baseline of initial conditions and a gauge for future treatment (Lewis and Miller, 2014).

While completing the dental chart, numbering systems are used to identify each tooth in the mouth. The Anatomical and Triadan Systems are most commonly used in veterinary dentistry and oral surgery (see Chapter 2 for detailed information). The Anatomical System uses the first letter of each tooth type along with its number according to its position within the mouth, counting teeth starting from the midline along the dental arch caudally (e.g. premolars: P1, P2, P3, P4). Lowercase letters are used for deciduous teeth and uppercase letters are used for permanent teeth. Placement of the number in the superscript or subscript position next to the letter designates whether it is located on the upper or lower jaw. Placement of the number to the left or right of the letter designates on which side of the mouth the tooth is located. For example, the permanent left maxillary fourth premolar tooth would be notated as ^{4}P, while the deciduous right mandibular canine tooth would be notated as c_1.

The Nomenclature Committee of the American Veterinary Dental College (AVDC) creates abbreviations of dental and oral pathology and diagnostics and treatment procedures in capital letters for use in dental charts (see https://www.avdc.org/Nomenclature/Nomen-Intro.html). It should be understood that determining and adopting nomenclature is an ongoing process, and clinicians should frequently check whether new abbreviations have been created and update their dental charts based on the most recent release of sets of abbreviations.

History-taking and general medical examination

As with all veterinary investigations, examination of the patient starts with history-taking and noting the signalment, including age, breed, sex and neutering status. Take the patient's history in regard to its general health. History pertinent to dentistry and oral surgery should be noted, in particular previously performed dental or oral surgical procedures. Enquire about clinical signs that may be suggestive of oral disease such as inappetence, dropping of or shying away from food, sneezing or snorting following eating and drinking, change from normal behaviour to aggressiveness when approached towards the face or mouth, and face rubbing or pawing at the mouth.

Find out about chewing habits, home care regimens, diet, treats and toys so that recommendations, whether new or corrective, can be made at the time of the appointment. If a home care regimen is currently in use, ask about the frequency of oral hygiene and what type of toothbrush, dentifrice and brushing methods are being used. If the client has not been successful, even though they attempted to perform home oral hygiene with their pet, a suggestion of alternative methods can be offered to solve the problem (see Chapter 13 for more detail). The veterinary surgeon should enquire about the type of diet (dry kibble, semi-moist or canned) and treats the pet is given, as some diets and treats contribute to dental and periodontal disease while others contribute to prevention of dental disease. Toys that the patient plays with may also be damaging to teeth, such as tennis balls that typically cause tooth abrasion or hard nylon toys, antlers and cow hooves that often cause tooth fracture.

The physical examination of the patient has to consider the patient as a whole, and should include as a minimum the assessment of mentation, bodyweight and condition, measurement of body temperature, basic cardiovascular and respiratory evaluation, and palpation of regional lymph nodes. Assessment of the patient's general health status is further completed by laboratory testing and diagnostic imaging as required, for example thoracic radiographs for a patient with cardiac or respiratory signs or oral cancer, and complete blood count and serum chemistry profile as pre-anaesthetic laboratory tests. Clotting profiles and/or tests for von Willebrand's disease may have to be run in patients of predisposed breeds or if a history of bleeding problems is present. Severely ill cats, including stomatitis patients, should be tested for feline leukaemia virus (FeLV) and feline immunodeficiency virus (FIV). Other preoperative tests to consider in cats with stomatitis include oral mucosal swabs for feline calicivirus (FCV) and feline herpes virus type 1 (FHV-1).

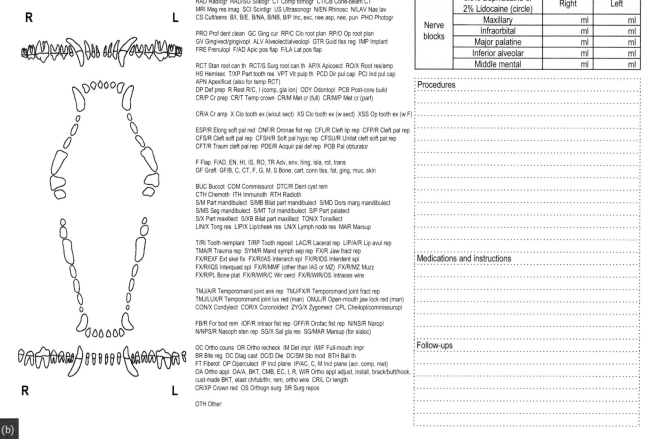

Penn Vet Dentistry/Oral Surgery Record Dog
Diagnosis in the Front, Procedures in the Back

Date:
Staff:
(circle primary clinician)
Chief Complaint:

Awake   Sedated   Anesthetized

Patient ID

R   L

MAL1/BV, DV, LABV, LV, MV, PV, CB/R, CB/C MAL2, MAL3, MAL4
DT Dec tooth DT/P Persist DT DTC Dent cyst

PD0, PD1, PD2, PD3, PD4 Norm, gingivitis, mild, mod, sev perio
GE, GH, GR Ging enl, hyp, rec ABE Alv bone exp ATE Abn tooth ext
CU Cont ulc PYO Pyo gran ST Stom ST/CS Cd stom TON/IN Tonsilli
CL/B, T Chew les (buc, subling) EOG/L, P, T Eos gran (lip, pal, tong)

OM Oral mass OM/AA, ADC, APN, APO, CE, FIO, FS, GCG, GCT, HS,
LS, MCT, MM, OO, OS, MTB, PAP, PCT, PNT, POF, SCC, UDN

AT Attr, AB Abr, E/D, E/H, E/HM Enam def, hyp, hypomin, CA Car
TR Tooth res RR Int res HC Hypercem
T/A, DEN, GEM, LUX, NE, NV, PE, SN, SR, U Tooth avul, dens invag,
gem, lux, near pulp exp, non-vit, pulp exp, super, super root, unerup
T/FX/EI, EF, CCF, UCF, CCRF, UCRF, RF Tooth fract (infract, enam,
comp crown, uncomp crown, comp crown-root, uncomp crown-root, root)
RCR Ret crown-root RTR Ret root

IOF Intraor fist OSS Osteoscler OST Osteomy
PA/A, C, G, P Periap absc, cyst, gran, path PU/M, S Pulp min, stone

LAC/B, G, L, O, P, T Lacerat (cheek, ging/alv, lip, tons/oroph, pal, tong)
LIP/A Lip avul TMA/B, E, BRN Ball, electr, burn trauma
MN/FX, MX/FX Mand, max fract SYM/S Mand symph sep

DMO Decr mouth op OMJL Open-mouth jaw lock FB For body
TMJ/A, D, FX, LUX Temporomand joint ank, dyspl, fract, lux

CFL, CFP, CFS, CFSH, CFSU, CFT, OAF, OFF, ONF, ESP, PDE Cleft
lip, cleft pal, cleft soft pal, soft pal hyp, unilat cleft soft pal, traum cleft
pal, orofac fist, oronas fist, elong soft pal, acquir pal def

N/NS, NPS, POL, SCC Naris sten, nasoph sten, nasoph pol, nas SCC
CMO Craniomand osteo CHO Calv hyperost FOD Fibr osteodyst
ENO Enopth EXO Exophth RBA Retrobul abs RPA Retrophar abs
LN/E Lym node enlarg MMM Mast mus myos

SG/ADC, ADS, IN, NEC Sal gla ADC, sialadeno, sialadeni, necr sialom
SG/MUC/S, P, C, SI Subling, phar, cerv sialoc, sialolith

OTH Other:

N A Extraoral/facial
N A Lymph nodes
N A Salivary glands
N A Oral mucosa
N A Tongue
N A Palate
N A Tonsils/pharynx

Tooth	M2	M1	P4	P3	P2	P1	C	I3	I2	I1	I1	I2	I3	C	P1	P2	P3	P4	M1	M2
Triadan	110	109	108	107	106	105	104	103	102	101	201	202	203	204	205	206	207	208	209	210
Mobility																				
Pocket																				
Recession																				
Furcation																				
Hyperplasia																				
Calculus																				
Plaque																				
Gingivitis																				

Tooth	M3	M2	M1	P4	P3	P2	P1	C	I3	I2	I1	I1	I2	I3	C	P1	P2	P3	P4	M1	M2	M3
Triadan	411	410	409	408	407	406	405	404	403	402	401	301	302	303	304	305	306	307	308	309	310	311
Mobility																						
Pocket																						
Recession																						
Furcation																						
Hyperplasia																						
Calculus																						
Plaque																						
Gingivitis																						

Completed ☐

MRCL category:

Right   Left

R   L

(a)

R   L

RAD Radiogr RAD/SG Sialogr CT Comp tomogr CT/CB Cone-beam CT
MRI Mag res imag SCI Scintigr US Ultrasonogr N/EN Rhinosc N/LAV Nas lav
CS Cult/sens B/I, B/E, B/NA, B/NB, B/P Inc, exc, nee asp, nee, pun PHO Photogr

PRO Prof dent clean GC Ging cur RP/C Clo root plan RP/O Op root plan
GV Gingivect/gingivopl ALV Alveolect/alveolopl GTR Guid tiss reg IMP Implant
FRE Frenulopl F/AD Apic pos flap F/LA Lat pos flap

RCT Stan root can th RCT/S Surg root can th AP/X Apicoect RO/X Root res/amp
HS Hemisec T/XP Part tooth res VPT Vit pulp th PCD Dir pul cap PCI Ind pul cap
APN Apexificat (also for temp RCT)
DP Def prep R Rest R/C, I (comp, gla ion) ODY Odontopl PCB Post-core build
CR/P Cr prep CR/T Temp crown CR/M Met cr (full) CR/M/P Met cr (part)

CR/A Cr amp X Clo tooth ex (w/out sect) XS Clo tooth ex (w sect) XSS Op tooth ex (w F)

ESP/R Elong soft pal red ONF/R Oronas fist rep CFL/R Cleft lip rep CFP/R Cleft pal rep
CFS/R Cleft soft pal rep CFSH/R Soft pal hypo rep CFSU/R Unilat cleft soft pal rep
CFT/R Traum cleft pal rep PDE/R Acquir pal def rep POB Pal obturator

F Flap F/AD, EN, HI, IS, RO, TR Adv, env, hing, isla, rot, trans
GF Graft GF/B, C, CT, F, G, M, S Bone, cart, conn tiss, fat, ging, muc, skin

BUC Buccot COM Commissurot DTC/R Dent cyst rem
CTH Chemoth ITH Immunoth RTH Radioth
S/M Part mandibulect S/MB Bilat part mandibulect S/MD Dors marg mandibulect
S/MS Seg mandibulect S/MT Tot mandibulect S/P Part palatect
S/X Part maxillect S/XB Bilat part maxillect TON/X Tonsillect
LIN/X Tong res LIP/X Lip/cheek res LN/X Lymph node res MAR Marsup

T/RI Tooth reimplant T/RP Tooth reposit LAC/R Lacerat rep LIP/A/R Lip avul rep
TMA/R Trauma rep SYM/R Mand symph sep rep FX/R Jaw fract rep
FX/REXF Ext skel fix FX/R/IAS Interarch spl FX/R/IDS Interdent spl
FX/R/IQS Interquad spl FX/R/MMF (other than IAS or MZ) FX/R/MZ Muzz
FX/R/PL Bone plat FX/R/WIR/C Wir cercl FX/R/WIR/OS Intraoss wire

TMJ/A/R Temporomand joint ank rep TMJ/FX/R Temporomand joint fract rep
TMJ/LUX/R Temporomand joint lux red (man) OMJL/R Open-mouth jaw lock red (man)
CON/X Condylect COR/X Coronoidect ZYG/X Zygomect CPL Cheilopl/commissuropl

FB/R For bod rem IOF/R Intraor fist rep OFF/R Orofac fist rep N/NS/R Naropl
N/NPS/R Nasoph sten rep SG/X Sal gla res SG/MAR Marsup (for sialoc)

OC Ortho couns OR Ortho recheck IM Det impr IM/F Full-mouth impr
BR Bite reg DC Diag cast DC/D Die DC/SM Sto mod BTH Ball th
FT Fiberot OP Operculect IP Incl plane IP/AC, C, M Incl plane (acr, comp, met)
OA Ortho appl OA/A, BKT, CMB, EC, I, R, WIR Ortho appl adjust, install, brack/butt/hook,
cust-made BKT, elast ch/tub/thr, rem, ortho wire CR/L Cr length
CR/XP Crown red OS Orthogn surg SR Surg repos

OTH Other:

Nerve blocks	0.5% Bupivacaine or 2% Lidocaine (circle)	Right	Left
	Maxillary	ml	ml
	Infraorbital	ml	ml
	Major palatine	ml	ml
	Inferior alveolar	ml	ml
	Middle mental	ml	ml

Procedures
....

Medications and instructions
....

Follow-ups
....

R   L

(b)

3.1 Examples of dental/oral surgical charts for dogs and cats. (a) Dog chart – 'Diagnosis'. (b) Dog chart – 'Procedures'. (continues) ▶
(Courtesy of Alexander M. Reiter, Dentistry and Oral Surgery Service, School of Veterinary Medicine, University of Pennsylvania)

Penn Vet Dentistry/Oral Surgery Record Cat
Diagnosis in the Front, Procedures in the Back

Date:
Staff:
(circle primary clinician)
Chief Complaint:

| Awake | Sedated | Anesthetized |

Patient ID

R **L**

MAL1/BV, DV, LABV, LV, MV, PV, CB/R, CB/C MAL2, MAL3, MAL4
DT Dec tooth DT/P Persist DT DTC Dent cyst

PD0, PD1, PD2, PD3, PD4 Norm, gingivitis, mild, mod, sev perio
GE, GH, GR Ging enl, hyp, rec ABE Alv bone exp ATE Abn tooth ext
CU Cont ulc PYO Pyo gran ST Stom ST/CS Cd stom TON/IN Tonsilli
CL/B, T Chew les (buc, subling) EOG/L, P, T Eos gran (lip, pal, tong)

OM Oral mass OM/AA, ADC, APN, APO, CE, FIO, FS, GCG, GCT, HS,
LS, MCT, MM, OO, OS, MTB, PAP, PCT, PNT, POF, SCC, UDN

AT Attr, AB Abr, E/D, E/H, E/HM Enam def, hyp, hymomin, CA Car
TR Tooth res RR Int res HC Hypercem
T/A, DEN, GEM, LUX, NE, NV, PE, SN, SR, U Tooth avul, dens invag,
gem, lux, near pulp exp, non-vit, pulp exp, super, super root, unerup
T/FX/EI, EF, CCF, UCF, CCRF, UCRF, RF Tooth fract (infract, enam,
comp crown, uncomp crown, comp crown-root, uncomp crown-root, root)
RCR Ret crown-root RTR Ret root

IOF Intraor fist OSS Osteoscler OST Osteomy
PA/A, C, G, P Periap absc, cyst, gran, path PU/M, S Pulp min, stone

LAC/B, G, L, O, P, T Lacerat (cheek, ging/alv, lip, tons/oroph, pal, tong)
LIP/A Lip avul TMA/B, E, BRN Bail, electr, burn trauma
MN/FX, MX/FX Mand, max fract SYM/S Mand symph sep

DMO Decr mouth op OMJL Open-mouth jaw lock FB For body
TMJ/A, D, FX, LUX Temporomand joint ank, dyspl, fract, lux

CFL, CFP, CFS, CFSH, CFSU, CFT, OAF, OFF, ONF, ESP, PDE Cleft
lip, cleft pal, cleft soft pal, soft pal hyp, unilat cleft soft pal, traum cleft
pal, orofac fist, oronas fist, elong soft pal, acquir pal def

N/NS, NPS, POL, SCC Naris sten, nasoph sten, nasoph pol, nas SCC
CMO Craniomand osteo CHO Calv hyperost FOD Fibr osteodyst
ENO Enopth EXO Exophth RBA Retrobul abs RPA Retrophar abs
LN/E Lym node enlarg MMM Mast mus myos

SG/ADC, ADS, IN, NEC Sal gla ADC, sialadeno, sialadeni, necr sialom
SG/MUC/S, P, C, SI Subling, phar, cerv sialoc, sialolith
OTH Other:

N A Extraoral/facial

N A Lymph nodes

N A Salivary glands

N A Oral mucosa

N A Tongue

N A Palate

N A Tonsils/pharynx

Tooth	M1	P4	P3	P2	C	I3	I2	I1	I1	I2	I3	C	P2	P3	P4	M1
Triadan	109	108	107	106	104	103	102	101	201	202	203	204	206	207	208	209
Mobility																
Recession																
Pocket																
Furcation																
Hyperplasia																
Calculus																
Plaque																
Gingivitis																

Tooth	M1	P4	P3		C	I3	I2	I1	I1	I2	I3	C		P3	P4	M1
Triadan	409	408	407		404	403	402	401	301	302	303	304		307	308	309
Mobility																
Recession																
Pocket																
Furcation																
Hyperplasia																
Calculus																
Plaque																
Gingivitis																

Right   Left

Completed ☐

MRCL
category:

R **L**

(c)

R **L**

RAD Radiogr RAD/SG Sialogr CT Comp tomogr CT/CB Cone-beam CT
MRI Mag res imag SCI Scintigr US Ultrasonogr N/EN Rhinosc N/LAV Nas lav
CS Cult/sens B/I, B/E, B/NA, B/NB, B/P Inc, exc, nee asp, nee, pun PHO Photogr

PRO Prof dent clean GC Ging cur RP/C Clo root plan RP/O Op root plan
GV Gingivect/gingivopl ALV Alveolect/alveolopl GTR Guid tiss reg IMP Implant
FRE Frenulopl F/AD Apic pos flap F/LA Lat pos flap

RCT Stan root can th RCT/S Surg root can th AP/X Apicoect RO/X Root res/amp
HS Hemisec T/XP Part tooth res VPT Vit pulp th PCD Dir pul cap PCI Ind pul cap
APN Apexificat (also for temp RCT)
DP Def prep R Rest R/C, I (comp, gla ion) ODY Odontopl PCB Post-core build
CR/P Cr prep CR/T Temp crown CR/M Met cr (full) CR/M/P Met cr (part)

CR/A Cr amp X Clo tooth ex (w/out sect) XS Clo tooth ex (w sect) XSS Op tooth ex (w F)

ESP/R Elong soft pal red ONF/R Oronas fist rep CFL/R Cleft lip rep CFP/R Cleft pal rep
CFS/R Cleft soft pal rep CFSH/R Soft pal hypo rep CFSU/R Unilat cleft soft pal rep
CFT/R Traum cleft pal rep PDE/R Acquir pal def rep POB Pal obturator

F Flap F/AD, EN, HI, IS, RO, TR Adv, env, hing, isla, rot, trans
GF Graft GF/B, C, CT, F, G, M, S Bone, cart, conn tiss, fat, ging, muc, skin

BUC Buccot COM Commissurot DTC/R Dent cyst rem
CTH Chemoth ITH Immunoth RTH Radioth
S/M Part mandibulect S/MB Bilat part mandibulect S/MD Dors marg mandibulect
S/MS Seg mandibulect S/MT Tot mandibulect S/P Part palatect
S/X Part maxillect S/XB Bilat part maxillect TON/X Tonsillect
LIN/X Tong res LIP/X Lip/cheek res LN/X Lymph node res MAR Marsup

T/RI Tooth reimplant T/RP Tooth reposit LAC/R Lacerat rep LIP/A/R Lip avul rep
TMA/R Trauma rep SYM/R Mand symph sep rep FX/R Jaw fract rep
FX/REXF Ext skel fix FX/R/IAS Interarch spl FX/R/IDS Interdent spl
FX/R/IQS Interquad spl FX/R/MMF (other than IAS or MZ) FX/R/MZ Muzz
FX/R/PL Bone plat FX/R/WIR/C Wir cercl FX/R/WIR/OS Intraoss wire

TMJ/A/R Temporomand joint ank rep TMJ/FX/R Temporomand joint fract rep
TMJ/LUX/R Temporomand joint lux red (man) OMJL/R Open-mouth jaw lock red (man)
CON/X Condylect COR/X Coronoidect ZYG/X Zygomect CPL Cheilopl/commissuropl

FB/R For bod rem IOF/R Intraor fist rep OFF/R Orofac fist rep N/NS/R Naropl
N/NPS/R Nasoph sten rep SG/X Sal gla res SG/MAR Marsup (for sialoc)

OC Ortho couns OR Ortho recheck IM Det impr IM/F Full-mouth impr
BR Bite reg DC Diag cast DC/D Die DC/SM Sto mod BTH Ball th
FT Fiberot OP Operculect IP Incl plane IP/AC, C, M Incl plane (acr, comp, met)
OA Ortho appl OA/A, BKT, CMB, EC, I, R, WIR Ortho appl adjust, install, brack/butt/hook,
cust-made BKT, elast ch/tub/thr, rem, ortho wire CR/L Cr length
CR/XP Crown red OS Orthogn surg SR Surg repos

OTH Other:

	0.5% Bupivacaine or 2% Lidocaine (circle)	Right	Left
Nerve blocks	Maxillary	ml	ml
	Infraorbital	ml	ml
	Major palatine	ml	ml
	Inferior alveolar	ml	ml
	Middle mental	ml	ml

Procedures

Medications and instructions

Follow-ups

R **L**

(d)

3.1 (continued) Examples of dental/oral surgical charts for dogs and cats. (c) Cat chart – 'Diagnosis'. (d) Cat chart – 'Procedures'.
(Courtesy of Alexander M. Reiter, Dentistry and Oral Surgery Service, School of Veterinary Medicine, University of Pennsylvania)

Equipment, instruments and materials

Oral examination procedures require a minimal investment of equipment, instruments and materials. To allow proper viewing, illumination from an overhead dental or surgical light that can be directed to focus on the intraoral structures is required. Surgical loupes with an attached head lamp may be used. The examiner should be sitting on a stool with wheels and adjustable seat height to enable positioning that facilitates proper ergonomics and reduces the risk of development of musculoskeletal disorders. A dental mirror, tongue depressor or Minnesota retractor is helpful to retract soft tissues for visualization of all oral structures. Lastly, the most important instruments used during the oral examination are the periodontal probe and dental explorer, often manufactured as one combined instrument (Pattison and Pattison, 1992; Nield-Gehrig, 2008). See Chapter 7 for more detailed information.

Mouth gags and wedge props

Gags and props may be used when the mouth needs to be held open and no hand is available to keep it open. They should be placed on the downwards side of the mouth, away from the viewing or working side. The devices are constructed of metal or made of a rubber-like material. The metal mouth gags have two small open rings that slip over the crowns of the maxillary and mandibular canine or other teeth, with a spring placed in between. A plastic covering of the rings is usually attached, preventing accidental fracture of the tooth. If the plastic is missing, the teeth should be protected with some gauze. The rubber wedge prop is shaped with ripples for holding the device in place between the maxillary and mandibular cheek teeth.

Prolonged wide mouth opening in cats (such as could occur during a procedure when using a spring-loaded mouth gag) has been reported to be associated with post-anaesthetic blindness (Stiles et al., 2012). Further investigation has determined that keeping the mouth open to the maximal range of motion causes decreased maxillary arterial blood flow (Barton-Lamb et al., 2013). A plastic syringe cap is an inexpensive alternative that can be cut with nail clippers to the desired length.

Dental mirror

A dental mirror provides several useful functions while working in the mouth of a veterinary patient. When used for indirect vision (Figure 3.2), it prevents the back and neck of the clinician from having to be strained and curved. The mirror provides the ability to maintain proper ergonomics, important in preventing workplace musculoskeletal disorders that have been known to cause forced early retirement of dentists and oral surgeons. The mirror is handy to use for retraction of the lips and tongue, especially during use of power scalers where heat from the tips may cause tissue trauma. A mirror may be used both for retraction and indirect vision, as in the case of holding the mirror caudal to the maxillary second molar to view the molars while retracting the cheek. Indirect illumination is another function of a dental mirror. When needing to focus on a particular area of a tooth, such as during scaling or root planing, the instrument can be held so as to bounce the overhead light off the mirror face and directly on to the tooth to achieve a bright focal spot. Dental mirrors are usually purchased with a separate handle and flat mirror face that is screwed into the

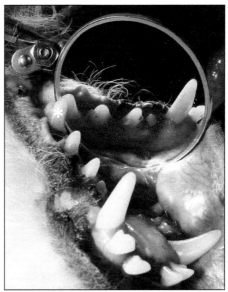

3.2 A dental mirror is used for indirect vision: holding it caudomedial to the right mandibular fourth premolar (✱ = tooth 408) allows visualization of the lingual aspects of the teeth.
(© Alexander M. Reiter)

handle. Mirror head sizes range from 16–32 mm (⅝ to 1¼ inches). The most useful for veterinary patients include size 3 (20 mm) for cats and small dogs and size 5 (24 mm) for medium and large dogs.

Dental explorer

A variety of design styles of dental explorers are available with differences in flexibility, shape and sharpness of the point (Figure 3.3). Some explorers are double-ended with contralateral curves, while others are single-ended. A shepherd's hook explorer is often paired with a Williams probe as a double-ended instrument. Though it is convenient to have the explorer handy while probing, the shepherd's hook is designed to be used only supragingivally, as it is inflexible, thick, bulky and not as sharp as others.

The explorer most suited for veterinary patients is the 11/12 ODU style. Having a very flexible and long shank makes this explorer adaptable for examining rostral and caudal teeth, and the small curved working ends are suitable for supragingival as well as subgingival use. The tip is

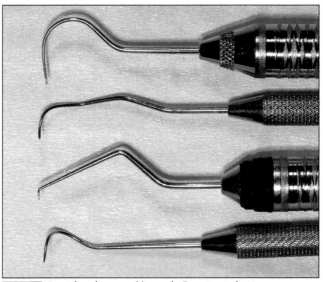

3.3 Dental explorer working ends. From top to bottom: shepherd's hook (number 23); 11/12 ODU; Orban (number 17); pigtail.
(© Bonnie Miller)

very fine and the point is sharp for better detection of surface defects. Other explorers available include the pigtail (sometimes referred to as cow-horn) and the Orban (number 17). The pigtail is thin and sharp; however, the curvature does not permit its use in deeper areas. The Orban is also sharp, and the 2 mm working end is bent at a 90-degree angle to the shank, allowing it to be inserted subgingivally without causing the gingiva to be distended during its use. The short working end of an Orban is a limitation for its use in deeper lesions.

Periodontal probe

The working end of a periodontal probe is either thin tapered, blunt rounded, or ball-ended. It is calibrated with markings (grooves or indentations) at various millimetre increments, and is either round, rod-shaped or flat. The grooves of some probes are colour-coded for easier reading. Several variations of marking increments are available; the most commonly used are the Williams and UNC probes (Figure 3.4).

The Williams probe has markings at 1, 2, 3, 5, 7, 8, 9 and 10 millimetres; the UNC probe does not skip any millimetre increments and is available with markings from 1 to 12 or 1 to 15 millimetres. For those working with feline patients or toy breed dogs, the Williams and UNC probes may be too thick in diameter to be easily inserted into a gingival sulcus. The Michigan-O probe is often preferred because it has a very thin working end. It typically is manufactured with markings at 3, 6 and 8 mm, which is not useful for examining feline teeth (it is best to have a groove at 1 mm). However, the Michigan-O probe can be obtained with Williams markings if specified at the time of ordering. The Nabers probe, used to assess the furcation area, has a curved blunt-tipped working end and is available with or without markings.

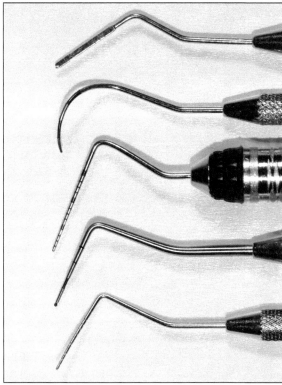

3.4 Periodontal probe working ends. From top to bottom: Goldman Fox (flat); Nabers furcation; UNC 15; World Health Organization (WHO); Williams.
(© Bonnie Miller)

Plaque disclosing solution

This is available as a single colour solution which stains plaque but not plaque-free enamel; the colour is usually red. Two-tone disclosing solutions are also available which stain older plaque blue and more recent plaque red. Disclosing solutions may be purchased as a liquid in bottle form, to be applied with a cotton bud, or with easy-to-use cotton-tip applicators with in-built disclosing solution. They are water-soluble and may stain fur and clothing temporarily but usually wash out. Likewise, staining of oral soft tissue might be noticed for some hours or days after application.

Extraoral examination

Each oral examination should begin with an extraoral examination. It is best to adopt a systematic approach, proceeding through the steps described below.

Observation

A patient with oral pain or discomfort may present with an abnormal head position. The head may be held abnormally low, or to one side. Ocular and neurological disorders may also be the cause of an abnormal head position. Drooling saliva is rarely the result of an excessive production of saliva but is more often the result of a reluctance to swallow because of oral pain (Harvey and Emily, 1993). History taking will inform if drooling is simply related to carsickness, or if breed conformation or previous oral surgeries are the cause of drooping of the lower lips. The examiner should also evaluate for facial symmetry, discharge from the nose, mouth or eyes, swellings, sinus tracts, and signs of dermatological disorders, in particular the lip folds of the skin adjacent to the lower lips and the ears. The anatomical position of the eyes should be evaluated, and the presence of exopthalmos or enopthalmos should be noted.

Malodour

Malodour emanating from the head of the patient may originate from the oral cavity (halitosis) or from extraoral sources, for example lip fold dermatitis, nasal foreign body or otitis externa. While most halitosis cases are caused by periodontal disease or oral tumours, oral malodour can also be caused by a number of other conditions (Figure 3.5) (Culham and Rawlings, 1998).

Source	Cause
Intraoral	• Plaque and calculus accumulation • Periodontal disease • Stomatitis • Osteomyelitis and osteonecrosis • Oral tumours • Foreign bodies • Oronasal communications • Non-healing oral wounds • Bacterial, viral and fungal infections
Extraoral	• Nasal, tracheal and lung disease • Cheilitis and lip fold dermatitis/pyoderma • Diabetic ketoacidosis • Uraemia/renal failure • Hepatic dysfunction causing hyperammonaemia • Gastro-oesophageal reflux, gastritis and vomiting • Pharyngeal, oesophageal and gastric tumours • Pharyngitis, laryngitis and tracheitis • Dietary indiscretion/consumption of spoiled food • Bronchitis and pneumonia

3.5 Intraoral and extraoral causes of malodour.

Nasal signs

Nasal signs may be unilateral or bilateral. They include sneezing, nasal discharge, epistaxis, and decreased patency of airflow. Due to the close anatomical relationship between the oral and nasal cavities, the possibility of a connection between nasal and oral conditions should be given consideration and may need to be investigated (Cohn, 2014). For example, a maxillary canine tooth with a deep periodontal pocket on its palatal aspect constitutes a primary oral condition (severe periodontitis resulting in alveolar bone loss) with a secondary nasal condition (rhinitis with unilateral nasal discharge due to oronasal fistula formation). The patency of nasal airflow is investigated by closing one nostril with a finger, then holding a light particle such as cotton wool or a few of the pet's hairs in front of the open nostril to observe air movement. Alternatively, a cooled microscopic slide may be held in front of the open nostril, and condensation of exhaled air, or lack thereof, observed. The same procedure is then repeated with the other nostril.

Palpation

Palpating the face helps to establish non-threatening contact with the dog or cat, and, in conjunction with calm talk, has a soothing effect on most patients. The palpable masticatory musculature includes the temporal, masseter and digastric muscles; the medial and lateral pterygoid muscles are located too deep for palpation. Masticatory muscles are evaluated for asymmetry, swelling, atrophy or pain. The ventral aspect of the mandibular bodies should be palpated from the mandibular symphysis to their angular processes. Similarly, the upper jaw (maxillofacial bones, the zygomatic arches and the bony orbital rims) is palpated from rostral to caudal. The lateral aspect of the temporomandibular joint can be felt immediately ventral to the caudal aspect of the zygomatic arch (Figure 3.6). While assessing bony structures, bear in mind that, in addition to looking for bony swellings, it is equally important to check for bony deficits, for example due to an invasive neoplastic lesion. A screening neurological assessment of the head can be performed next (Figure 3.7) (Oliver *et al.*, 1997).

The mandibular and sublingual salivary glands are caudal to the angular process of each mandible. The parotid salivary gland is V-shaped and located around the base of each ear. The mandibular lymph nodes are found caudomedial to the anguglar processes of the mandibles and ventrorostral to the mandibular and sublingual salivary glands; if lymphadenomegaly is found, the examiner should determine whether it is unilateral or bilateral, soft or firm, mobile or fixed, consistent or fluctuant, and non-painful or painful. Other superficial lymph nodes

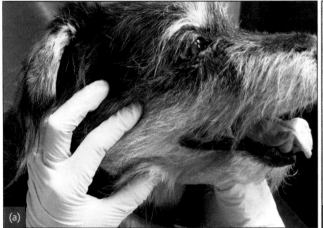
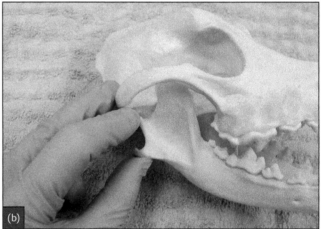

3.6 To palpate the lateral aspect of the temporomandibular joint, position the index finger ventral to the caudal end of the zygomatic arch. Demonstration on (a) the head of a crossbreed dog and (b) a dog skull.

Characteristic	Reflex testing (if applicable)	Corresponding cranial nerve (CN)
Facial symmetry	–	Facial nerve (CN VII)
Symmetry of eye position and pupils	–	Oculomotor nerve (CN III), trochlear nerve (CN IV), abducens nerve (CN VI) and sympathetic nerves
Eye (vision and lid function)	Menace gesture (blink provoked)	Optic nerve (CN II) and facial nerve (CN VII)
Eyelid (sensory and motor function)	Medial and lateral canthus touched (blink provoked)	Trigeminal nerve (CN V; ophthalmic and maxillary branches) and facial nerve (CN VII)
Eye movement	Observation of vestibular eye movements while head being turned from side to side	Oculomotor nerve (CN III), trochlear nerve (CN IV), abducens nerve (CN VI) and vestibulocochlear nerve (CN VIII; vestibular branch)
Pupil	Pupillary light reflex	Optic nerve (CN II) and oculomotor nerve (CN III)
Facial and lingual sensitivity	Touch or pinching of nose, jaws and tongue (eliciting facial or behavioural movements)	Trigeminal nerve (CN V; maxillary and mandibular branches) and facial nerve (CN VII)
Masticatory muscles	Evaluation of jaw tone	Trigeminal nerve (CN V; mandibular branch) Except caudal belly of the digastric muscle: facial nerve (CN VII)
Pharynx	Gag reflex upon touch	Glossopharyngeal nerve (CN IX) and vagus nerve (CN X)
Tongue symmetry and motor action	Observation and rubbing of nose to elicit licking	Hypoglossal nerve (CN XII)

3.7 Screening neurological examination of the head.

should also be palpated to rule out generalized lymphadenopathy. The parotid, lateral and medial retropharyngeal lymph centres are not normally palpable, even if significant changes such as neoplastic metastasis are present. Their evaluation by cytological (after CT or ultrasound guided needle biopsy) or histological (after excisional biopsy) techniques may therefore have to be considered in staging of oral and maxillofacial neoplasia patients (Herring *et al.*, 2002).

Gentle retropulsion of the globes of the eyes should be performed by placing both thumbs or index fingers over the closed eyelids and pressing inwards lightly; subjectively assess the degree of resistance, while comparing left and right (Figure 3.8). Differential diagnoses for decreased and increased retropulsion of the eye globes are listed in Figure 3.9 (Stades and Boevé, 1995).

Dynamic evaluation of mouth opening and closing

The examiner should evaluate for signs of restricted mouth opening, resistance, pain, crepitus or clicking noises, or an inability to close the mouth. Pain on opening of the mouth can be caused by intraoral causes, bone fractures, temporomandibular joint disorders, craniomandibular osteopathy, masticatory muscle inflammation, ear disease and space-occupying lesions in the orbit (Figure 3.10). The examiner should also distinguish whether an inability or an unwillingness to open or close the mouth is present. If an animal is unable to close its mouth, it should be established whether there is a mechanical obstacle (as with open-mouth jaw locking) or whether the jaw can be closed with gentle pressure (such as in bilateral fracture of the lower jaw or mandibular neurapraxia) (Harvey and Emily, 1993).

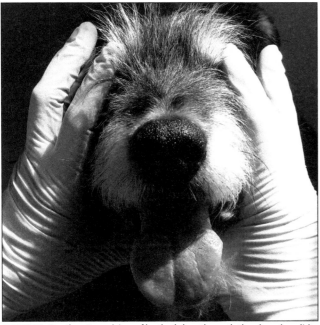

3.8 Gentle retropulsion of both globes through the closed eyelids; many pets are amenable to this, provided there is no painful disorder.

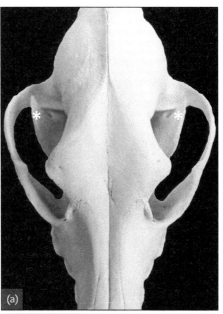

(a)

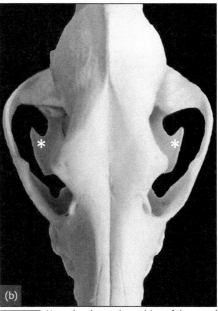

(b)

3.10 Note the change in position of the mandibular coronoid processes (∗) within the orbits of a dog skull when the mouth is (a) closed and (b) open. When the mouth is opened, the coronoid processes experience a forward movement towards the retrobulbar spaces.

Finding	Aetiology	Possible causes
Decreased retropulsion (may present as exophthalmos)	Retrobulbar space-occupying lesion (can potentially originate from or involve the oral cavity)	Neoplasia Haemorrhage Abscess, inflammation Foreign body Cyst Temporomandibular joint luxation with rostrodorsal displacement of the mandibular condyle
	Increased intraocular pressure or increased size of the globe	Glaucoma Neoplasia Abscess, inflammation Congenital macrophthalmos or acquired buphthalmos
Increased retropulsion (may present as enophthalmos)	Decreased intraocular pressure or decreased size of the globe	Loss of aqueous fluid Microphthalmos
	Atrophy of extraocular structures	Atrophy of extraocular muscles Atrophy of masticatory muscles

3.9 Differential diagnoses for increased and decreased ocular retropulsion.

Intraoral examination

Practical considerations in the conscious cat or dog

The clinician needs to gather as much information as possible with the patient awake to be able to formulate a preliminary diagnostic and treatment plan. The client must be made aware that the dog or cat must be under general anaesthesia at some point to allow for completion of a thorough oral examination and provision of an accurate estimate of the costs of recommended procedures. A preliminary estimate may have to be updated, once the diagnostics have been completed under anaesthesia. This, however, has the disadvantage of potentially prolonging the time spent under anaesthesia for the patient. A better alternative may be the provision of a wide, bracketed estimate at the time of the preoperative consultation.

The majority of dogs and cats will be sufficiently cooperative for a conscious intraoral examination. The best opportunity for the initial occlusal assessment of the patient is in the conscious or sedated patient, with the patient's mouth closed. Aspects that need to be considered for a successful examination are listed below:

- Gather as much information as possible by retracting the lips and cheeks and examining the labial and buccal aspects of the teeth, the oral vestibule and the occlusion while the mouth is still closed. This is important because cats and dogs may become agitated and evasive once the mouth is forced open
- Lift the lips gently by the margins, to avoid accidentally touching a painful lesion such as mucosal ulcers
- In dogs, avoid pushing on the sensitive nasal planum. Even careful lifting of the lips close to the nasal planum is tolerated only for a few seconds and followed by sneezing and/or evasive movements
- In cats, the general rule applies that minimal restraint results in less defensive behaviour. Consider approaching the patient from caudolaterally, instead of the front. A frontal approach is more threatening to the cat and renders the clinician at greater risk of feline defensive behaviour. Repeated stroking of the head prior to the intraoral examination helps to calm the cat. Gentle front leg restraint by an assistant may be helpful in some cases, in particular during the relatively short moment of opening the mouth
- In cats, for opening the mouth, the head should be held by the zygomatic arches with one hand, and the lower jaw is gently pushed ventrally with the index finger of the other hand positioned at the mandibular incisors. This way the buccal mucosa does not have to be touched at all. Look for areas that cannot be seen when the mouth is closed, i.e. the tongue, palate, lingual and palatal aspects of the teeth.
- In dogs, opening of the mouth is achieved by holding around the muzzle with one hand, placing two fingers on or immediately behind the canine teeth. With the other hand, press gently down on the mandibular incisor teeth. Most dogs respond well to affirmative talk to achieve sufficient masticatory muscle relaxation so that the mouth can be opened. Be prepared that only a few seconds may be available for the viewing of palatal, lingual and occlusal aspects of the oral cavity
- In most cats and dogs, it should be possible to view the sublingual space and ventral aspect of the tongue briefly by opening the mouth calmly, then pushing a free finger of the hand that holds on to the patient's

lower jaw into the intermandibular space through the ventral skin. This will lift the tongue up sufficiently to allow the observation of this otherwise hidden area (Harvey and Emily, 1993)
- If a dog strongly resents the opening of the mouth for behavioural reasons, the occlusal, lingual and palatal aspects of the oral cavity might be partially viewed while the dog is panting. A torch light or an examination light carried on the examiner's forehead is required for this
- In more aggressive dogs, if safe to do so, the owner may be able to assist in lifting the dog's lips and opening its mouth. In small-breed dogs with defensive biting behaviour, a wooden tongue depressor may be used to lift the lips (Figure 3.11). A tie muzzle may be placed, enabling lifting of the lips rostrally and caudally to the tie while an assistant restrains the dog's body and front limbs. This technique will work better in small-breed dogs, but may not be safe to use in large, strong, aggressive dogs
- In very fractious cats, a limited glimpse of the lingual and palatal aspect of the teeth, the tongue and palate is possible while the cat is hissing. This may be viewed very briefly with the animal restrained by an assistant with the necessary handling precautions (towel wrapping, gauntlets, etc.). This technique is not suitable, however, for the evaluation of the labial and buccal aspects of the teeth, and prolonged handling that is antagonizing to the cat should be avoided prior to induction of anaesthesia.

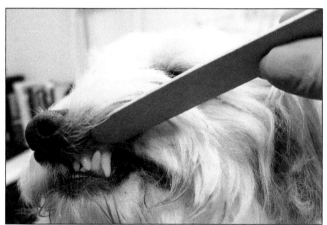

3.11 Demonstration of the lifting of the upper lip of a small crossbreed dog with the aid of a wooden tongue depressor. This technique may be helpful if an assistant is able to safely hold the body, neck and the caudal part of the head of an aggressive dog.

Guide to the intraoral examination

Completion of the steps of the oral assessment should be performed in the same order for each patient so that a routine will be developed and important areas are not inadvertently overlooked. The following descriptions of the intraoral examination suppose that the patient is under general anaesthesia. A fair percentage of the structures to be viewed can be seen in the conscious cat or dog as well, and the following lists may serve as a guide for what to look out for in the conscious oral examination. However, much of the detailed examination will be possible only in the anaesthetized patient. All findings will be noted on the dental chart. They may also be drawn on to the chart if appropriate and photographed for additional documentation. An intraoral examination is rarely complete without further diagnostic imaging, in particular dental radiography (see Chapter 4 for more detailed information).

Assessment of occlusion

Occlusion assessment is made during the conscious oral examination. The patient's mouth should be closed and the lips lifted; it should be viewed from both sides as well as the front. The examination can also be performed on the sedated patient. The tongue tends to protrude more rostrally in patients under chemical restraint, thus getting in between the teeth and making occlusal assessment more difficult. In an anaesthetized patient, assessment of occlusion may be accomplished by temporary extubation. One could also detach the endotracheal tube from the anaesthesia machine, deflate its cuff, and then insert the tube slightly further down the trachea until complete closure of the mouth is possible. Pre-measurement of the total length of the endotracheal tube is important with this technique to ensure that pushing the tube 2–3 cm further caudally would not cause its tip to impinge on the bronchial carina. Finally, the endotracheal tube can be positioned so that it emerges from the mouth immediately caudal to a maxillary canine tooth, often allowing satisfactory closure of a mouth.

Dogs and cats have anisognathism of their jaws, with their maxillary dental arch usually being wider than the mandibular dental arch.

Normal occlusion in dogs: Viewed from the sides, the mandibular canine tooth should occlude in the space between the maxillary canine and third incisor teeth. The maxillary and mandibular premolar teeth exhibit an interdigitation that approximates a 'zigzag pattern', and the premolar teeth should be visible without overlap with opposing teeth. The maxillary fourth premolar teeth occlude buccally to the mandibular first molar teeth, working together as shearing teeth in a 'scissor action'. A slight buccal overlap between the mandibular fourth premolar and first molar teeth is almost always present, and expert opinion is divided over whether to term this 'normal' or 'abnormal' for dogs. The mandibular incisor teeth should occlude slightly palatally to the maxillary incisor teeth, their incisal edges resting on the cingula of the maxillary counterparts. The incisor teeth should form a closed and slightly curved arch. Viewed from the front, the midlines of the upper and lower jaws (between the maxillary and mandibular first incisors) should line up. The mandibular canine teeth should just about touch, but not dig into the gingiva between the maxillary canine and third incisor teeth. The alignment of the teeth between the mandibular canine teeth and mandibular molar teeth should be a fairly straight line. The maxillary molar teeth tend to be positioned on a slight inwards arch towards the palate.

Normal occlusion in cats: The incisors are aligned in a straight or slightly curved line with minimal contact of the incisal edges or in scissor bite (see Chapters 2 and 10). The mandibular fourth premolar tooth almost always overlaps slightly on the buccal aspect of the mandibular first molar tooth. The rudimentary maxillary first molar tooth is positioned distopalatally to the maxillary fourth premolar tooth and can rarely be seen during a conscious oral examination (unless the mouth can be opened for a length of time). Other aspects of normal occlusion are similar to in the dog.

Malocclusion: This can be either pathological or 'accepted breed standard'. Examine for any deviation from the normal occlusion, such as abnormal tilting or rotation of individual teeth or jaw-length discrepancies. Malocclusions are discussed in more detail in Chapter 10. From the perspective of a complete oral examination, pay particular attention to malocculding teeth that may impinge on soft tissue or rub against other teeth during occlusion, thereby causing trauma to oral mucosa and skin or abnormal tooth wear (attrition), respectively. The documentation of malocclusion should include notes on the dental chart, photographs, and – in some cases – full-mouth impressions, bite registration and stone models.

Non-periodontal soft tissues of the mouth

Equipment requirements for oral soft tissue examination include a good light source (for example, an operating light or focused light source on the operator's forehead), a periodontal probe (good for the exploration of sinus tracts and other soft tissue defects), surgical instruments for tissue sampling, diagnostic imaging, and the cautious use of a mouth gag or wedge prop. For operator safety, the examiner should ensure sufficient depth of general anaesthesia prior to inserting fingers for palpation of soft tissue structures inside the mouth. Mouth closure of a patient under light anaesthesia can be unexpected and forceful and could result in bite injury to the operator.

Lips and mucocutaneous junction: If depigmentation, inflammation, erosions or ulcers are present, also inspect other mucocutaneous junctions for similar signs that could be indicative of autoimmune disease or immune-mediated diseases (see Chapter 8). In cats with ulcerative lip lesions, eosinophilic granuloma is often encountered, and a thorough dermatological assessment should be completed. Deep palpation of the lip tissues should be performed to evaluate the presence of abnormal thickenings.

Labial and buccal mucosa: Presence of petechiae, pallor or jaundice should be recognized during the preoperative examination, since further pre-anaesthetic diagnostics would be indicated. Under anaesthesia, examine the mucosa for signs of generalized or focal inflammation, ulceration, mass lesions or destructive lesions. All abnormalities should be noted on the dental chart, and adjacent teeth serve as landmarks for the description of the lesion location. Note whether ulcers or lacerations are in an area that is normally in contact with a tooth surface or might get caught between teeth, creating inadvertent self-trauma. A mild form of trauma-induced mucosal hyperplasia is common along the bite planes of the caudal cheek teeth. The lesions typically start at the level of the carnassial teeth, involving the buccal mucosa just caudal to the lip commissure or the sublingual mucosa, and tend to be fairly symmetrical bilaterally (Figure 3.12). This condition is well tolerated and does not usually require treatment. However, inspect the lesions carefully for signs of inflammation or asymmetry, and take a biopsy if in doubt. Healed inflammatory lesions of oral mucosa may be visible in patients with otherwise pigmented mucosa as areas of depigmentation (Figure 3.13). Further, closely inspect the mucogingival junction for sinus tracts. The mucogingival junction is the thinnest and weakest part of the oral mucosa; thus, any inflammatory exudate is likely to find its draining path at this point (Figure 3.14).

Gingiva in edentulous areas: Gingivitis at the site of a previously lost or extracted tooth may be an indication that an infected root remnant is present, and a sinus tract may be identified with the blunt tip of a periodontal probe.

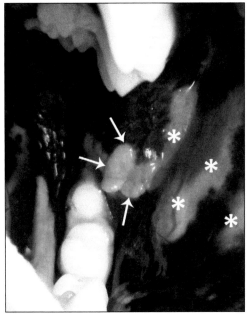

3.12 Depigmented hyperplastic lesions (arrowed) and thickened areas (*) of buccal mucosa secondary to chronic trauma of soft tissues along bite planes in a 9-year-old male Cocker Spaniel.

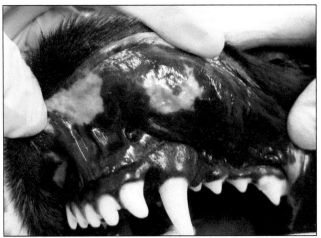

3.13 Partial depigmentation in areas of healed inflammatory lesions in a 9-year-old male Cocker Spaniel with a history of stomatitis. The patient's signs had been medically controlled at the time the photograph was taken. Note that the areas of depigmentation are in the labial and buccal mucosa which makes contact with tooth surfaces when the lips are in their natural position.

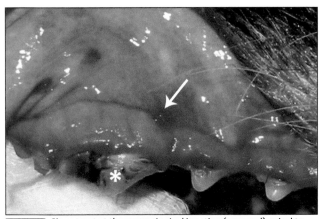

3.14 Sinus tract at the mucogingival junction (arrowed) apical to the mesial aspect of the right maxillary fourth premolar (* = tooth 108). Gentle use of the tip of a periodontal probe will confirm the presence of an opening at this location.

Hard palate: The roof of the mouth should be evaluated for defects, depigmentation, erosions, ulcers, mass lesions and the presence of foreign bodies. Congenital cleft palate can be very obvious or hidden from view; probing with a periodontal probe is required along the midline of the palate if the clinical presentation is indicative of the condition, as the fully epithelialized mucosal edges are often found to be apposing each other (see Chapter 10). Acquired hard palate defects may be longitudinal, as in a traumatic split palate along the midline as part of high-rise syndrome in cats, or the defect may be round or ovoid in shape and more randomly located if oronasal communications are caused by other types of trauma, inflammatory or neoplastic lesions. Complex fractures of the maxillofacial bones may present with any distortion or separation of the palate, depending on the fracture lines and the degree of dislocation of the fracture fragments. The hard palate mucosa has a pattern of transverse palatine rugae, which form ridges, and variably deep infoldings, which are particularly deep in brachycephalic breeds and may entrap hair and debris. The impacted material attracts formation of plaque that can lead to oral malodour and inflammation. The rostral portion of the palatal mucosa often appears 'puffy', as though sitting on a cushion of air. The rich vascularization of this area as well as the tissues filling the palatine fissures (i.e. incisive duct of the vomeronasal organ, connective tissue, vessels and nerves) are responsible for this effect. The unpaired incisive papilla immediately caudal to the maxillary incisors may be mistaken for a mass lesion (see Chapter 2). Ulcerative lesions should be examined to determine whether they are round and circumscript or longitudinal. The latter points towards ingestion-related injury, and similar lesions may be found on the tongue. In case of palatal mass lesions, nasal involvement or nasal origin of the lesion should be suspected, and further diagnostics that include the nasal cavity should be considered.

Soft palate: The size of the soft palate should be assessed just prior to intubation; there should be minimal overlap of the caudal edge of the soft palate with the tip of the epiglottis. Congenital clefts of the soft palate are present concomitantly with or independently from hard palatal defects. The nasopharyngeal meatus overlying the soft palate should be palpated, since a nasopharyngeal mass lesion (e.g. nasopharyngeal polyp in cats), when present, may be felt in this area. The mucosa of the oral side of the soft palate should be evaluated for the presence of erosions or ulcerations.

Palatine tonsils: These should be examined for signs of inflammation, change in size or mass lesions, discharge, and presence of foreign bodies in the tonsillar crypts. The tonsillar fold should be gently and atraumatically deflected with an instrument for full evaluation of the fossa and tonsil.

Tongue: The size of the tongue should be evaluated to exclude the presence of macroglossia or microglossia. Its dorsal and ventral surfaces are then inspected for the loss of papillae and the presence of ulcers, wounds, mass lesions and scars from healed wounds. The examiner should check for swellings and mass lesions in the sublingual region; mucosal hyperplasia may be present when tissue gets trapped along the bite planes of cheek teeth. One should also look for lacerations or sinus tracts in cases of suspected penetration injuries with sticks or other sharp pointed foreign bodies. Finally, the tongue is palpated to detect foreign bodies, abscesses or internal mass lesions.

Pharynx: The palatoglossal folds form the lateral borders of the entrance to the oropharynx. The examiner should observe whether inflammation and/or mass lesions are present. Proliferative space-occupying changes are common in cats with chronic gingivostomatitis. The roof of the oropharynx is formed by the soft palate and its floor by the caudodorsal base of the tongue. The nasopharynx is situated dorsal to the soft palate, and may have to be viewed by means of flexible endoscopy or by manual rostroflexion of the soft palate in order to look for the presence of foreign bodies, such as blades of grass, or other lesions, such as nasopharyngeal polyps. The examiner may also palpate the nasopharyngeal meatus by dorsal manipulation of the soft palate with a middle finger. The ventral surface of the tympanic bulla may be palpated if the finger is pushed slightly more caudally and laterally. Caudal to the soft palate is the common pharynx, leading into the larynx.

Larynx: Observe the larynx for any signs of abnormality. This is usually done at the time of intubation of the patient, using a laryngoscope with a bright light.

Teeth

Equipment requirements for proper dental examination include a good light source, mouth gag, pointed dental explorer, dental mirror and dental radiography. The dental explorer is used to assess the topography of the surface of the clinical crown but is also useful to detect subgingival dental abnormalities that are not clinically visible. Explorers are also used to determine the presence of pulp exposure and carious lesions and to assess the thoroughness of treatment following calculus removal or restoration placement. Explorers have a flexible wire-like working end that tapers to a sharp point. The terminal 2 mm of the working end located directly behind the point is called the tip. As the side of the point is dragged across the tooth surface, irregularities, such as calculus deposits and defects created by tooth resorption, will cause the tip to vibrate. When explorers are held with a very relaxed modified pen grasp, the vibrations will travel from the tip to the handle to be felt by the clinician, as the point encounters subtle defects. Development of this tactile sensitivity is critical to locating irregularities of the tooth surface. A sharp tactile sense will be developed as the clinician becomes more experienced. After lightly grasping the explorer and establishing an intraoral finger rest close to the tooth to be explored, the exploratory stroke is a light 'feeling' stroke, using a pushing or pulling motion while moving the tip in either a vertical, oblique or horizontal direction with short overlapping strokes. Use caution when moving the tip in a horizontal direction as the point can be hazardous to the junctional epithelium.

Chapter 5 describes dental abnormalities in detail; the list below focuses on lesions for which exploration is required as part of the diagnostic process.

- First of all, the teeth need to be counted, and any missing teeth must be marked on the dental chart. The examiner must indicate whether there are any deciduous or supernumerary teeth present. Each tooth is then inspected for the presence of structural defects, discoloration, abnormal size or shape. Any visible lesion is explored by running the explorer tip over it.
- The crowns of each tooth are evaluated for any structural deficit, which often manifests as loss of the most coronal portion of the crown in a more or less

transverse pattern, but it can also present as a slab fracture where the side of the tooth is injured. The maxillary fourth premolar teeth have a higher incidence of slab fracture compared with any other teeth. A fractured maxillary fourth premolar tooth may be overlooked, as it is often still considerably larger than the adjacent third premolar tooth, even when fractured. However, comparison with the other side will help to reveal that some crown structure is indeed missing. A slab fracture of a mandibular first molar tooth can be difficult to diagnose in a conscious dog, as the fracture tends to occur on the lingual aspect, and the dog's tongue has to be pushed aside to view the fracture site. A recently fractured tooth surface has jagged, sharp enamel edges. Corresponding lacerations of the gingiva, alveolar mucosa, labial and buccal mucosa or the tongue might be present adjacent to the tooth fracture. With time, an older crown fracture can obtain rounded edges and will be harder to distinguish from a worn crown. Pulp exposure in a fractured or worn tooth can be confirmed by exploration if it is not obvious on inspection. This may also be required to differentiate it from tertiary dentine. In a fractured tooth with pulp exposure, the tip of the explorer sinks through an opening into the pulp chamber of the crown (Figure 3.15). This should not be attempted in the conscious patient, as it can be difficult to predict whether or not viable nerve tissue might still be in the pulp cavity. Worn tooth surfaces with tertiary dentine, in contrast, have a hard, closed and even surface. The explorer would not sink in or catch. Rarely, an older fracture might undergo dense concrete-like debris impaction into the open pulp chamber, mimicking a closed surface.
- Caries is occasionally found in dogs and typically located on occlusal surfaces of molar teeth, but can sometimes also be present on smooth surfaces of the crowns of any teeth. The point of the explorer will 'stick' in enamel and dentine softened by the disease process. Differentiate this from the much more common occlusal food staining in the occlusal pit of the maxillary first molar tooth. The point of the explorer

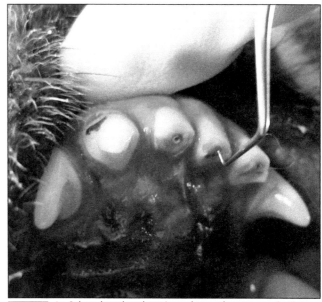

3.15 An Orban dental explorer is used to explore an opening into the pulp chamber of the fractured left maxillary first incisor (tooth 201) in an 8-year-old crossbreed dog. The right maxillary first incisor (tooth 101) and left maxillary second incisor (tooth 202) also have complicated crown fractures.

would not 'stick' while examining the surface of a stained tooth. Be careful of overzealous exploring of areas of tertiary dentine. Place the side of the point in contact with the surface, not the point itself, as dentine is soft enough to permit some scratching of its surface if the point is pushed in strongly. With experience, the difference between this and true deep 'sticking' of the explorer in a carious lesion will be learned.

- Abrasion is caused by gradual wear against external objects such as sticks or tennis balls. Attrition is caused by rubbing of teeth against each other with resultant gradual development of wear-facets. These conditions are bracketed together here as their appearance is similar. The defects of the crowns have smooth margins, as opposed to the sharp, jagged-edged margins of a fresh fracture, and the surface of a wear-facet has a smooth polished appearance. Frequently, there is presence of discolored dentine in the centre of the defect, where the pulp had been located before it began receding; here, tertiary dentine has been formed by pulpal odontoblasts as a response to the chronic traumatic stimulus. It does not have the same orderly crystalline structure as primary or secondary dentine, resulting in beige to brown discoloration. As mentioned above, the explorer should not find an opening into the pulp chamber. However, some dogs wear their teeth faster than tertiary dentine can be formed, resulting in pulp exposure due to abnormal tooth wear.
- Tooth resorption that is located externally on the crown and the most coronal aspect of the root is usually accessible to palpation with a sharp dental explorer. Subgingival exploration is an important part of the oral examination, especially in cats; however, it has to be performed with utmost care, as subgingival soft tissues are easily damaged. Tooth resorption (particularly when originating internally) requires dental radiography for diagnosis. Clinical detection or confirmation of tooth resorption is by tactile sensation of dropping of the explorer tip into the hard-walled defect. The edges of lesions (particularly when originating externally) often have enamel 'overhangs', under which the explorer tip readily catches. The examiner should be aware that presence of subgingival calculus can mimic the tactile sensation of early tooth resorption. If in doubt, the exploration is repeated after subgingival scaling of the suspect area.

Periodontal tissues

Incomplete periodontal examination may lead to inappropriate treatment. For example, overlooking moderate to advanced periodontal disease (as is often the case with anaesthesia-free dental procedures offered at grooming services) might result in supragingival scaling only rather than the required subgingival debridement. Evaluation of the periodontium will detect signs of gingival inflammation, gingival enlargement or recession, attachment loss, periodontal pocket formation, furcation involvement, and the presence of tooth mobility. Equipment requirements include a good light source, mouth gag, blunt periodontal probe, dental mirror and dental radiography. Probing should be performed routinely, as it is the most reliable method of detecting periodontal pockets and determining furcation involvement. It should be viewed as the minimum standard of care in small animal practices that offer dental and oral surgical procedures to their clients. The list below focuses on lesions for which probing is required as part of the diagnostic process.

- Calculus (tartar): Although a number of scoring systems exist, they are probably more research-oriented and of less interest to the practitioner. Documenting the presence of calculus is important as a highly visible indicator of where plaque has been allowed to accumulate abundantly and subsequently has mineralized to become calculus. This will indicate a number of possible conditions to the clinician. For example, calculus on the fractured surface of a tooth indicates that the fracture is not recent, but might be older. The presence of calculus also highlights areas that have been neglected (avoiding chewing on teeth that are painful will lead to increased calculus build-up) or insufficiently cleansed (by toothbrushing or other home oral hygiene methods). Abundant calculus can hide the dental and periodontal structures beneath, and its removal might be required prior to being able to proceed with the periodontal evaluation. Photographic documentation is fast, and images 'before-and-after' professional dental cleaning can be educational and motivational for the pet owner (see Chapter 13).
- Plaque: Many plaque scoring systems exist that are more of interest to researchers than to practitioners. Plaque is the primary causative factor of periodontal disease. However, dental charting will record the effects of periodontal disease in terms of other parameters (see below) rather than the presence of plaque. The presence of subgingival plaque in any periodontal pocket prior to treatment is a given fact, hence does not necessarily require separate recording. Note that some older texts describe abundant subgingival plaque as 'pyorrhoea', which is an outdated term and a misnomer because plaque is not pus, although it might look and smell similar at times. Plaque disclosing solutions are useful particularly at re-examinations and, similar to photographic documentation of calculus accumulation, can be educational and motivational for the pet owner (see Chapter 13). Because thin layers of plaque tend to be transparent and mucoid, they are easily missed in a conscious patient and become more visible once stained with disclosing solution. A thicker creamy beige matter, known as materia alba, is often abundant and more readily visible. Thinner layers of plaque can be detected under anaesthesia by running the periodontal probe over the tooth surface, leaving a visible trace behind in the plaque deposit, with the working end of the probe picking up some of the mucoid matter.
- Gingivitis and gingival bleeding: The gingiva is evaluated for the degree of inflammation and bleeding. Healthy gingival tissues should appear stippled, contoured to follow the curvature of the cementoenamel junction, tapered to a thin gingival margin and pink (or brown to black, in animals with pigmented oral mucosa) in colour. For each tooth, subsequent to probing of the gingiva, observe changes in colour, shape, consistency and bleeding.
- Gingival recession: This is measured in millimetres with a periodontal probe from the cementoenamel junction of the exposed neck of the tooth to the gingival margin. Record the measurement at the point of most severe recession, and mark the location on the tooth (for example, 'GR 6D' for 6 mm of gingival recession at the distal aspect of the tooth). Be aware that periodontal pockets may be present in addition to gingival recession. To calculate total attachment loss, the measurements for gingival recession extent and periodontal pocket depth are added together for the position around the tooth that exhibits the greatest loss of attachment.

- Gingival enlargement: This presents as gingival over-growth on to areas of the crown that would not normally be covered by gingiva. Knowledge of the normal gingival contour and location is required for the clinician to measure the degree of enlargement. The free gingival margin normally apposes the crown about 0.5 mm in cats and 1–3 mm in dogs beyond the cementoenamel junction. Adjacent teeth that may have less or no gingival enlargement may serve to help the clinician to estimate where the gingival contour should be. The term enlargement is a clinical term and could encompass benign and malignant causes for excess gingiva or gingiva-like tissue. Gingival hyperplasia is a common cause of gingival enlargement. Vertically enlarging gingival tissue can form a 'pseudopocket' (or gingival pocket) where the periodontal probe discovers a pocket, but periodontal attachment to the cementoe-namel junction may still be intact. Differential diagnosis should also include gingival oedema, which accompa-nies gingivitis. If gingivectomy is performed in case of an oedematous lesion, gingival recession may develop following resolution of inflammation. Pseudopockets invite accumulation of plaque, hair and debris, and they may therefore contribute to future attachment loss, in which case a pseudopocket and a true periodontal pocket combine to form one deeper pocket.
- Periodontal pocket: Each healthy tooth is surrounded by a gingival sulcus that should be no deeper than 0.5 mm in cats and 3 mm in dogs (depth variations exist depending on the size of teeth and animals). Once this measurement is exceeded, it is considered to be pathological and termed a periodontal pocket (i.e. the gingival attachment migrates apically along the root surface) (Figure 3.16). Good probing technique is important to avoid iatrogenic damage. It is important to master the modified pen grasp to obtain sufficient control over the tip of the instrument. The measurement of the depth of the gingival sulcus or periodontal pocket is as follows:
    - Heavy calculus deposits may impede the accuracy of measurements; therefore, a gross dental scaling may be required prior to probing
    - The probe is inserted below the gingival margin into the space between the free gingiva and the tooth, with the side of the probe tip in contact with the tooth
    - The probe is gently advanced apically to the junctional epithelium
    - The base of the sulcus or pocket will feel soft, spongy and resilient. Clinicians who are heavy handed may cause the probe tip to pierce the attachment
    - Using a light amount of pressure (10–20 grams), a 'walking' stroke is used to move the probe around the circumference of the base of the sulcus or pocket of each tooth. To practice the appropriate amount of pressure needed for probing, hold the end of a probe at a 90-degree angle to the fat pad of your thumb and press until the skin indents approximately 2 mm
    - The up-and-down bobbing movement of a walking stroke should be 1–2 mm in height, touching the junctional epithelium every 1 mm as the probe tip is advanced around the tooth. With each upward movement, the probe does not need to be completely removed from the sulcus or pocket
    - While probing around the tooth, the side of the working end should be kept at an angle of less than 10 degrees in relation to the long axis of the tooth to avoid inaccuracy of measurement

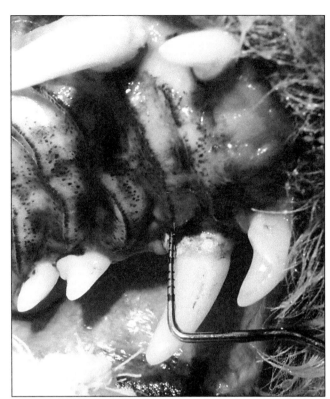

3.16 A UNC 15 periodontal probe is used to evaluate the palatal aspect of the left maxillary canine (tooth 204) in a dog. Note the presence of a 6 mm deep periodontal pocket, calculus attached to the cervical aspect of the tooth and bleeding from the probing site.
(© Alexander M. Reiter)

  - The deepest measurement per tooth that is not within normal limits of 3 mm in dogs and 0.5 mm in cats and the location of the pocket for comparison during subsequent visits (e.g. 5M notates a pocket of 5 mm depth at the mesial surface of the tooth) are recorded.
- Furcation involvement: The periodontal health assessment of multi-rooted teeth should include an examination of the bone support in the furcation areas. A periodontal probe is held at a 90-degree angle to the tooth to check for furcation involvement (Figure 3.17). A probe specially designed for furcation assessment is the curved Nabers probe. Its use minimizes the amount of tissue distension at the gingival margin compared with a straight probe. Assessment should be made from the labial/buccal surfaces and also from the lingual/palatal surfaces. Furcation scores indicate the extent of the loss of bone in the furcation area (Figure 3.18).
- Tooth mobility: To measure the amount of horizontal mobility of each individual tooth, the tip and sides of the periodontal probe are used to push and pull the crown of the tooth in an alternating labial/buccal–lingual/palatal direction. Due to the elasticity of the periodontal ligament that connects the root to the alveolar bone, a very slight amount of movement is considered to be physiological. Vertical tooth mobility may be assessed by using the broad end of a probe to exert pressure on an incisal edge or occlusal surface towards the apex of the tooth. Record the mobility score for each tooth (Figure 3.19). Be aware that healthy mandibular incisor teeth in many dogs, particularly in smaller breeds, have significantly increased horizontal mobility. This alone is not an indication for extraction, unless other periodontal disease parameters such as gingival recession or periodontal pockets are present.

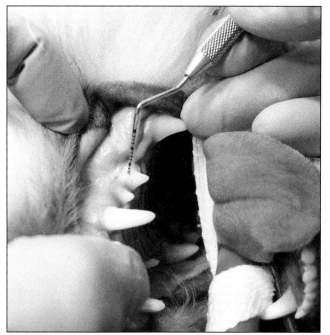

3.17 A UNC 15 periodontal probe is used to palpate the furcation area of the left maxillary second premolar (tooth 206) in a 6-month-old crossbreed dog. The periodontal probe is held with the modified pen grasp (see Chapter 7 for more detail). Note that the maxillary third premolar (tooth 207) is also missing.

Stage	Description
Stage 1 (F1, furcation involvement)	Periodontal probe extends less than half way under the crown in any direction of a multi-rooted tooth with attachment loss
Stage 2 (F2, furcation involvement)	Periodontal probe extends greater than half way under the crown of a multi-rooted tooth with attachment loss, but not through and through
Stage 3 (F3, furcation exposure)	Periodontal probe extends under the crown of a multi-rooted tooth, through and through from one side of the furcation and out the other

3.18 Furcation involvement (according to the American Veterinary Dental College).

Stage	Description
Stage 0 (M0)	Physiological mobility up to 0.2 mm
Stage 1 (M1)	Increased mobility in any direction other than axial over a distance of more than 0.2 mm and up to 0.5 mm
Stage 2 (M2)	Increased mobility in any direction other than axial over a distance of more than 0.5 mm and up to 1 mm
Stage 3 (M3)	Increased mobility in any direction other than axial over a distance exceeding 1 mm or any axial (up or down) movement

3.19 Tooth mobility (according to the American Veterinary Dental College).

Information obtained as listed above will be further enhanced with dental radiography (see Chapter 4). Once periodontal attachment loss has been measured with a combination of periodontal probing and dental radiography, the percentage attachment loss is calculated to stage the severity of periodontal disease (Figure 3.20).

Stage	Brief description	Attachment loss	Radiographic signs
Normal (PD0)	Clinically normal	None	None
Stage 1 (PD1)	Gingivitis only without attachment loss	None	None
Stage 2 (PD2)	Early periodontitis	Less than 25% of attachment loss or stage 1 furcation involvement in a multi-rooted tooth	Early radiographic signs of bone loss
Stage 3 (PD3)	Moderate periodontitis	25-50% of attachment loss or stage 2 furcation involvement in a multi-rooted tooth	Moderate radiographic signs of bone loss
Stage 4 (PD4)	Advanced periodontitis	More than 50% of attachment loss or stage 3 furcation involvement in a multi-rooted tooth	Advanced radiographic signs of bone loss

3.20 Periodontal disease classification (according to the American Veterinary Dental College). The degree of severity of periodontal disease relates to a single tooth; a patient may have teeth that have different stages of periodontal disease. The loss of periodontal attachment is determined by probing of the clinical attachment level and radiographic determination of the distance of the alveolar margin from the cementoenamel junction relative to the length of the root.

Assessment of veterinary products' effectiveness and efficacy

Veterinary Oral Health Council

Many companies have been marketing veterinary products with claims of reducing plaque and/or calculus accumulation. Prior to the launch of the Veterinary Oral Health Council (VOHC) in 1997, there were no standardized independent product review systems in place. The VOHC established an endorsement system based on its positive review of specific criteria used in protocols that are designed to provide objective data. Originally established in the USA at the University of Pennsylvania, the VOHC is now recognized worldwide. Veterinary clients seeking to purchase products that have been awarded the VOHC Seal of Acceptance can be confident that the marketing claims are credible. A full list of these products may be found on the VOHC website (www.vohc.org).

Various methods of objectively assessing periodontal disease have been utilized in studies that evaluated the effectiveness/efficacy of veterinary products. These epidemiological indices are used during clinical trials to quantify clinical conditions in populations of animals. The most commonly used indices measure plaque and calculus accumulations, gingival inflammation, and the amount of alveolar bone loss. Rather than measuring the indices on every tooth in the mouth, scoring performed on subsets of specific teeth has been shown to be reliable in making an assumption of the overall disease presence (Harvey *et al.*, 2012).

Numerical scales are used to measure the extent of a surface area of the tooth (normally the labial and buccal surface) that is covered by plaque and calculus. To identify the location of the plaque, disclosing agents are frequently used during scoring procedures in product evaluation studies. Among several different types of solutions, including iodine, mercurochrome and Bismarck brown, erythrosin is the most common dye utilized today. For veterinary practice, a liquid disclosing agent is applied with a cotton swab or squirted on to the teeth with care taken so adjacent tissues and fur are not stained.

The scoring systems mentioned below have been developed for human dentition, where there is not a wide degree of variance between circumference sizes and root lengths of teeth, unlike veterinary patients, in which there is variation both within one mouth and between breed types. The Total Mouth Periodontal Scoring (TMPS) system takes into account the differences in shape, size and number of roots within the mouth of dogs and cats to give weighting factors that more accurately describe the influence each tooth has in determining the presence of periodontal disease. The TMPS system, developed at the University of Pennsylvania in 2008, separates the assessment of gingivitis (TMPS-G) from the assessment of periodontitis (TMPS-P) (Harvey *et al.*, 2008; Harvey, 2010; Harvey *et al.*, 2012). While the below-mentioned indices are used in research studies for assessment of product claims, the general practitioner can utilize such data collected from their patients for purposes of determining the need of periodontal therapy.

Plaque index

Ramfjord (1959) developed the first periodontal index used in human patients to measure the extent of plaque covering the crowns of interproximal, lingual and facial surfaces of the six teeth that he selected for his test subset. After staining the teeth with a Bismarck brown solution (substituted today with a red erythrosin dye solution), Ramfjord used a 0–3 scale to measure the presence of plaque. Shick and Ash (1961) modified Ramfjord's criteria by changing the measurement area to include only the gingival half of the crowns of the index teeth. The patient's plaque score is obtained by adding together the individual tooth scores and dividing by the number of teeth scored.

Greene and Vermillion (1960) developed a plaque and calculus scoring method, the Oral Hygiene Index (OHI), which was the first to utilize a dental explorer rather than use of a stain. It was later simplified to include only six tooth surfaces and is now known as the Simplified Oral Hygiene Index (OHI-S) (Greene and Vermillion, 1964). It divides the crown into horizontal thirds (incisal, middle, and gingival sections). The per-person score is obtained by adding together all tooth scores and dividing by the number of tooth sections examined.

Quigley and Hein (1962) used a 0–5 plaque scoring method that only examined the gingival third of the crowns of the teeth using a disclosing solution. Later, Turesky, Gilmore and Glickman (1970) modified the Quigley–Hein Plaque Index by scoring the entire crown surface, dividing it into horizontal thirds and using a 0–5 scale while placing more emphasis on the gingival third. The Turesky–Gilmore–Glickman modification of the Quigley–Hein Plaque Index (Figure 3.21) has been widely accepted and used in human and veterinary studies. Logan and Boyce (1994) modified it for use in veterinary studies that measured the effectiveness/efficacy of products in reducing plaque accumulation. The Logan and Boyce Plaque Index (Figure 3.22) measured horizontal halves of the crown surface, assessing amounts of coverage and thickness of plaque accumulated on each half. The colour intensity of the dye set the criteria for numerical assignment of the thickness score (light, medium or dark). On each half, the coverage score is multiplied by

Grade	Description
0	No plaque
1	Separate flecks of plaque at the cervical margin of the tooth
2	A thin, continuous band of plaque (up to 1 mm) at the cervical margin
3	A band of plaque wider than 1 mm but covering less than one-third of the crown
4	Plaque covering at least one-third but less than two-thirds of the crown
5	Plaque covering two-thirds or more of the crown

3.21 Turesky–Gilmore–Glickman modification of the Quigley–Hein Plaque Index.

Grade	Description
Coverage scores	
0	No observable plaque
1	Less than 25% coverage
2	25% to 49% coverage
3	50% to 74% coverage
4	75% and more coverage
Thickness scores	
1	Light (pink to light red)
2	Medium (red)
3	Heavy (dark red)

3.22 Original Logan and Boyce Plaque Index.

the thickness score, then each half score is added to the other for a total tooth score. The mouth score is the mean of all tooth scores. This method quickly became popular among veterinary researchers until it was determined that the Logan and Boyce methods have poor intra- and inter-examiner reproducibility. A modification was proposed to include the use of anatomical tooth landmarks when dividing the crown into halves and use of dye colour references that remove some of the subjectivity in colour determinations (Hennet *et al.*, 2006).

Calculus index

A variety of indices have been used to evaluate the accumulation or reduction of amounts of calculus deposits while testing effectiveness/efficacy of products. The Calculus Surface Index (CSI) only assesses the presence or absence of deposits, while the Calculus Surface Severity Index (CSSI) uses numerical criteria and also divides the crown surfaces into longitudinal sections (Ennever *et al.*, 1961). The frequently used Marginal Line Calculus Index divides the crown horizontally into thirds and was developed to assess only the supragingival calculus accumulated on the gingival third of the tooth (Mühlemann and Villa, 1967). The total tooth score is achieved after vertically dividing the horizontal gingival third and measuring each gingival half. Currently, the VOHC will not accept longitudinal segmentation in trials for the acceptance seal: 'Either whole tooth or horizontally segmented tooth surfaces can be used for scoring. Only the scores from the gingival half of the tooth are to be considered in the analysis when horizontal segmentation is used.'

The Ramfjord Calculus Index (Figure 3.23) is a quick and easy way for general practitioners to quantify and document in the dental chart the calculus accumulations of their patients (Ramfjord, 1959).

Grade	Description
0	No calculus present
1	Supragingival calculus covering not more than one-third of the exposed tooth surface
2	Supragingival calculus covering more than one-third but not more than two-thirds of the exposed tooth surface, or presence of individual flecks of subgingival calculus around the cervical portion of the tooth, or both
3	Supragingival calculus covering more than two-thirds of the exposed tooth surface, or a continuous heavy band of subgingival calculus around the cervical portion of the tooth, or both

3.23 Ramfjord Calculus Index.

Gingival index

Several gingival bleeding indices have been described with criteria that indicate the presence of gingival inflammation. One of the most commonly used gingival indices is the Löe and Silness Gingival Index (Löe and Silness, 1963) (Figure 3.24). Besides indicating the presence of bleeding, it assesses the severity of gingivitis by examining colour changes that indicate the initial stages of inflammation when bleeding may not be present. A blunt instrument, such as a periodontal probe, is used to palpate the soft tissue lining of the gingival margin.

Grade	Definition	Description
0	Normal gingiva	–
1	Mild inflammation	Slight change in colour and oedema; no bleeding on probing
2	Moderate inflammation	Redness, oedema and glazing; bleeding on probing
3	Severe inflammation	Marked redness and oedema; ulceration; tendency to spontaneous bleeding

3.24 Löe and Silness Gingival Index.

References and further reading

Barton-Lamb AL, Martin-Flores M, Scrivani PV et al. (2013) Evaluation of maxillary arterial blood flow in anesthetized cats with the mouth closed and open. The Veterinary Journal 196, 325–331

Cohn LA (2014) Canine nasal disease. Veterinary Clinics of North America: Small Animal Practice 44, 75–89

Culham N and Rawlings JM (1998) Oral malodour and its relevance to periodontal disease in the dog. Journal of Veterinary Dentistry 15, 165–168

Ennever J, Sturzenberger OP and Radike AW (1961) The calculus surface index method for scoring clinical calculus studies. Journal of Periodontology 32, 54–57

Greene JC and Vermillion JR (1960) Oral hygiene index: a method for classifying oral hygiene status. Journal of the American Dental Association 61, 172

Greene JC and Vermillion JR (1964) The simplified oral hygiene index. Journal of the American Dental Association 68, 7–13

Harvey CE (2010) Total mouth periodontal score system in cats. Proceedings of the 19th European Congress of Veterinary Dentistry, p. 117

Harvey CE and Emily PP (1993) Small Animal Dentistry, pp. 20–23. Mosby, St Louis

Harvey CE, Laster L, Shofer F et al. (2008) Scoring the full extent of periodontal disease in the dog: development of a total mouth periodontal score (TMPS) system. Journal of Veterinary Dentistry 25, 176–180

Harvey CE, Laster L and Shofer FS (2012) Validation of use of subsets of teeth when applying the total mouth periodontal score (TMPS) system in dogs. Journal of Veterinary Dentistry 29, 222–226

Hennet P, Servet E, Salesse H et al. (2006) Evaluation of the Logan and Boyce plaque index for the study of dental plaque accumulation in dogs. Research in Veterinary Science 80, 175–180

Herring ES, Smith MM and Robertson JL (2002) Lymph node staging of oral and maxillofacial neoplasms in 31 dogs and cats. Journal of Veterinary Dentistry 19, 122–126

Lewis JR and Miller BR (2014) Veterinary dentistry. In: McCurnin's Clinical Textbook for Veterinary Technicians, 8th edn, ed. JM Bassert and JA Thomas, pp. 1297–1331. Elsevier Saunders, St Louis

Löe H and Silness J (1963) Periodontal disease in pregnancy. Acta Odontologica Scandinavica 21, 533–551

Logan EI and Boyce EN (1994) Oral health assessment in dogs: parameters and methods. Journal of Veterinary Dentistry 11, 58–63

Mühlemann HR and Villa PR (1967) The marginal line calculus index. Helvetica Odontologica Acta 11, 175–179

Nield-Gehrig JS (2008) In: Fundamentals of Periodontal Instrumentation and Advanced Root Instrumentation, 6th edn, pp. 219–230, 245–248. Lippincott Williams and Wilkins, Philadelphia

Oliver JE, Lorenz MD and Kornegay JN (1997) Handbook of Veterinary Neurology, 3rd edn, pp. 9–10. WB Saunders, Philadelphia

Pattison AM and Pattison GL (1992) Periodontal Instrumentation, 2nd edn, pp. 4, 5, 17–19, 93–95. Appleton and Lange, Norwalk

Quigley GA and Hein JW (1962) Comparative cleansing efficiency of manual and power brushing. Journal of the American Dental Association 65, 26–29

Ramfjord SP (1959) Indices for prevalence and incidence of periodontal disease. Journal of Periodontology 30, 51–59

Shick RA and Ash MM (1961) Evaluation of the vertical method of toothbrushing. Journal of Periodontology 32, 346

Stades FC and Boevé MH (1995) Eyes. In: Medical History and Physical Examination in Companion Animals, ed. A Rijnberk and HW de Vries, pp. 234–235. Kluwer Academic Publishers, Dordrecht/Boston/London

Stiles J, Weil AB, Packer RA et al. (2012) Post anesthetic cortical blindness in cats: twenty cases. The Veterinary Journal 193, 367–373

Turesky S, Gilmore ND and Glickman I (1970) Reduced plaque formation by the chloromethyl analogue of vitamin C. Journal of Periodontology 41, 41–43

Useful websites

American Veterinary Dental College: www.avdc.org

European Veterinary Dental College: www.evdc.org

Veterinary Oral Health Council: www.vohc.org

Chapter 4

Dental and oral diagnostic imaging and interpretation

Helena Kuntsi, Tobias Schwarz, Wilfried Mai and Alexander M. Reiter

Radiography is the most commonly utilized diagnostic imaging tool in veterinary practice and is used in the work-up of all parts of the body in dogs and cats. Before the advent of modern cross-sectional imaging modalities such as ultrasonography, computed tomography (CT) and magnetic resonance imaging (MRI), radiography was the only diagnostic imaging tool available for the head (apart from fluoroscopic swallowing studies) and was therefore used widely. However, due to the problems of structure superimposition and poor sensitivity for soft tissue and fluid-based lesions, it is a relatively unrewarding technique. In the past, many specific positioning and contrast procedures were developed that provided moderately better results, but these are still inferior in diagnostic yield to intraoral radiography for dental assessment, CT for general imaging of the head and MRI for imaging of soft tissue structures, in particular the neurocranium and eyes. Functional imaging modalities such as scintigraphy and positron emission tomography can be used to localize sources of pain and metastases and to monitor tumour behaviour and fracture healing.

Dental radiography

Principles

Radiography plays an essential part in the diagnosis and treatment of dental and oral surgical disorders. Intraoral radiographs provide superior detail compared with head radiographs. Indications for obtaining dental radiographs include clinical evidence of periodontitis (periodontal pocket, gingival recession, furcation exposure, and increased tooth mobility), pulp pathology (crown discoloration, displacement of a tooth) and dental defects (wear, fracture, caries, tooth resorption) or missing teeth. Radiographs should always be obtained before extraction of a tooth and, if necessary, to confirm complete extraction. Full-mouth dental radiographs are necessary for all periodontal patients, for trauma cases (e.g. jaw fractures) and whenever there is evidence of a generalized oral problem (Tsugawa and Verstraete, 2000).

However, dental radiography may be indicated in all dental patients, regardless of clinical appearance of dental and periodontal structures, as it has been demonstrated to greatly improve the diagnostic yield and reveal clinically important information in most patients (Verstraete et al., 1998a,b). Despite being useful for obtaining a panoramic overview of the teeth, periodontal tissues and jaws in humans, orthopantomography is not yet practical in veterinary dentistry due to the variability in size and shape of the head in dogs and cats. Cone-beam and multi-slice CT allow for the production of curvilinear reconstruction images of both jaws, which may be useful in veterinary practice.

Equipment

Dental X-ray machine

The dental X-ray machine consists of a generator, tube head, image capturing system and control panel. The X-ray beam is modified by altering its energy (kVp), exposure length (time), exposure tube current (mA), beam shape (collimator) and film–focus distance. Some dental X-ray machines use a preset energy (usually between 60 and 90 kVp) and tube current (mA) and only allow selection of different settings of exposure time (in seconds), while others contain an anatomically based selection for exposure energy, electric current and time. A collimator reduces the size of the X-ray beam and therefore the volume of irradiated tissue in the patient. Scatter radiation in dental X-ray machines is typically very low, and general safety advice is to stand at least 1.8 metres (6 feet) from the patient, at an angle of 90 to 135 degrees to the central ray of the X-ray beam. The X-ray machine should be mounted near the treatment table so that it will reach the patient during treatment. The machine can be mounted on the ceiling or a wall (Figure 4.1) or on a stand with wheels (the use of mobile stands may not be permitted in some countries). Portable handheld systems are also available (Figure 4.2). Safety regulations for the use of these systems vary between different countries.

Dental radiographic films

Traditionally, dental radiographs have been obtained with dental films, of which the most commonly used sizes in veterinary dentistry are numbers 2 (31 x 41 mm; 1¼ x 1⅝ inches) and 4 (57 x 76 mm; 2¼ x 3 inches). Numbers 0 (22 x 35 mm; ⅞ x 1⅜ inches) and 1 (24 x 40 mm; 1⁹⁄₁₆ x 1⁵⁄₁₆ inches) films are good for obtaining radiographs of cheek teeth in cats, and number 3 (27 x 54 mm; 1¹⁄₁₆ x 2⅛ inches) films are useful for obtaining radiographs of cheek teeth in small dogs (Figure 4.3). Dental films also come in different speeds, determining the amount of radiation required to produce an image on the film. The faster the

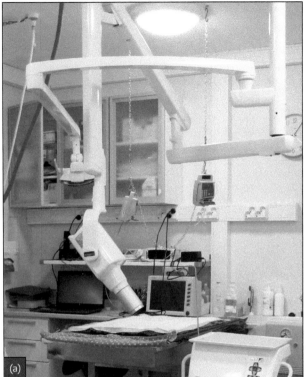

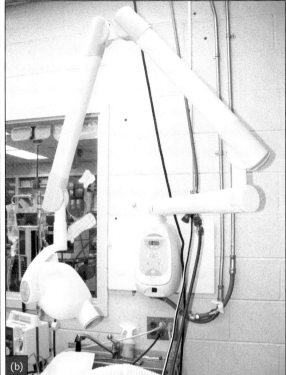

4.1 (a) Ceiling-mounted and (b) wall-mounted dental X-ray machines.
(a, © Dr Alexander M. Reiter)

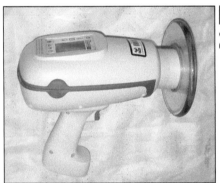

4.2 Handheld dental X-ray device.
(© Dr Alexander M. Reiter)

film speed, the less exposure is required. Films with speeds D (ultra-speed) or E (Ekta-speed; faster than D, thus requiring less exposure time, but resulting in an image with decreased resolution) are appropriate for intraoral radiography. The films come in packages containing an outer plastic wrap, lead sheet and paper around the film (Figure 4.4). A small dimple is situated in one corner of the film package and the film to aid orienting the radiographic image. The convexity of the dimple must face the X-ray beam during exposure.

Several systems are available for developing films:

- Small ready-to-use containers with developer and fixer fluids in which the films are dipped in a darkroom

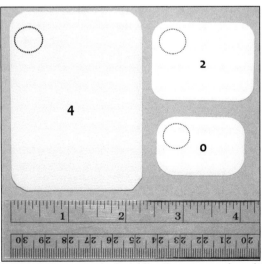

4.3 Sizes 0, 2 and 4 dental film; the convex surface of the dimple (circled) must face the X-ray beam during exposure.
(© Dr Alexander M. Reiter)

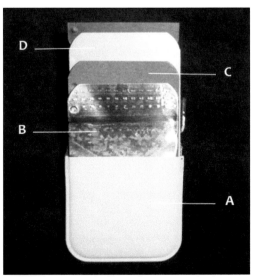

4.4 Content of a film pack: A = outer plastic wrap; B= lead sheet; C = dark paper around the film ; D = film.

- Chairside processor (a small darkroom) with containers of developer, water and fixer fluids, a light-filtering lid and lightproof portals for inserting films into the containers (Figure 4.5)
- Automatic processors, which also dry the films during exit.

Single film clips to dip the films in each container and multiple film hangers to dry processed and rinsed films of a single patient will be needed for the first two systems (Figure 4.6).

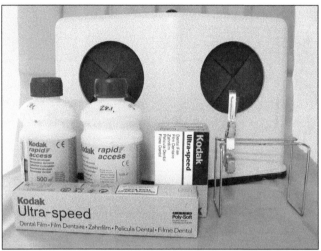

4.5 Chairside processor with solutions for developing and fixing. Note also the packages of dental film and a stand for drying processed film.

Sensor pads and phosphor plates

Digital systems have gained popularity in dental radiography, carrying many advantages over radiographic films. The dental X-ray machine is the same as that used with radiographic films (as long as it is capable of short-enough exposure times), but the films are replaced either by a sensor pad that is attached to a computer either with a cable (Figure 4.7) or wirelessly (direct digital radiography), or by phosphor plates from which the latent images are transferred on to a computer through a scanning device (computed radiography, also called indirect digital radiography) (Figure 4.8). The advantages of digital radiography include speed of image creation, elimination of developing and fixing chemicals, digital enhancement of images, less need for radiation, and digital storage of images. Disadvantages include higher initial cost at the time of investment compared with standard radiographic systems, and the expense of replacing a sensor pad (which is significantly more expensive for direct systems) in the case of damage from biting on to it. If the latter complication can be avoided, the total cost will even out over time, since cost per digital exposure is less in both digital systems compared with using radiographic films. The phosphor plates used in an indirect digital system are as thin as radiographic films and are available in different sizes (sizes 0, 1, 2, 3, 4 and other specially designed plates), while sensor pads may occasionally appear to be too thick in a small mouth and are available in a limited number of sizes. The lack of a sensor size number 4, in particular, makes direct systems inferior for obtaining images of larger teeth (such as canine teeth in dogs) because the entire tooth cannot be captured in one image. In addition, important pathology such as unerupted teeth, oral and maxillofacial tumours and jaw fractures are much more difficult to evaluate or may be left undiagnosed when using size 0 or 2 sensor pads.

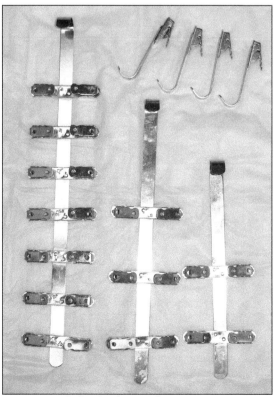

4.6 Single film clips (top right) and various sizes of film hangers.
(© Dr Alexander M. Reiter)

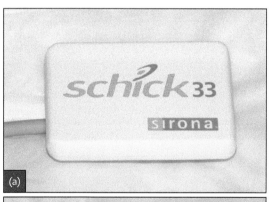

(a)

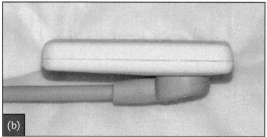

(b)

4.7 Size 2 sensor pad for use in direct digital radiography. (a) Front view. Note the cord which attaches the sensor pad to a computer. (b) Side view. Note the thickness of the sensor pad.
(© Dr Alexander M. Reiter)

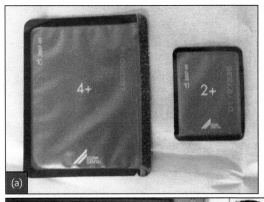

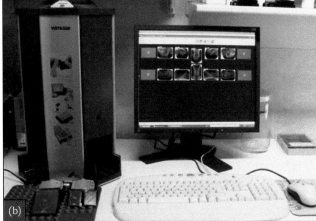

4.8 (a) Phosphor plates within disposable plastic sleeves. (b) Scanning (laser reader) machine used to transfer latent images on to a computer.

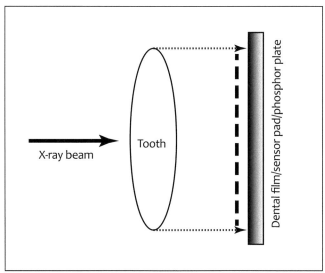

4.9 Parallel technique. The plane of the radiographic film and the long axis of the teeth of interest are parallel to each other, and the X-ray beam is aimed perpendicular to them.
(© Dr Alexander M. Reiter)

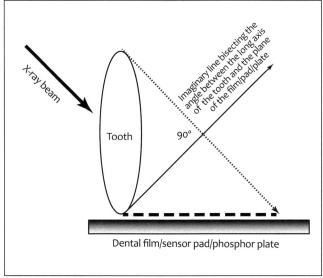

4.10 Bisecting angle technique. The radiographic film is placed at an angle to the long axis of the teeth of interest, and the X-ray beam is aimed perpendicular to an imaginary line bisecting that angle.
(© Dr Alexander M. Reiter)

Dental radiographic techniques

A full-mouth set of radiographs of a dog or cat typically includes 10–14 views and should show all the teeth with 2–3 mm of periapical area visible for each root. The use of a number 4 film/plate size is advisable to ensure capturing of large teeth or voluminous pathology in one image. An intraoral technique allows superimposition of the contralateral jaw to be avoided and is therefore the technique of choice for imaging most areas. However, an extraoral technique may provide additional information for teeth and surrounding tissues situated in the caudal maxilla of cats and brachycephalic dogs. The goal is to obtain an image with each tooth as near to actual size and shape as possible. In the mid to caudal mandibular body, this is achieved using a parallel technique (Figure 4.9), but in all other areas a bisecting angle technique is necessary (Figure 4.10) (Operative Techniques 4.1 and 4.2).

Mounting and storage of films and images

Regardless of whether using radiographic films or a digital radiography system, films/images should be organized appropriately for viewing and establishing a diagnosis (Tsugawa and Verstraete, 2000). 'Labial mounting' refers to organizing films/images so that the crowns of the maxillary teeth point downwards and those of the mandibular teeth point upwards. The incisor teeth are positioned towards the middle and the molar teeth, towards the periphery. The teeth of the left side of the mouth are positioned to the right of the viewer, and those of the right side of the mouth are positioned to the left of the viewer, as if the operator is facing the patient (Figure 4.11). With radiographic films, the convex dimple in the corner of the film must face the viewer. In digital radiography, the software allows the images to be organized in labial mounting, either automatically or manually (Figure 4.12).

Radiographic films can be stored in specific paper or plastic envelopes that can hold multiple films. To avoid artefacts forming during storage, care must be taken to thoroughly rinse out fixer and completely dry the films before storing them in the envelopes. One of the advantages of digital radiography is space-saving and thus easier storage of images. However, one must ensure access to a large enough digital storage space and an automatic back-up system for saving images as part of the medical record of each patient.

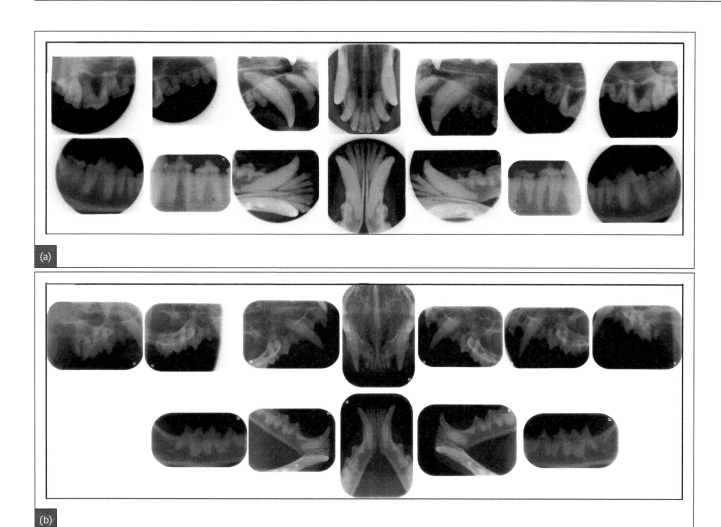

4.11 Labial mounting of processed dental X-ray films of the dentition of (a) a dog and (b) a cat.

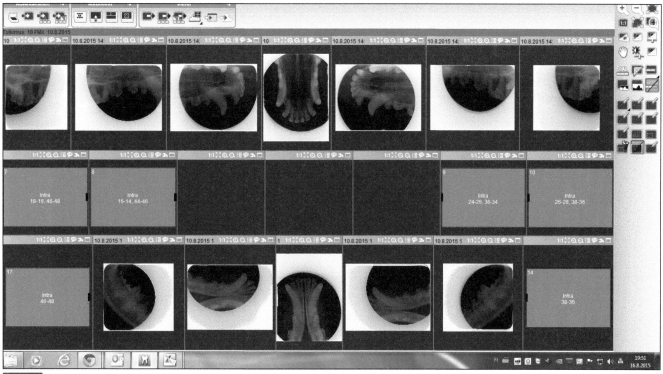

4.12 In digital radiography, the software allows images to be organized in labial mounting, either automatically or manually.

Head radiography

Principles

A general radiographic examination of the head may still be performed in dogs and cats with dental, oral and maxillofacial problems if other options are not available and to triage for the most appropriate further imaging modality.

Equipment

A standard X-ray unit with conventional films and processing techniques, indirect digital radiography with phosphor plates or direct digital radiography with sensor pads should ensure sufficient image quality. Digital radiography allows faster imaging with a lower likelihood of under- or overexposure. The image quality depends on the technology used and the ability of the software system to adjust the image-processing settings to the needs of the imaged anatomy.

Patient preparation and radiographic views

For reasons of operator safety and image quality, it is recommended that head radiographs are obtained only in sedated or anaesthetized patients. Radiolucent positioning aids and mouth gags of different sizes are needed for most views. Exact positioning in cats can be challenging. Head radiographs can be performed using tabletop equipment to minimize any undesirable magnification effects.

To obtain an understanding of the anatomy, at least two orthogonal views of the head should be obtained. Additional oblique views are specific for some areas and need to be performed for each side separately. All radiographic views are labelled according to the point of entrance of the central X-ray beam into the head and its exit point. Further specifics of radiographic anatomical nomenclature can be found elsewhere (Smallwood *et al.*, 1985; Dennis, 2006).

Dorsoventral views

The dorsoventral (DV) view is relatively easy to obtain in dogs and cats. The patient is placed in sternal recumbency and the head positioned with both mandibles firmly anchored to the supporting surface. The central X-ray beam should be vertical and placed at the level of the eyes (Figure 4.13). If an endotracheal tube is in place, it should be positioned in between the incisor teeth, unless it hampers visualization of a specific area. Using an intraoral cassette, an intraoral DV view of the rostral upper jaw can be obtained in anaesthetized animals. To maximize the imaged field, the cassette should be placed with the corner inserted into the mouth and supported to keep it parallel to the table (Figure 4.14).

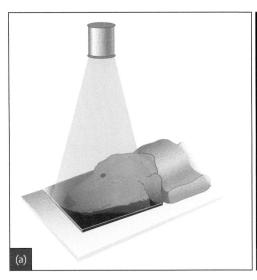

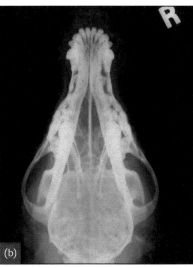

4.13 (a) Positioning of a dog for a dorsoventral head radiograph. The head should be symmetrically anchored on the supporting surface and the central beam aligned between the eyes. Side markers should always be used. (b) Resulting radiographic image. The superimposition of the jaw bones limits dental and periodontal assessment.

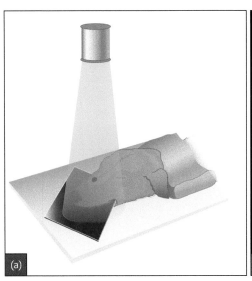

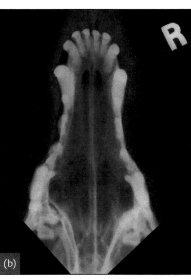

4.14 (a) Positioning of a dog for a dorsoventral intraoral view of the upper jaw and nose. Maximal cassette coverage can be achieved by inserting it diagonally into the mouth. The beam should be aligned halfway between the nostrils and the eyes. Side markers should always be used. (b) Resulting radiographic image.

Ventrodorsal views

A ventrodorsal (VD) view of the head is more difficult to perform with perfect symmetry than a DV view, but it may be needed, for example, in the case of extensive mandibular trauma. A towel or positioning sponge should be placed below the neck to help to extend the neck, stabilize the head and keep the hard palate parallel to the table. The central X-ray beam should be centred halfway between the mandibular symphysis and the angular processes of the mandibles (Figure 4.15). If an endotracheal tube is in place, it should be positioned in between the incisor teeth, unless it hampers visualization of a specific area. Using an intraoral cassette, an intraoral VD view of the rostral lower jaw can be obtained in anaesthetized animals. To maximize the imaged field, the cassette should be placed with the corner inserted into the mouth and supported to keep it parallel to the table (Figure 4.16).

Lateral views

Lateral views can be obtained with the animal in either left or right lateral recumbency. The head should be positioned moderately extended. The central X-ray beam should be centred at the caudal hard palate (or zygomatic arch at the level of the eyes). The dorsal surface of the head should be assessed for median axis symmetry (dorsal midline at equal distance to the supporting surface rostrally and caudally) and transverse axis symmetry (maxillary teeth should cast a perfect shadow on to contralateral teeth when the lips are retracted upwards) (Figure 4.17). Positioning sponges may be placed under the muzzle to slightly elevate the nose and chin and help obtain the ideal position. It is often useful to perform a closed- and an open-mouth view. Radiolucent gags should be used, such as plastic syringes. If only one view is performed, it is useful to have the mouth slightly open.

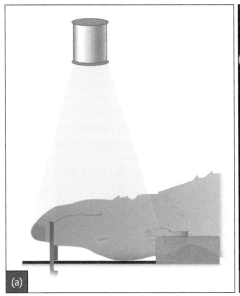
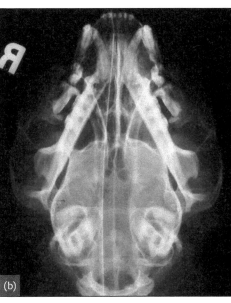

4.15 (a) Positioning of a dog for a ventrodorsal head radiograph. The head should be symmetrically positioned and the central beam aligned half way between the mandibular symphysis and angular processes of the mandibles. Side markers should always be used. (b) Resulting radiographic image of the head in a cat.

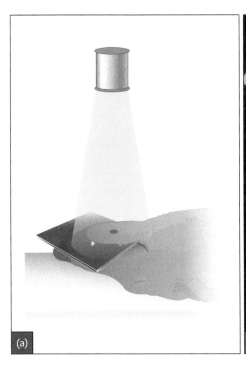
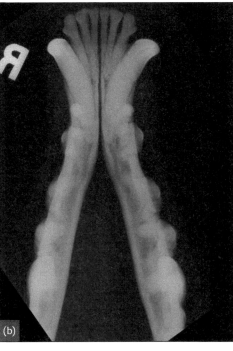

4.16 (a) Positioning of a dog for a ventrodorsal intraoral view of the lower jaw. Maximal cassette coverage can be achieved by inserting it diagonally into the mouth. The beam should be aligned halfway between the chin and the eyes. Side markers should always be used. (b) Resulting radiographic image; the mandibular second and third molar teeth could not be included with this technique.

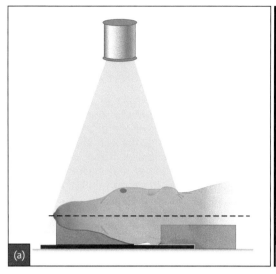

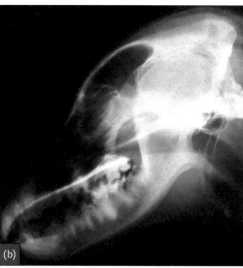

4.17 (a) Positioning of a dog for a lateral head radiograph. The head should be supported with radiolucent foam wedges to be perfectly parallel with the supporting surface in both dimensions. The central beam should be aligned on the zygomatic arch at the level of the eyes (or caudal hard palate). (b) Resulting radiographic image.

Oblique view of the upper jaw

To obtain a view of one maxillary quadrant free from superimposition of contralateral and ventral structures, the thorax, head and neck are positioned in between dorsal and lateral recumbency, with the target maxillary quadrant closest to the supporting surface. The head is extended and the mouth opened maximally with a radiolucent mouth gag. The tongue and endotracheal tube are positioned as ventral as possible and secured in this position. It is sometimes helpful to pull the tongue rostrally as well. The head should be rotated approximately 30 degrees from lateral recumbency towards dorsal recumbency. The central X-ray beam should be centred on the maxillary third premolar tooth of the maxilla closest to the supporting surface (Figure 4.18). If tabletop cassettes are used, it can be helpful to angle the X-ray beam slightly caudally into the mouth by no more than 10 degrees. It can be difficult to achieve this view with the entire maxillary quadrant displayed without superimposition of ventral and contralateral

structures, particularly in brachycephalic dogs and in cats. The incisor teeth cannot usually be visualized. This view needs to be performed for each side separately.

Oblique view of the lower jaw

To obtain a view of one mandibular quadrant free from superimposition of contralateral and dorsal structures, the thorax, head and neck are positioned in a half sternal, half lateral recumbency, with the target mandible closest to the supporting surface on a small block. The head is extended and the mouth opened maximally with a radiolucent mouth gag. The tongue and endotracheal tube are positioned as contralateral and as dorsal as possible and are secured in this position. The head should be rotated from sternal recumbency approximately 30 degrees towards lateral recumbency. The central X-ray beam should be centred on the mandibular third premolar tooth of the mandible closest to the supporting surface (Figure 4.19). If tabletop cassettes are used, it can be helpful to

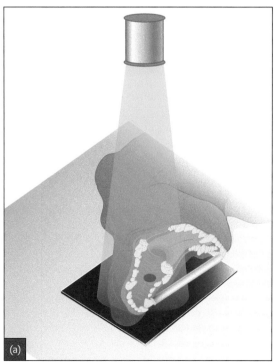

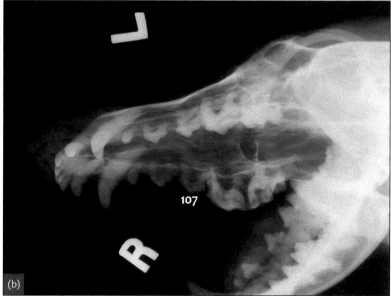

4.18 (a) Positioning of a dog for an open-mouth oblique view of the right upper jaw. The head should be rotated from right lateral recumbency approximately 30 degrees towards dorsal recumbency. The mouth must be maximally opened with a radiolucent mouth gag. The central beam should be centred on tooth 107. Side markers should be put at the level of each maxilla. (b) Resulting radiographic image.

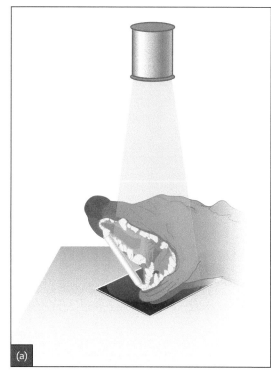

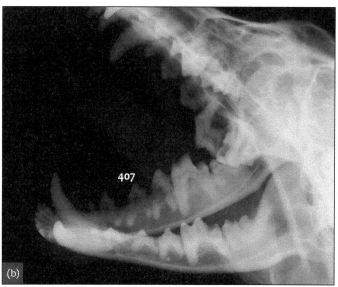

4.19 (a) Positioning of a dog for an open-mouth oblique view of the right lower jaw. The head should be rotated from ventral recumbency approximately 30 degrees towards right lateral recumbency. The mouth must be maximally opened with a radiolucent mouth gag. The central beam should be centred on tooth 407. Side markers should be put at the level of each mandible. To view the right mandibular teeth without foreshortening, ensure that the head is rotated far enough. (b) Resulting radiographic image; teeth 410 and 411 are obscured by maxillary teeth.

angle the X-ray beam slightly caudally into the mouth by no more than 10 degrees. This view is even more difficult to achieve than the maxillary oblique view and only works reasonably well in dolichocephalic dogs. The incisor teeth cannot usually be visualized. This view needs to be performed for each side separately.

Oblique view of the canine temporomandibular joint

The patient is positioned in lateral recumbency with the head extended and symmetrical as described for the lateral view. A slight open-mouth position is beneficial. The tip of the nose is now elevated from the supporting surface by 10 degrees (dolichocephalic), 15 degrees (mesaticephalic) or 25–35 degrees (brachycephalic) for the respective head type conformations (Figure 4.20). An additional 5–10 degree rotation of the head from lateral

recumbency towards dorsal recumbency can be helpful to view the temporomandibular joint (TMJ) rostrally and ventrally, free from superimposition of other head structures (Morgan, 1993). The central X-ray beam should be centred slightly rostral to the palpable 'upper' TMJ (the one that is further away from the supporting surface). The view needs to be performed for each side separately.

Oblique view of the feline temporomandibular joint

In the cat, the most successful way to free-view one TMJ is an oblique view along the median plane. The cat is positioned in lateral recumbency, and the head is extended and positioned as described for a lateral view, with the target TMJ on the supporting surface. Now the head is rotated by 20 degrees from lateral recumbency towards dorsal recumbency (Figure 4.21) (Ticer and Spencer, 1978). An additional 5–10 degree elevation of the tip of the nose from the

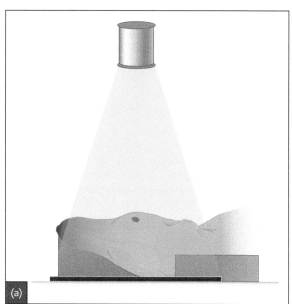

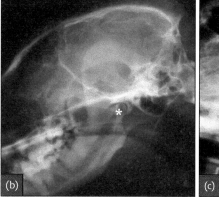

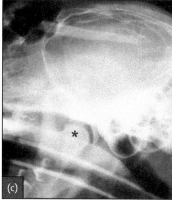

4.20 (a) Positioning of a mesaticephalic dog for an oblique view of the left temporomandibular joint (TMJ). The head is positioned in left lateral recumbency with the tip of the nose elevated by 15 degrees. In addition, the head can be rotated from left lateral recumbency by 5 degrees towards dorsal recumbency. The central beam should be centred slightly rostral to the palpable right TMJ. Side markers should always be used. (b) Resulting radiographic image, (∗) indicates the mandibular condyle. (c) In skeletally immature dogs the mandibular condyle (∗) is wider in shape and less sharply marginated which is a normal feature.

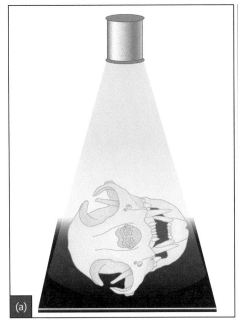

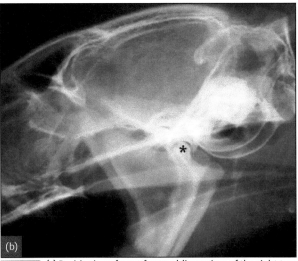

4.21 (a) Positioning of a cat for an oblique view of the right temporomandibular joint (TMJ). The head is rotated from right lateral recumbency by 20 degrees towards dorsal recumbency. In addition the nose tip can be elevated by 5–10 degrees. The central beam should be centred slightly rostral to the palpable left TMJ. Side markers should always be used. (b) Resulting radiographic image, (*) indicates the condyle.

supporting surface can be helpful (Meomartino *et al.*, 1999). The central X-ray beam should be centred slightly rostral to the palpable 'upper' TMJ. This view needs to be performed for each side separately and is technically challenging.

Ultrasonography

Ultrasonography utilizes high-frequency sound waves (typically of the order of a few megahertz in frequency) to image internal anatomy in real time. It is based on the reflection of sound from the internal structures of the body. It provides cross-sectional images in any orientation. Ultrasonography typically does not require sedation or anaesthesia, though these may be necessary in fractious patients and when interventional procedures are performed. Another advantage of ultrasonography is that it allows insertion of needles into organs and lesions under direct visual guidance to obtain samples for cytopathology or histopathology. The inability of ultrasonography to image through air-filled spaces or bony structures makes it unsuitable for imaging areas such as the lungs or skeleton, but it is an excellent non-invasive modality for soft tissue organs.

Both linear and curvilinear transducers are suitable to image structures in the head and neck; higher-frequency transducers (10–12 MHz or higher) are usually preferred, given the relatively superficial location of most structures imaged with ultrasonography in this area. It is important to clip the hair in the region being examined and to apply acoustic gel to optimize image quality. Ultrasonography provides excellent soft tissue contrast, higher than that of radiography or CT. For example, fluid is readily identified on ultrasonography due to its completely black appearance ('anechoic'). Soft tissue parenchymal lesions (which would be invisible on radiographs) are typically readily visible with ultrasonography; mineralization and air pockets or bubbles also have typical and easily recognizable ultrasonographic features.

Ultrasonography of the canine and feline head has a number of limited applications for examination of the orbital cavity, the brain (via an open fontanelle), the middle ear, regional lymph nodes (Figure 4.22), salivary glands, the intermandibular space and the tongue. The ventral

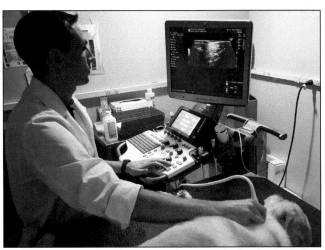

4.22 Ultrasound machine; a transducer is applied to the skin in the neck area to image the medial retropharyngeal lymph nodes.

intermandibular approach allows quick and painless extraoral access to assess abscesses, other masses and suspected foreign bodies of the tongue. The retromandibular ventral or ventrolateral windows can be used to evaluate other soft tissue structures such as the mandibular and retropharyngeal lymph nodes, mandibular and sublingual salivary glands, and peripharyngeal tissues.

Computed tomography

Principles

CT is a cross-sectional imaging modality that uses ionizing radiation (X-rays). While it allows detailed assessment of all body parts, it is particularly useful for the diagnosis and treatment planning for various conditions of the head such as ear disease, lesions of the nasal cavity and sinuses, intracranial lesions, ocular and orbital disease, TMJ disease, salivary gland and lymph node pathology, and oral and maxillofacial trauma and neoplasia (Forrest and Schwarz, 2011; Nemec *et al.*, 2015). Tooth fractures, root remnants and odontogenic cysts can be diagnosed with CT; it also allows assessment of the pulp cavity but is probably not sensitive enough for assessment of individual root canals. Endodontic filling material is very dense and often causes artefacts in CT images. Gas can be seen in the pulp cavity with infection or trauma, as well as in larger caries-related crown defects. CT is a sensitive technique for detecting alveolar bone resorption associated with periapical disease. Diffuse loss of alveolar bone and periosteal reactions can be seen in severe periodontitis cases. Use of intravenous iodine-based contrast medium is helpful in delineating oral soft tissue masses, inflammation and oedema. However, radiography is still the gold standard for diagnosing dental and periodontal disease.

Equipment

The patient is positioned on a couch that moves through the centre of a rotating gantry, which houses an X-ray tube. Modern CT machines have a helical acquisition mode where the patient bed moves through the gantry while the X-ray tube is spinning around it (Figure 4.23). Multiple rows of detectors allow faster acquisitions with maximal image detail. A new type of smaller CT unit that is already used extensively in human dental imaging is cone-beam CT. These units are an offshoot of digital X-ray technology, where the X-ray tube and image receptor are mounted on a C-arm that rotates around the patient. These units hold some future promise for veterinary dentistry and oral surgery, as they can have a very good image resolution for bone and teeth (Figure 4.24).

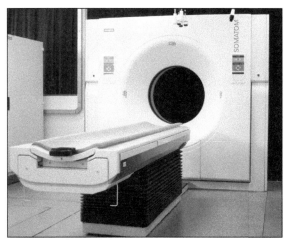

4.23 Multi-slice helical computed tomography scanner, with the patient couch in the foreground and gantry at the back.

Magnetic resonance imaging

Principles

MRI uses the magnetic properties of hydrogen nuclei (protons), which are very abundant in biological tissues, to obtain images of high contrast. Soft tissue contrast is much higher with MRI than with CT. Other advantages of MRI compared with CT are that it allows images to be obtained in any orientation (transverse, sagittal, dorsal or oblique) and that it does not utilize ionizing radiation. Drawbacks include longer acquisition (and therefore anaesthesia) times, lower availability and higher cost.

The high soft tissue contrast of MRI is due to the fact that signal intensity (brightness) of a tissue depends on its concentration of protons (especially those contained in water), their physicochemical environment (what molecules they are in, and what atoms and molecules surround them), as well as the image acquisition parameters (referred to as an 'MRI pulse sequence'). For example, pure fluids are usually bright ('hyperintense') on T2-weighted pulse sequences, whereas they are dark ('hypointense') on T1-weighted pulse sequences. The MRI pulse sequence determines contrast and signal-to-noise ratio in the images. Important information about the nature of tissues can be obtained by imaging the same body region with various pulse sequences and observing the changes in signal. In addition, specific pulse sequences can be used to suppress the signal given from tissues such as water or fat, thereby changing the relative contrast in the images.

As with CT, increased vascularization or abnormal (leaky) vessels associated with pathology can be detected with MRI using contrast material (gadolinium), although contrast uptake is not specific for the nature of the lesion. Due to its superior soft tissue contrast, MRI is a good technique for evaluating the extent of soft tissue disease. When comparing MRI and CT images, soft tissue lesions almost always appear more extensive with MRI due to its inherent higher sensitivity to changes in chemical composition of tissues compared with CT, which relies mostly on the enhancement of lesions following administration of contrast medium to identify the boundaries of the disease process. CT remains better than MRI at detecting early bony involvement secondary to soft tissue lesions; however, significant bone involvement can also be identified with MRI. The choice between MRI and CT will therefore depend upon the anticipated diagnosis and location of the disease process, whether the primary process is thought to affect soft tissue or bone, and whether subtle bone involvement carries important diagnostic or prognostic value.

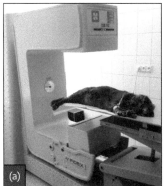
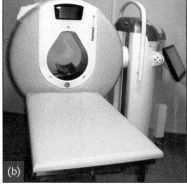
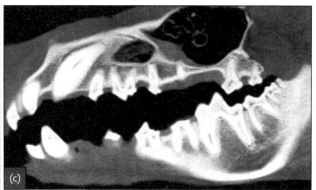

4.24 Small animal dedicated cone-beam computed tomography (CT) units. The X-ray tube and image receptors are housed in a C-shaped arm that rotates around the patient. (a) The unit requires neither an external cooling system nor three-phase power supply, unlike a conventional CT unit. (b) In this model, the tunnel part can also be rotated horizontally. (c) Sagittal image of a canine mouth and nose generated from 0.46 mm slice width revealing high anatomical dental and periodontal detail.
(a, c, Courtesy of Animage, LLC Pleasanton, CA, USA; www.animage.com)

With MRI, enamel and dentine appear black because of a lack of unbound protons. The pulp cavity, containing nerves, blood vessels and connective tissue within the teeth, usually appears white or grey. In the upper and lower jaws the cortical bone surrounding the teeth looks dark and the bone marrow bright. Although not the preferred technique for evaluating the teeth and periodontal tissues in dogs and cats, significant disease can be detected with MRI. Periapical disease appears as rounded lesions around tooth roots, typically hypointense on T1-weighted images, hyperintense on T2-weighted images and showing a rim-enhancement pattern after gadolinium injection with non-enhancing central regions (corresponding to the periapical granuloma, cyst or abscess).

Equipment

The basic components of an MRI scanner (Figure 4.25) are the magnet, the coil and the control panel. MRI magnets are basically classified as low-field (usually around 0.2 tesla) or high-field (1.5 tesla and above). Low-field scanners are more affordable and use permanent magnets that do not require liquid helium and are therefore also much cheaper to maintain. High-field scanners are superconducting magnets that require the active elements to be maintained at a very low temperature, requiring the use of liquid helium, which needs to be replenished on a regular basis. The purchase and maintenance costs of these scanners are much higher; however, due to their higher magnetic field strength, they provide much better resolution and signal-to-noise ratio. The receiving coil is another important part of the equipment, and use of coils that are adapted to the anatomy of interest is important. For head imaging, head coils with a birdcage design are often used. However, for imaging of small specific parts of the head, such as the TMJs, small surface coils can also be employed.

MRI acquisition times require the use of general anaesthesia, with another requirement being that the equipment used must be MRI compatible. For head imaging the patient should be placed in sternal recumbency with the long axis of the body parallel to the long axis of the gantry. The head should be placed perfectly symmetrically within the coil so that exact symmetry is achieved when imaging in the transverse plane; the hard palate should be parallel to the table. This often requires the use of pads and tape to maintain the head in the appropriate position.

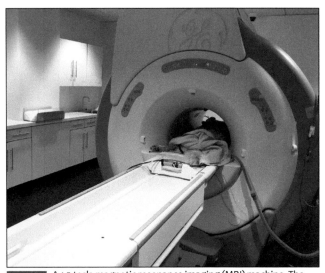

4.25 A 1.5 tesla magnetic resonance imaging (MRI) machine. The patient is in the gantry of the magnet that contains the high magnetic field. All anaesthesia equipment used must be MRI compatible.

Principles of radiological interpretation

Orientation and anatomy

For establishing orientation and making a diagnosis when evaluating dental radiographic films/images, it is important to recognize certain anatomical landmarks and understand the direction of the X-ray beam. An obvious landmark in the upper jaw is the hard palate and in the lower jaw, the mandibular canal (Figure 4.26).

In addition to using the bisecting angle technique, the tube head can also be moved horizontally so that the X-ray beam comes from a slightly rostral or caudal direction. For recognizing and separating the superimposed mesiobuccal and mesiopalatal roots of the maxillary fourth premolar (Figure 4.27), the Clark's or SLOB (Same Lingual, Opposite Buccal) rule can be helpful. Basically, an object placed lingual to a reference point moves to the direction of the incoming beam. On the contrary, an object placed buccal to a reference point moves opposite to the direction of the incoming beam. When applied to the maxillary fourth premolar tooth, the rule translates into 'the mesiopalatal root moves to the direction of the incoming beam'. If the beam comes from a rostral direction, the mesiopalatal root is positioned more rostral than the mesiobuccal root on the film/image. If the beam comes from a caudal direction, the mesiopalatal root is positioned more caudal than the mesiobuccal root on the film/image (Figure 4.28). Furthermore, if the beam comes from a rostral direction, the distal root of the maxillary

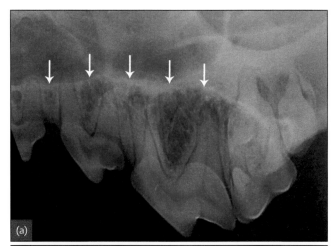

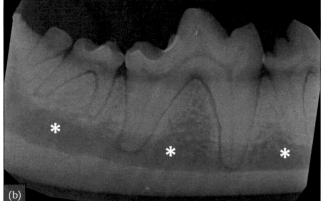

4.26 Dental radiographs taken in a dog showing (a) the left maxillary cheek teeth (arrows depict the line of conjunction between the vertical body of the maxilla and its palatine process) and (b) the right mandibular cheek teeth, (∗) indicates the mandibular canal.

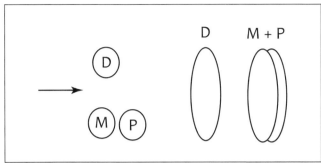

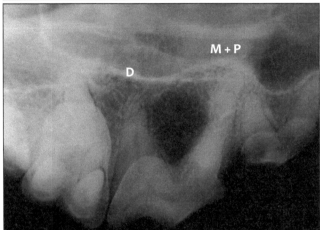

4.27 Radiograph of the right maxillary fourth premolar tooth in a dog. The X-ray beam is coming from a lateral direction (arrowed), resulting in superimposition of the mesiobuccal (M) and mesiopalatal (P) roots. The distal root (D) is clearly visible.
(© Dr Alexander M. Reiter)

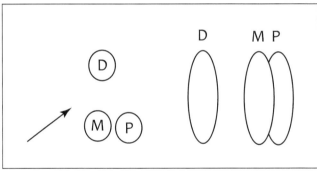

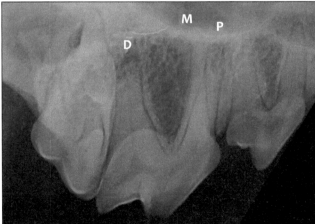

4.28 Radiograph of the right maxillary fourth premolar tooth in a dog. The X-ray beam is coming from a rostral direction (arrowed), resulting in the mesiopalatal root (P) being positioned more rostral than the mesiobuccal root (M) and the distal root (D) starting to overlap with the maxillary first molar tooth.
(© Dr Alexander M. Reiter)

fourth premolar tooth 'moves' caudally and overlaps with the maxillary first molar tooth. If the beam comes from a caudal direction, the mesial roots of the maxillary fourth premolar tooth 'move' rostrally and overlap with the maxillary third premolar tooth (Figure 4.29). To avoid superimposition of nearby teeth and correctly access all three roots, therefore, two views are often necessary.

The important radiographic structures of the tooth and surrounding area are presented in Figure 4.30. When evaluating radiographs, one must first check that the images are technically adequate and diagnostic. All teeth and 2–3 mm periapical tissue for each root should be visible. Each tooth should be captured entirely in at least one image. Furthermore, the images should be free from artefacts that might hinder evaluation. Artefacts could be due to a technical problem in the film, sensor pad or phosphor

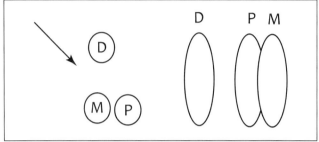

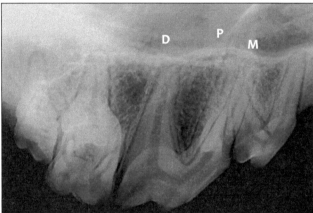

4.29 Radiograph of the right maxillary fourth premolar tooth in a dog. The X-ray beam is coming from a caudal direction (arrowed), resulting in the mesiopalatal root (P) being positioned more caudal than the mesiobuccal root (M) which is overlapping with the distal root (D) of the maxillary third premolar tooth.
(© Dr Alexander M. Reiter)

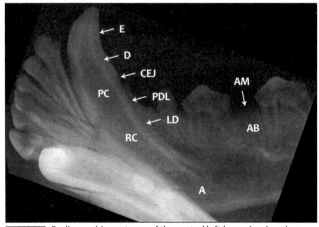

4.30 Radiographic anatomy of the rostral left lower jaw in a dog. A = apex; AB = alveolar bone; AM = alveolar margin; CEJ = cementoenamel junction; D = dentine; E = enamel; LD = lamina dura; PC = pulp chamber; PDL = periodontal ligament space; RC = root canal.

plate (fingerprints, bends and scratches) or errors in the developing process (splashes of developer or fixer) or digital systems (technical problems with the software or the digital reader, such as a broken prism). The films/images are then evaluated systematically, paying attention to findings in all different categories: anatomical abnormalities, signs of periodontal and endodontic disease, structural tooth defects, etc.

Röntgen signs

The Röntgen signs are a list of diagnostic imaging characteristics that should be checked for every structure of interest during the reviewing process. They include size, shape, opacity, location and number. This can be applied to all structures of the head including the dentition and the jaws.

Size

Enlargement of oral and maxillofacial structures would include macrodontia, macroglossia, enlargement of structures of the skull due to periosteal reaction such as in craniomandibular osteopathy, periosteal reaction of tumour-affected bone, and swelling of soft tissues due to inflammatory or neoplastic conditions. Abnormally small structures include, for example, underdeveloped teeth and atrophied masticatory muscles.

Shape

Shape abnormalities are often the most relevant findings in dentistry and oral surgery and include abnormally formed teeth, altered periodontal structures, worn and fractured teeth, jaw fractures, oral and maxillofacial masses, and osteolytic changes and periosteal reactions of facial bones.

Opacity

The teeth are the hardest and most mineralized structures of the body, and loss of radiographic opacity of hard tissues (teeth, bone) is always a significant finding. Developmental abnormalities such as enamel hypoplasia and enamel hypomineralization may be due to a systemic insult (such as with distemper) or result from local trauma, infection and inflammation during the time when enamel is developing in a tooth that has not yet erupted. More severe insult may lead to odontodysplasia, i.e. deformation of the entire tooth.

Damage to the hard tissues (enamel, dentine and cementum) of erupted teeth can be caused by fracture, resorption, erosion, attrition, abrasion, caries and neoplasia. With metabolic conditions such as primary or secondary hyperparathyroidism there is often osteopenia, with preferential demineralization of the alveolar bone of the upper and lower jaws leading to the radiographic appearance of freely floating teeth. Osteolysis is the process of active bone destruction through an aggressive infectious or neoplastic disease. Other causes of abnormally reduced opacity include abnormal gas accumulation, for instance in an infected root canal. This is relatively subtle and identified on CT.

Periosteal and endosteal lesions are reactive changes of bone resulting from a chronic insult and manifest as increased bone opacity. Condensing osteitis is excessive bone mineralization around the apex of a non-vital tooth caused by long-standing exudation of low toxicity from an infected pulp (requiring endodontic therapy). Osteosclerosis is excessive bone mineralization around the apex of a vital

tooth caused by low-grade pulp irritation (asymptomatic; not requiring endodontic therapy). Similar responses occur in and around the affected tooth (Figure 4.31).

Pulp stones are foci of mineralization in the dental pulp; they are asymptomatic, and their only clinical relevance is that insertion of endodontic files may be made more difficult, if not impossible, during root canal therapy (Figure 4.32). Diffuse pulpal mineralization resulting in pulp cavity obliteration, however, may be either age-related or due to a chronic insult to the pulp.

The periodontal ligament is a soft tissue structure that is evident as a thin radiolucent rim between the lamina dura of the alveolar bone and the cementum of the root. Widening of this rim may signify bone resorption, normally of peridontal (starting at the alveolar margin) or endodontic (initially centred around the tooth apex) origin. However, variations in size of the periodontal ligament space around the roots of a tooth, and even along the same root, are common and pathology should be diagnosed based on multiple factors (e.g. concomitant absence of the lamina dura in the same location, comparison with the corresponding tooth on the opposite side, anatomical location, root shape). Radiographic loss of the periodontal ligament space and lamina dura, on the other hand, almost inevitably indicates an area of fusion between the tooth and bone (dentoalveolar ankylosis).

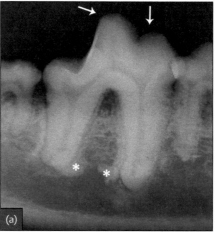

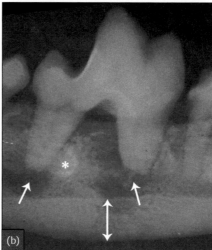

4.31 Radiographs of the right mandibular first molar tooth in two dogs. (a) There is osteosclerosis near the mesial and distal roots (*) and structural deficits of the cusps of the crown (arrowed). (b) There is condensing osteitis (*) near the distal root, apical root resorption and periapical lucencies (arrowed) and thickening of the ventral mandibular cortex (double-ended arrow).
(© Dr Alexander M. Reiter)

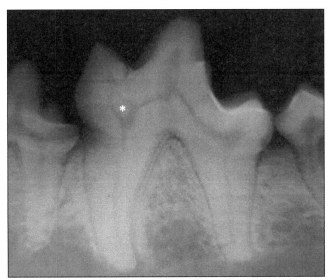

4.32 Radiograph of a left mandibular first molar tooth in a dog, showing a pulp stone (∗) in the mesial aspect of the tooth's pulp chamber.
(© Dr Alexander M. Reiter)

Changes in opacity of the soft tissues of the head include mineralization (often seen in neoplasia), chronic infection, and metabolic and idiopathic conditions such as calcinosis circumscripta.

Location and number

Location and number changes are particularly relevant for the dentition and include missing and supernumerary teeth or additional tooth roots, as well as abnormal tooth locations leading to malocclusion (Figure 4.33). Congenitally

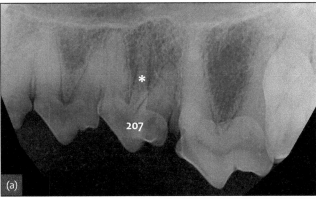

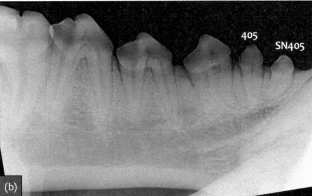

4.33 Radiographs of (a) the left upper jaw in a dog, showing an extra root (∗) at the left maxillary third premolar tooth (207), and (b) the right lower jaw in a dog, showing the presence of two right mandibular first premolar teeth (405 and SN405), one of which is supernumerary (SN).

absent teeth can be differentiated from recently extracted or lost teeth by the complete absence of an alveolar socket and slightly lower than usual alveolar margin height. After a certain period of time following extraction or tooth loss, though, the radiographic appearance may be similar.

Teeth and periodontal tissues

Periodontal disease

Intraoral radiography is the mainstay of detailed imaging of the teeth and periodontal tissues (Tsugawa et al., 2003). However, CT and cone-beam CT can be valuable additional techniques (Doring et al., 2018; Soukup et al., 2015). CT can now provide a spatial image resolution of about two line pairs per mm, although this is still coarser than dedicated digital dental radiography, which has up to 30 line pairs per mm. However, CT overcomes the problems of angle-dependent image distortion and superimposition inherent to all radiographic techniques. It also provides a very accurate display of the entire masticatory apparatus in a very time-efficient way. The use of curvilinear image reconstructions allows assessment of all teeth in conjunction but also individually for each root (Figure 4.34).

The focus of radiographic investigation is on changes in the alveolar bone and periodontal ligament space. In a tooth with healthy periodontal tissues, the alveolar margin should lie within 2 mm of the cementoenamel junction. In horizontal bone loss, which is the most common feature of periodontitis, the alveolar bone has recessed horizontally, the furcation (where roots join in multi-rooted teeth) becomes exposed, and a suprabony pocket is present (Figure 4.35) (Lommer and Verstraete, 2001). In vertical bone loss, the bottom of the bony pocket is somewhat oblique to the surrounding alveolar margin, forming an infrabony pocket. A typical finding in cats (and occasionally also in dogs) is alveolar bone expansion, which most commonly affects the canine teeth; the alveolar bone on the labial aspect of the canine tooth appears enlarged, often is less radiopaque and may have detached from the root surface. This can be accompanied by abnormal extrusion or – with progressive attachment loss – infrabony pocketing and luxation of the affected tooth (Figure 4.36).

Structural tooth defects

Tooth wear

Attrition (caused by tooth-to-tooth contact) and abrasion (caused by contact of the tooth with non-dental material) appear radiographically as a smooth wearing of the cusps of involved teeth. The crowns will be shorter, and the radiopaque enamel absent on involved surfaces. A number of adjacent teeth may show tooth wear. Changes in the pulp cavity of a still vital tooth include narrowing of the pulp chamber and root canal (pulpal sclerosis) due to odontoblastic stimulation to produce more dentine.

Tooth fracture

Crown fractures usually result in radiographically detectable loss of enamel and dentine. The crown of a fractured maxillary fourth premolar tooth no longer has a rounded main cusp, but a pointed roof-like appearance (Figure 4.37). In crown and crown-root fractures, a fracture line may be visible between the tooth and a piece of the tooth that has not yet fully detached. A root fracture may occur

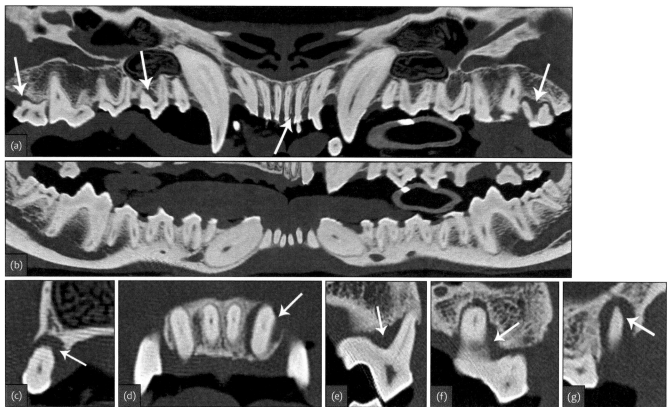

4.34 Computed tomographic images of a dog with periodontal disease. (a, b) The curvilinear reconstruction images of both jaws allow for assessment of all teeth and roots, both simultaneously and individually. Obvious loss of alveolar bone (arrowed) is present at the right maxillary second premolar and second molar teeth and the left maxillary second incisor and second molar teeth (106, 110, 202 and 210). (c–g) Transverse slice images provide more detail for individual teeth. Loss of alveolar bone is arrowed.

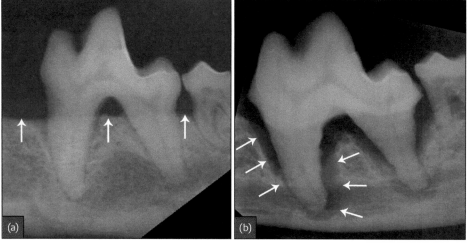

4.35 Radiographs of the left mandibular first molar tooth in two different dogs. Note the loss of alveolar bone (arrowed) in (a) the horizontal and (b) the vertical direction.

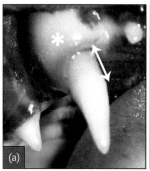
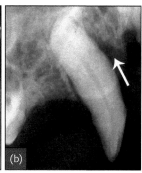
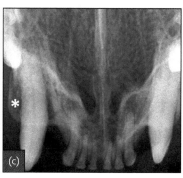

4.36 (a) Clinical photograph and (b, c) radiographs in a cat, showing abnormal extrusion of the right maxillary canine tooth (double-ended arrow indicating root surface exposure) and associated vertical bone loss (arrowed) and alveolar bone expansion (∗).

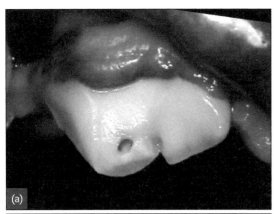

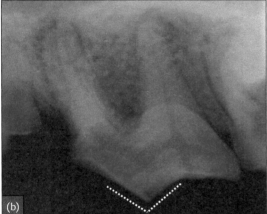

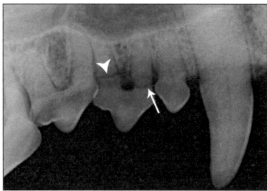

4.37 (a) Clinical photograph and (b) radiograph of a left maxillary fourth premolar tooth in a dog with a complicated crown-root fracture; note the pointed appearance of the tooth's main cusp (dotted lines) and periapical radiolucencies.
(© Dr Alexander M. Reiter)

4.38 Radiograph of the right maxillary second premolar tooth in a dog with fracture of the distal (arrowhead) and mesial (arrowed) roots. Alveolar bone loss adjacent to the affected tooth can also be noted.

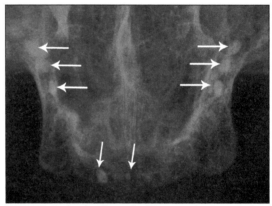

4.39 Occlusal radiograph of the upper jaw in a cat, showing multiple root remnants (arrowed).
(© Dr Alexander M. Reiter)

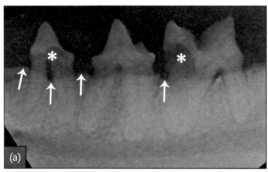

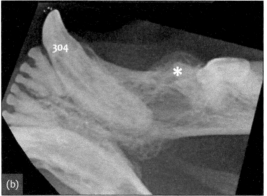

4.40 Radiographs of two cats. (a) Inflammatory resorption (type 1 resorption) affecting the left mandibular third premolar and first molar teeth (*). The periodontal ligament space is visible along the roots. Note alveolar bone loss adjacent to the affected teeth (arrowed). (b) Non-inflammatory resorption (type 2 resorption) of the left mandibular canine (304) and third premolar teeth (*). Note the lack of periodontal ligament space and bone proliferation, rather than resorption, adjacent to affected teeth.

at any level of the tooth. When the X-ray beam falls parallel with the plane of a root fracture, the site of the fracture appears as a sharp radiolucent line between tooth fragments (Figure 4.38). If the X-ray beam orientation is more oblique to the fracture plane, some of the tooth structure superimposes over the fracture, and the fracture appears as a poorly defined grey shadow or may not be visible at all. Root fractures are usually transverse and oblique and are more commonly noticed on incisor teeth. Longitudinal crown-root fractures are relatively uncommon. Root remnants are a common radiographic finding in dogs and cats (Farcas et al., 2014). On occlusal radiographs, root remnants are often found as round opaque structures with a variously sized central lucency (the root canal) (Figure 4.39).

Resorption

Radiographically detectable external resorption may be inflammatory (AVDC type 1 resorption) or non-inflammatory (AVDC type 2 resorption) in nature (Figure 4.40). The latter is also referred to as replacement resorption, in which the periodontal ligament space and lamina dura disappear in some or several areas around the root due to fusion between the root and alveolar bone (dento–alveolar ankylosis) and the resorbing tooth substance is replaced by new bone (Peralta et al., 2010a, b). Ankylosis is radiographically evident mostly on mesial and distal (rather than on lingual/palatal and labial/buccal) root surfaces; in addition, the trabecular pattern of alveolar bone often camouflages small areas of ankylosis and root resorption. Generally, the root will have a moth-eaten appearance in the area affected by type 2 resorption. Unlike type 1 resorption, the adjacent bone is not resorbed, so radiolucencies are not found in the bone adjacent to the affected root (Lommer and Verstraete, 2000). Both types are often diagnosed in teeth of cats. According to the AVDC classification, a tooth receives the designation of a type 3 resorption if both types of resorption (1 and 2) are found together in the same tooth. In dogs, type 2 tooth resorption is much more frequently diagnosed than type 1 tooth resorption. The severity of external tooth resorption is staged according to loss of tooth substance. External surface resorption is also relatively common in dogs. It affects cementum and dentine and is often considered a self-limiting process. Radiographically, the affected root appears irregularly shaped, with one or more resorption lacunae but normally corresponding periodontal ligament space and lamina dura (Peralta *et al.*, 2010a).

Radiographically detectable internal resorption presents as a fairly uniform, oval-shaped radiolucent enlargement of the pulp cavity. The original outline of the root canal or pulp chamber is distorted (Figure 4.41). Unlike external root resorption, resorption of the adjacent bone does not occur. Observation of radiographs taken at different angles should give a fairly good indication of whether a resorptive defect is internal or external. A lesion of internal origin appears close to the root canal whatever the angle of the radiograph. On the other hand, a defect on the external aspect of the root moves away from the canal as the angulation changes. In internal resorption, the outline of the root canal is usually distorted, and the root canal and the radiolucent resorptive defect appear contiguous. When the defect is external, the root canal outline appears normal and can usually be seen running through the radiolucent defect. External inflammatory root resorption is always accompanied by resorption of alveolar bone, with radiolucencies apparent in the root and the adjacent bone. Internal root resorption does not usually involve the bone and, as a rule, the radiolucency is confined to the root. On rare occasions, the internal defect perforates the root and the bone adjacent to it is resorbed and appears radiolucent on the radiograph.

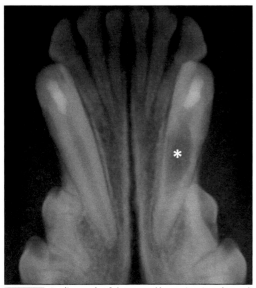

4.41 Radiograph of the rostral lower jaw in a dog, whose mandibular canine teeth had been treated with crown reduction and vital pulp therapy. Internal resorption (*) resulted in an oval-shaped lucency in the root canal of the left mandibular canine tooth.

Caries

Caries is uncommon in dogs and rarely diagnosed in cats. It causes destruction of the tooth substance, as well as extending into the pulp resulting in endodontic and periapical disease. Radiographically caries appears as loss of tooth substance, most commonly on the occlusal surfaces of the maxillary and mandibular molars (Figure 4.42).

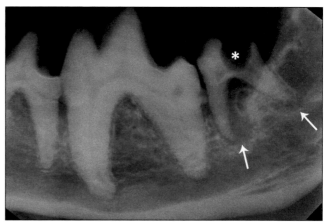

4.42 Radiograph of the caudal left lower jaw in a dog, showing a crater-shaped crown defect (*) and periapical disease around the root apices (arrowed) of the left mandibular second molar tooth affected by caries.

Endodontic disease

Intraoral radiography is also paramount for the diagnosis and treatment of endodontic and periapical disease. Endodontic findings include those that relate to pathology of the pulp–dentine complex. When the pulp becomes necrotic for various reasons (tooth wear, fracture), odontoblasts will no longer produce pre-dentine along the inner dentinal walls of the affected tooth. Therefore, a tooth that has been non-vital for some time has thinner dentinal walls and a larger pulp cavity compared with a vital tooth in the same animal; diagnosis is facilitated by obtaining radiographs of the contralateral tooth for comparison of root canal widths between teeth (Figure 4.43). Inflammatory endodontic findings include internal resorption, in which an area of the pulp cavity is larger, and external resorption, in which the apex of a root appears shorter and more irregular. Cone-beam CT has been experimentally demonstrated to be more accurate than radiography in diagnosing periapical lesions in dogs (De Paula-Silva, 2009; Lopez *et al.*, 2014).

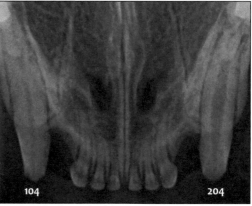

4.43 Radiograph of the rostral upper jaw in a cat. Note the difference in width of the root canal between the vital right maxillary canine (104) and the non-vital left maxillary canine tooth (204).

Periapical disease

The periodontal ligament should follow the root in close proximity, but a chevron artefact is often present, surrounding the apex of incisor and canine teeth. This is a tunnel-shaped widening of the periodontal ligament space that follows the shape of the root and is part of normal radiographic variation (Figure 4.44).

On the contrary, a bullous radiolucency surrounding the apex of a root is a sign of periapical disease that usually originates from a diseased pulp. A radiolucency surrounding the root apex with loss of lamina dura is usually related to the presence of a chronic periapical abscess or a periapical granuloma (Figure 4.45); its border varies from a well defined sclerotic band to a diffuse region that blends into adjacent bone. A periapical cyst may be radiographically indistinguishable from a granuloma, though often it is more apt to have a thin hyperostotic (radiopaque) border compared with a granuloma (Figure 4.46). An acute periapical

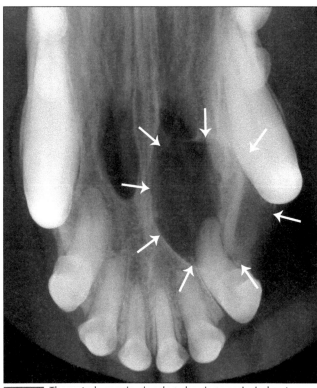

4.46 The rostral upper jaw in a dog, showing a periapical cyst (arrowed) associated with a left maxillary third incisor tooth.
(© Dr Alexander M. Reiter)

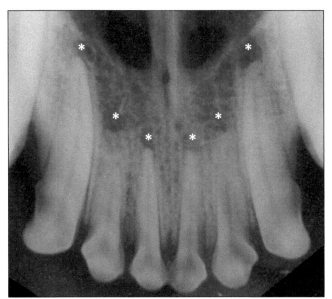

4.44 Chevron artefacts (*) surrounding the root apices of vital maxillary incisor teeth of a dog.
(© Dr Alexander M. Reiter)

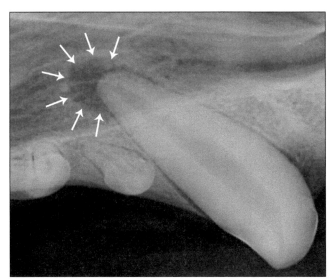

4.45 Right maxillary canine tooth in a dog with periapical lesion compatible with a granuloma or an abscess (arrowed), characterized by a radiolucent halo and loss of lamina dura around the root apex.

abscess, even if very painful clinically, may be unremarkable radiographically; the periodontal ligament may be within normal limits or only slightly widened with a relatively normal (or slightly thickened) lamina dura. A phoenix abscess is an acute exacerbation of a periapical granuloma and is radiographically indistinguishable from it (Figure 4.47). If the inflammation exceeds the periapical area, more widespread involvement of the bone and bone marrow (osteomyelitis) will occur.

Combined endodontic and periodontal lesions

Combined lesions show components of both periodontal and endodontic pathology. An 'endo-perio' lesion initially starts as pulpitis that extends periapically and then further coronally along the periodontal ligament space, causing periodontitis. A 'perio-endo' lesion initially starts as periodontitis that extends apically and then further into the pulp through apical foramina, causing pulpitis (Figure 4.48). In a 'true combined lesion', endodontic and periodontal diseases develop independently of each other.

Tooth displacement injuries

Traumatic tooth displacement may present as luxation (displacement of the tooth within the alveolus) or avulsion (the tooth is no longer in the alveolus). The most common tooth displacement injury is lateral luxation of the maxillary canine tooth (Figure 4.49), which involves alveolar bone fracture (often with the crown displaced labially and the root being pushed towards the nasal cavity). The associated fracture of alveolar bone may be difficult to see on radiographs.

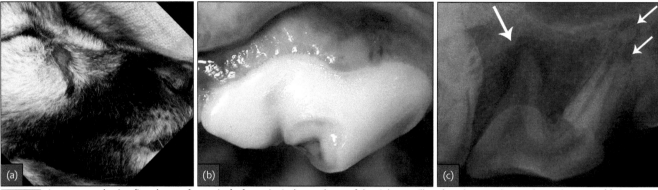

4.47 Acute exacerbation (i.e. abscess formation) of a periapical granuloma of the right maxillary fourth premolar tooth in a dog. Note (a) the cutaneous draining tract below the medial canthus of the eye, (b) the complicated crown fracture, and (c) radiolucencies (arrowed) around the root apices of the tooth.

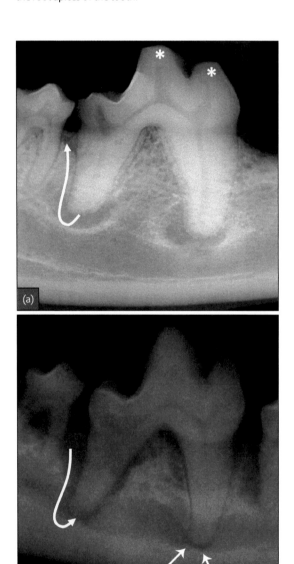

4.48 Combined endodontic and periodontal lesions of the right mandibular first molar tooth in two different dogs (the curved arrows show the direction of disease progression). (a) In the type 1 endo-perio lesion, note the structural deficits (*) of the cusps of the crown, resulting in a primary endodontic lesion with secondary periodontal involvement. (b) In the type 2 perio-endo lesion, there is a primary periodontal lesion with secondary endodontic involvement. Note the development of periapical disease at the mesial root (short arrows), which is less affected by bone loss compared with the distal root.
(© Dr Alexander M. Reiter)

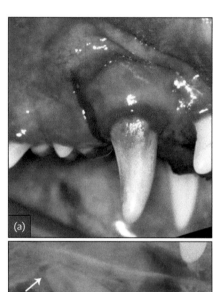

4.49 Lateral luxation of a right maxillary canine tooth in a dog. Note (a) the mucosal laceration and (b) the widened periodontal ligament space (arrowed).
(© Dr Alexander M. Reiter)

Assessment of treatment and outcome

Intraoral radiography is a valuable and often necessary tool for decision-making in dentistry and oral surgery. Evaluation of instrumentation during root canal therapy, identification of fractured roots and assessment of jaw fracture reduction are common indications for intraoperative radiographs. Postoperative radiographs are routinely obtained in many cases, such as after crown amputation and intentional retention of resorbing root tissue, postoperative evaluation of endodontic treatment, advanced periodontal surgery, jaw fracture repair, tumour excision, and confirmation of complete tooth extraction in complicated cases.

Evaluation of root canal therapy, including the assessment of shaping, obturation, compaction and restoration, and of the short- and long-term outcome, is mostly based on radiographs. A tooth treated with successful root canal therapy will have maintained a normal width of the periodontal ligament space, and previously present periapical findings will either not have progressed or may have disappeared. If a periapical lucency has decreased or remained the same and apical resorption has not progressed, the treatment outcome is defined as 'no evidence of failure' (Figure 4.50). If a periapical lucency or apical resorption has developed subsequent to treatment, or if a periapical lucency has increased in size and apical resorption has progressed, the outcome is defined as 'failure'.

Evaluation of the outcome of vital pulp therapy also includes the assessment of signs of the continued presence of pulp vitality, including continued tooth development (root lengthening and apical closure in immature teeth; progressive thickening of the dentinal walls and narrowing of the pulp cavity in mature teeth) and absence of internal or external root resorption (Figure 4.51). Occasionally, chronic pulpitis may result in diffuse pulpal mineralization (Figure 4.52), which, if occurring after vital pulp therapy, would be considered a treatment failure. Traditionally, formation of an irregular dentinal bridge between the pulp capping material and the underlying pulp has been considered as a sign of successful vital pulp therapy, but more recent studies show that a dentinal bridge is not significantly associated with increased or decreased odds of treatment failure (Luotonen et al., 2014).

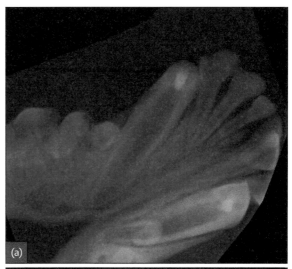
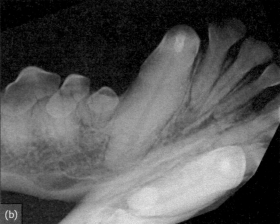

4.51 Radiographs of the rostral lower jaw in a dog (a) prior to and (b) 5 years after successful vital pulp therapy of both mandibular canine teeth. Note the continued root development with continued apposition of dentine and apical closure.

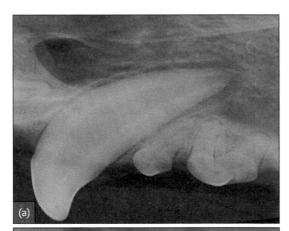
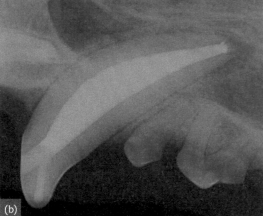

4.50 Radiographs of a left maxillary canine tooth (a) prior to and (b) several months after root canal therapy. Note that the previously widened periodontal ligament space and the periapical lucency have decreased.

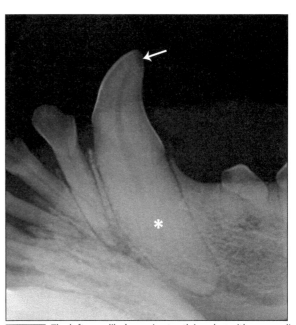

4.52 The left mandibular canine tooth in a dog with uncomplicated crown fracture (arrowed) and stricture of the root canal (*) due to diffuse pulpal mineralization.

Jaws and temporomandibular joints

Odontogenic cysts

Cysts in the jaws are most commonly diagnosed in the tooth-bearing region, as they originate from rests of odontogenic epithelium that remain within bone after tooth formation. Radiography and particularly CT are very sensitive to detect and monitor cysts. The typical radiographic appearance of a cyst is a round or oval radiolucent area, surrounded by a thin opaque lining. Occasionally, cysts are multilocular, with several radiolucent areas separated by bony walls. Cysts may cause displacement or resorption of adjacent teeth and, if present in the upper jaw, could cause nasal airway obstruction. The dentigerous cyst is most commonly diagnosed in the area of an unerupted mandibular first premolar tooth in brachycephalic dogs. It is initially attached to the cementoenamel junction of the unerupted tooth; however, with continued enlargement it will completely enclose the tooth within its lumen. The second most common odontogenic cyst is the periapical cyst.

Malocclusions and malformations

Radiography can also be useful for documenting dental and skeletal malocclusions and general malformations of the head such as brachycephalism. One of the consequences of brachycephalism can be overcrowding of teeth with associated tooth eruption disorders and malocclusion as well as upper airway problems.

Asynchronous growth of the skull bones is often assumed in dogs and cats with marked head asymmetry and is best assessed with CT. In cats a slightly curved nasal septum and intranasal obstructing hypertrophic turbinates are common incidental findings. A curved nasal septum is also commonly seen in brachycephalic dogs where it may be quite prominent, contributing to the obstructive airway conditions these patients often have. Premature closure of the bony sutures of the zygomatic arch may also cause maxillofacial asymmetry and open-mouth jaw locking.

Inflammatory, metabolic and osteoproliferative conditions

Osteomyelitis and osteonecrosis of skull bones are rare conditions that most commonly affect young adult to middle-aged, large-breed dogs. The radiographic appearance includes generalized and palisading periosteal reaction, osteolysis, and soft tissue swelling indicating cellulitis around affected skull bones. Intraoral dental radiography and CT are helpful to characterize the extent and location of inflammation (Figure 4.53).

Penetrating foreign bodies often enter the soft tissues of the head via the oral cavity and lead to infection and abscessation of the retrobulbar space, masticatory muscles, tongue, periaural space, salivary glands and retropharyngeal region. Both contrast-enhanced CT and MRI are very sensitive for tracking inflammation and infection, although the visibility of the foreign body depends on the material, with plant materials often being difficult to see. Bite injuries and other wounds also lead to tissue changes that can be visualized accurately using similar techniques.

Fibrous osteodystrophy (Figure 4.54) is a form of osteopenia and periosteal reaction due to primary or secondary

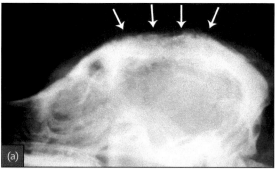
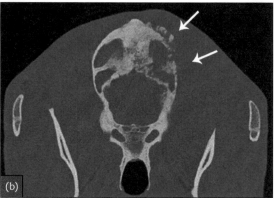

4.53 (a) Lateral head radiograph and (b) computed tomographic image of two young dogs with osteomyelitis of the calvarium. There is marked irregular periosteal reaction and osteolysis of the calvarium (arrowed), but the facial bones are relatively spared.

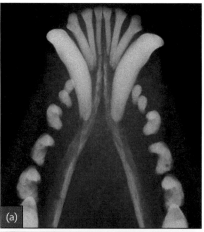
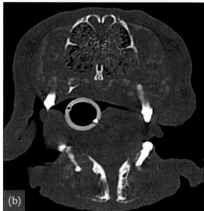

4.54 (a) Ventrodorsal intraoral radiograph of the lower jaw of a 6-year-old Keeshond dog with fibrous osteodystrophy, showing marked osteopenia and a 'floating teeth' appearance due to secondary renal hyperparathyroidism. (b) Computed tomographic image of a dog with fibrous osteodystrophy due to primary hyperparathyroidism, showing marked mandibular and maxillary osteopenia and fibrous tissue proliferation.

hyperparathyroidism. Calcium is absorbed preferentially from the bones of the jaw to aid in blood calcium homeostasis, causing replacement of bone by fibrous tissue. The teeth are not affected, resulting in a radiographic appearance of 'floating teeth' within thickened fibrous tissue.

Craniomandibular osteopathy (Figure 4.55) is an osteoproliferative disorder of unknown aetiology seen in young dogs, particularly in West Highland White, Scottish and Cairn Terriers. Radiographic features typically include marked palisading periosteal new bone formation of the mandibles, which can extend to the tympanic bullae and calvarium. The condition is usually but not always bilateral. Affected dogs have pain and exhibit an inability to open their mouth. Often they present with fever and severe depression.

A related condition is idiopathic calvarial hyperostosis in young Bullmastiffs, which causes similar clinical signs (fever, depression and pain on mouth opening), as well as head swelling and nasal discharge. Radiography or CT show marked thickening and sclerosis of the calvarial bones (Figure 4.56). Affected animals can also have palisading new bone formation in the antebrachium, similar to hypertrophic osteodystrophy.

Periostitis ossificans usually presents with a unilateral swelling of the caudal mandibular body in puppies with mixed dentition. Radiographs typically show a double-cortex appearance at the ventral, lingual or buccal aspect of the affected mandible. The condition often resolves spontaneously (Blazejewski et al., 2010).

Jaw fractures

Intraoral dental radiographic techniques are superior in the detection of many maxillary and mandibular fracture lines compared with head radiography, particularly if they are located in the rostral to mid-portions of the jaws. Head radiography becomes more useful in the case of fractures of the caudal upper and lower jaw, zygomatic arch, TMJ and calvarium. Radiography in general appears to be more sensitive than CT in the detection of non-displaced fractures of the mandibular body. CT, however, allows for a quick and detailed assessment of many dental, osseous and soft tissue structures of the head, thus facilitating decision-making for treatment and prognosis of the oral and maxillofacial trauma patient (Bar-Am et al., 2008) (Figure 4.57).

The radiographic characterization of jaw fractures includes description of the fracture line: whether it is vertical, horizontal or oblique, closed or open, non-displaced or displaced, and simple or comminuted. The fracture lines are usually sharply defined and radiolucent. A cortical discontinuity will become evident if there is displacement of fracture segments. Particularly for mandibular fractures, the fracture margins may overlap each other, resulting in radiopaque lines at the fracture site. The presence and involvement of teeth in or near the fracture line must also be recorded.

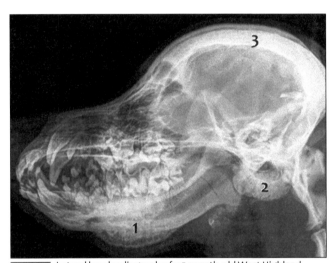

4.55 Lateral head radiograph of a 5-month-old West Highland White Terrier with craniomandibular osteopathy. There is marked enlargement of the mandibles (1), tympanic bullae (2) and calvarium (3) with palisading new bone formation.

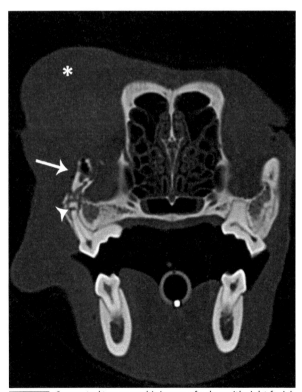

4.57 Computed tomographic image of a dog with right facial trauma after being kicked by a horse. Note the right periorbital swelling (*), comminuted zygomatic arch fracture containing gas (arrowed), and an apical fracture of the distobuccal root of the right maxillary first molar tooth (arrowhead).

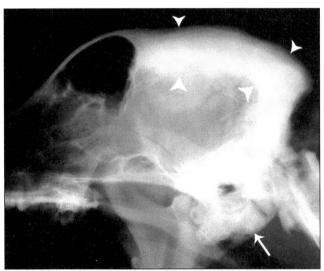

4.56 Lateral head radiograph of a 7-month-old Bullmastiff with calvarial hyperostosis. There is marked enlargement of the calvarium (arrowheads) and tympanic bullae (arrowed). The mandibles are usually not affected.

Temporomandibular joint disorders

CT is faster and more accurate than radiography for assessing TMJ pathology for aetiology, treatment planning and prognosis (Schwarz *et al.*, 2002; Schwarz, 2011; Arzi *et al.*, 2013). Although CT and radiography have been the traditional methods for imaging the TMJ, MRI can also be used and provides excellent anatomical assessment of the mandibular condyle and mandibular fossa (Figure 4.58). With optimal settings, the TMJ disc can be imaged in most dogs using a sagittal plane T1-weighted image aligned with the mandibular condyle in an open-mouth position (Macready *et al.*, 2010). In cats, the TMJ disc cannot be visualized with current MRI techniques. The angulation of the mandibular condyle in relation to the mandibular ramus can be measured accurately with CT and MRI, with the normal range being between 70.2 and 83 degrees in dogs (Macready *et al.*, 2010). This measurement is relevant in the diagnostic work-up of dogs with open-mouth jaw locking.

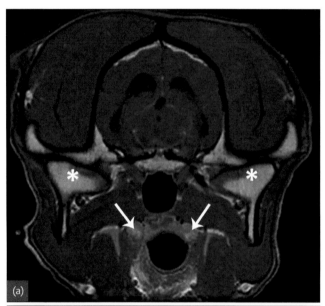

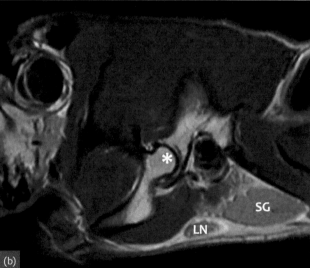

4.58 (a) Transverse T1-weighted post-contrast and (b) para-sagittal T1-weighted magnetic resonance images in two normal dogs showing the anatomy of the temporomandibular joints. The relationship between the mandibular condyle (∗) and mandibular fossa can readily be assessed with magnetic resonance imaging due to the ability to image in any plane. In (a), normal palatine tonsils are visible (arrowed). In (b), a normal mandibular salivary gland (SG) and one mandibular lymph node (LN) are also visible.

Osteoarthritis and cyst-like lesions

Osteoarthritis of the TMJ (Figure 4.59) is a relatively common condition in dogs and cats, characterized by cartilage erosion and osteophytosis (Arzi *et al.*, 2013). CT is sensitive for the detection of subchondral bony changes including cyst-like lesions (Figure 4.60). The relationship between the mandibular condyle and mandibular fossa can also be readily assessed with MRI due to its multiplanar imaging capabilities. However, with modern multi-detector CT scanners, excellent quality reformatted images can be obtained in any plane, allowing superb morphological assessment. Subchondral cysts in the mandibular condyle can also be identified with MRI, as can other conditions such as incongruence, luxation, fracture, infection or degenerative changes.

Fracture and ankylosis

Non-displaced fractures of the mandibular condyle may be difficult to detect on lateral oblique radiographic views and are best demonstrated on DV (or VD) views (Figure 4.61) or CT images. Excessive new bone formation after trauma can lead to TMJ ankylosis particularly in immature, adolescent and young adult cats and dogs (Figure 4.62).

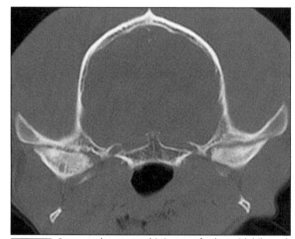

4.59 Computed tomographic image of a dog with bilateral temporomandibular joint osteoarthritis. There is marked subchondral bone erosion.

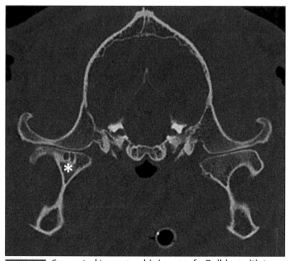

4.60 Computed tomographic image of a Bulldog with two subchondral bone cyst-like lesions in the right mandibular condyle (∗). Note also the baroque shape of the bones forming the temporomandibular joints, consistent with dysplasia.

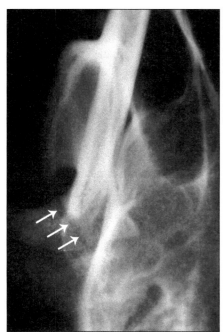

4.61 Close-up image of a dorsoventral radiograph of a dog with a sagittal mandibular condyle fracture. The fracture line is barely visible (arrowed).

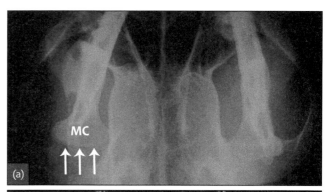

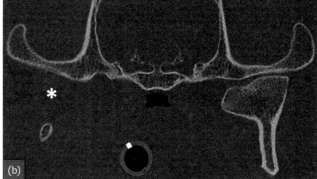

4.63 (a) Dorsoventral radiograph and (b) computed tomographic image of a Boxer with temporomandibular joint luxation. The right mandibular condyle (MC) is luxated rostrally (arrowed). The space where the mandibular condyle should be situated in the mandibular fossa is empty (*).

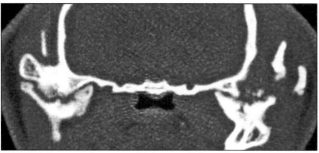

4.62 Computed tomographic image of bilateral temporomandibular joint ankylosis in a cat.

The clinically important distinction between uni- and bilateral ankylosis can be very difficult to make without appropriate diagnostic imaging. Difficulty in opening the mouth can be caused by intracapsular ankylosis of the TMJ (true ankylosis) or be due to extracapsular restrictive structures (false ankylosis) such as jaw and zygomatic arch fractures/calluses and congenital and developmental skull deformations. Other causes of restricted mouth opening include tetanus and retrobulbar, periaural, salivary, masticatory muscle or bone mass lesions. CT with the mouth closed and maximally opened is the imaging modality of choice for investigating all of these causes.

Subluxation and luxation

Subluxation of the TMJ can be caused by trauma, joint dysplasia, mandibular symphyseal laxity, skull deformities and TMJ osteoarthritis. TMJ luxation (Figure 4.63) is commonly the consequence of severe head trauma, with the mandibular condyle usually luxating in a rostrodorsal direction and causing the lower jaw to shift to the opposite side. Caudal luxation of the mandibular condyle is usually accompanied by fracture of the retroarticular process (a caudoventral extension of the mandibular fossa of the temporal bone). Radiographic diagnosis of TMJ displacement requires perfect positioning of the patient under general anaesthesia and at least DV and lateral oblique views. Compared with radiography, CT allows the detection of more subtle changes.

Dysplasia and open-mouth jaw locking

TMJ dysplasia is a poorly understood condition that comes in two forms. Many chondrodystrophic dog breeds, such as Dachshunds, Cavalier King Charles Spaniels and Pekingese dogs have a grossly misshapen, but not necessarily shallow, mandibular condyle and mandibular fossa; these dogs usually do not have any associated clinical signs. Another subset of dogs, particularly Irish Setters and Basset Hounds, may have a less congruent mandibular condyle, shallower mandibular fossa and blunted retroarticular process. It is only the latter type of dog that has a tendency for TMJ subluxation.

In open-mouth jaw locking (Figure 4.64) the mandibular coronoid process of the mandible impinges on or is locked ventrolateral to the zygomatic arch, thus keeping the mouth wide open. DV radiographic views are usually sufficient to diagnose contact of the coronoid process with the zygomatic arch. CT is not necessary to diagnose coronoid impingement itself; however, particularly when performed with the jaw in the locked open position, it allows investigation of the many possible causes such as mandibular symphyseal laxity, developmental or traumatic abnormalities of the zygomatic arch such as premature zygomaticotemporal suture synostosis (Ryan et al., 2013), maxillofacial fractures, TMJ dysplasia and subluxation.

Oral and maxillofacial tumours

Intraoral radiography is an essential part of the diagnosis and treatment of oral and maxillofacial tumours. It provides important initial information on the nature of the tumour, serves in the staging of the disease, helps determine surgical margins, and supports the planning of medical or radiation therapy. Several views, including all

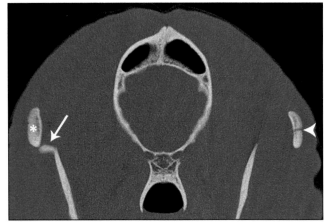

4.64 Computed tomographic image of a 1-year-old German Shorthaired Pointer with a history of open-mouth jaw locking. The tip of the coronoid process of the right mandible is fractured (arrowed) due to impingement on the right zygomatic arch, which has a closed zygomaticotemporal suture and adjacent sclerosis consistent with premature zygomaticotemporal synostosis (*) and is situated more medial than the left zygomatic arch. For comparison, the left zygomatic arch has an open zygomaticotemporal suture (arrowhead), which is normal for a dog of this age.

margins of the suspect area and comparison with the contralateral side, are necessary for proper radiographic evaluation. Radiographic description of a tumour includes information about its location, size, shape (for example round, oval or multilobular), opacity (radiolucent, radiopaque, or both), and effect on the adjacent bone (new bone formation, bony destruction, or both) and teeth (displacement or resorption).

Radiographic characteristics

In rare cases, the radiographic appearance is so unique that a diagnosis can be made according to imaging findings. A compound odontoma with numerous rudimentary tooth structures is radiographically very distinct. Other radiographically distinct tumours are the complex odontoma, presenting as a large, irregular mineralized mass, and the peripheral odontogenic fibroma, when it shows focal mineralization surrounded by soft tissue.

Benign tumours are typically smooth, round or oval in shape and may be radiolucent, mixed radiolucent and radiopaque, or radiopaque. While both benign and malignant masses may appear radiolucent, radiopacity and internal mineralization are usually signs of a benign lesion. Benign lesions often exert slow pressure on adjacent tissues, thus allowing them to respond; the adjacent teeth and cortical bone may be displaced, and the cortex maintains its integrity by remodelling, which may appear as bowing. On the contrary, malignant tumours often grow rapidly, causing destruction of surrounding structures. Typical radiographic findings for malignant tumours are ill-defined, invasive borders followed by bone lysis, cortical thinning and tooth resorption; they may or may not be surrounded by periosteal reaction, which sometimes has a laminated or sunburst pattern. Malignant radiographic signs also include multifocal periapical lesions, tooth displacement in an occlusal direction and floating (very mobile) teeth. Malignant tumours tend to invade by means of the easiest route, such as the periodontal ligament space and neurovascular canals, resulting in their irregular widening.

Odontogenic tumours

With the exception of peripheral odontogenic fibromas and acanthomatous ameloblastomas in dogs, odontogenic tumours are infrequently observed in domestic carnivores. The fibromatous and ossifying epulides are now called peripheral odontogenic fibromas, which arise from periodontal ligament stroma and show minimal or no osteolysis on radiographs (Figure 4.65). The ossifying type differs from the fibromatous type by having a distinct focus of mineralization within the soft tissue mass. The acanthomatous epulis is now called acanthomatous ameloblastoma, which is a locally aggressive and bone-invasive tumour in dogs that has not been reported to spread to regional or distant sites (Figure 4.66). Radiographic features of odontomas include an expansile oral soft tissue mass with a bony rim containing rudimentary teeth (compound odontoma) or unorganized dental tissues (complex odontoma) (Figure 4.67) (Walker et al., 2009).

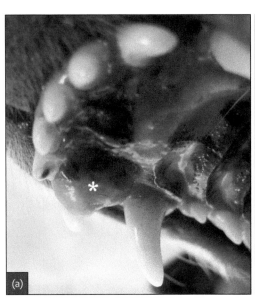

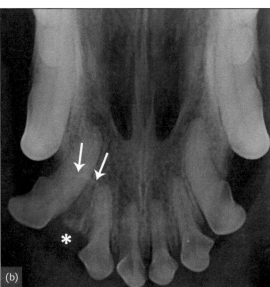

4.65 (a) Clinical photograph and (b) radiograph of a peripheral odontogenic fibroma (fibromatous type) in the rostral upper jaw in a dog. Note the soft tissue swelling (*) between the right maxillary second and third incisor teeth, resulting in increased interproximal spacing between the two teeth, and subtle radiolucency with a well defined, mildly sclerotic margin (arrowed).

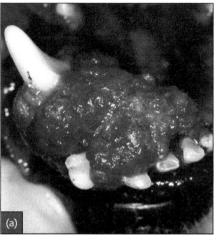
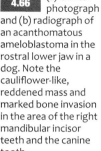

4.66 (a) Clinical photograph and (b) radiograph of an acanthomatous ameloblastoma in the rostral lower jaw in a dog. Note the cauliflower-like, reddened mass and marked bone invasion in the area of the right mandibular incisor teeth and the canine tooth.
(© Dr Alexander M. Reiter)

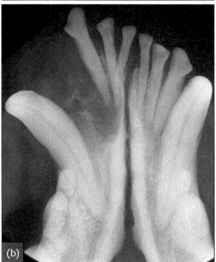

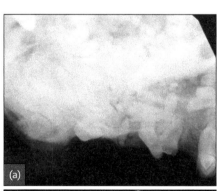

4.67 (a) Intraoral lateral oblique radiograph of a left maxillary compound odontoma in a dog. (b) Numerous tooth-like structures were removed from this lesion.
(Courtesy of Frank J. M. Verstraete, University of California-Davis)

Bone tumours

Benign bone tumours such as osteomas are very rare but most commonly seen in old cats, presenting as smooth homogeneous osseous masses arising from the skull (Figure 4.68). Radiographically, malignant primary bone tumours such as osteosarcoma and chondrosarcoma are often osteolytic with varying degrees of osteoproductive changes or mineralization (Figure 4.69). The multilobular tumour of bone (osteochondrosarcoma, chondroma rodens) presents as a coarse granular mass. It arises from the flat bones of the skull, usually without much osteolysis but with pressure resorption of adjacent bone. Even though it is mostly expansile in nature, infiltrative growth into the cranial cavity is possible (Figure 4.70).

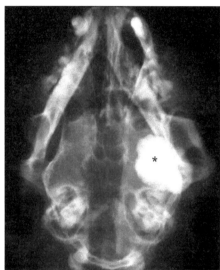

4.68 Ventrodorsal radiograph of the head of a 14-year-old cat with a benign mandibular osteoma (∗). The mass is smoothly marginated and shows no sign of osteolysis.

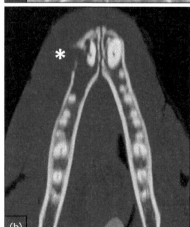

4.69 (a) Dorsoventral radiograph of the head of a dog with a caudal maxillary osteosarcoma. There is a very irregular periosteal reaction and osteolysis (arrowed). (b) Computed tomographic image of a rostral mandibular osteosarcoma in a dog. The image shows the aggressive osteolytic nature (∗) of this primary bone tumour. Note that there is no invasion of the opposite mandible.

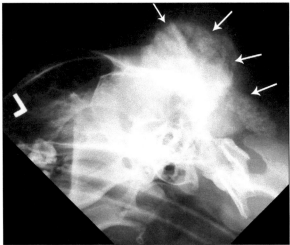

4.70 Oblique lateral radiograph of the head of a dog with a multilobular tumour of the calvarium (arrowed). This tumour arises from flat bones of the skull and has both expansile and infiltrative behaviour.

Soft tissue tumours

Oral soft tissue neoplasms such as fibrosarcoma, malignant melanoma and squamous cell carcinoma cause oral soft tissue swelling and adjacent periosteal reaction and varying degrees of local osteolysis, which is not restrained by bone margins.

Advanced imaging of tumours

Radiography is usually inadequate to fully assess oral and maxillofacial neoplasia located on the caudal mandible, mid to caudal maxilla, nasal cavity, caudal oral cavity, pharynx, larynx and cranial neck of the animal. Advanced cross-sectional imaging such as CT and MRI is required to assess the extent of the disease process and plan for surgical removal and/or radiation therapy (Amory *et al.*, 2014). While CT is preferred for the assessment of bone involvement (Figure 4.71), the soft tissue margins are usually more visible on MRI than CT due to the inherent higher soft tissue contrast of MRI (Figure 4.72). The

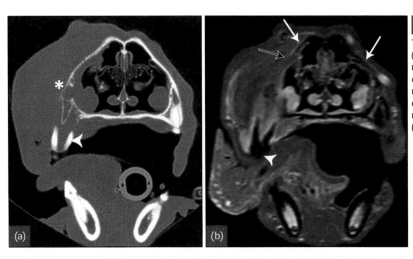

4.71 (a) Transverse computed tomographic (CT) image in a bone algorithm and (b) transverse T1-weighted post-contrast magnetic resonance imaging (MRI) of a dog with a squamous cell carcinoma of the right maxilla. While the bone destruction is readily appreciated on CT (∗), it can also be identified on MRI, where the normal dark signal from the cortical bone (arrowed) has disappeared in the region of the mass (black arrow). Tooth roots are visibly embedded in the neoplastic mass (arrowhead).

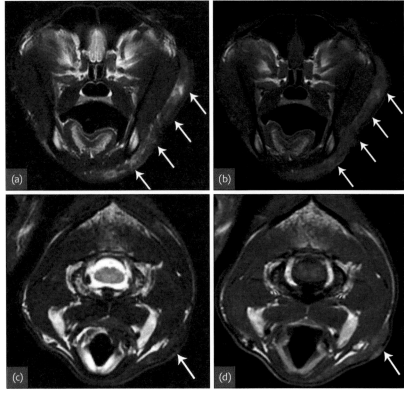

4.72 (a, c) T2-weighted and (b, d) T1-weighted post-contrast magnetic resonance images of a cat with a focal and poorly marginated left-sided facial swelling that was diagnosed as mast cell tumour. (a, b) These images have been obtained at the level of the palpated mass and show diffuse swelling along the left side of the face (arrowed) that is (a) heterogeneously T2-hyperintense and (b) enhances strongly after gadolinium injection. These images show that the neoplastic tissue extends far more caudally than clinically perceived. (c) The T2-weighted image at the level of C1 (first vertebra) still shows abnormal thickened tissue along the left ventrolateral aspect of the neck (arrowed), which was (d) enhanced and represented extensive neoplastic infiltration.

appearance of oral and maxillofacial masses on CT or MRI is not specific for tumour type; however, osteosarcomas have been reported to appear on MRI as very mottled, multiloculated masses, with intensely hyperintense, 'popcorn-like' pockets of fluid accumulation apparent on T2-weighted images (Kafka *et al*., 2004). Multilobular tumours of bone may have a similar appearance on MRI (Lipsitz *et al*., 2001).

Regional lymph nodes

Computed tomography and magnetic resonance imaging

Another advantage of CT and MRI is the assessment of regional lymph nodes for metastasis. Three lymph centres should be assessed (although the parotid and lateral retropharyngeal lymph nodes are not regularly visible on CT or MRI in normal or diseased dogs (and never in cats)):

- Parotid lymph nodes (one to three on each side, bean-shaped, at the caudal aspect of the zygomatic arch and masseter muscle, at the rostral base of the ear, under the rostrodorsal margin of the parotid gland)
- Mandibular lymph nodes (two to five on each side, oval-shaped, adjacent to the linguofacial vein and rostral to the mandibular salivary glands) (Figure 4.73)
- Retropharyngeal lymph nodes (medial node: caudomedial to the mandibular salivary gland, elongated, transversely compressed, bounded by the digastricus muscle cranially, longus colli muscle dorsally, sternocephalic muscle caudolaterally, and pharynx and larynx medially; lateral node: not seen in about one-third of dogs, much smaller and rounded, covered by or at the caudal margin of the parotid gland).

Normal lymph nodes on MRI are hypointense to surrounding fat on T1-weighted images, and slightly hypointense to surrounding fat on T2-weighted images (Kneissl and Probst, 2006). After gadolinium injection, normal nodes enhance so that they become isointense to the

surrounding fat on post-contrast T1-weighted series. No definitive criteria have been developed to differentiate lymphadenopathy of reactive or malignant origin. However, as has been described with other imaging modalities, significant node enlargement, rounded appearance and heterogeneous contrast enhancement with loss of margination are all features that increase the suspicion of malignancy. Comparison between the left and right side is often used to detect asymmetrical enlargement of lymph nodes.

Ultrasonography

Ultrasonography is not commonly used for the imaging of oral and maxillofacial conditions in dogs and cats. However, in certain applications it can be useful especially for the assessment and ultrasound-guided sampling of regional lymph nodes for cancer staging (Wisner *et al*., 1991). There are no clear criteria allowing ultrasonographic differentiation between reactive lymphadenitis and metastatic disease. Abnormal lymph nodes are enlarged and hypoechoic or heterogeneous. Loss of the oval shape to a more rounded shape, irregular/fuzzy margins, strong nodal hypoechogenicity and increased echogenicity of the perinodal fat have been reported to be present more commonly with neoplastic conditions. However, these features can also be seen with severe lymphadenitis (Lurie *et al*., 2006). Metastatic disease can also be present even in the absence of these ultrasonographic criteria. For these reasons, ultrasound-guided aspiration of suspect lymph nodes is an important part of cancer staging (Figure 4.74).

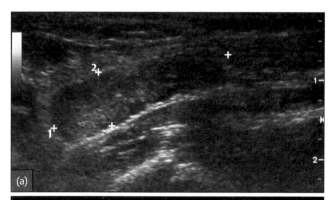

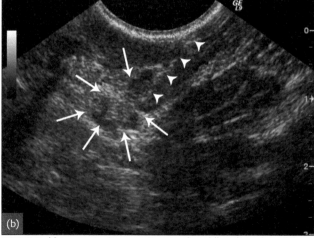

4.74 (a) Long-axis ultrasound image of a mildly enlarged medial retropharyngeal lymph node (between callipers) in a dog with sialadenitis. The node has mildly irregular margins, heterogeneous echostructure, and the perinodal fat is hyperechoic (reactive lymphadenitis on cytology). (b) Ultrasound-guided aspiration of a medial retropharyngeal lymph node in a dog. The needle is visible (arrowheads), as it is guided to the node (arrowed) for aspiration.

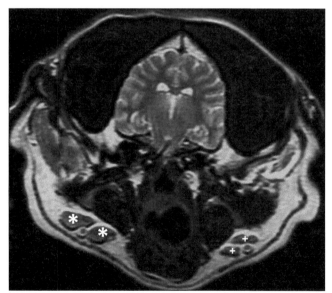

4.73 Transverse T2-weighted magnetic resonance image at the level of the mandibular lymph nodes in a dog with a squamous cell carcinoma along the right maxilla (same dog as in Figure 4.71). The right mandibular lymph nodes (∗) are enlarged compared to the left lymph nodes (+); they were aspirated and found to contain metastases.

The mandibular lymph nodes are easily accessible for blind fine-needle aspiration. Due to its deep location and proximity of vital structures such as vessels and nerves (common carotid artery, internal jugular vein, hypoglossal nerve, vagus nerve, and sympathetic nerves), blind aspiration of the medial retropharyngeal node is not warranted. This node, however, can be easily imaged with ultrasonography. Regardless of bodyweight or age, the average width in dogs is 1 cm (up to 2 cm), height is 0.5 cm (up to 1 cm) and length is 2.5 cm (up to 5 cm) (Burns et al., 2008). Useful landmarks to identify this node are the longus colli muscle, mandibular salivary gland, and common carotid artery. The node appears as an elongated (in a craniodorsal to caudoventral orientation), transversely compressed structure that is hypoechoic to the surrounding fat and salivary gland with a relatively homogeneous echostructure.

Palatine tonsils

The palatine tonsils can be readily assessed with MRI or CT. They are located at the lateral walls of the pharynx near the base of the tongue. On transverse MR images they appear as small protuberances that are mildly hyperintense to muscles on T2 and T1-weighted images (see Figure 4.58), and usually strongly enhance after contrast administration. It is easier to differentiate the tonsils from surrounding tissues with MRI than with CT. In the case of tonsillitis there is usually bilateral enlargement of the tonsils (Figure 4.75); with neoplasia, irregular asymmetrical enlargement is visible with extension of abnormal tissue beyond the normal anatomical boundaries often associated with marked retropharyngeal lymphadenopathy (Thierry et al., 2017).

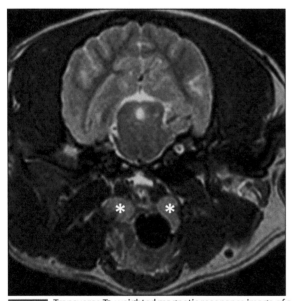

4.75 Transverse T2-weighted magnetic resonance image of a dog with tonsillitis. Both palatine tonsils (*) are swollen, protruding and hyperintense, consistent with oedema or inflammation.

Tongue

Besides using MRI, tongue conditions can be assessed with ultrasonography using a submental approach via a ventral, intermandibular window (Solano and Penninck, 1996). The mylohyoid and the geniohyoid muscles are identified as poorly echogenic structures ventral to the

tongue, though it is usually impossible to differentiate between these two muscles. The normal tongue is homogeneously finely echogenic. In cross-section (transverse plane) its shape varies from ovoid to bilobed. The left and right lingual arteries can be seen during parasagittal scanning as two anechoic to hypoechoic tubular structures with highly echogenic walls in the ventral third of the tongue; pulsating flow can be demonstrated on Doppler examination. At the caudal margin of the tongue the basihyoid bone creates a distinct acoustic shadow, and caudal to this the air in the pharynx obscures the area of the tonsils, which cannot therefore be readily assessed.

Ultrasonographic examination of the tongue may characterize tumours by revealing architecture, size and extension of a lesion (Figure 4.76). Although malignant and inflammatory lesions of the tongue are usually hypoechoic and occasionally cystic, hyperechoic lingual neoplasms have also been reported; therefore, diagnostic cytology or histopathology are necessary. Ultrasonography can also differentiate between solid versus fluid-filled lesions, such as abscesses, and can help identify foreign bodies due to their hyperechoic structure and associated acoustic shadowing. Response to treatment such as radiation therapy can also be monitored with ultrasonography. Sampling of small lesions is easily performed under ultrasonic guidance to obtain a cytopathological diagnosis.

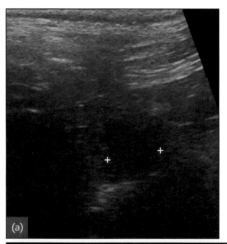

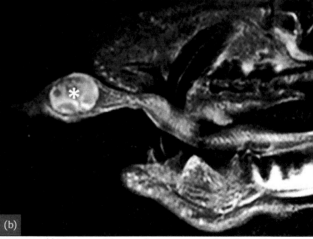

4.76 (a) Ultrasound image of a tongue mass in a Chow Chow, acquired using a ventral intermandibular approach. The hypoechoic mass (between callipers) stands out from the surrounding lingual muscles. (b) Sagittal T2-weighted magnetic resonance image of a haemangiosarcoma (*) in the tongue of a dog. The excellent soft tissue contrast of magnetic resonance imaging provides clear delineation of the tumour margin within the tongue, even before the use of contrast material.

Neuromuscular conditions

An animal presenting with a so-called dropped lower jaw cannot actively close the mouth, but an examiner can do so. This condition may be due to bilateral trigeminal neuropathy (mandibular neurapraxia) or bilateral mandibular fracture. Rarer causes include intracranial neoplasia such as lymphoma or meningioma affecting both trigeminal nerves, botulism, and a specific juvenile masticatory myositis in Cavalier King Charles Spaniels (Pitcher and Hahn, 2007). MRI is the imaging modality of choice to assess the brain and trigeminal nerves.

Masticatory muscle myositis (also called masticatory myositis) is an autoimmune disease against 2M fibres of the temporal, masseter and medial and lateral pterygoid muscles seen mostly in middle-aged, large-breed dogs. In the acute phase there is pain and muscle swelling; in chronic stages dogs present with inability to open their mouth and muscle atrophy. Both CT and MRI show characteristic findings of inflamed and fibrosed muscles with typical contrast enhancement and can be used for biopsy location guidance (Reiter and Schwarz, 2007). Although CT has proven quite useful in the diagnosis of neuromuscular diseases, MRI might be superior to CT due to its higher sensitivity to soft tissue changes (Bishop *et al.*, 2008; Cauduro *et al.*, 2013). On T2-weighted series, multifocal to coalescing, ill-defined and poorly marginated, hyperintense lesions can be seen in temporal, masseter and medial and lateral pterygoid muscles of dogs with masticatory muscle myositis. On T1-weighted images these lesions are usually isointense to normal muscle and enhance moderately to strongly after intravenous injection of gadolinium (Figure 4.77). Depending on the chronicity of the lesions, the muscles can be either enlarged or atrophied.

Salivary glands

The only contrast radiographic procedure that is still commonly performed on the head is sialography (Figure 4.78). This technique may be used to identify diseases of the salivary glands and their ducts. The patient needs to be anaesthetized, and survey head radiographs should be performed first. These are screened for areas of soft tissue swelling and mineralized sialoliths. The ducts of the zygomatic, parotid and mandibular glands can be cannulated; however, the duct of the sublingual gland, which is often of clinical interest, can be difficult to cannulate. Furthermore, it can have a common papilla (duct opening) with the mandibular duct. Iodine-based aqueous contrast medium is injected, and DV and lateral radiographs are obtained immediately afterwards. Radiographic interpretation is based on the assessment of ductal, parenchymal and extraglandular contrast uptake.

The same technique can also be used for CT sialography, which allows accurate assessment of ducts, glands and their connection to possible fluid-filled structures (sialoceles). Survey CT is important for scrutinizing

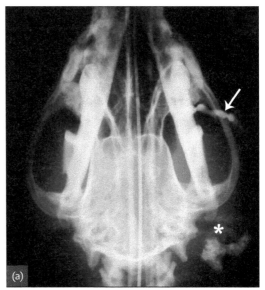

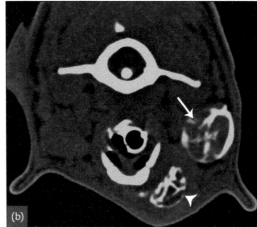

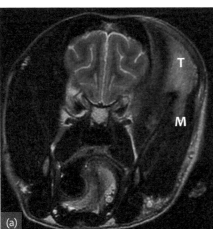

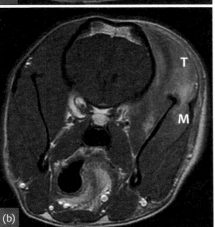

4.77 (a) Transverse T2-weighted and (b) T1-weighted post-contrast magnetic resonance images of a dog with masticatory muscle myositis. Note the areas of hyperintensity on the T2-weighted image in the left temporal (T) and masseter (M) muscles consistent with oedema, and the intense patchy contrast enhancement after gadolinium injection.

4.78 (a) Dorsoventral radiograph obtained following right zygomatic and parotid sialogram of a Border Collie with right facial swelling. The zygomatic duct (arrowed) is distended and irregularly shaped, and there is incomplete filling of the parotid gland (*). The diagnosis was zygomatic and parotid sialadenitis. (b) Sublingual and mandibular computed tomography sialography in a Labrador Retriever with a left-sided sublingual sialocele (ranula). The left mandibular gland (arrowed) shows normal contrast filling, whereas the left sublingual duct injection filled a sublingual sialocele (arrowhead).

the salivary ducts for obstructive sialoliths and the periglandular fat for oedematous changes with infection. The salivary duct can be obstructed or ruptured, neoplasia, cysts and abscesses can cause parenchymal filling defects, and contrast medium can extend through defects of the gland or duct into submucosal or subcutaneous spaces. In limbic epilepsy, salivary glands are often enlarged and asymmetrical but otherwise normal (consider the presence of sialadenosis). Intravenous contrast medium administration can reveal non-enhancing parenchyma consistent with a cyst, abscess or central necrosis (e.g. necrotizing sialometaplasia). Differentiation between neoplastic and inflammatory/infectious conditions is not always possible.

Due to the excellent soft tissue contrast obtained with MRI, the salivary glands are clearly differentiated from the adjacent fat and muscles even without gadolinium injection. Normal salivary glands are mildly to moderately hyperintense compared with muscles on T1-weighted pre-contrast and T2-weighted series and typically show moderate homogeneous contrast enhancement after gadolinium injection. The paired major salivary glands can routinely be evaluated with MRI. The parotid gland is located at the base of the ear ventral to the horizontal portion of the ear canal; it is V-shaped and has a lobulated appearance. The mandibular gland is ventral and medial to the parotid gland, oval-shaped and smoothly marginated. A hypointense hilus is usually seen in the mid-portion of the gland. The monostomatic part of the sublingual gland is intimately associated with the mandibular gland; its polystomatic part consists of several smaller glandular structures that surround the duct as it runs rostrally. The zygomatic gland is located caudal to the eye in the retrobulbar space; it is adjacent and immediately lateral to the medial pterygoid muscle, and in the transverse plane it is rectangular, trapezoid or triangular in shape with well defined borders and slightly lobulated margins. It is surrounded by hyperintense orbital fat (Figure 4.79).

Sialadenitis

Sialadenitis can be assessed with ultrasonography when inflammation affects an easily accessible gland such as the mandibular gland. When using ultrasonography, an inflamed gland appears enlarged, heterogeneous and is surrounded by hyperechoic heterogeneous tissue that often has a striated pattern due to oedema/cellulitis in the periglandular fat. Hypoechoic areas in an affected gland can represent regions of necrosis or abscessation (Figure 4.80). The zygomatic glands are better assessed with CT or MRI (Cannon *et al.*, 2011). When using MRI, an inflamed gland appears enlarged with fuzzy margins. It is hypointense on T1-weighted pre-contrast images, hyperintense on T2-weighted series and shows significant contrast enhancement on T1-weighted series after gadolinium injection (Figure 4.81). The enhancement is often heterogeneous, with non-enhancing areas that can correspond to areas of necrosis or sialocele formation as a result of the inflammation. The eye is frequently displaced by an enlarged zygomatic gland. Like CT, MRI provides more information than ultrasonography in the case of zygomatic sialadenitis. Although a retrobulbar mass can be detected with ultrasonography, it is usually not possible to confirm that the lesion originates from the salivary gland because of attenuation by the inflamed tissues and bony boundaries. The exact extent of the disease can be clearly defined with MRI, whereas it is impossible to do so with

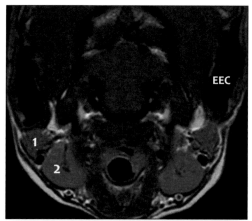

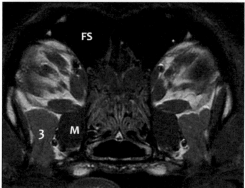

4.79 Transverse T1-weighted images in two dogs showing the normal magnetic resonance imaging appearance of the salivary glands. 1 = right parotid salivary gland; 2 = right mandibular salivary gland; 3 = right zygomatic salivary gland; EEC = left external ear canal; FS = right frontal sinus; M = medial pterygoid muscle.

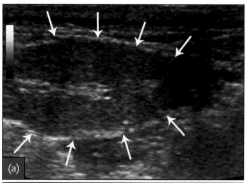

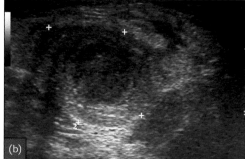

4.80 Long-axis ultrasonograms of the normal and inflamed mandibular salivary glands in a dog with mandibular sialadenitis. At histopathology, there was chronic active severe pyogranulomatous and fibrosing sialadenitis and cellulitis. (a) The normal gland (arrowed) is oval-shaped, has a well defined margin, a hypoechoic homogeneous parenchyma and a normal hyperechoic hilus. (b) The inflamed gland (between callipers) is enlarged, with a hyperechoic capsule and a hypoechoic core consistent with abscessation or necrosis. There is severe hyperechogenicity of the periglandular fat and soft tissues, with a striated pattern suggesting oedema/cellulitis.

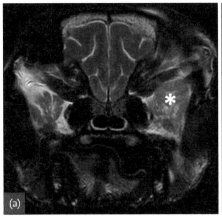 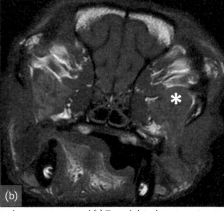 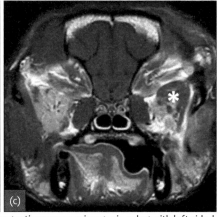

4.81 Transverse (a) T2-weighted, (b) T1-weighted pre-contrast and (c) T1-weighted post-contrast magnetic resonance images in a dog with left-sided zygomatic sialadenitis. Compared with the normal right gland, the affected gland (*) is enlarged, (a) T2-hyperintense, (b) contains patchy areas of T1-hypointensities on the T1-weighted pre-contrast series, and (c) after contrast administration contains patchy areas of enhancement, while some areas are not enhanced in comparison with similar regions of the normal contralateral gland, indicating areas of necrosis or infarction.

ultrasonography. Sialadenitis can affect other glands such as the mandibular glands, and MRI signs are similar (gland enlargement, changes in signal, heterogeneous signal enhancement and periglandular oedema/cellulitis often with satellite lymphadenitis) (Figure 4.82).

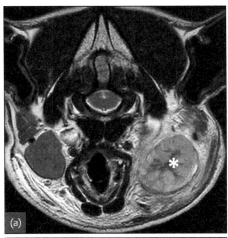

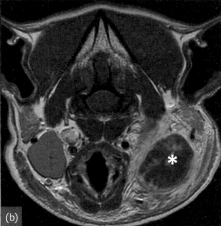

4.82 (a) T2-weighted and (b) T1-weighted post-contrast transverse magnetic resonance images in a dog with left-sided mandibular sialadenitis. The left salivary gland (*) is severely enlarged, T2-hyperintense and after gadolinium injection there are patchy areas of enhancement and hypointense non-enhancing areas (compared with the normal gland), consistent with areas of necrosis or infarction. At histopathology, there was severe diffuse necrotizing and pyogranulomatous sialadenitis with multifocal fibrinoid vasculitis (infarcts). Culture of biopsy samples grew *Enterococcus faecium* and *Staphylococcus simulans*.

Salivary mucocele

Salivary mucoceles (sialoceles) most commonly affect the sublingual salivary gland–duct complex in dogs. The zygomatic and parotid glands are rarely affected. A salivary mucocele is a collection of saliva that has leaked from a damaged salivary gland or its duct, resulting in accumulation of saliva in the deeper structures of the intermandibular space, angle of the lower jaw, pterygopalatine fossa or the upper cervical region, depending on the origin of the leakage. Possible causes include blunt trauma, foreign bodies and sialoliths, but sometimes the cause is not clear. Ultrasonography is a good imaging tool for investigating the source of the swelling. The appearance of a sialocele on ultrasonography varies depending on the age of the lesion (Torad and Hassan, 2013). Between 2 weeks and 1 month from the onset of clinical signs, a cervical mucocele appears as a round echogenic structure with a large volume of central anechoic content and a clearly identified hyperechoic rim surrounding the gland. Between 1 and 2 months from the onset of clinical signs, the volume of anechoic material appears less than that seen in the acute cases, and the overall appearance of the lesion is heterogeneous. In cases older than 2 months, the mass appears more grainy or mottled due to the presence of amorphous material, with a heterogeneous appearance and a further decrease in anechoic content.

Salivary gland tumours

It is not clear if MRI has superior diagnostic value compared with CT in the case of salivary gland tumours. Affected glands appear significantly enlarged with irregular margins and possible extension of the disease into the adjacent soft tissues. Signal intensity is heterogeneous on all pulse sequences, and patchy contrast enhancement is usually seen.

Foreign bodies

Foreign bodies typically penetrate areas in the sublingual area, palatoglossal fold, soft palate, palatine tonsil, floor of the orbit, or pharyngeal wall and can create deep and contaminated wounds. Ultrasonography, CT or MRI should be utilized to verify their exact location and facilitate foreign body removal (Figure 4.83).

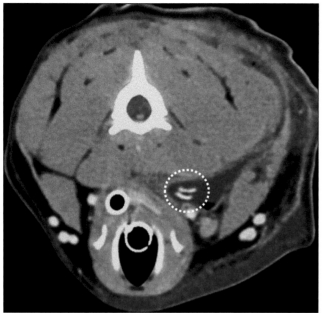

4.83 Intravenous contrast-enhanced computed tomographic image of a dog with a retropharyngeal stick injury. Two pieces of wood (within dotted circle), adjacent fluid and gas within an abscess capsule can be seen in the left retropharyngeal space.

References and further reading

Amory J, Reetz JA, Sanchez MD *et al.* (2014) Computed tomographic imaging characteristics of odontogenic neoplasms in dogs. *Veterinary Radiology and Ultrasound* **55**, 147–158

Arzi B, Chissell DD, Verstraete FJ *et al.* (2013) Computed tomographic findings in dogs and cats with temporomandibular joint disorders: 58 cases (2006–2011). *Journal of the American Veterinary Medical Association* **242**, 69–75

Bar-Am Y, Pollard RE, Kass PH *et al.* (2008) The diagnostic yield of conventional radiographs and computed tomography in dogs and cats with maxillofacial trauma. *Veterinary Surgery* **37**, 294–299

Bishop TM, Glass EN, De Lahunta A *et al.* (2008) Masticatory muscle myositis in a young dog. *Veterinary Radiology and Ultrasound* **49**, 270–272

Blazejewski SW, Lewis JR, Gracis M *et al.* (2010) Self-resolving mandibular swellings indicative of periostitis ossificans in immature large breed dogs: 5 cases (1999–2006). *Journal of Veterinary Dentistry* **27**, 148–159

Burns GO, Scrivani PV, Thompson MS *et al.* (2008) Relation between age, body weight, and medial retropharyngeal lymph node size in apparently healthy dogs. *Veterinary Radiology and Ultrasound* **49**, 277–281

Cannon MS, Paglia D, Zwingenberger AL *et al.* (2011) Clinical and diagnostic imaging findings in dogs with zygomatic sialadenitis: 11 cases (1990–2009). *Journal of the American Veterinary Medical Association* **239**, 1211–1218

Cauduro A, Paolo F and Asperio RM (2013) Use of MRI for the early diagnosis of masticatory muscle myositis. *Journal of the American Animal Hospital Association* **49**, 347–352

Dennis R (2006) Skull – general. In: *BSAVA Manual of Canine and Feline Musculoskeletal Imaging*, ed. FJ Barr and RM Kirberger, pp. 173–191. BSAVA Publications, Gloucester

De Paula-Silva FW, Wu MK, Leonardo MR *et al.* (2009) Accuracy of periapical radiography and cone-beam computed tomography scans in diagnosing apical periodontitis using histopathological findings as a gold standard. *Journal of Endodontics* **35**, 1009–1012

Doring S, Arzi B, Hatcher DC *et al.* (2018) Evaluation of the diagnostic yield of dental radiography and cone-beam computed tomography for the identification of dental disorders in small to medium-sized brachycephalic dogs. *American Journal of Veterinary Research* **79**, 62–72

Farcas N, Lommer MJ, Kass PH *et al.* (2014) Dental radiographic findings in cats with chronic gingivostomatitis (2002–2012). *Journal of the American Veterinary Medical Association* **244**, 339–345

Forrest L and Schwarz T (2011) Oral cavity, mandible, maxilla and dental apparatus. In: *Veterinary Computed Tomography*, ed. T Schwarz and J Saunders, pp. 111–124. Wiley-Blackwell, Ames

Kafka UCM, Carstens A, Steenkamp G *et al.* (2004) Diagnostic value of magnetic resonance imaging and computed tomography for oral masses in dogs. *Journal of the South African Veterinary Association* **75**, 163–168

Kneissl S and Probst A (2006) Magnetic resonance imaging features of presumed normal head and neck lymph nodes in dogs. *Veterinary Radiology and Ultrasound* **47**, 538–541

Lipsitz D, Levitski RE and Berry WL (2001) Magnetic resonance imaging features of multilobular osteochondrosarcoma in three dogs. *Veterinary Radiology and Ultrasound* **42**, 14–19

Lommer MJ and Verstraete FJ (2000) Prevalence of odontoclastic resorption lesions and periapical radiographic lucencies in cats: 265 cases (1995–1998). *Journal of the American Veterinary Medical Association* **217**, 1866–1869

Lommer MJ and Verstraete FJ (2001) Radiographic patterns of periodontitis in cats: 147 cases (1998–1999). *Journal of the American Veterinary Medical Association* **218**, 230–234

Luotonen N, Kunsti-Vaattovaara H, Sarklala-Kessel E *et al.* (2014) Vital pulp therapy in dogs: 190 cases (2001–2011). *Journal of the American Veterinary Medical Association* **244**, 449–459

Lurie DM, Seguin B, Schneider PD *et al.* (2006) Contrast-assisted ultrasound for sentinel lymph node detection in spontaneously arising canine head and neck tumors. *Investigative Radiology* **41**, 415–421

Macready DM, Hecht S, Craig LE *et al.* (2010) Magnetic resonance imaging features of the temporomandibular joint in normal dogs. *Veterinary Radiology and Ultrasound* **51**, 436–440

Meomartino L, Fatone G, Brunetti A *et al.* (1999) Temporomandibular joint ankylosis in the cat: a review of seven cases. *Journal of Small Animal Practice* **40**, 7–10

Morgan JP (1993) Radiography of the head. In: *Techniques of Veterinary Radiography, 5th edn*, ed. JP Morgan, pp. 121–133. Iowa State Press, Ames

Nemec A, Daniaux L, Johnson E *et al.* (2015) Craniomaxillofacial abnormalities in dogs with congenital palatal defects: computed tomographic findings. *Veterinary Surgery* **44**, 417–422

Peralta S, Verstraete JF and Kass PH (2010a) Radiographic evaluation of the types of tooth resorption in dogs. *American Journal of Veterinary Research* **71**, 784–793

Peralta S, Verstraete JF and Kass PH (2010b) Radiographic evaluation of the classification of the extent of tooth resorption in dogs. *American Journal of Veterinary Research* **71**, 794–798

Pitcher GDC and Hahn CN (2007) Atypical masticatory muscle myositis in three Cavalier King Charles Spaniel littermates. *Journal of Small Animal Practice* **48**, 226–228

Reiter AM and Schwarz T (2007) Computed tomographic appearance of masticatory myositis in dogs: seven cases (1999–2006). *Journal of the American Veterinary Medical Association* **231**, 924–930

Ryan JM, Fraga-Manteiga E, Schwarz T *et al.* (2013) Unilateral synostosis of the zygomaticotemporal suture associated with mandibular coronoid process impingement in a dog. *Veterinary Comparative Orthopaedics and Traumatology* **26**, 421–424

Schwarz T (2011) Temporomandibular joint and masticatory apparatus. In: *Veterinary Computed Tomography*, ed. T Schwarz and J Saunders, pp. 125–136. Wiley-Blackwell, Ames

Schwarz T, Weller R, Dickie AM *et al.* (2002) Imaging of the canine and feline temporomandibular joint: a review. *Veterinary Radiology and Ultrasound* **43**, 85–97

Seiler G, Rossi F, Vignoli M *et al.* (2007) Computed tomographic features of skull osteomyelitis in four young dogs. *Veterinary Radiology and Ultrasound* **48**, 544–549

Smallwood JE, Shively MJ, Rendano VT *et al.* (1985) A standardized nomenclature for radiographic projections used in veterinary medicine. *Veterinary Radiology* **26**, 2–9

Soukup JW, Drees R, Koening LJ *et al.* (2015) Comparison of the diagnostic image quality of the canine maxillary dentoalveolar structures obtained by cone beam computed tomography and 64-multidetector row computed tomography. *Journal of Veterinary Dentistry* **32**, 80–86

Solano M and Penninck DG (1996) Ultrasonography of the canine, feline and equine tongue: normal findings and case history reports. *Veterinary Radiology and Ultrasound* **37**, 206–213

Thierry F, Longo M, Pecceu E *et al.* (2017) Computed tomographic appearance of canine tonsillar neoplasia: 14 cases. *Veterinary Radiology and Ultrasound*, doi: 10.111/vru.12561

Ticer JW and Spencer CP (1978) Injury of the feline temporomandibular joint: radiographic signs. *Veterinary Radiology* **19**, 146–156

Torad FA and Hassan EA (2013) Clinical and ultrasonographic characteristics of salivary mucoceles in 13 dogs. *Veterinary Radiology and Ultrasound* **54**, 293–298

Tsugawa AJ and Verstraete FJ (2000) How to obtain and interpret periodontal radiographs in dogs. *Clinical Techniques in Small Animal Practice* **15**, 204–210

Tsugawa AJ, Verstraete FJ, Kass PH *et al.* (2003) Diagnostic value of the use of lateral and occlusal radiographic views in comparison with periodontal probing for the assessment of periodontal attachment on the canine teeth in dogs. *American Journal of Veterinary Research* **64**, 255–261

Verstraete FJ, Kass PH and Terpak CH (1998a) Diagnostic value of full-mouth radiography in dogs. *American Journal of Veterinary Research* **59**, 686–691

Verstraete FJ, Kass PH and Terpak CH (1998b) Diagnostic value of full-mouth radiography in cats. *American Journal of Veterinary Research* **59**, 692–695

Walker KS, Lewis JR, Durham AC *et al.* (2009) Diagnostic imaging in veterinary dental practice: Odontoma and impacted premolar. *Journal of the American Veterinary Medical Association* **253**, 1279–1281

Wisner ER, Mattoon JS, Nyland TG *et al.* (1991) Normal ultrasonographic anatomy of the canine neck. *Veterinary Radiology and Ultrasound* **32**, 185–190

OPERATIVE TECHNIQUE 4.1

Full-mouth dental radiographs in the dog

INDICATIONS

Diagnostic imaging of teeth, periodontal tissues and jaws.

POSITIONING

- Views 1–7: Sternal recumbency, ensuring the head is straight and the hard palate is parallel to the table when looking from the front and the side.
- Views 8–14: Dorsal recumbency, ensuring the head is straight and the hard palate parallel to the table when looking from the front and the side.
- The same views can also be obtained with the animal in lateral recumbency and the head and/or X-ray beam rotated as needed.

ASSISTANT

May be needed for film processing.

TECHNIQUE

General

In all views, bring the cone of the dental X-ray machine as close to the target as possible, ensuring the beam captures the desired teeth and periapical bone by centring the film/sensor pad/phosphor plate within the circumference of the cone. If necessary, use sponges or rubber tubes to keep the dental film/sensor pad/phosphor plate in the desired position. Wooden sticks or other instruments may be used to aid in visualizing the beam and bisecting angle. For any view, it is recommended that the cusps of the target teeth are placed close to the margin of the film (or sensor pad/phosphor plate) to increase the area of visualization and decrease the risk of projecting the root apices beyond the opposite border of the film.

> ### Key to coloured lines in figures
> - Yellow: X-ray beam
> - Blue: Long axis of the tooth
> - White: Plane of the dental film/sensor pad/phosphor plate
> - Red: Angle bisected between the blue and white lines.

View 1: Occlusal view of maxillary incisor and canine teeth

- Place the film horizontally on to the crowns of the maxillary canines and against the hard palate, ensuring that the film is inserted as caudally as possible in the mouth while the incisal edge of the incisor teeth is level with the margin of the film.
- Looking from the side, bisect the angle between the long axis of the canine teeth and the plane of the film.
- The beam should be perpendicular to the bisecting line.

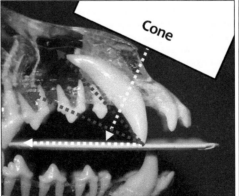
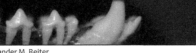
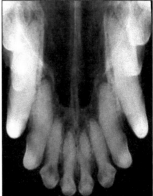

©Dr Alexander M. Reiter

→ OPERATIVE TECHNIQUE 4.1 CONTINUED

Views 2 and (for the opposite side; not shown) 3: Lateral views of maxillary canine teeth

- Place the film horizontally on to the crowns of the maxillary canine teeth and against the hard palate, ensuring that the tip of the canine tooth of the side of interest is placed close to the ipsilateral rostral corner of the film (right side is shown).
- Looking from the front, bisect the angle between the long axis of the canine tooth of the side of interest and the plane of the film.
- The beam should be perpendicular to the bisecting line.

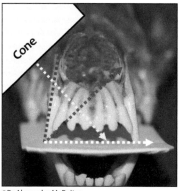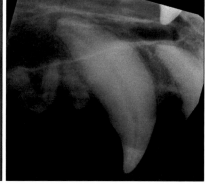

©Dr Alexander M. Reiter

Views 4 and (for the opposite side; not shown) 5: Lateral views of rostral maxillary cheek teeth

- Place the film as close to the hard palate as possible (often similar film position as for views 2 and 3; right side is shown).
- Looking from the front, bisect the angle between the long axis of the second or third premolar teeth of the side of interest and the plane of the film.
- The beam should be perpendicular to the bisecting line.
- Maxillary canine and rostral premolar teeth can often be visualized on the same view.

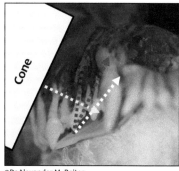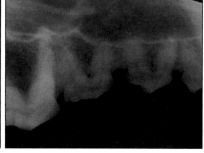

©Dr Alexander M. Reiter

Views 6 and (for the opposite side; not shown) 7: Lateral views of caudal maxillary cheek teeth

- Place the film as close to the hard palate as possible (right side is shown).
- Looking from the front, bisect the angle between the long axis of the mesiobuccal root of the fourth premolar tooth and the plane of the film. A slightly different angle may be necessary to correctly visualize the roots of the molar teeth.
- The beam should be perpendicular to the bisecting line.
- To correctly visualize all roots of three-rooted teeth, additional radiographs may have to be taken, slightly angling the beam rostrally or caudally from the initial position.

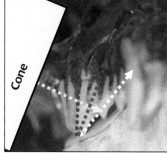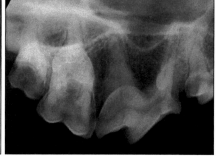

©Dr Alexander M. Reiter

View 8: Occlusal view of mandibular incisor and canine teeth

- Place the film on to the crowns of the canine teeth after rolling the tongue out of the way and into the pharynx, ensuring that the film is inserted as caudally as possible in the mouth while the incisal edge of the incisor teeth is level with the margin of the film.
- Looking from the side, bisect the angle between the long axis of the canine teeth and the plane of the film.
- The beam should be perpendicular to the bisecting line.

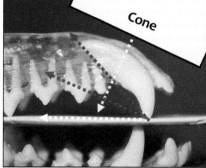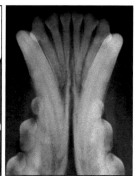

©Dr Alexander M. Reiter

→ **OPERATIVE TECHNIQUE 4.1 CONTINUED**

Views 9 and (for the opposite side; not shown) 10: Lateral views of mandibular canine and incisor teeth

- Place the film on to the crowns of the canine teeth after rolling the tongue out of the way and into the pharynx, ensuring that the tip of the canine tooth of the side of interest is placed close to the ipsilateral rostral corner of the film (left side is shown).
- Looking from the front, bisect the angle between the long axis of the canine tooth of the side of interest and the plane of the film.
- In some individuals, the beam may have to be slightly more vertical than perpendicular to the bisecting line to avoid superimposition of the canine tooth apex over the mandibular symphysis.

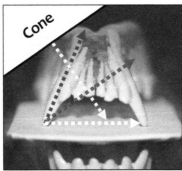
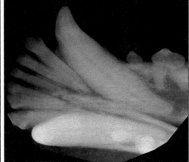

©Dr Alexander M. Reiter

Views 11 and (for the opposite side; not shown) 12: Lateral views of rostral mandibular cheek teeth

- Place the film as close to the mandible as possible and rostral enough to capture the first premolar tooth (often similar position as for views 9 and 10; left side is shown).
- Looking from the front, bisect the angle between the long axis of the first, second or third premolar teeth of the side of interest and the plane of the film.
- The beam should be perpendicular to the bisecting line.
- Mandibular canine and rostral premolar teeth can often be visualized on the same view.

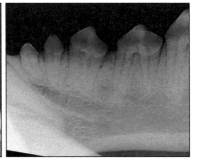
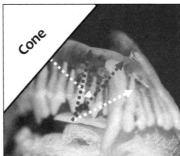

©Dr Alexander M. Reiter

Views 13 and (for the opposite side; not shown) 14: Lateral views of caudal mandibular cheek teeth

- Place the film between the mandible and tongue, as close as possible to the bone and as parallel as possible to the long axis of the mandibular body (left side is shown).
- Centre the beam on the mandibular first molar tooth.
- The beam should be perpendicular to the film.

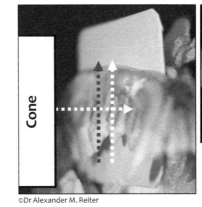
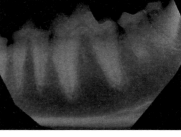

©Dr Alexander M. Reiter

OPERATIVE TECHNIQUE 4.2

Full-mouth dental radiographs in the cat

INDICATIONS

Diagnostic imaging of teeth, periodontal tissues and jaws.

POSITIONING

- Views 1–5: Sternal recumbency, ensuring the head is straight and the hard palate parallel to the table when looking from the front and the side.
- Views 6 and 7: Lateral recumbency, rotating the head slightly towards dorsal recumbency or the X-ray beam in the opposite direction.
- Views 8–12: Dorsal recumbency, ensuring the head is straight and the hard palate parallel to the table when looking from the front and the side.
- The same views can also be obtained with the animal in lateral recumbency and the head and/or X-ray beam rotated as needed.

ASSISTANT

May be needed for film processing.

TECHNIQUE

General

In all views, bring the cone of the dental X-ray machine as close to the target as possible, ensuring the beam captures the desired teeth and periapical bone by centring the film/sensor pad/phosphor plate within the circumference of the cone. If necessary, use sponges or rubber tubes to keep the dental film/sensor pad/phosphor plate in the desired position. Wooden sticks or other instruments may be used to aid in visualizing the beam and bisecting angle. For any view, it is recommended that the cusps of the target teeth are placed close to the margin of the film (or sensor pad/phosphor plate) to increase the area of visualization and decrease the risk of projecting the root apices beyond the opposite border of the film.

> #### Key to coloured lines in figures
> - Yellow: X-ray beam
> - Blue: Long axis of the tooth
> - White: Plane of the dental film/sensor pad/phosphor plate
> - Red: Angle bisected between the blue and white lines.

View 1: Occlusal view of maxillary incisor and canine teeth

- Place the film horizontally on to the crowns of the maxillary canine teeth and against the hard palate, ensuring that the film is inserted as caudally as possible in the mouth while the incisal edge of the incisor teeth is level with the margin of the film.
- Looking from the side, bisect the angle between the long axis of the canine teeth and the plane of the film.
- The beam should be perpendicular to the bisecting line.

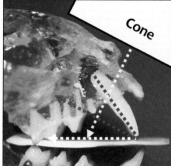
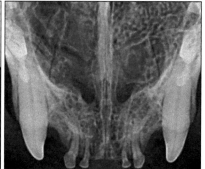

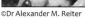
©Dr Alexander M. Reiter

→ **OPERATIVE TECHNIQUE 4.2 CONTINUED**

Views 2 and (for the opposite side; not shown) 3: Lateral views of the maxillary canine teeth

- Place the film horizontally on to the crowns of the maxillary canine teeth and against the hard palate, ensuring that the tip of the canine tooth of the side of interest is placed close to the ipsilateral rostral corner of the film (right side is shown).
- Looking from the front, bisect the angle between the long axis of the canine tooth of the side of interest and the plane of the film.
- The beam should be perpendicular to the bisecting line.

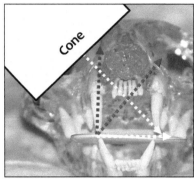
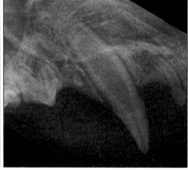

©Dr Alexander M. Reiter

Views 4 and (for the opposite side; not shown) 5: Lateral views of the maxillary cheek teeth

- Place the film on to the cusps of the maxillary second, third and fourth premolar teeth and first molar tooth of the side of interest and as close to the hard palate as possible (right side is shown; note the zygomatic arch overlapping the teeth).
- Looking from the front, bisect the angle between the long axis of the fourth premolar tooth and the plane of the film.
- The beam should be perpendicular to the bisecting line.

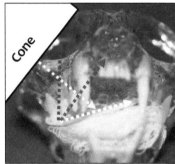
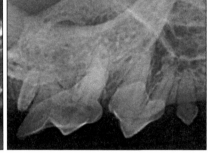

©Dr Alexander M. Reiter

Views 6 and (for the opposite side; not shown) 7: Extraoral views of the contralateral maxillary cheek teeth

This view reduces superimposition by the zygomatic arch, improving visualization of the dental roots (right side is shown; the yellow dot overlies the mesial aspect of the fourth premolar tooth).

- Open the cat's mouth with a plastic, radiolucent gag and place the film on the table under the head and parallel to the roots of the teeth to be radiographed.
- Slightly rotate the head of the patient ventrodorsally or the beam in a ventral direction.
- The beam should avoid crossing the crowns of the premolar teeth closer to the cone and run through the apex of the mesiopalatal root of the fourth premolar tooth closer to the table.

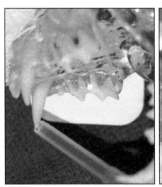
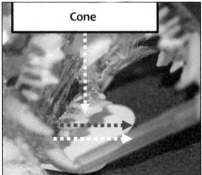
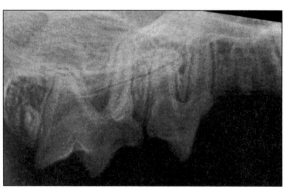

©Dr Alexander M. Reiter

→ **OPERATIVE TECHNIQUE 4.2 CONTINUED**

View 8: Occlusal view of mandibular incisor and canine teeth

- Place the film on to the crowns of the canine teeth after rolling the tongue out of the way and into the pharynx, ensuring that the film is inserted as caudally as possible in the mouth.
- Looking from the side, bisect the angle between the long axis of the canine teeth and the plane of the film.
- The beam should be perpendicular to the bisecting line.

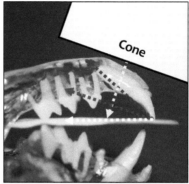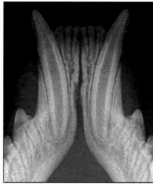

©Dr Alexander M. Reiter

Views 9 and (for the opposite side; not shown) 10: Lateral views of the mandibular canine teeth

- Place the film on to the crowns of the canine teeth after rolling the tongue out of the way and into the pharynx, ensuring that the tip of the canine tooth of the side of interest is placed close to the ipsilateral rostral corner of the film (left side is shown).
- Looking from the front, bisect the angle between the long axis of the canine tooth of the side of interest and the plane of the film.
- The beam should be slightly more vertical than perpendicular to the bisecting line to avoid superimposition of the canine tooth apex over the mandibular symphysis.

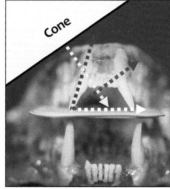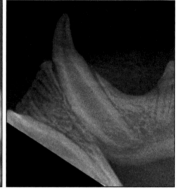

©Dr Alexander M. Reiter

Views 11 and (for the opposite side; not shown) 12: Lateral views of the mandibular cheek teeth

- Place the film between the mandible and tongue, as close as possible to the bone and as parallel as possible to the long axis of the mandibular body (left side is shown). The film should be pushed ventrally to visualize the ventral mandibular cortex.
- The beam should be perpendicular to the film. In some cats, the third premolar tooth cannot be correctly visualized with this view because the mandibular symphysis may impede the correct placement of the film. If this is the case, the bisecting angle technique shown in views 9 and 10 should be used instead.

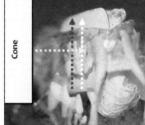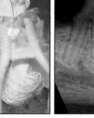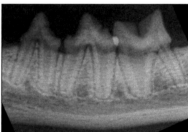

©Dr Alexander M. Reiter

Chapter 5

Commonly encountered dental and oral pathologies

Alexander M. Reiter

This chapter provides information about dental and oral pathologies commonly encountered in cats and dogs. The information is deliberately kept brief for conditions that are covered in greater detail in other chapters.

Periodontal disease

The periodontium is a functional unit consisting of the gingiva, periodontal ligament, alveolar bone and cementum. Periodontal disease is inflammation and infection of the periodontium by plaque bacteria and the host's response to the bacterial insult. Small dog breeds and older animals have a higher risk of developing periodontal disease (Harvey *et al.*, 1994; Holmstrom, 2012).

Types of periodontal disease
Gingivitis

Gingivitis is inflammation of the gingiva. It presents clinically as reddening and oedema of the tissue, initially starting at the gingival margin and later progressing to visible ulceration with spontaneous bleeding (Figure 5.1). It does not inevitably progress to periodontitis, but gingivitis always precedes periodontitis (Reiter *et al.*, 2012). With continued inflammation, the gingiva detaches from the tooth (Figure 5.2), creating a periodontal pocket. A shift occurs in the gingival flora from a Gram-positive aerobic to a Gram-negative anaerobic spectrum. The release of

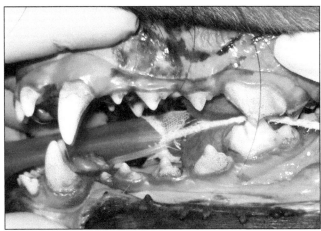

5.1 Generalized, marginal gingivitis with mild to moderate plaque and calculus accumulation in a dog.
(© Dr Alexander M. Reiter)

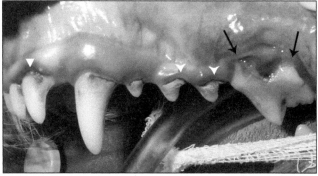

5.2 Gingivitis with mild (arrowheads) and severe (arrowed) gingival recession in a dog with moderate plaque and calculus accumulation.
(© Dr Alexander M. Reiter)

endotoxins and enzymes from the bacteria and white blood cells is destructive to the tissues. Gingivitis is treated by plaque control; professional dental cleaning followed by home oral hygiene (such as daily toothbrushing) can resolve gingivitis (Reiter *et al.*, 2012).

Periodontitis

Periodontitis is the more severe form of periodontal disease, which also affects the non-gingival components of the periodontium (i.e. the periodontal ligament, cementum and alveolar bone). It results in loss of attachment and recession of the gingiva (root surface exposure caused by apical migration of the gingival margin or loss of gingiva), furcation exposure, formation of periodontal pockets and loss of alveolar bone (Lommer and Verstraete, 2001; Rawlinson and Reiter, 2005; Reiter and Harvey, 2010) (Figure 5.3). With increasing bone loss, the tooth becomes mobile and ultimately exfoliates (Harvey, 2005). Bacterial infection of the pulp is possible in areas devoid of cementum and through apical and non-apical ramifications. Periodontitis probably exists (or has previously occurred, because the actual inflammation may have ceased) when gingival recession exposes part of the root, a periodontal probe detects a periodontal pocket apical to the cemento-enamel junction, the tooth is mobile, and radiographs show horizontal or vertical alveolar bone loss (Harvey, 1998, 2005; Reiter and Harvey, 2010) (Figure 5.4). The goals of treatment are elimination of supra- and subgingival plaque and its associated microflora, and surgical reduction of periodontal pockets. Teeth should be extracted if they cannot be salvaged.

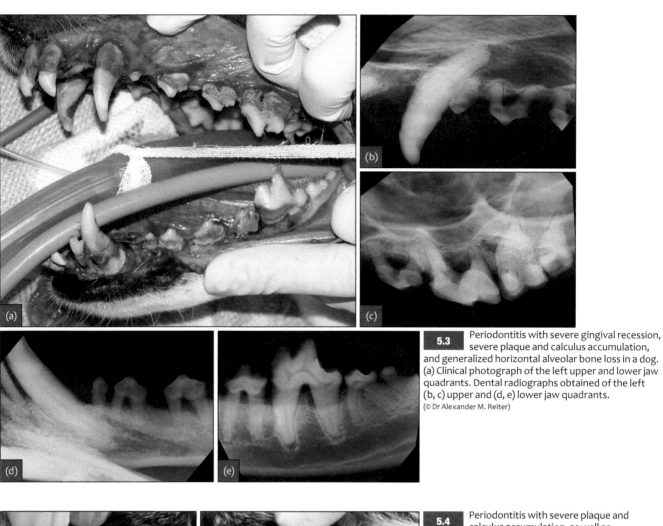

5.3 Periodontitis with severe gingival recession, severe plaque and calculus accumulation, and generalized horizontal alveolar bone loss in a dog. (a) Clinical photograph of the left upper and lower jaw quadrants. Dental radiographs obtained of the left (b, c) upper and (d, e) lower jaw quadrants.
(© Dr Alexander M. Reiter)

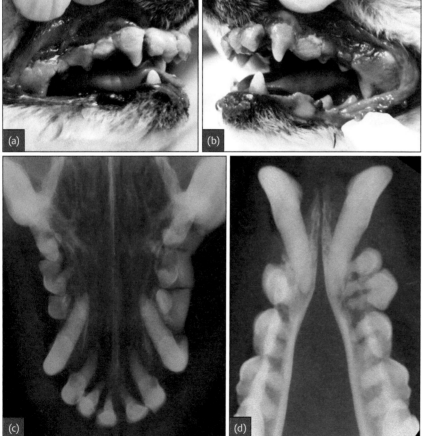

5.4 Periodontitis with severe plaque and calculus accumulation, as well as generalized horizontal and vertical alveolar bone loss in a dog. (a, b) Clinical photographs and (c, d) dental radiographs.
(© Dr Alexander M. Reiter)

Causes of periodontal disease

Plaque

A biofilm develops within hours on a clean tooth surface following professional dental cleaning. When home oral hygiene is insufficient or infrequent, dental plaque thickens and matures. Aerobic bacteria in deeper parts of the plaque layer consume any remaining oxygen, creating an anaerobic environment that is favourable for the development of anaerobic periodontopathogens (Reiter and Harvey, 2010). Aerobic cocci initially colonize the pellicle, which is a glycoprotein layer deposited on the surface of teeth after evaporation of the salivary fluid. Aerobic rods then adhere to the coccal layer. Both aerobic cocci and rods multiply, decreasing the available oxygen in the deeper layers of the plaque, and obligate anaerobes start growing. With continued plaque maturation (enriched by inflammatory products), periodontopathogens begin to thrive in an environment that is anoxic and rich in nutrients. This process can take less than 24 hours (Hennet and Harvey, 1992; Reiter and Harvey, 2010).

Periodontopathogens

Periodontopathogens are bacteria that can:

- Be cultured more readily from diseased individuals than from non-diseased individuals and from diseased areas of the mouth than from healthy areas in the same individual
- Produce toxins or tissue-destructive enzymes (e.g. matrix metalloproteinases)
- Show cytotoxic effects on tissue culture
- Reveal other 'virulent factors' (Reiter and Harvey, 2010).

The Gram-negative anaerobic rod *Porphyromonas gingivalis* is considered to be the key human periodontopathogen. A catalase-positive form of *P. gingivalis*, called *P. gulae*, can be found in dogs and cats (Fournier *et al.*, 2001). There are several other bacteria (including spirochaetes) that are recognized as periodontopathogens in small companion animals (Harvey *et al.*, 1995; Valdez *et al.*, 2000; Love *et al.*, 2002; Hardham *et al.*, 2005; Radice *et al.*, 2006; Hamada *et al.*, 2008; Nordhoff *et al.*, 2008; Booij-Vrieling *et al.*, 2010; Kato *et al.*, 2011; Riggio *et al.*, 2011; Senhorinho *et al.*, 2011; Dahlen *et al.*, 2012; Yamasaki *et al.*, 2012; Pérez-Salcedo *et al.*, 2013; Khazandi *et al.*, 2014; Pérez-Salcedo *et al.*, 2015).

The host's response

Neutrophils are attracted to the site of bacterial infection, engulfing, ingesting and digesting the plaque bacteria, with this process manifesting clinically as gingivitis. 'Bursting' neutrophils release bacterial toxins and destructive enzymes, which cause the breakdown of connective tissue integrity, and pro-inflammatory cytokines which propagate the inflammatory response (Reiter and Harvey, 2010). The epithelium within the gingival sulcus becomes ulcerated and the gingival connective tissue is exposed to direct bacterial invasion. As the infection and inflammation continue into deeper layers of the periodontium, periodontitis develops with resorption of alveolar bone. If the process continues without intervention, the tooth becomes mobile and eventually exfoliates (Reiter and Harvey, 2010).

Systemic effects of periodontal disease

Bacteraemia secondary to periodontal disease occurs frequently in patients with periodontal disease. In otherwise healthy patients, it is rapidly cleared by the reticuloendothelial system (Silver *et al.*, 1975; Reiter *et al.*, 2012). Thus, perioperative use of antibiotics is only required in patients with pre-existing conditions that could worsen during or after the dental or oral surgical procedure (see Chapter 13). In addition to bacteraemia, there is a chronic release of inflammatory mediators, immune complexes and by-products of bacterial and cellular degradation into the blood and lymph vessels, which may produce direct or immune-mediated distant organ pathology (Reiter *et al.*, 2012).

The systemic effects of periodontal disease have been well documented in humans (heart disease and stroke, diabetes, respiratory disease, and an increased risk of premature delivery and low birth weight infants) (Wolf *et al.*, 2005) and are being increasingly investigated in dogs and cats (DeBowes *et al.*, 1996; DeBowes, 1998; Pavlica *et al.*, 2008; Glickman *et al.*, 2009; Peddle *et al.*, 2009; Glickman *et al.*, 2011; Rawlinson *et al.*, 2011; Cave *et al.*, 2012; Kouki *et al.*, 2013; Nemec *et al.*, 2013; O'Neill *et al.*, 2013). It has recently been shown that cats with periodontal disease are at an increased risk of developing chronic kidney disease, and that this risk increases with severity of the dental disease (Trevejo *et al.*, 2018).

Diagnosis of periodontal disease

The diagnosis of periodontal disease (including the use of instruments to measure gingival sulcus, gingival and periodontal pocket depths, as well as score tooth mobility, furcation exposure, plaque index, calculus index and gingival index, and periodontal disease classification along with radiographic examination of the teeth and alveolar bone) is described in Chapter 3 (see also Boyce and Logan, 1994; Hefferren *et al.*, 1994; Logan and Boyce, 1994; Hennet, 1999; Harvey *et al.*, 2008; Scherl *et al.*, 2009; Harvey *et al.*, 2012). Quantitative light-induced fluorescence (QLF™) was recently determined to be a reliable, reproducible method for the assessment of plaque deposition in cats (Marshall-Jones *et al.*, 2017).

Treatment of periodontal disease

Professional dental cleaning refers to scaling (supragingival and subgingival plaque and calculus removal) and polishing of the teeth with power/hand instrumentation performed by a trained veterinary healthcare provider under general anaesthesia. Closed periodontal therapy focuses on root planing, gingival curettage and the local administration of antiseptics/antibiotics. Open periodontal therapy is accomplished after the creation of periodontal flaps, thus allowing osseous and regenerative surgery. Home oral hygiene refers to measures taken by pet owners that are aimed at controlling or preventing plaque and calculus accumulation (Reiter *et al.*, 2012). For detailed information about the treatment of periodontal disease and home oral hygiene, see Chapters 7 and 13.

Gingival enlargement

Gingival enlargement is a clinical term that refers to the overgrowth or thickening of gingiva in the absence of a histological diagnosis (Figure 5.5). It is often due to gingival hyperplasia (a histological term referring to an abnormal

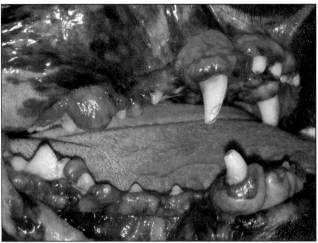

5.5 Generalized gingival enlargement in a dog.
(© Dr Alexander M. Reiter)

increase in the number of normal cells in a normal arrangement). Gingival hyperplasia manifests clinically as gingival enlargement and the formation of gingival pockets (or pseudopockets) (Lewis and Reiter, 2005). Gingival hyperplasia may affect genetically predisposed individuals or can be caused by gingivitis, hormonal changes and the administration of anticonvulsants, ciclosporin and calcium-channel blockers (Nam *et al.*, 2008; Thomason *et al.*, 2009; Pariser and Berdoulav, 2011; Namikawa et al., 2012).

Juvenile hyperplastic gingivitis occurs in adolescent cats after eruption of the permanent dentition at about 6 to 8 months of age, with the inflamed gingiva being enlarged to such a degree that it can cover the crowns of the teeth (Figure 5.6). It is not known whether juvenile hyperplastic

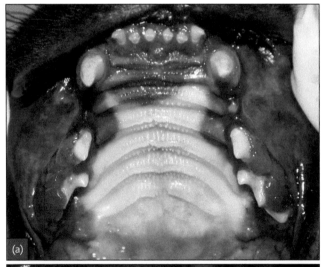

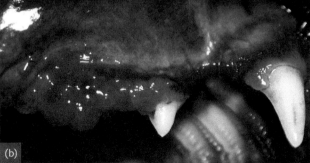

5.6 (a) Occlusal and (b) lateral views of the teeth in a 6-month-old cat with juvenile hyperplastic gingivitis.
(© Dr Margherita Gracis)

gingivitis is a precursor to a more severe oral inflammation that progresses to stomatitis in the adult cat (Reiter, 2012).

Treatment of gingival enlargement involves cessation of its cause and removal of excess gingiva. Gingivectomy is the gross removal of excess gingiva, while gingivoplasty is a form of gingivectomy performed to restore the physiological contours of the gingiva. Because most cat teeth have less than 2 mm of attached gingiva, gingival surgery should be carefully executed in this species and is often reserved for canine teeth and teeth with significant gingival enlargement (Reiter, 2012). See Chapter 7 for detailed information about the diagnosis and treatment of gingival enlargement.

Oral soft tissue and bone inflammation

Oral soft tissue inflammation

Contact mucositis and contact mucosal ulceration are lesions in susceptible individuals that are secondary to mucosal contact with a tooth surface bearing the causative irritant, allergen or antigen. They have also been called 'contact ulcers' and 'kissing lesions' and are more often recognized in dogs (Figure 5.7) (Lommer, 2013). More widespread oral inflammation is primarily seen in adult cats and is characterized by persistent chronic inflammation of the oral mucosa. The aetiology of feline stomatitis is poorly understood, but feline calicivirus and possibly other viruses are suspected to play an important role. Affected cats are often presented with a long history of halitosis, drooling of saliva, pawing at the face, pain upon eating and drinking, difficulty swallowing and weight loss. Oral lesions appear as focal or diffuse inflammation involving the gingiva, alveolar mucosa, labial and buccal mucosa, sublingual mucosa, and the mucosal region lateral to the palatoglossal folds (Figure 5.8) (Lommer, 2013).

The goals of treatment are to remove the inciting causes, control oral plaque accumulation and decrease the inflammatory and immunological responses of the host. Medicinal treatment options include local and systemic administration of immunosuppressive, immunomodulatory and immunostimulatory, anti-inflammatory, analgesic, antiseptic and/or antibiotic medications. Surgical treatment options include partial and full-mouth tooth extraction and

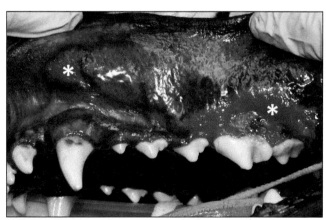

5.7 Gingivitis and contact mucosal inflammation (contact mucositis) in a dog. The area of alveolar, labial and buccal mucosa that would be in contact with the plaque-laden tooth surfaces is ulcerated (*).
(© Dr Alexander M. Reiter)

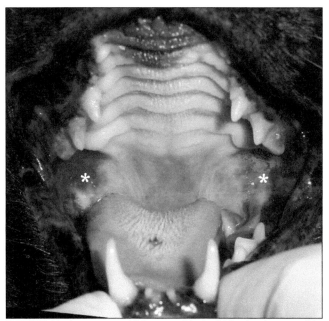

5.8 Moderate stomatitis in a cat with gingivitis, alveolar mucositis and inflammation of the mucosa of the caudal oral cavity (∗). Note also the missing incisor teeth, gingival recession at the mandibular canine teeth, and severe plaque and calculus accumulation at the maxillary cheek teeth. The palatal mucosa, however, is devoid of inflammation.
(© Dr Alexander M. Reiter)

laser surgery (Jennings *et al.*, 2015). For detailed information about the diagnosis and treatment of oral soft tissue inflammation, see Chapter 8.

Osteomyelitis and osteonecrosis

Osteomyelitis is a local or generalized inflammation of bone and bone marrow, usually resulting from bacterial or, less commonly, fungal infection. Osteomyelitis can arise from an endodontic infection, an infection through the periodontal ligament space, an extraction wound, open jaw fracture or spread from a local or remote area of infection. If untreated, the acute form may progress to a chronic form, eventually leading to bone necrosis. Treatment involves tooth extraction, aggressive soft and hard tissue debridement, and administration of systemic antibiotics (Peralta *et al.*, 2015). Osteonecrosis of jaw bones may also be caused after radiation therapy of nasal (Adams *et al.*, 2005) and oral tumours (Nemec *et al.*, 2015). See Chapter 8 for detailed information about the diagnosis and treatment of osteomyelitis and osteonecrosis.

Autoimmune conditions affecting the mouth and masticatory apparatus

Pemphigus vulgaris is an autoimmune disease characterized histologically by intraepithelial blister formation (after the breakdown or loss of intercellular adhesion), biochemically by evidence of circulating autoantibodies against components of the epithelial desmosome–tonofilament complexes, and clinically by the presence of vesiculobullous and/or ulcerative oral and mucocutaneous lesions (Figure 5.9) (Lommer, 2013; Rybníček and Hill, 2007).

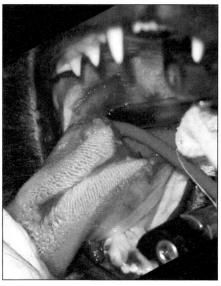

5.9 Pemphigus vulgaris in a cat with inflammation of the dorsal surface of the tongue and palatoglossal folds.
(© Dr Alexander M. Reiter)

Bullous pemphigoid is an autoimmune disease characterized histologically by subepithelial clefting (separation at the epithelium–connective tissue interface), biochemically by evidence of circulating autoantibodies against components of the basement membrane, and clinically by the presence of erythematous, erosive, vesiculobullous and/or ulcerative oral lesions (Figure 5.10) (Lommer, 2013).

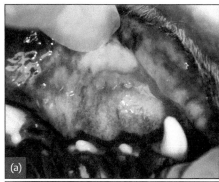
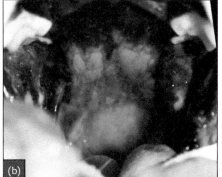
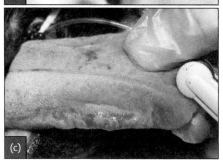

5.10 Bullous pemphigoid in a dog with inflammation of the (a) mucocutaneous junction and labial/buccal mucosa, (b) mucosa at the transition between the hard and soft palate and (c) dorsolateral tongue surface.
(© Dr Alexander M. Reiter)

Lupus erythematosus is an autoimmune disease characterized histologically by basal cell destruction, hyperkeratosis, epithelial atrophy, subepithelial and perivascular lymphocytic infiltration and vascular dilatation with submucosal oedema, biochemically by evidence of circulating autoantibodies against various cellular antigens in both the nucleus and cytoplasm, and clinically by the presence of acute lesions (systemic lupus erythematosus) on the skin, mucosa and multiple organs, or chronic lesions (discoid lupus erythematosus) mostly confined to the skin of the face and mucosa of the oral cavity (Lommer, 2013; Olivry *et al.*, 2015).

Masticatory muscle myositis is an autoimmune disease affecting the temporal, masseter, and medial and lateral pterygoid muscles of the dog. The term masticatory myositis is an acceptable alternative (Reiter and Schwarz, 2007). For detailed information about the diagnosis and treatment of these conditions, the reader is referred to Chapter 8.

Abnormal number, size and morphology of teeth

A persistent deciduous tooth is a primary tooth that is present when it should have exfoliated (Figure 5.11). A supernumerary tooth is an extra tooth (also called hyperdontia) (Figure 5.12). Hypodontia is the developmental absence of a few teeth, while oligodontia is the developmental absence of numerous teeth and anodontia is a failure of all teeth to develop. These terms must not be used for unerupted teeth or those that are missing as a result of exfoliation or extraction (Verhaert, 2007).

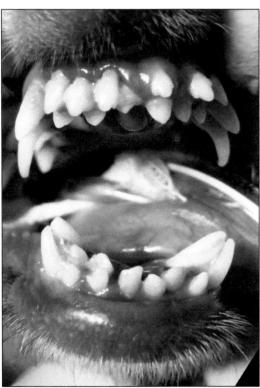

5.11 Persistence of multiple deciduous teeth in a young adult dog. Crowding of teeth led to entrapment of debris, plaque and calculus accumulation, and early onset of periodontal disease.
(© Dr Alexander M. Reiter)

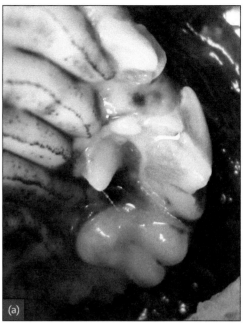

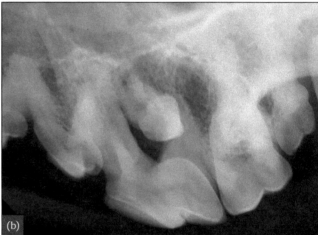

5.12 (a) Clinical photograph and (b) dental radiograph showing a supernumerary tooth palatal to the left maxillary fourth premolar tooth in a dog. There was severe bone loss noted upon periodontal probing with discharge of mucopurulent material.
(© Dr Alexander M. Reiter)

Macrodontia refers to a tooth that is larger than normal, and microdontia refers to a tooth that is smaller than normal. Fusion is the combining of adjacent tooth germs, resulting in partial or complete union of the developing teeth. Concrescence is the fusion of the roots of two or more teeth at the cementum level. Fused roots are the fusion of roots of the same tooth. Gemination (also called twinning) is a single tooth bud's attempt to divide partially (cleft of the crown) or completely (presence of an identical supernumerary tooth) (Verhaert, 2007).

A supernumerary root refers to the presence of an extra root (Figure 5.13). Dilaceration is a disturbance in tooth development, causing the crown or root to be abruptly bent or crooked. Dens invaginatus (also called dens in dente) refers to an invagination of the outer surface of a tooth into the interior, occurring in either the crown (involving the pulp chamber) or the root (involving the root canal). An enamel pearl is a small, nodular growth on the root of a tooth made of enamel with or without a small dentine core and sometimes a covering of cementum (Verhaert, 2007). For detailed information about the diagnosis and treatment of developmental abnormalities of teeth, see Chapter 10.

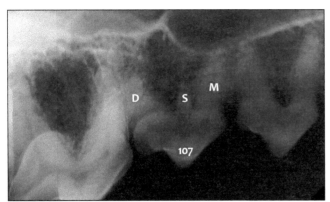

5.13 Supernumerary root (S) in between the mesial (M) and distal (D) roots of the right maxillary third premolar tooth (107) in a dog.
(© Dr Alexander M. Reiter)

Abnormal eruption of teeth

Eruption is sometimes delayed for weeks and occasionally for months (Hoffman, 2008). Familial delayed eruption occurs in Tibetan and Wheaten Terriers and probably also in other dog breeds. Delayed eruption of deciduous and permanent teeth has also been observed in dogs affected by myotonia congenita (Gracis *et al.*, 2000). Folliculitis is inflammation of the follicle of a developing tooth. Pericoronitis is inflammation of the soft tissues surrounding the crown of a partially erupted tooth. Transposition refers to two teeth that have exchanged position.

An unerupted tooth is a tooth that has not perforated the oral mucosa (Figure 5.14). An embedded tooth is an unerupted tooth whose eruption is compromised by lack of eruptive force. An impacted tooth is an unerupted tooth

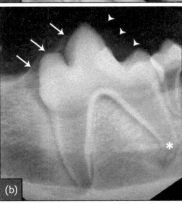

5.14 (a) Delayed eruption of the permanent left canine (204 and 304) and carnassial (208 and 309) teeth in a young adult dog. (b) The dental radiograph of the unerupted permanent left mandibular first molar tooth shows bony (arrowed) and fibrous (arrowheads) tissue surrounding its crown. Note also the dilaceration (*) at the apex of the distal root of the unerupted tooth.
(© Dr Alexander M. Reiter)

whose eruption is prevented by contact with a physical barrier (Edstrom *et al.*, 2013; Carle and Shope, 2014).

A dentigerous cyst is an odontogenic cyst (also called a follicular or tooth-containing cyst) initially formed around the crown of an unerupted tooth (Figure 5.15). Bone and root resorption accompany cystic enlargement and may lead to severe jaw weakening. Therefore, unerupted teeth should be extracted utilizing an open extraction technique and any epithelial cyst lining should be carefully curetted out to avoid recurrence. The lining has also been reported to be able to undergo neoplastic metaplasia; even though evidence for this is limited, it is advisable to submit the removed tissues for histopathological examination (Gioso and Carvalho, 2003; D'Astous, 2011; Verstraete *et al.*, 2011; MacGee *et al.*, 2012; Kim *et al.*, 2013; Babbitt *et al.*, 2016; Thatcher, 2017). The reader is referred to Chapter 10 for detailed information about the diagnosis and treatment of tooth eruption abnormalities.

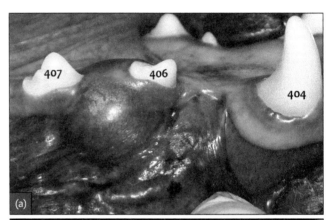

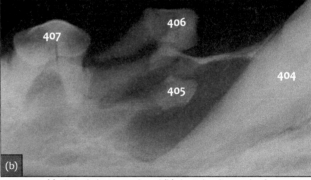

5.15 (a) Clinical photograph and (b) dental radiograph of a dentigerous cyst with significant bone loss between the right mandibular canine (404) and third premolar (407) teeth in an adult dog. The cyst originates from the unerupted first premolar tooth (405). The second premolar tooth (406) is displaced and the roots are partially resorbed by the pressure exerted from the cystic lesion.
(© Dr Alexander M. Reiter)

Malocclusion

Malocclusion refers to any deviation from normal occlusion and may be due to abnormal positioning of a tooth or teeth (dental malocclusion) or due to asymmetry or other deviation of bones that support the dentition (skeletal malocclusion) (AVDC, 2017).

Dental malocclusion

Neutroclusion (class 1 malocclusion) refers to malposition of one or more individual teeth. This may be present with or without skeletal malocclusion. A tooth may be in its anatomically correct position in the dental arch but is abnormally angled in a distal (distoversion), mesial (mesioversion), lingual (linguoversion), palatal (palatoversion), labial (labioversion) or buccal (buccoversion) direction. Crossbite describes a dental malocclusion in which one or more mandibular teeth have a more labial (rostral crossbite) or buccal (caudal crossbite) position than one or more antagonist maxillary teeth (AVDC, 2017).

Skeletal malocclusion
Symmetrical skeletal malocclusion

Mandibular distocclusion (class 2 malocclusion) refers to an abnormal rostrocaudal relationship between the dental arches in which the lower arch occludes caudal to its normal position relative to the upper arch. Mandibular mesiocclusion (class 3 malocclusion) refers to an abnormal rostrocaudal relationship between the dental arches in which the lower arch occludes rostral to its normal position relative to the upper arch (AVDC, 2017).

Asymmetrical skeletal malocclusion

Maxillomandibular asymmetry (class 4 malocclusion) refers to asymmetry in a rostrocaudal, side-to-side or dorsoventral direction (AVDC, 2017).

- Maxillomandibular asymmetry in a rostrocaudal direction occurs when mandibular mesiocclusion or distocclusion is present on one side of the face while the contralateral side retains normal dental alignment.
- Maxillomandibular asymmetry in a side-to-side direction occurs when there is loss of the midline alignment of the maxilla and mandible.
- Maxillomandibular asymmetry in a dorsoventral direction results in an open bite, which is defined as an abnormal vertical space between opposing dental arches when the mouth is closed.

Management of malocclusion

Preventive orthodontics are procedures undertaken in anticipation of a problem developing (AVDC, 2017). It requires knowledge of the development of the dentition and maxillofacial structures, and includes the diagnostic procedures undertaken to predict malocclusion and the therapeutic procedures instituted to prevent its onset. Examples of preventive procedures include:

- Client education about timetables for exfoliation of deciduous teeth and eruption of permanent teeth
- Fibrotomy (severing of gingival fibres around a permanent tooth to prevent its relapse after corrective orthodontics)
- Operculectomy (surgical removal of an operculum to enable eruption of a permanent tooth)
- Extraction of a tooth that, if left, could result in the development of malocclusion.

Interceptive orthodontics is concerned with the elimination of a developing or established malocclusion. Interceptive procedures are typically undertaken in the growing patient (AVDC, 2017). Examples of interceptive procedures include:

- Crown reduction of a permanent tooth in malocclusion
- Extraction of a tooth in malocclusion.

Corrective orthodontics is concerned with the correction of malocclusion without loss of the maloccluded tooth or part of its crown. This is accomplished by means of tooth movement (AVDC, 2017). Examples of corrective procedures include:

- Surgical repositioning of a tooth
- Orthognathic surgery to treat skeletal malocclusion
- Passive movement of a tooth using an inclined plane
- Active movement of a tooth using an elastic chain.

See Chapter 10 for detailed information about the diagnosis and treatment of malocclusion.

Defects of dental hard tissues
Tooth resorption

Tooth resorption refers to resorption of dental hard tissue. Internal resorption is tooth resorption that originates from within the pulp cavity (Figure 5.16). External resorption is tooth resorption that originates from the outside surface of the tooth. It is classified based on the severity of the resorption (stages 1–5) (Figure 5.17) and on the radiographic appearance of the resorption (types 1–3) (Figure 5.18) (AVDC, 2017).

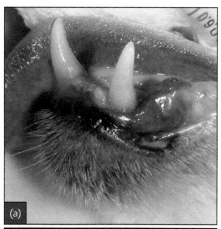

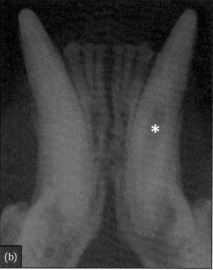

5.16 (a) Both mandibular canine teeth in this cat appeared unremarkable on clinical oral examination. (b) However, a dental radiograph shows internal resorption (∗) of the root of the left mandibular canine tooth.
(© Dr Alexander M. Reiter)

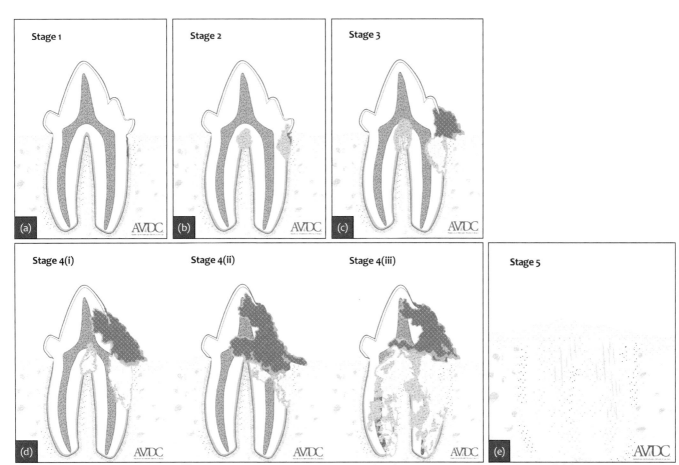

5.17 Stages of tooth resorption. (a) In stage 1, there is mild dental hard tissue loss (cementum or cementum and enamel). (b) In stage 2, there is moderate dental hard tissue loss (cementum or cementum and enamel with loss of dentine that does not extend to the pulp cavity. (c) In stage 3, there is deep dental hard tissue loss (cementum or cementum and enamel with loss of dentine that extends to the pulp cavity); most of the tooth retains its integrity. (d) In stage 4, there is extensive hard tissue loss (cementum or cementum and enamel with loss of dentine that extends to the pulp cavity); most of the tooth has lost its integrity. (i) The crown and the root may be affected equally, (ii) the crown may be more severely affected than the root, (iii) or the root may be more severely affected than the crown. (e) Remnants of dental hard tissue visible only as irregular radiopacities; complete gingival covering.
(© AVDC® used with permission)

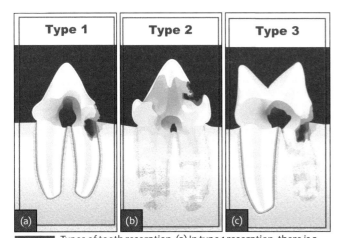

5.18 Types of tooth resorption. (a) In type 1 resorption, there is a focal or multifocal radiolucency present in a tooth with otherwise normal radiopacity and normal periodontal ligament space. This type is also known as inflammatory resorption. (b) In type 2 resorption, there is narrowing or disappearance of the periodontal ligament space in at least some areas, and decreased radiopacity of the tooth. This type is also known as replacement resorption. (c) Features of both type 1 and type 2 resorption in the same tooth are present in type 3 resorption. A tooth with this appearance has areas of normal and narrow or lost periodontal ligament space, and there is focal or multifocal radiolucency in the tooth and decreased radiopacity in other areas of the tooth.
(© AVDC® used with permission)

Tooth resorption is very common in cats and usually involves multiple teeth in more than one jaw quadrant (Reiter and Mendoza, 2002). It is increasingly noted in dogs (Peralta *et al.*, 2010ab; Roux *et al.*, 2011; Nemec *et al.*, 2012a). Chronic excessive dietary intake of vitamin D has been proposed to play a role in the development of tooth resorption in cats (Reiter *et al.*, 2005ab). Pathognomonic of inflammatory resorption is that alveolar bone adjacent to root resorption also gets resorbed because of periodontal or endodontic disease (Figure 5.19). Dentoalveolar ankylosis and replacement resorption occur when the root surfaces fuse with surrounding alveolar bone, thus including the tooth in the normal remodelling process of bone (Figure 5.20). When replacement resorption occurs or progresses coronally towards the gingival attachment apparatus, an inflammatory component may join the initially non-inflammatory lesion so that both replacement resorption and inflammatory resorption are present on the same tooth (Figure 5.21) (Reiter *et al.*, 2005ab).

Tooth resorption is asymptomatic as long as the resorption process does not involve inflammatory cells, remains below the gingival attachment (where it is not exposed to oral bacteria) and does not affect the pulp. Inflammatory resorption, however, may cause oral pain, manifesting as dropping of food while eating, reluctance to eat hard food and spontaneous repetitive lower jaw

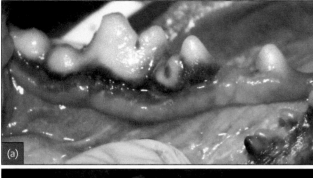

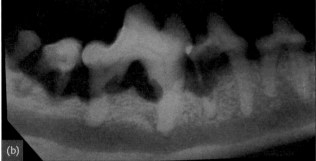

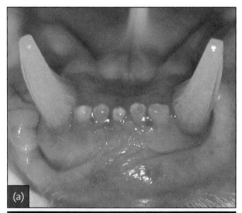

5.19 (a) Clinical photograph and (b) dental radiograph of inflammatory resorption of the right mandibular cheek teeth and adjacent alveolar bone in a dog.
(© Dr Alexander M. Reiter)

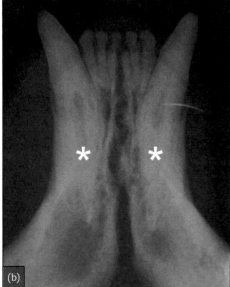

5.20 (a) Clinical photograph and (b) dental radiograph of dentoalveolar ankylosis and replacement resorption (*) of the mandibular canine teeth in a cat.
(© Dr Alexander M. Reiter)

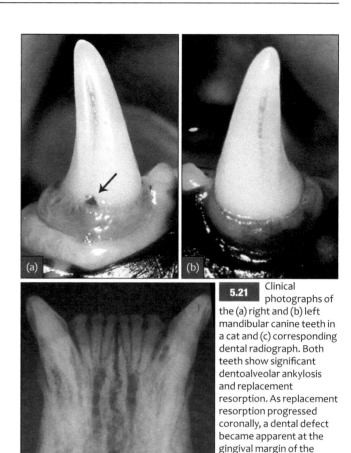

5.21 Clinical photographs of the (a) right and (b) left mandibular canine teeth in a cat and (c) corresponding dental radiograph. Both teeth show significant dentoalveolar ankylosis and replacement resorption. As replacement resorption progressed coronally, a dental defect became apparent at the gingival margin of the labial aspect of the right mandibular canine tooth (arrowed), causing an inflammatory component to join the initially non-inflammatory lesion.
(© Dr Alexander M. Reiter)

motions. In advanced stages of tooth resorption the crown fractures off, leaving an open wound behind (Figure 5.22) (Reiter and Mendoza, 2002).

Some cats show abnormally extruded canine teeth, accompanied by thickening of the alveolar bone (Figure 5.23). Abnormal tooth extrusion refers to an increase in clinical crown length not related to gingival recession or lack of tooth wear. Alveolar bone expansion is a thickening of alveolar bone at labial and buccal aspects of teeth (Bell and Soukup, 2015). An association has been reported between tooth resorption and abnormal tooth extrusion and/or alveolar bone expansion (Figure 5.24) (Lewis *et al.*, 2008).

Teeth with inflammatory resorption, those with excessive extrusion, and root remnants should be extracted. Ankylosed teeth and those with roots undergoing replacement resorption may be treated by means of crown amputation and intentional root retention (Reiter, 2012). See Chapter 12 for further information about the removal of teeth affected by resorption.

Enamel hypoplasia and enamel hypomineralization

Enamel hypoplasia refers to inadequate deposition of enamel matrix. This can affect one or several teeth and may be focal or multifocal. The crowns of affected teeth can have areas of normal enamel next to areas of hypoplastic or missing enamel. Enamel hypomineralization

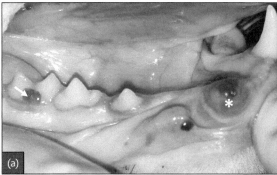
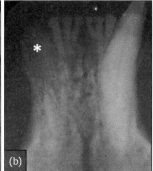
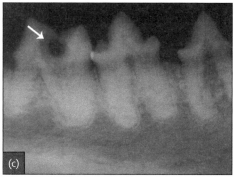

5.22 (a) Clinical photograph and (b, c) dental radiographs of the right mandibular teeth in a cat. The crown of the canine tooth has fractured off, leaving an open wound behind (*). There is radiographic evidence of significant root replacement resorption. The first molar tooth shows an obvious defect filled with granulation tissue that manifests radiographically as a spherical lucency (arrowed). There is increased gingival inflammation at the third premolar tooth whose furcation appears to reveal early signs of resorption in addition to loss of periodontal ligament space.
(© Dr Alexander M. Reiter)

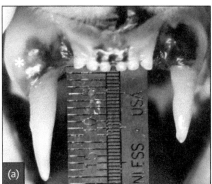
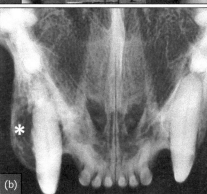

5.23 (a) Clinical photograph and (b) dental radiograph of an abnormally extruded right maxillary canine tooth, accompanied by thickening of the alveolar bone (*).
(© Dr Alexander M. Reiter)

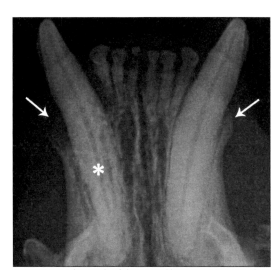

5.24 Radiograph of the rostral lower jaw in a cat, showing bilateral alveolar bone expansion (arrowed) on the labial aspects of the canine teeth. The right mandibular canine tooth shows signs of dentoalveolar ankylosis and replacement resorption (*).
(© Dr Alexander M. Reiter)

refers to inadequate mineralization of enamel matrix. This often affects several or all teeth. The crowns of affected teeth are covered by soft enamel that may be worn rapidly (Boy *et al.*, 2016). For detailed information about the diagnosis and treatment of enamel hypoplasia and hypomineralization, see Chapter 10.

Caries and erosion

Caries is rare in dogs and clinically not relevant in cats (Hale, 1998). It tends to develop on cariogenic tooth surfaces such as pits and fissures (although dogs with smooth-surface caries have been reported) in the presence of cariogenic bacteria (belonging to the mutans group of streptococci) in animals fed a cariogenic diet (containing highly refined carbohydrates such as sugar). Bacterial fermentation of carbohydrates creates lactic, acetic and propionic acids that demineralize the enamel.

A carious lesion advances along the course of enamel rods to the dentinoenamel junction, spreads at the junction, and then continues to advance along the course of dentinal tubules towards the pulp. Thus, a small enamel opening in pit and fissure caries may actually be leading to a much larger dentine defect. Visible marks on the tooth surface should be examined using a sharp dental explorer (Figure 5.25). If the explorer sticks in the affected area, drops into a cavity or the surface feels softened, then there is probably a carious lesion. Conversely, smooth-surface caries is largest at the surface and becomes progressively smaller as it penetrates deeper into the enamel (Figure 5.26) (Reiter, 1998).

Tooth erosion is not the same as caries. Erosion refers to demineralization of tooth substance due to external acids (Reiter and Harvey, 2010). Erosion is rarely seen in the teeth

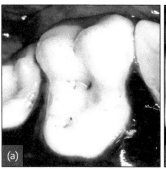
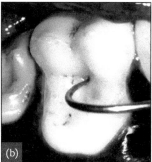

5.25 (a) The occlusal surface of the right maxillary first molar tooth in a dog shows a dark spot suggestive of caries. (b) This should be examined using a sharp dental explorer.
(© Dr Alexander M. Reiter)

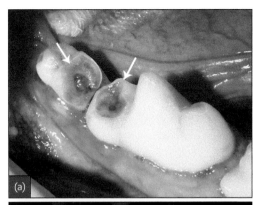

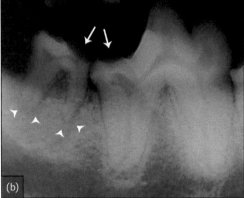

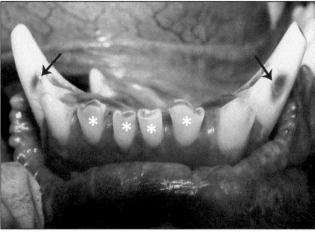

5.28 Tooth attrition affecting the mandibular incisor and canine teeth in a dog with mandibular mesiocclusion and level bite. Note the exposed and discolored dentine on the worn occlusal surfaces of the affected incisor teeth (∗) and the mesial aspects of the canine teeth (arrowed).
(© Dr Alexander M. Reiter)

5.26 (a) Clinical photograph and (b) radiograph of the right mandibular first and second molar teeth with carious lesions (arrowed). The second molar tooth shows pulp exposure, and there are subtle signs of periapical lucencies around its root apices (arrowheads).
(© Dr Alexander M. Reiter)

of cats and dogs. Treatment of caries and erosion includes cessation of their causes, sealing of the dental crowns, defect restoration, endodontic therapy and tooth extraction.

Tooth wear

Abrasion is tooth wear caused by contact of a tooth with a non-dental material (such as a tennis ball or cage bars) (Figure 5.27). Attrition is tooth wear caused by contact of a tooth with another tooth (such as when a maloccluding tooth contacts another tooth) (Figure 5.28) (Reiter *et al.*,

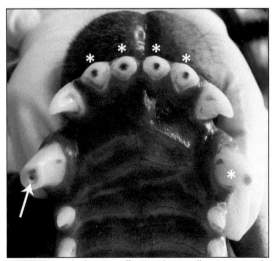

5.27 Tooth abrasion affecting the maxillary incisor and canine teeth in a dog. Note the tertiary dentine on the worn occlusal surfaces of the affected teeth (∗) and pulp exposure on the right maxillary canine tooth (arrowed).
(© Dr Alexander M. Reiter)

2012). Tertiary dentine is produced as a result of a local insult such as tooth wear. It can be reactionary (produced by existing odontoblasts) or reparative (produced by odontoblast-like cells that have differentiated from pulpal stem cells). Sclerotic dentine is somewhat transparent dentine characterized by mineralization of the dentinal tubules as a result of an insult or normal aging. If tooth wear removes enamel and dentine faster than odontoblasts of the pulp can form dentine, the pulp may either succumb to prolonged chronic inflammation or become exposed, inflamed and necrotic (Reiter and Harvey, 2010). See Chapter 9 for detailed information about diagnosis and treatment of tooth wear.

Tooth fracture

Tooth fractures are classified based on the fracture location (crown, crown-root or root) and whether the pulp is exposed (uncomplicated or complicated) (Figure 5.29). Enamel infraction refers to an incomplete fracture (crack) of the enamel without loss of tooth substance (Figure 5.30). An enamel fracture is a fracture with loss of crown substance confined to the enamel only; the consequences are usually minimal, depending on the patient's age (thickness of dentine) and extent of enamel loss (Figure 5.31) (Reiter and Harvey, 2010).

An uncomplicated crown fracture refers to a fracture of the crown that does not expose the pulp (Figure 5.32). Near pulp exposure means that a thin layer of dentine separates the pulp from the outer tooth surface. If dentine is exposed but not yet the pulp, odontoblasts may react by producing tertiary dentine. It is also possible for bacteria to pass through the dentinal tubules to the pulp and cause an infection of the pulp tissue. A complicated crown fracture is a fracture of the crown that exposes the pulp (Figure 5.33). A crown-root fracture is a fracture that involves the crown and root(s) of the tooth; it can be uncomplicated (Figure 5.34) or complicated (Figure 5.35). A root fracture is a fracture involving the root (far more common with pulp exposure than without) (Reiter and Harvey, 2010). There is debate about whether the current nomenclature should be amended, as the term 'uncomplicated' could be mistakenly interpreted as that there are no negative consequences for endodontic health and that treatment may not be needed.

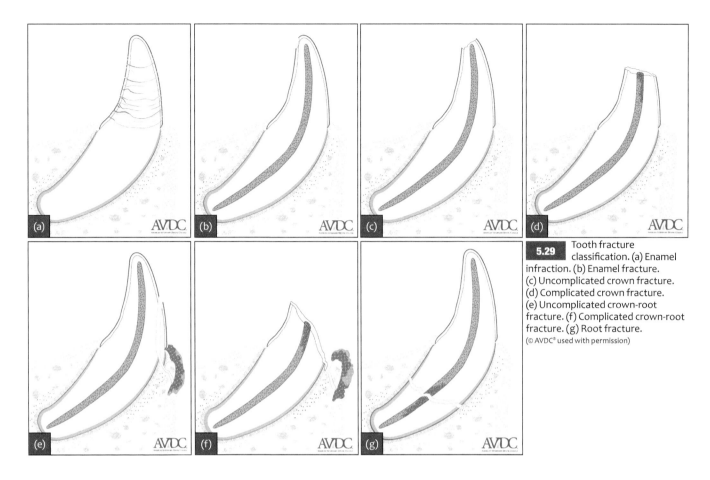

5.29 Tooth fracture classification. (a) Enamel infraction. (b) Enamel fracture. (c) Uncomplicated crown fracture. (d) Complicated crown fracture. (e) Uncomplicated crown-root fracture. (f) Complicated crown-root fracture. (g) Root fracture.
(© AVDC® used with permission)

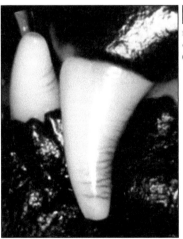

5.30 Enamel infraction of left maxillary and mandibular canine teeth in a dog.
(© Dr Alexander M. Reiter)

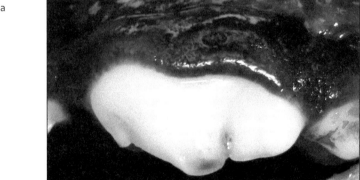

5.32 Uncomplicated crown fracture of the left maxillary fourth premolar tooth in a dog.
(© Dr Alexander M. Reiter)

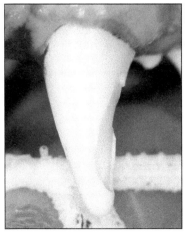

5.31 Enamel fracture of the left maxillary canine tooth in a dog.
(© Dr Alexander M. Reiter)

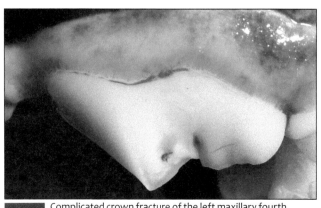

5.33 Complicated crown fracture of the left maxillary fourth premolar tooth in a dog.
(© Dr Alexander M. Reiter)

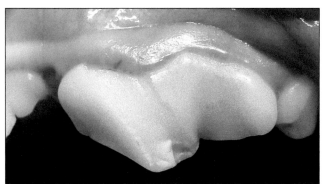

5.34 Uncomplicated crown-root fracture of the left maxillary fourth premolar tooth in a dog.
(© Dr Alexander M. Reiter)

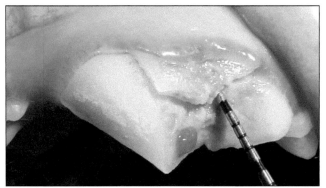

5.35 Complicated crown-root fracture of the left maxillary fourth premolar tooth in a dog.
(© Dr Alexander M. Reiter)

Canine tooth fractures are usually due to trauma from road traffic accidents, falls from heights, or kicks and hits. Certain working dogs are more prone to fracture of canine teeth if their distal tooth surfaces are weakened by wear from chewing on cage bars (Figure 5.36). Carnassial tooth

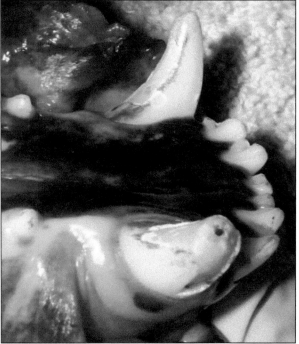

5.36 Metal staining and worn distal surfaces of the mandibular canine teeth in a dog. Note the complicated crown fracture of the right mandibular canine tooth.
(© Dr Alexander M. Reiter)

fractures (primarily the maxillary fourth premolar teeth and less so the mandibular first molar teeth) in dogs are often caused by chewing on very hard objects. Tooth resorption is typically the cause of crown fracture in cats, with crown-root or root remnants being retained in the alveoli (Reiter and Lewis, 2011). The reader is referred to Chapter 9 for detailed information about diagnosis and treatment of tooth fractures.

Endodontic and periapical disease

Pulpitis and pulp necrosis

Pulpitis can either be reversible or irreversible. Dystrophic mineralization of the pulp may occasionally occur as a result of pulpitis, leading to regional narrowing or complete disappearance of the pulp cavity. This should not be confused with pulp stones, which are intrapulpal mineralized structures unrelated to current disease (Reiter and Harvey, 2010). Pulp necrosis is a sequel to untreated irreversible pulpitis, a traumatic injury, or events that cause long-term interruption of the blood supply to the pulp. A tooth with necrotic pulp is called a non-vital tooth. Infection and inflammation of the pulp can spread through the apical and non-apical ramifications into the periapical region, furcation area, and other areas of the periodontal ligament space. Blunt trauma may lead to endodontic disease and result in crown discoloration (pink, red, purple, grey or brown) (Figure 5.37). One study revealed that over 90% of teeth with crown discoloration are non-vital because of pulpal oedema and haemorrhage causing increased pressure within the pulp cavity and obliterating its blood vessels (Hale, 2001).

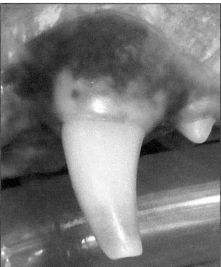

5.37 Purplish discoloration of the coronal third of the fractured or worn crown of the left maxillary canine tooth in a dog.
(© Dr Alexander M. Reiter)

Periapical pathology

A periapical cyst (also known as a radicular cyst) is an odontogenic cyst formed around the apex of a tooth after stimulation and proliferation of epithelial rests in the periodontal ligament (Figure 5.38). If such a tooth is extracted without removing the cyst lining around the root apex, a residual cyst remains (Reiter and Harvey, 2010).

A periapical granuloma refers to chronic apical periodontitis with an accumulation of mononuclear inflammatory

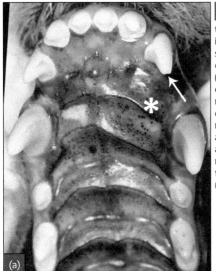

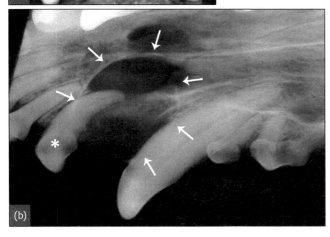

5.38 (a) Swelling (∗) palatal to the left maxillary third incisor tooth that shows a barely visible crown fracture (arrowed). (b) The dental radiograph reveals a well demarcated radiolucency (arrowed) associated with the apex of the left maxillary third incisor tooth (∗).
(© Dr Alexander M. Reiter)

cells and an encircling aggregation of fibroblasts and collagen that appears radiographically as a diffuse or circumscribed radiolucent lesion, which may be indistinguishable from a periapical abscess (Reiter and Harvey, 2010).

A periapical abscess is an acute or chronic inflammation of the periapical tissues characterized by localized accumulation of suppuration (Figure 5.39). Clinical signs include facial swelling, sinus tracts, pain and fever and general malaise in more acute or advanced cases. An intraoral sinus tract is a pathological communication between the tooth, bone or soft tissue and the oral cavity. An orofacial sinus tract is a pathological communication between the oral cavity and the face. A phoenix abscess is an acute exacerbation of chronic apical periodontitis (Reiter and Harvey, 2010).

Hypercementosis refers to excessive deposition of cementum around the root of a tooth. This is frequently seen in cats and may be associated with or have the same cause as tooth resorption (Figure 5.40) (Reiter et al., 2005a). Osteosclerosis is excessive bone mineralization around the apex of a vital tooth caused by low-grade pulp irritation. The affected tooth is asymptomatic and does not require endodontic therapy.

Condensing osteitis is excessive bone mineralization around the apex of a non-vital tooth caused by longstanding and low-toxic exudation from an infected pulp. An affected tooth requires endodontic therapy. Alveolar osteitis is inflammation of the bone in immediate proximity to the alveolus and may occur when a blood clot dislodges in an unsutured tooth extraction site. Osteomyelitis and osteonecrosis refer to localized or widespread infection and necrosis of the bone and bone marrow, respectively (Reiter and Harvey, 2010). See Chapters 4 and 9 for detailed information about diagnosis and treatment of endodontic and periapical disease.

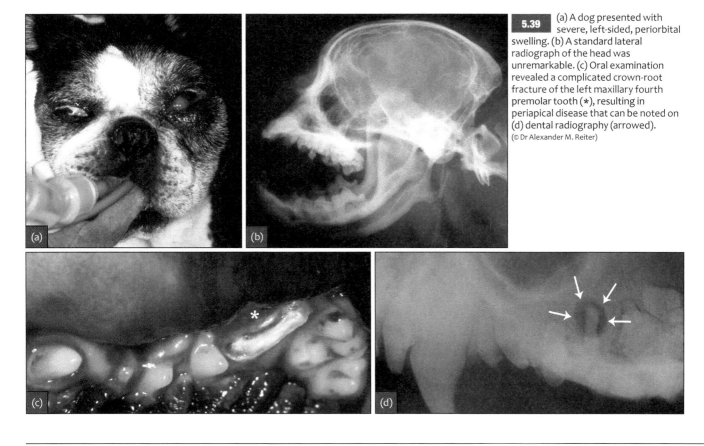

5.39 (a) A dog presented with severe, left-sided, periorbital swelling. (b) A standard lateral radiograph of the head was unremarkable. (c) Oral examination revealed a complicated crown-root fracture of the left maxillary fourth premolar tooth (∗), resulting in periapical disease that can be noted on (d) dental radiography (arrowed).
(© Dr Alexander M. Reiter)

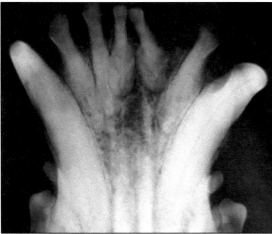

5.40 Hypercementosis of the mandibular incisor teeth in a dog. Note that the left mandibular second incisor tooth is missing.
(© Dr Alexander M. Reiter)

Tooth displacement injury

Tooth luxation refers to clinically or radiographically evident displacement of the tooth within its alveolus, while tooth avulsion is a complete extrusive luxation with the tooth out of its alveolus (Gracis, 2012). Lateral and incomplete extrusive luxation in dogs is typically associated with alveolar fracture (Ulbricht et al., 2004), while in cats it usually occurs after alveolar bone expansion, infrabony pocket formation and abnormal tooth extrusion (Figure 5.41), eventually causing inability to fully close the mouth (Figure 5.42).

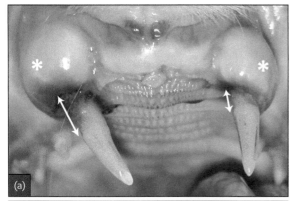

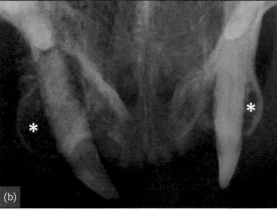

5.41 (a) Clinical photograph and (b) dental radiograph showing lateral luxation of the right maxillary canine tooth in a cat associated with alveolar bone expansion (∗), infrabony pocket formation and abnormal tooth extrusion (double-ended arrows), which are present bilaterally. Incisor tooth root remnants are visible on the radiograph.
(© Dr Alexander M. Reiter)

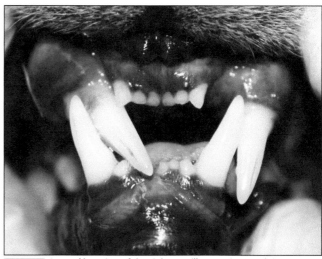

5.42 Lateral luxation of the right maxillary canine tooth in a cat, causing inability to fully close the mouth.
(© Dr Alexander M. Reiter)

Intrusive luxation of canine teeth into the nasal cavity may sometimes occur in patients with severe periodontal disease following mild trauma (Figure 5.43) (Edstrom et al., 2015).

Tooth repositioning is the manual repositioning of a displaced tooth. Tooth reimplantation is the manual reimplantation of an avulsed tooth. The success of reimplantation of an avulsed tooth is greatly influenced by the length of time that the tooth is out of the alveolar socket. An avulsed tooth should be placed in fresh milk, in which periodontal ligament fibres may remain vital for 3 to 6 hours. Luxated and avulsed teeth require immediate repositioning, stabilization and root canal therapy due to the likely loss of blood supply to the pulp (Gracis and Orsini, 1998). For detailed information about the diagnosis and treatment of teeth with displacement injuries, see Chapter 9.

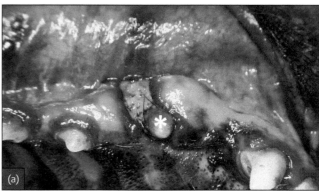

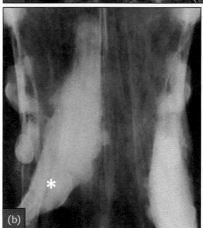

5.43 (a) Clinical photograph and (b) dental radiograph showing intrusion of the right maxillary canine tooth (∗) into the nasal cavity of a dog. Only the tip of the crown of the intruded tooth is visible on oral examination. Note also the gingivitis, gingival cleft formation, alveolar bone exposure, and alveolar and labial mucositis.
(© Dr Alexander M. Reiter)

Jaw fracture

Traumatic jaw fractures occur after motor vehicle trauma, falls, kicks, gunshots and fights with other animals. Pathological jaw fractures are often secondary to periodontal disease, less often due to oral neoplasia, and rarely caused by metabolic abnormalities.

Jaw fracture location

A mandibular fracture is a fracture of the lower jaw (mandible). The line of a favourable mandibular body fracture runs in a rostroventral direction, resulting in a more stable compression of the fracture segments upon contraction of the masticatory muscles that close the mouth (Figure 5.44). The line of an unfavourable mandibular fracture runs in a caudoventral direction, resulting in a more unstable separation of the fracture segments upon contraction of the masticatory muscles that close the mouth (Figure 5.45). Common sites for mandibular fracture in dogs are the premolar/molar region and the area distal to the canine tooth (Figure 5.46). Mandibular symphysis separation and fracture of the parasymphyseal or ramus areas are more often seen in cats (Figure 5.47). Unilateral mandibular fractures often result in deviation of

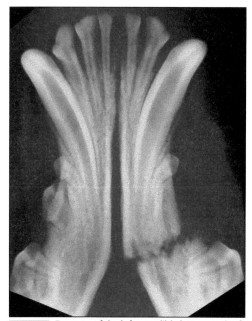

5.46 Fracture of the left mandible between the first and third premolar teeth in a dog. The second premolar tooth was missing prior to fracture.
(© Dr Alexander M. Reiter)

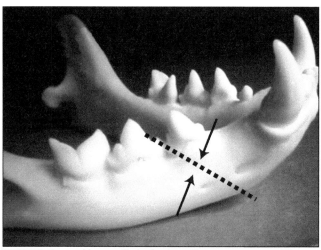

5.44 Favourable mandibular fracture. The arrows represent the forces exerted on the fracture line upon contraction of the masticatory muscles that close the mouth.
(© Dr Alexander M. Reiter)

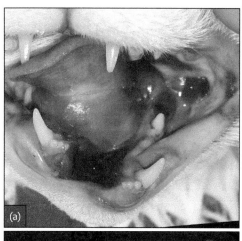

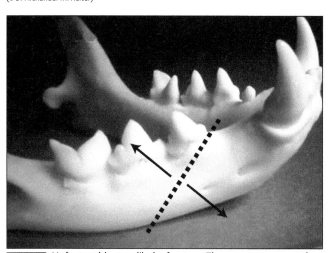

5.45 Unfavourable mandibular fracture. The arrows represent the forces exerted on the fracture line upon contraction of the masticatory muscles that close the mouth.
(© Dr Alexander M. Reiter)

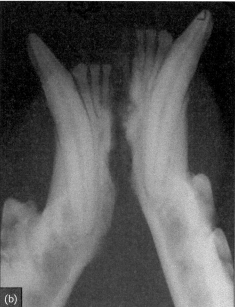

5.47 (a) Clinical photograph and (b) dental radiograph showing symphysis separation in a cat.
(© Dr Alexander M. Reiter)

the lower jaw towards the side of injury, causing malocclusion. Bilateral mandibular fractures may cause a dropped lower jaw appearance (Reiter and Lewis, 2011).

A maxillary fracture is a fracture of the upper jaw (maxilla and other facial bones). Fractures of the upper jaw are often multiple. Epistaxis, facial swelling, pain and asymmetry are the usual physical findings, with or without crepitus and subcutaneous emphysema (Figure 5.48). Airway obstruction caused by displaced bones, swelling or blood can be life-threatening. Cats with head trauma commonly present with an acute cleft palate, zygomatic arch fracture or separation of the temporal bone from the parietal bone; the latter may often go unnoticed (Figure 5.49) (Reiter and Lewis, 2011).

Diagnostic imaging should be performed to assess tooth injuries and define fracture sites. Dental radiography is usually sufficient for rostrally located mandibular and maxillary fractures and fractures involving the premolar/molar tooth-bearing part of the mandibular body. Computed tomography (CT) should be employed for assessment of more complex oral and maxillofacial trauma (Reiter and Lewis, 2011).

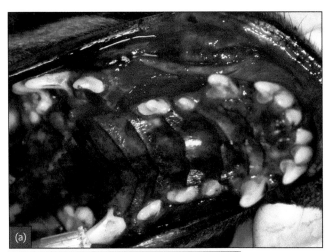

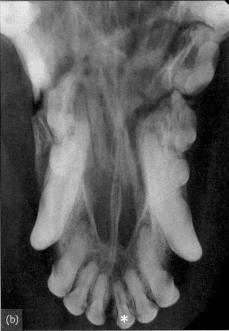

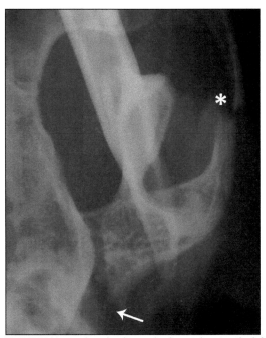

5.49 Ventrodorsal radiograph of a cat showing the left temporomandibular joint area obtained with a dental film and extraoral film placement. There is a fracture of the left zygomatic arch (∗) and separation of the left temporal bone from the parietal bone (arrowed).
(© Dr Alexander M. Reiter)

5.48 (a) Clinical photograph and (b) dental radiograph showing maxillary fractures in a dog. Note that the left maxillary first incisor tooth (∗) has a wider pulp cavity compared with the other incisor teeth, indicating that the loss of pulp vitality is unrelated to the recent motor-vehicle trauma that caused the maxillary fractures.
(© Dr Alexander M. Reiter)

Management of teeth in jaw fracture lines

Jaw fracture stabilization and postoperative occlusion are unfavourably influenced by extraction of structurally intact teeth associated with fracture lines. These teeth can contribute to proper alignment of fracture segments and provide anchorage for fracture repair devices (Shetty and Freymiller, 1989). Extraction of a tooth entails further trauma to, and weakening of, the bone and also presents technical difficulties when the bone fragments are highly mobile. The complication rate with regards to bone fracture healing is not necessarily lower following extraction of teeth located in fracture lines (Thaller and Mabourakh, 1994; Gerbino et al., 1997; Ellis, 2002). However, if teeth within fracture lines extending along the periodontal ligament space towards the root apex are retained, they should be carefully monitored for evidence of periodontal or endodontic pathology, and appropriate treatment must be instituted as soon as either is recognized (Kamboozia and Punnia-Moorthy, 1993).

Overview of treatment for jaw fractures

There are various ways to repair jaw fractures, including maxillomandibular fixation (e.g. muzzling, labial reverse sutures through buttons, interarch bonding between maxillary and mandibular canine teeth), circumferential wiring (e.g. mandibular symphysis wire cerclage), interquadrant fixation (e.g. for traumatic cleft palate with wide separation in the midline), interdental wiring with intraoral composite splinting (e.g. when teeth can be used as anchor points), intraosseous wiring (e.g. in edentulous areas), external skeletal fixation (e.g. in cases with missing bone fragments, severe comminution and edentulous bone segments), bone plating (e.g. utilizing mini-, intermediate and microplates) and partial mandibulectomy or maxillectomy (e.g. when tissues are already necrotic) (Reiter and Lewis, 2011). See Chapter 9 for detailed information about the diagnosis and treatment of jaw fractures.

Temporomandibular joint pathology

Fracture of the temporomandibular joint (TMJ) involves breaking of one or more of the bony structures forming the TMJ. A conservative approach (anticipating healing as a pain-free and functional non-union) is often chosen over surgical intervention (condylectomy) in cases where normal occlusion is maintained (Reiter and Lewis, 2011). However, trauma to the TMJ (or adjacent structures such as the mandibular ramus and zygomatic arch) can occasionally lead to ankylosis and progressive inability to open the mouth (particularly in young animals). Treatment of ankylosis consists of condylectomy and excision of all associated osteophytes (Strøm *et al.*, 2016).

Luxation of the TMJ is often confused with open-mouth jaw locking. Both conditions may present with inability to close the mouth, but their causes, manifestations and treatments differ. A diagnosis is made by means of clinical examination and radiography (e.g. dorsoventral view) or CT. Rostrodorsal luxation of the TMJ can usually be resolved by placing a pencil between the ipsilateral maxillary and mandibular carnassial teeth and then closing the mouth. However, this treatment would cause further trauma and pain in a patient with open-mouth jaw locking, which is treated by means of partial zygomectomy, partial coronoidectomy or a combination of both procedures (Reiter and Lewis, 2011). For detailed information about the diagnosis and treatment of TMJ pathology, the reader is referred to Chapter 9.

Oral soft tissue injury

Bite wound

A laceration resulting from a bite comprises a tear or cut in the gingiva/alveolar mucosa, tongue/sublingual mucosa, lip skin/labial mucosa, cheek skin/buccal mucosa, palatal mucosa or palatine tonsil/oropharyngeal mucosa (Figure 5.50). A chewing lesion is a mucosal or cutaneous lesion resulting from self-induced bite trauma on the cheek, lip, palate or tongue/sublingual region (Figure 5.51) (Lewis and Reiter, 2011; Durand and Smith, 2015).

Foreign body

A penetrating oral foreign body is an object that originates outside the body and enters oral tissue to create deep and contaminated wounds in the sublingual area, palatoglossal fold, soft palate, palatine tonsil and tonsillar fold, floor of the orbit or pharyngeal wall. A retrobulbar abscess develops behind the globe of the eye, while a retropharyngeal abscess is located behind the pharynx. Foreign bodies can also be caught around the tongue, sawing their way into the lingual frenulum, be stuck in between teeth (Figure 5.52), causing inflammation of the surrounding soft tissue, or be trapped in a salivary gland duct, resulting in facial swelling (Goldsworthy *et al.*, 2013; Robinson *et al.*, 2014; Tremolada *et al.*, 2015; Voelter-Ratson *et al.*, 2015).

Burns

A burn is an injury to the skin, mucosa or other body part due to fire, heat, radiation, electricity or a caustic agent. Thermal burns result from exposure to hot items and can

be seen on the nasal planum, lips, labial mucosa, tongue and palate. Chemical burns result from exposure to corrosive materials (Lewis and Reiter, 2011).

Electrical injury refers to physical trauma to the skin, mucosa or other tissues that occurs when they come into direct contact with an electrical current. Life-threatening complications from electrical injury are related to neurogenic pulmonary oedema and smoke inhalation. The lips, labial and buccal mucosa, alveolar mucosa, gingiva, the tongue and palate are usually affected. More extensive burns also affect teeth and bones (Lewis and Reiter, 2011).

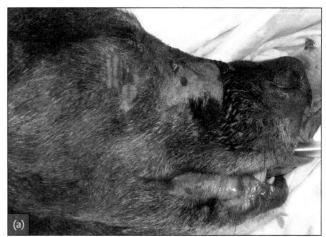
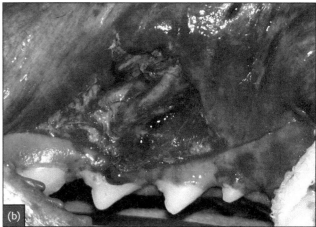

5.50 (a) Extraoral and (b) intraoral bite wounds in a dog.
(© Dr Alexander M. Reiter)

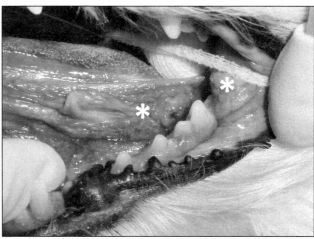

5.51 Proliferative chewing lesions in the left sublingual and buccal mucosa (∗) resulting from self-induced bite trauma in a dog.
(© Dr Alexander M. Reiter)

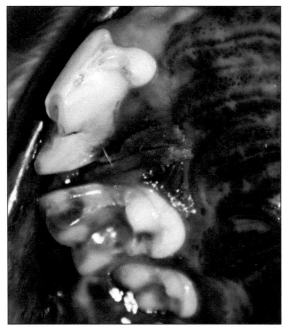

5.52 A wooden foreign body is stuck between the right maxillary fourth premolar and first molar teeth in a dog.
(© Dr Alexander M. Reiter)

Ballistic trauma

Ballistic trauma refers to physical trauma sustained from a projectile that was launched through space, most commonly by a weapon such as a gun or a bow (Figure 5.53). Arrow injuries may contain razor-sharp triangular projections deeply seated in delicate tissues that are surrounded by important neurovascular structures (Figure 5.54) (Lewis and Reiter, 2011).

Lip avulsion

Lip avulsion can occasionally be seen in cats and dogs after motor vehicle trauma (lower or upper lip is affected) (White, 2010), in cats whose lip has been stepped on by a person (lower lip is usually affected) or dogs being grasped at the muzzle, held up and shaken by a larger animal (upper lip is usually affected). For detailed information about the diagnosis and treatment of oral soft tissue injuries, see Chapter 9.

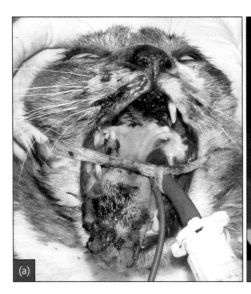
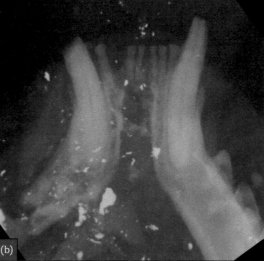

5.53 (a) Gunshot trauma causing multiple soft and hard tissue injuries in a cat. (b) Dental radiograph of the rostral lower jaw in the same cat, revealing symphysis separation, parasymphyseal fracture, right mandibular body fracture, fractured teeth and numerous pieces of the impacting projectile.
(© Dr Alexander M. Reiter)

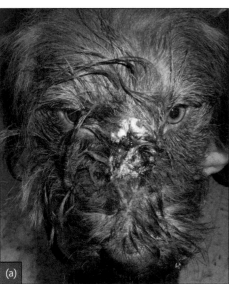
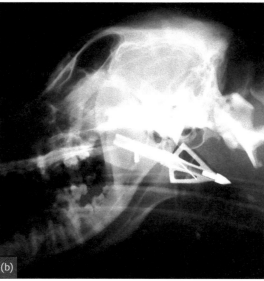

5.54 (a) Entrance wound of a hunting arrow at the dorsum of the nose in a dog. (b) Corresponding radiograph of the head in the same dog, showing the arrow pathway with its remaining carbon-fibre shaft and three-bladed broadhead tip.
(© Dr Alexander M. Reiter)

Abnormalities of the palate

Abnormalities of the palate primarily include communications between the oral/oropharyngeal and nasal/nasopharyngeal cavities along the hard or soft palate, which may be congenital or acquired after birth, and soft palate elongations, which are congenital.

Congenital palate defects

Congenital palate defects involve the primary and/or secondary palate. A cleft lip is a longitudinal defect of the upper lip, or the upper lip, the alveolar process and most rostral hard palate. A cleft palate is a longitudinal defect in the midline of the hard and soft palate. A cleft soft palate is a longitudinal defect in the midline of the soft palate only. A unilateral soft palate defect is a longitudinal defect of the soft palate on one side only. Soft palate hypoplasia refers to a decrease in normal length of the soft palate (Reiter and Holt, 2012). The reader is referred to Chapter 10 for detailed information about the diagnosis and treatment of congenital palate defects.

Acquired palate defects

A traumatic cleft palate is a longitudinal defect in the midline of the hard and/or soft palate resulting from trauma (often associated with falling from a height or hit-by-car trauma in cats) (Bonner et al., 2012). An oronasal fistula is a communication between the oral and nasal cavities along the upper dental arch, usually due to severe periodontal disease of a maxillary tooth (Figure 5.55). Other palate defects may result from electrical cord injury, gunshot trauma, animal bites, foreign body penetration, maloccluding teeth, eosinophilic granuloma and iatrogenic trauma (e.g. following improper extraction of maxillary teeth or inadequate wound closure after excision of maxillary tumours) (Reiter and Lewis, 2011). See Chapter 9 for detailed information about the diagnosis and treatment of acquired palate defects.

Elongated soft palate

An elongated soft palate refers to a congenital increase in length of the soft palate. This is commonly seen in brachycephalic dogs in conjunction with stenotic nares, a

shortened nose, the presence of rhinopharyngeal turbinates, relative macroglossia, everted and enlarged palatine tonsils and laryngeal saccules, collapse or paralysis of the laryngeal cartilages, narrow trachea and bronchial collapse. As the respiratory effort increases, the elongated soft palate may secondarily become thickened and hyperplastic (Reiter and Holt, 2012). For detailed information about the diagnosis and treatment of brachycephalic obstructive airway syndrome, see Chapter 10.

Oral and maxillofacial tumours

Odontogenic tumours

A peripheral odontogenic fibroma (POF) is a benign mesenchymal odontogenic tumour associated with the gingiva and believed to originate from the periodontal ligament. It is characterized by varying amounts of inactive-looking odontogenic epithelium embedded in a mature, fibrous stroma, which may undergo osseous metaplasia. Historically it has been referred to as fibromatous epulis or – when bone or tooth-like hard tissue is present within the lesion – ossifying epulis. The use of the term 'epulis' (plural 'epulides') is discouraged, as it is a general term referring to a gingival mass lesion of any type (benign or malignant) (Figure 5.56) (Fiani et al., 2011b). In cats, POFs typically present as multiple gingival masses (Colgin et al., 2001).

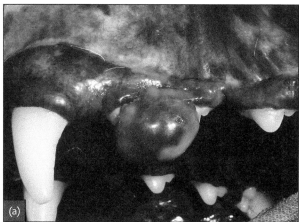

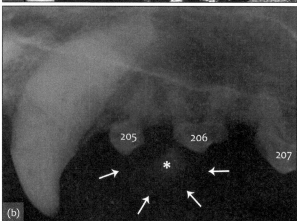

5.56 (a) Peripheral odontogenic fibroma centred between the left maxillary first and second premolar teeth in a dog. (b) The corresponding dental radiograph shows hard tissue (∗) within the soft tissue contours of the tumour (arrowed). The root resorption associated with the first and second premolar teeth (205 and 206) is probably unrelated to the tumour, as it can also be seen on the third premolar (207) which is not affected by the tumour.
(© Dr Alexander M. Reiter)

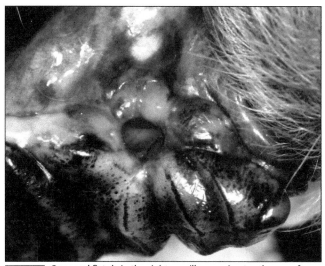

5.55 Oronasal fistula in the right maxillary canine tooth area of a dog with missing teeth.
(© Dr Alexander M. Reiter)

A canine acanthomatous ameloblastoma is a typically benign, but aggressive, histological variant of a group of epithelial odontogenic tumours known collectively as ameloblastomas, which have a basic structure resembling the enamel organ (suggesting derivation from amelo-blasts). The acanthomatous histological designation refers to the central cells within nests of odontogenic epithelium that are squamous and may be keratinized, rather than stellate (Figure 5.57) (Fulton *et al.*, 2014).

An amyloid-producing odontogenic tumour is a benign epithelial odontogenic tumour affecting both dogs and cats and is characterized by the presence of odontogenic epithelium and extracellular amyloid (Hirayama *et al.*, 2010). A feline inductive odontogenic tumour is a benign tumour unique to adolescent and young adult cats, typically affecting the maxilla and showing characteristic, spherical condensations of fibroblastic connective tissue associated with islands of odontogenic epithelium (Sakai *et al.*, 2008). It has also been incorrectly called inductive fibroameloblastoma. A cementoma is a rare benign odontogenic neoplasm of mesenchymal origin, consisting of cementum-like tissue deposited by cells resembling cementoblasts (Villamizar-Martinez *et al.*, 2016).

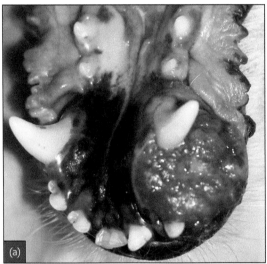

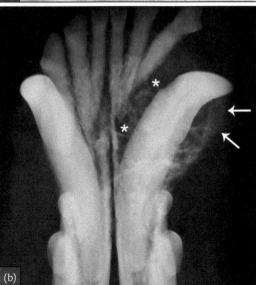

5.57 (a) Acanthomatous ameloblastoma centred between the left mandibular third incisor and canine teeth in a dog. (b) The corresponding dental radiograph shows displacement of teeth, bone lysis (∗) and a sunburst pattern (arrowed).
(© Dr Alexander M. Reiter)

Benign non-odontogenic tumours

A papilloma is an exophytic, pedunculated, cauliflower-like benign neoplasm of the epithelium. Canine papillomatosis is thought to be due to infection with canine papillomavirus and is typically seen in young dogs. Severe papillomatosis may be recognized in older dogs that are immunocompromised (Figure 5.58) (Sancak *et al.*, 2015).

An adenoma is a benign epithelial tumour in which the cells form recognizable glandular structures or in which the cells are derived from glandular epithelium. A lipoma is a benign mesenchymal neoplasm of lipocytes. An osteoma is a benign neoplasm of bone consisting of mature, compact or cancellous bone (Figure 5.59) (Fiani *et al.*, 2011a).

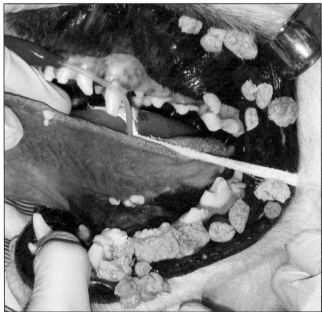

5.58 Severe oral papillomatosis in a geriatric dog with malignant lymphoma treated with chemotherapy.
(© Dr Alexander M. Reiter)

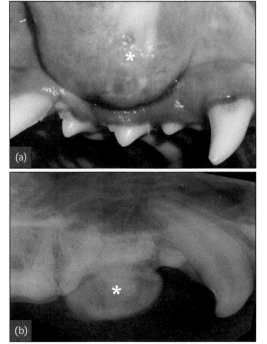

5.59 (a) Clinical photograph and (b) dental radiograph of an osteoma (∗) centred over the right maxillary second and third premolar teeth in a dog.
(© Dr Alexander M. Reiter)

A giant cell granuloma is a benign, tumour-like growth consisting of multinucleated giant cells within a background stroma on the gingiva (peripheral giant cell granuloma) or within bone (central giant cell granuloma); it is also called a giant cell epulis (de Bruijn *et al.*, 2007; Desoutter *et al.*, 2012). A plasma cell tumour is a proliferation of plasma cells, commonly occurring on the gingiva or dorsum of the tongue; it is also called a plasmacytoma (Figure 5.60) (Smithson *et al.*, 2012). A granular cell tumour is a benign tumour of the skin or mucosa with uncertain histogenesis, most commonly occurring in the tongue; it is also called a myoblastoma (Suzuki *et al.*, 2015).

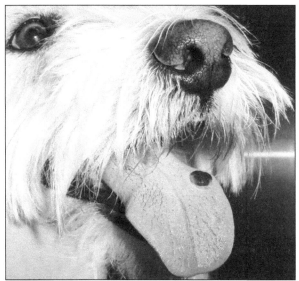

5.60 Plasma cell tumour on the dorsal aspect of the tongue in a dog.
(© Dr Alexander M. Reiter)

Malignant non-odontogenic tumours

A malignant melanoma is an invasive malignant neoplasm of melanocytes or melanocyte precursors that may or may not be pigmented (amelanotic); it is also called a melanosarcoma (Figure 5.61). A squamous cell carcinoma is an invasive malignant epithelial neoplasm of the oral epithelium with varying degrees of squamous differentiation

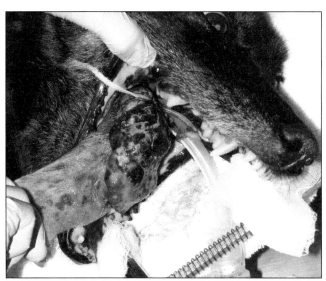

5.61 Malignant melanoma on the dorsal aspect of the tongue in a dog.
(© Dr Alexander M. Reiter)

(Figure 5.62) (Supsavhad *et al.*, 2016). A fibrosarcoma is an invasive malignant mesenchymal neoplasm of fibroblasts; a distinct histologically low-grade, biologically high-grade variant is often found in the oral cavity of young adult large-breed dogs (Figure 5.63) (Frazier *et al.*, 2012; Gardner *et al.*, 2015). A peripheral nerve sheath tumour is a group of neural tumours arising from Schwann cells or perineural fibroblasts (or a combination of both cell types) of the cranial nerves, spinal nerve roots or peripheral nerves; they may be classified as histologically benign or malignant (Figure 5.64) (Boonsriroj *et al.*, 2014).

An osteosarcoma is a locally aggressive malignant mesenchymal neoplasm of primitive bone cells that has the ability to produce osteoid or immature bone (Figure 5.65) (Coyle *et al.*, 2015). A multilobular tumour of bone is a potentially malignant and locally invasive neoplasm of bone that more commonly affects the mandible, hard palate and flat bones of the cranium (Figure 5.66). It has a multilobular histological pattern of bony or cartilaginous matrix surrounded by a thin layer of spindle cells that gives it a near pathognomonic radiographic 'popcorn ball' appearance. This type of neoplasm is also known as a multilobular osteochondrosarcoma, multilobular osteoma, multilobular chondroma, chondroma rodens or multilobular osteosarcoma (Rosselli *et al.*, 2017).

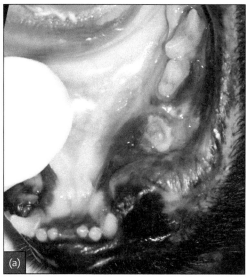

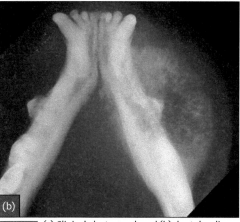

5.62 (a) Clinical photograph and (b) dental radiograph of a squamous cell carcinoma affecting the left lower jaw in a cat. Note the resorption of the left mandibular third premolar tooth and bone lysis with transportation of bony spicules to the periphery of the expanding tumour.
(© Dr Alexander M. Reiter)

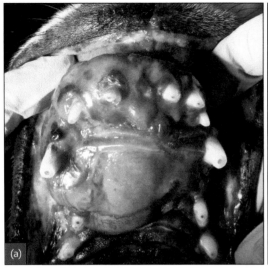

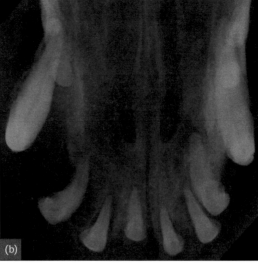

5.63 (a) Clinical photograph and (b) dental radiograph of a fibrosarcoma affecting the rostral upper jaw in a dog. Note the bone lysis and widening of the interproximal spaces in between the teeth.
(© Dr Alexander M. Reiter)

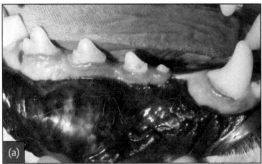

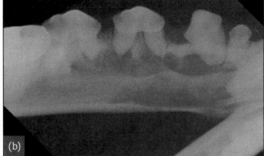

5.64 (a) Clinical photograph and (b) radiograph of a malignant peripheral nerve sheath tumour affecting the right lower jaw in a dog. Note the bone lysis within the mandibular canal and thinning of the ventral mandibular cortex.
(© Dr Alexander M. Reiter)

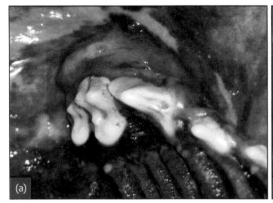

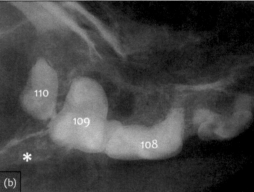

5.65 (a) Clinical photograph and (b) radiograph of an osteosarcoma affecting the caudal right upper jaw in a dog. Note the bone lysis of the maxilla (around teeth 108, 109 and 110) and zygomatic arch (*).
(© Dr Alexander M. Reiter)

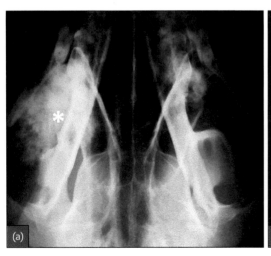

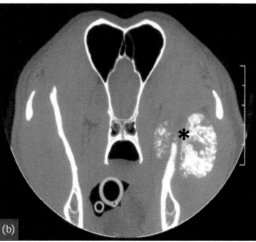

5.66 (a) Dorsoventral head radiograph and (b) computed tomographic scan of a multilobular tumour of bone affecting the coronoid process of the left mandible (*) in a dog.
(© Dr Alexander M. Reiter)

An adenocarcinoma is an invasive malignant epithelial neoplasm derived from glandular tissue from the oral cavity, nasal cavity or salivary tissue (major or accessory) (Döring and Arzi, 2015). A haemangiosarcoma is a malignant neoplasm of vascular endothelial origin characterized by extensive metastasis; it has been reported in the gingiva, tongue and hard palate (Burton *et al.*, 2014). A rhabdomyosarcoma is a malignant neoplasm of skeletal muscle or embryonic mesenchymal cells (Brockus and Myers, 2004).

A mast cell tumour is a local aggregation of mast cells forming a nodular tumour that has the potential to become malignant; it is also called a mastocytoma (Figure 5.67) (Elliott *et al.*, 2016). A lymphosarcoma is a malignant neoplasm defined by a proliferation of lymphocytes within solid organs such as the lymph nodes, tonsils, bone marrow, liver and spleen. The disease may also occur in the eye, skin, nasal cavity, oral cavity and gastrointestinal tract; it is also known as a lymphoma (Nemec *et al.*, 2012b).

An anaplastic neoplasm is a malignant neoplasm whose cells are generally undifferentiated and pleomorphic (displaying variability in size, shape and pattern of cells and/or their nuclei). An undifferentiated neoplasm is a malignant neoplasm whose cells are generally immature and lack distinctive features of a particular tissue type (AVDC, 2017).

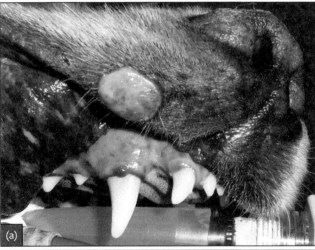

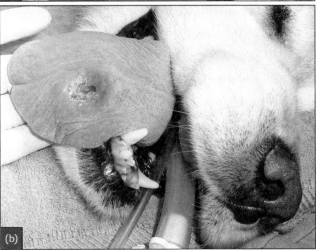

5.67 Mast cell tumour affecting the (a) right upper lip and (b) tongue in two dogs.
(© Dr Alexander M. Reiter)

Diagnosis and treatment of oral and maxillofacial tumours

Staging refers to determining the extent and spread of a neoplasm. This can be accomplished by obtaining tissue samples from the primary tumour (e.g. incisional biopsy) and regional lymph nodes (e.g. needle biopsy), as well as performing diagnostic imaging of local and distant sites (e.g. dental radiography, CT, thoracic radiography, abdominal ultrasonography). Regional metastasis is neoplastic spread to regional lymph node(s) confirmed by biopsy. Distant metastasis is neoplastic spread to distant sites confirmed by biopsy or diagnostic imaging (AVDC, 2017).

Lymph node resection or lymphadenectomy is the surgical removal of a lymph node. Buccotomy refers to an incision through the cheek (e.g. to gain access for an intraoral procedure). Commissurotomy refers to an incision through the lip commissure (e.g. to obtain access to an intraoral procedure). Cheiloplasty/commissuroplasty is a reconstructive surgery of the lip/lip commissure. Glossectomy refers to removal of tongue tissue, and lip and cheek resection is the surgical removal of lip and cheek tissue (which can involve the mucosa, musculature, neurovascular tissue and skin) (AVDC, 2017).

Partial mandibulectomy refers to the surgical removal (*en bloc*) of part of the mandible and surrounding soft tissues. A dorsal marginal mandibulectomy (also called a marginal mandibulectomy or mandibular rim excision) is a form of partial mandibulectomy in which the ventral border of the mandible is maintained. A segmental mandibulectomy is a form of partial mandibulectomy in which a full dorsoventral segment of the mandible is removed. A bilateral partial mandibulectomy refers to the surgical removal of part of both the left and right mandible and surrounding soft tissues. A total mandibulectomy is the surgical removal of one mandible and surrounding soft tissues. A partial maxillectomy refers to the surgical removal (*en bloc*) of part of the maxilla and/ or other facial bones and surrounding soft tissues. A bilateral partial maxillectomy includes the surgical removal of part of both the left and right maxilla and/or other facial bones and surrounding soft tissues. A partial palatectomy involves partial resection of the palate (AVDC, 2017; Sarowitz *et al.*, 2017).

Radiotherapy (also called radiation therapy) uses ionizing radiation to control or kill tumour cells (Kawabe *et al.*, 2015). Chemotherapy uses cytotoxic anti-neoplastic drugs (chemotherapeutic agents) to control or kill tumour cells. Immunotherapy uses the immune system to control or kill tumour cells (Boston *et al.*, 2014). See Chapter 11 for detailed information about the diagnosis and treatment of oral and maxillofacial tumours.

Salivary gland pathology

Ptyalism

Ptyalism (also called sialorrhoea, hypersalivation and hypersialism) refers to an excessive production and flow of saliva. It is rare as a primary salivary gland abnormality in cats and dogs. Drooling (the discharge of saliva from the mouth) may be noted due to an abnormal conformation of the lower lips in giant-breed dogs, Cocker Spaniels and other breeds. Treatment consists of bilateral mandibular and sublingual duct ligation or gland resection, lip fold resection, cheiloplasty or a combination of these procedures. If drooling saliva results from difficulty swallowing, the underlying problem (such as oral pain, mass lesion, foreign body, inability to close the mouth and oesophageal disease) must be resolved.

Sialocele

A sialocele (or salivary mucocele) is a clinical swelling caused by an accumulation of saliva that has leaked from a salivary duct or gland capsule (mucus extravasation phenomenon) into subcutaneous or submucosal tissue (Smith and Reiter, 2015). A sublingual sialocele (also called a ranula) is a mucus extravasation phenomenon manifesting in the sublingual region. A pharyngeal sialocele manifests in the pharyngeal region and a cervical sialocele in the intermandibular or cervical region. These often originate from the sublingual or mandibular salivary glands. A parotid sialocele presents over the lateral aspect of the face (Proot et al., 2016). A mucus retention cyst refers to an intraductal mucus accumulation with duct dilatation, resulting from obstruction of salivary flow (e.g. due to a sialolith or other foreign body). The ductal obstruction may lead to inflammation of the glandular tissue (Smith and Reiter, 2015).

Sialadenitis

Sialadenitis is the inflammation of a salivary gland, typically seen in middle-aged to older dogs. The zygomatic gland is most often affected (Boland et al., 2013). The patient may present with a painful swelling in the area of the affected gland, exophthalmos, lymphadenopathy, difficulty opening the mouth and fever. Sialolithiasis, characterized by the presence of one or more sialoliths in the salivary duct or gland, may be a contributing factor.

Sialadenosis and necrotizing sialometaplasia

Sialadenosis (also called sialosis) is a non-inflammatory, non-neoplastic enlargement of a salivary gland. There are no obvious cytological or histological abnormalities. Necrotizing sialometaplasia (salivary gland necrosis or infarction) refers to the squamous metaplasia of the salivary gland ducts and lobules with ischaemic necrosis of the salivary gland lobules (Spangler and Culbertson, 1991). Both conditions occur most often in the mandibular glands of young adult to middle-aged, small-breed dogs (e.g. terriers). Both disorders have a similar history and clinical presentation, but it remains speculative whether sialadenosis can progress to necrotizing sialometaplasia (Smith and Reiter, 2015). See Chapter 8 for detailed information about the diagnosis and treatment of these conditions.

Salivary gland neoplasia

Neoplasia of salivary glands is uncommon in cats and dogs. The mandibular salivary gland appears to be most often affected, with adenocarcinoma most commonly diagnosed (Hammer et al., 2001). Staging according to the tumour, node and metastasis (TNM) system will permit formulation of a treatment plan. Complete surgical excision of malignant tumours is difficult because of their invasive characteristics and the proximity of neural and vascular structures in the salivary gland region. Radiation therapy, with or without surgical intervention, may be an alternative to surgery alone (Brocks et al., 2008; Kim et al., 2008; Volmer et al., 2009; Lenoci and Ricciardi, 2015; Nakahira et al., 2017).

Other oral and maxillofacial pathology

Eosinophilic granuloma refers to conditions affecting the lip/labial mucosa, hard/soft palate, tongue/sublingual mucosa and skin that are characterized histopathologically by the presence of an eosinophilic infiltrate (Figure 5.68) (Bredal et al., 1996; Wildermuth et al., 2012). A pyogenic granuloma is a mucosal inflammatory proliferation most often developing buccal to the mandibular first molar tooth (in the cat probably due to malocclusion and secondary

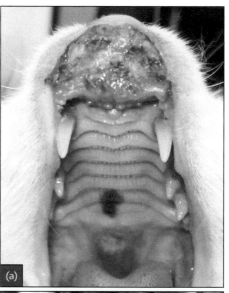

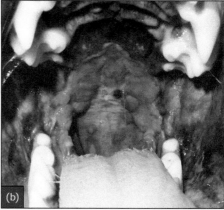

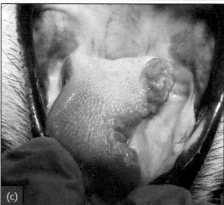

5.68 Eosinophilic granuloma affecting (a) the upper lip and rostral soft palate in a cat, (b) the caudal hard palate, tonsillar region, soft palate and palatoglossal folds in a dog, and (c) the lateral aspect of the tongue in a cat.
(© Dr Alexander M. Reiter)

traumatic contact of these tissues by the ipsilateral maxillary fourth premolar tooth) (Figure 5.69) (Riehl *et al.*, 2014; Gracis *et al.*, 2015). Erythema multiforme is a typically drug-induced hypersensitivity reaction characterized by erythematous, vesiculobullous and/or ulcerative oral and skin lesions (Figure 5.70) (Nemec *et al.*, 2012b; Lommer, 2013). Calcinosis circumscripta refers to circumscribed areas of mineralization characterized by deposition of calcium salts (e.g. in the tip of the tongue of young large-breed dogs) (Figure 5.71) (Tafti *et al.*, 2005; Mouzakitis *et al.*, 2015).

Craniomandibular osteopathy is a disease characterized by cyclical resorption of normal bone and excessive replacement by immature bone along mandibular, temporal and other bone surfaces in immature and adolescent dogs (Padgett and Mostosky, 1986; Pettitt *et al.*, 2012). Calvarial hyperostosis is a disease characterized by irregular, progressive proliferation and thickening of the cortex of the bones forming the calvarium in adolescent dogs (Pastor *et al.*, 2000; McConnell *et al.*, 2006). Fibrous osteodystrophy is a disease characterized by the formation of hyperostotic bone lesions, in which deposition of unmineralized osteoid by hyperplastic osteoblasts and production of fibrous connective tissue exceed the rate of bone resorption; it usually develops due to primary or secondary hyperparathyroidism and results in softened, pliable and distorted bones of the face ('rubber jaw') (Reinhart *et al.*, 2015). Periostitis ossificans refers to

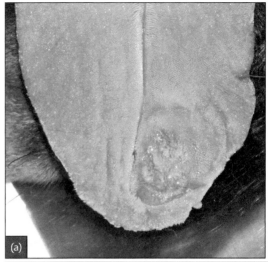
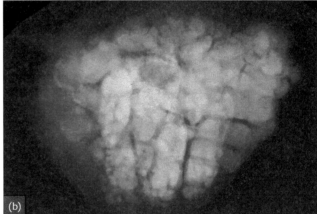

5.71 (a) Clinical photograph and (b) radiograph of calcinosis circumscripta affecting the apex of the tongue in a young dog.
(© Dr Alexander M. Reiter)

periosteal new bone formation in immature dogs, manifesting clinically as (usually) unilateral swelling of the mid to caudal body of the mandible and radiographically as a two-layered (double) ventral mandibular cortex (Blazejewski *et al.*, 2010). For detailed information about the diagnosis and treatment of these conditions, the reader is referred to Chapters 8 and 10.

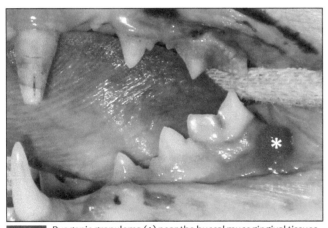

5.69 Pyogenic granuloma (∗) near the buccal mucogingival tissues of the left mandibular first molar tooth in a cat.
(© Dr Alexander M. Reiter)

References and further reading

Adams WM, Bjorling DE, McAnulty JE *et al.* (2005) Outcome of accelerated radiotherapy alone or accelerated radiotherapy followed by exenteration of the nasal cavity in dogs with intranasal neoplasia: 53 cases (1990–2002). *Journal of the American Veterinary Medical Association* **227**, 936–941

AVDC (2017) *Nomenclature*. American Veterinary Dental College (www.avdc.org)

Babbitt SG, Krakowski Volker M and Luskin IR (2016) Incidence of radiographic cystic lesions associated with unerupted teeth in dogs. *Journal of Veterinary Dentistry* **33**, 226–233

Bell CM and Soukup JW (2015) Histologic, clinical and radiologic findings of alveolar bone expansion and osteomyelitis of the jaws in cats. *Veterinary Pathology* **52**, 910–918

Blazejewski SW, Lewis JR, Gracis M *et al.* (2010) Mandibular periostitis ossificans in immature large breed dogs: five cases (1999–2006). *Journal of Veterinary Dentistry* **27**, 148–159

Boland L, Gomes E, Payen G *et al.* (2013) Zygomatic salivary gland diseases in the dog: three cases diagnosed by MRI. *Journal of the American Animal Hospital Association* **49**, 333–337

Bonner SE, Reiter AM and Lewis JR (2012) Orofacial manifestations of high-rise syndrome: a retrospective study of 84 cats (2000–2010). *Journal of Veterinary Dentistry* **29**, 10–18

Booij-Vrieling HE, van der Reijden WA, Houwers DJ *et al.* (2010) Comparison of periodontal pathogens between cats and their owners. *Veterinary Microbiology* **144**, 147–152

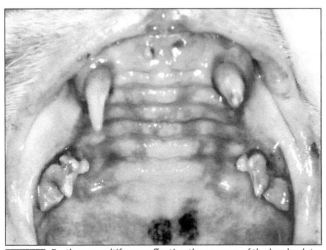

5.70 Erythema multiforme affecting the mucosa of the hard palate in a cat.
(© Dr Alexander M. Reiter)

Boonsriroj H, Kimitsuki K, Akagi T *et al.* (2014) Malignant epithelioid schwannoma of the oral cavity in a cat. *Journal of Veterinary Medical Science* **76**, 927–930

Boston SE, Lu X, Culp WT *et al.* (2014) Efficacy of systemic adjuvant therapies administered to dogs after excision of oral malignant melanomas: 151 cases (2001–2012). *Journal of the American Veterinary Medical Association* **245**, 401–407

Boy S, Crossley D and Steenkamp G (2016) Developmental structural tooth defects in dogs – Experience from veterinary dental referral practice and review of the literature. *Frontiers in Veterinary Science* doi: 10.3389/fvets.2016.00009

Boyce EN and Logan EI (1994) Oral health assessment in dogs: study design and results. *Journal of Veterinary Dentistry* **11**, 64–70

Bredal WP, Gunnes G, Vollset I *et al.* (1996) Oral eosinophilic granuloma in three Cavalier King Charles Spaniels. *Journal of Small Animal Practice* **37**, 499–504

Brocks BA, Peeters ME and Kimpfler S (2008) Oncocytoma in the mandibular salivary gland of a cat. *Journal of Feline Medicine and Surgery* **10**, 188–191

Brockus CW and Myers RK (2004) Multifocal rhabdomyosarcomas within the tongue and oral cavity of a dog. *Veterinary Pathology* **41**, 273–274

Burton JH, Powers BE and Biller BJ (2014) Clinical outcome in 20 cases of lingual hemangiosarcoma in dogs: 1996–2011. *Veterinary Comparative Oncology* **12**, 198–204

Carle D and Shope B (2014) Soft tissue tooth impaction in a dog. *Journal of Veterinary Dentistry* **31**, 96–105

Cave NJ, Bridges JP and Thomas DG (2012) Systemic effects of periodontal disease in cats. *Veterinary Quarterly* **32**, 131–144

Colgin LM, Schulman FY and Dubielzig RR (2001) Multiple epulides in 13 cats. *Veterinary Pathology* **38**, 227–229

Coyle VJ, Rassnick KM, Borst LB *et al.* (2015) Biological behaviour of canine mandibular osteosarcoma. A retrospective study of 50 cases (1999–2007). *Veterinary Comparative Oncology* **13**, 89–97

Dahlen G, Charalampakis G, Abrahamsson I *et al.* (2012) Predominant bacterial species in subgingival plaque in dogs. *Journal of Periodontal Research* **47**, 354–364

D'Astous J (2011) An overview of dentigerous cysts in dogs and cats. *Canadian Veterinary Journal* **52**, 905–907

DeBowes LJ (1998) The effects of dental disease on systemic disease. *Veterinary Clinics of North America: Small Animal Practice* **28**, 1057–1062

DeBowes LJ, Mosier D, Logan E *et al.* (1996) Association of periodontal disease and histologic lesions in multiple organs from 45 dogs. *Journal of Veterinary Dentistry* **13**, 57–60

de Bruijn ND, Kirpensteijn J, Neyens IJ *et al.* (2007) A clinicopathological study of 52 feline epulides. *Veterinary Pathology* **44**, 161–169

Desoutter AV, Goldschmidt MH and Sánchez MD (2012) Clinical and histologic features of 26 canine peripheral giant cell granulomas (formerly giant cell epulis). *Veterinary Pathology* **49**, 1018–1023

Döring S and Arzi B (2015) Diagnostic imaging in veterinary dental practice. Oral adenocarcinoma. *Journal of the American Veterinary Medical Association* **247**, 601–603

Durand C and Smith MM (2015) Excision of sublingual granuloma. *Journal of Veterinary Dentistry* **32**, 266–270

Edstrom EJ, Smith MM and Taney K (2013) Extraction of the impacted mandibular canine tooth in the dog. *Journal of Veterinary Dentistry* **30**, 56–61

Edstrom EJ, Smith MM, Taney K *et al.* (2015) Traumatic intrusion of a maxillary canine tooth: three cases. *Journal of Veterinary Dentistry* **32**, 41–53

Elliott JW, Cripps P, Blackwood L *et al.* (2016) Canine oral mucosal mast cell tumours. *Veterinary Comparative Oncology* **14**, 101–111

Ellis E (2002) Outcomes of patients with teeth in the line of mandibular angle fractures treated with stable internal fixation. *Journal of Oral and Maxillofacial Surgery* **60**, 863–865

Fiani N, Arzi B, Johnson EG *et al.* (2011a) Osteoma of the oral and maxillofacial regions in cats: seven cases (1999–2009). *Journal of the American Veterinary Medical Association* **238**, 1470–1475

Fiani N, Verstraete FJ, Kass PH *et al.* (2011b) Clinicopathologic characterization of odontogenic tumors and focal fibrous hyperplasia in dogs: 152 cases (1995–2005). *Journal of the American Veterinary Medical Association* **238**, 495–500

Fournier D, Mouton C, Lapierre P *et al.* (2001) *Porphyromonas gulae* sp. nov., an anaerobic, Gram-negative coccobacillus from the gingival sulcus of various animal hosts. *International Journal of Systematic and Evolutionary Microbiology* **51**, 1179–1189

Frazier SA, Johns SM, Ortega J *et al.* (2012) Outcome in dogs with surgically resected oral fibrosarcoma (1997–2008). *Veterinary Comparative Oncology* **10**, 33–43

Fulton A, Arzi B, Murphy B *et al.* (2014) The expression of calretinin and cytokeratins in canine acanthomatous ameloblastoma and oral squamous cell carcinoma. *Veterinary Comparative Oncology* **12**, 258–265

Gardner H, Fidel J, Haldorson G *et al.* (2015) Canine oral fibrosarcomas: a retrospective analysis of 65 cases (1998–2010). *Veterinary Comparative Oncology* **13**, 40–47

Gerbino G, Tarello F, Fasolis M *et al.* (1997) Rigid fixation with teeth in the line of mandibular fractures. *International Journal of Oral and Maxillofacial Surgery* **26**, 182–186

Gioso MA and Carvalho VG (2003) Maxillary dentigerous cyst in a cat. *Journal of Veterinary Dentistry* **20**, 28–30

Glickman LT, Glickman NW, Moore GE *et al.* (2009) Evaluation of the risk of endocarditis and other cardiovascular events on the basis of the severity of periodontal disease in dogs. *Journal of the American Veterinary Medical Association* **234**, 486–494

Glickman LT, Glickman NW, Moore GE *et al.* (2011) Association between chronic azotemic kidney disease and the severity of periodontal disease in dogs. *Preventive Veterinary Medicine* **99**, 193–200

Goldsworthy SJ, Burton C and Guilherme S (2013) Parotid duct foreign body in a dog diagnosed with CT. *Journal of the American Animal Hospital Association* **49**, 250–254

Gracis M (2012) Management of periodontal trauma. In: *Oral and Maxillofacial Surgery in Dogs and Cats, 1st edn*, ed. FJM Verstraete and MJ Lommer, pp. 201–215. Saunders Elsevier, Edinburgh

Gracis M, Keith D and Vite CH (2000) Dental and craniofacial findings in eight Miniature Schnauzer dogs affected by myotonia congenita: preliminary results. *Journal of Veterinary Dentistry* **17**, 119–127

Gracis M, Molinari E and Ferro S (2015) Caudal mucogingival lesions secondary to traumatic dental occlusion in 27 cats: macroscopic and microscopic description, treatment and follow-up. *Journal of Feline Medicine and Surgery* **17**, 318–328

Gracis M and Orsini P (1998) Treatment of traumatic dental displacement in dogs: six cases of lateral luxation. *Journal of Veterinary Dentistry* **15**, 65–72

Hale FA (1998) Dental caries in the dog. *Journal of Veterinary Dentistry* **15**, 79–83

Hale FA (2001) Localized intrinsic staining of teeth due to pulpitis and pulp necrosis in dogs. *Journal of Veterinary Dentistry* **18**, 14–20

Hamada N, Takahashi Y, Watanabe K *et al.* (2008) Molecular and antigenic similarities of the fimbrial major components between *Porphyromonas gulae* and *P. gingivalis*. *Veterinary Microbiology* **128**, 108–117

Hammer A, Getzy D, Ogilvie G *et al.* (2001) Salivary gland neoplasia in the dog and cat: survival times and prognostic factors. *Journal of the American Animal Hospital Association* **37**, 478–482

Hardham J, Dreier K, Wong J *et al.* (2005) Pigmented-anaerobic bacteria associated with canine periodontitis. *Veterinary Microbiology* **106**, 119–128

Harvey CE (1998) Periodontal disease in dogs – etiopathogenesis, prevalence, and significance. *Veterinary Clinics of North America: Small Animal Practice* **28**, 1111–1128

Harvey CE (2005) Management of periodontal disease: understanding the options. *Veterinary Clinics of North America: Small Animal Practice* **31**, 819–836

Harvey CE, Laster L, Shofer F *et al.* (2008) Scoring the full extent of periodontal disease in the dog: development of a total mouth periodontal score (TMPS) system. *Journal of Veterinary Dentistry* **25**, 176–180

Harvey CE, Laster L and Shofer FS (2012) Validation of use of subsets of teeth when applying the total mouth periodontal score (TMPS) system in dogs. *Journal of Veterinary Dentistry* **29**, 222–226

Harvey CE, Shofer FS and Laster L (1994) Association of age and body weight with periodontal disease in North American dogs. *Journal of Veterinary Dentistry* **11**, 94–105

Harvey CE, Thornsberry C and Miller BR (1995) Subgingival bacteria – comparison of culture results in dogs and cats with gingivitis. *Journal of Veterinary Dentistry* **12**, 147–150

Hefferren JJ, Schiff TG and Smith MR (1994) Assessment methods and clinical outcomes: chemical and microbial composition, formation, and maturation dynamics of pellicle, plaque, and calculus. *Journal of Veterinary Dentistry* **11**, 75–79

Hennet P (1999) Review of studies assessing plaque accumulation and gingival inflammation in dogs. *Journal of Veterinary Dentistry* **16**, 23–29

Hennet PR and Harvey CE (1992) Natural development of periodontal disease in the dog: a review of clinical, anatomical and histological features. *Journal of Veterinary Dentistry* **9**, 13–19

Hirayama K, Miyasho T, Ohmachi T *et al.* (2010) Biochemical and immunohistochemical characterization of the amyloid in canine amyloid-producing odontogenic tumor. *Veterinary Pathology* **47**, 915–922

Hoffman S (2008) Abnormal tooth eruption in a cat. *Journal of Veterinary Dentistry* **25**, 118–122

Holmstrom SE (2012) Veterinary dentistry in senior canines and felines. *Veterinary Clinics of North America: Small Animal Practice* **42**, 793–808

Jennings MW, Lewis JR, Soltero-Rivera MM *et al.* (2015) Effect of tooth extraction on stomatitis in cats: 95 cases (2000–2013). *Journal of the American Veterinary Medical Association* **246**, 654–660

Kamboozia AH and Punnia-Moorthy A (1993) The fate of teeth in mandibular fracture lines. A clinical and radiographic follow-up study. *International Journal of Oral and Maxillofacial Surgery* **22**, 97–101

Kato Y, Shirai M, Murakami M *et al.* (2011) Molecular detection of human periodontal pathogens in oral swab specimens from dogs in Japan. *Journal of Veterinary Dentistry* **28**, 84–89

Kawabe M, Mori T, Ito Y *et al.* (2015) Outcomes of dogs undergoing radiotherapy for treatment of oral malignant melanoma: 111 cases (2006–2012). *Journal of the American Veterinary Medical Association* **247**, 1146–1153

Khazandi M, Bird PS, Owens J *et al.* (2014) *In vitro* efficacy of cefovecin against anaerobic bacteria isolated from subgingival plaque of dogs and cats with periodontal disease. *Anaerobe* **28**, 104–108

Kim CG, Lee SY, Kim JW *et al.* (2013) Assessment of dental abnormalities by full-mouth radiography in small breed dogs. *Journal of the American Animal Hospital Association* **49**, 23–30

Kim H, Nakaichi M, Itamoto K *et al.* (2008) Malignant mixed tumor in the salivary gland of a cat. *Journal of Veterinary Science* **9**, 331–333

Kouki MI, Papadimitriou SA, Kazakos GM *et al.* (2013) Periodontal disease as a potential factor for systemic inflammatory response in the dog. *Journal of Veterinary Dentistry* **30**, 26–29

Lenoci D and Ricciardi M (2015) Ultrasound and multidetector computed tomography of mandibular salivary gland adenocarcinoma in two dogs. *Open Veterinary Journal* **5**, 173–178

Lewis JR, Okuda A, Pachtinger G *et al.* (2008) Significant association between tooth extrusion and tooth resorption in domestic cats. *Journal of Veterinary Dentistry* **25**, 86–95

Lewis JR and Reiter AM (2005) Management of generalized gingival enlargement in a dog – case report and review of the literature. *Journal of Veterinary Dentistry* **22**, 160–169

Lewis JR and Reiter AM (2011) Trauma-associated soft tissue injury to the head and neck. In: *Manual of Trauma Management in the Dog and Cat*, ed. K Drobatz, MW Beal and RS Syring, pp. 279–292. Wiley-Blackwell, Chichester

Logan EI and Boyce EN (1994) Oral health assessment in dogs: parameters and methods. *Journal of Veterinary Dentistry* **11**, 58–63

Lommer MJ (2013) Oral inflammation in small animals. *Veterinary Clinics of North America: Small Animal Practice* **43**, 555–571

Lommer MJ and Verstraete FJ (2001) Radiographic patterns of periodontitis in cats: 147 cases (1998–1999). *Journal of the American Veterinary Medical Association* **218**, 230–234

Love DN, Redwin J and Norris JM (2002) Cloning and expression of the superoxide dismutase gene of the feline strain of *Porphyromonas gingivalis*: immunological recognition of the protein by cats with periodontal disease. *Veterinary Microbiology* **86**, 245–256

MacGee S, Pinson DM and Shaiken L (2012) Bilateral dentigerous cysts in a dog. *Journal of Veterinary Dentistry* **29**, 242–249

Marshall-Jones ZV, Wallis CV, Allsopp JM *et al.* (2017) Assessment of dental plaque coverage by Quantitative Light-induced Fluorescence (QLF) in domestic short-haired cats. *Research in Veterinary Science* **111**, 99–107

McConnell JF, Hayes A, Platt SR *et al.* (2006) Calvarial hyperostosis syndrome in two bullmastiffs. *Veterinary Radiology and Ultrasound* **47**, 72–77

Mouzakitis E, Papazoglou LG, Loukopoulos PG *et al.* (2015) Carbon dioxide laser excision of lingual calcinosis circumscripta in a dog. *Journal of Veterinary Dentistry* **32**, 177–179

Nakahira R, Michishita M, Kato M *et al.* (2017) Oncocytic carcinoma of the salivary gland in a dog. *Journal of Veterinary Diagnostic Investigation* **29**, 105–108

Nam HS, McAnulty JF, Kwak HH *et al.* (2008) Gingival overgrowth in dogs associated with clinically relevant cyclosporine blood levels: observations in a canine renal transplantation model. *Veterinary Surgery* **37**, 247–253

Namikawa K, Maruo T, Honda M *et al.* (2012) Gingival overgrowth in a dog that received long-term cyclosporine for immune-mediated hemolytic anemia. *Canadian Veterinary Journal* **53**, 67–70

Nemec A, Arzi B, Hansen K *et al.* (2015) Osteonecrosis of the jaws in dogs in previously irradiated fields: 13 cases (1989–2014). *Frontiers in Veterinary Science* doi: 10.3389/fvets.2015.00005

Nemec A, Arzi B, Murphy B *et al.* (2012a) Prevalence and types of tooth resorption in dogs with oral tumors. *American Journal of Veterinary Research* **73**, 1057–1066

Nemec A, Verstraete FJ, Jerin A *et al.* (2013) Periodontal disease, periodontal treatment and systemic nitric oxide in dogs. *Research in Veterinary Science* **94**, 542–544

Nemec A, Zavodovskaya R, Affolter VK *et al.* (2012b) Erythema multiforme and epitheliotropic T-cell lymphoma in the oral cavity of dogs: 1989 to 2009. *Journal of Small Animal Practice* **53**, 445–452

Nordhoff M, Ruhe B, Kellermeier C *et al.* (2008) Association of *Treponema* spp. with canine periodontitis. *Veterinary Microbiology* **127**, 334–342

Olivry T, Rossi MA, Banovic F *et al.* (2015) Mucocutaneous lupus erythematosus in dogs (21 cases). *Veterinary Dermatology* **26**, 256-e55

O'Neill DG, Elliott J, Church DB *et al.* (2013) Chronic kidney disease in dogs in UK veterinary practices: prevalence, risk factors, and survival. *Journal of Veterinary Internal Medicine* **27**, 814–821

Padgett GA and Mostosky UV (1986) The mode of inheritance of craniomandibular osteopathy in West Highland White terrier dogs. *American Journal of Medical Genetics* **25**, 9–13

Pariser MS and Berdoulav P (2011) Amlodipine-induced gingival hyperplasia in a Great Dane. *Journal of the American Animal Hospital Association* **47**, 375–376

Pastor KF, Boulay JP, Schelling SH *et al.* (2000) Idiopathic hyperostosis of the calvaria in five young bullmastiffs. *Journal of the American Animal Hospital Association* **36**, 439–445

Pavlica Z, Petelin M, Juntes P *et al.* (2008) Periodontal disease burden and pathological changes in organs of dogs. *Journal of Veterinary Dentistry* **25**, 97–105

Peddle GD, Drobatz KJ, Harvey CE *et al.* (2009) Association of periodontal disease, oral procedures, and other clinical findings with bacterial endocarditis in dogs. *Journal of the American Veterinary Medical Association* **234**, 100–107

Peralta S, Arzi B, Nemec A *et al.* (2015) Non-radiation-related osteonecrosis of the jaws in dogs: 14 cases (1996–2014). *Frontiers in Veterinary Science* **2**, doi: 10.3389/fvets.2015.00007

Peralta S, Verstraete FJ and Kass PH (2010a) Radiographic evaluation of the classification of the extent of tooth resorption in dogs. *American Journal of Veterinary Research* **71**, 794–798

Peralta S, Verstraete FJ and Kass PH (2010b) Radiographic evaluation of the types of tooth resorption in dogs. *American Journal of Veterinary Research* **71**, 784–793

Pérez-Salcedo L, Herrera D, Esteban-Saltiveri D *et al.* (2013) Isolation and identification of *Porphyromonas* spp. and other putative pathogens from cats with periodontal disease. *Journal of Veterinary Dentistry* **30**, 208–213

Pérez-Salcedo L, Laguna E, Sánchez MC *et al.* (2015) Molecular identification of black-pigmented bacteria from subgingival samples of cats suffering from periodontal disease. *Journal of Small Animal Practice* **56**, 270–275

Pettitt R, Fox R, Comerford EJ *et al.* (2012) Bilateral angular carpal deformity in a dog with craniomandibular osteopathy. *Veterinary and Comparative Orthopaedics and Traumatology* **25**, 149–154

Proot JL, Nelissen P, Ladlow JF *et al.* (2016) Parotidectomy for the treatment of parotid sialocoele in 14 dogs. *Journal of Small Animal Practice* **57**, 79–83

Radice M, Martino PA and Reiter AM (2006) Evaluation of subgingival bacteria in the dog and their susceptibility to commonly used antibiotics. *Journal of Veterinary Dentistry* **23**, 219–224

Rawlinson JE, Goldstein RE, Reiter AM *et al.* (2011) Association of periodontal disease with systemic health indices in dogs and the systemic response to periodontal treatment. *Journal of the American Veterinary Medical Association* **238**, 601–609

Rawlinson JE and Reiter AM (2005) Repair of a gingival cleft associated with a maxillary canine tooth in a dog. *Journal of Veterinary Dentistry* **22**, 234–242

Reinhart JM, Nuth EK, Byers CG *et al.* (2015) Pre-operative fibrous osteodystrophy and severe, refractory, post-operative hypocalcemia following parathyroidectomy in a dog. *Canadian Veterinary Journal* **56**, 867–871

Reiter AM (1998) Tooth caries in animals. *Proceedings of the 12th Annual Veterinary Dental Forum*, New Orleans, Louisiana, USA, pp. 321–326

Reiter AM (2012) Dental and oral diseases. In: *The Cat: Clinical Medicine and Management*, ed. SE Little, pp. 329–370. Saunders, St. Louis

Reiter AM and Harvey CE (2010) Periodontal and endodontic disease. In: *Mechanisms of Disease in Small Animal Surgery, 3rd edn*, ed. MJ Bojrab and E Monnet Jackson, pp. 125–128. NewMedia, Teton

Reiter AM and Holt D (2012) Palate surgery. In: *Veterinary Surgery: Small Animal*, ed. KM Tobias and SA Johnston, Elsevier, St. Louis pp. 1707–1717

Reiter AM and Lewis JR (2011) Trauma-associated musculoskeletal injuries of the head. In: *Manual of Trauma Management in the Dog and Cat*, ed. K Drobatz, MW Beal and RS Syring, pp. 255–278. Wiley-Blackwell, Chichester

Reiter AM, Lewis JR and Harvey CE (2012) Dentistry for the surgeon. In: *Veterinary Surgery: Small Animal*, ed. KM Tobias and SA Johnston, pp. 1037–1053. Elsevier, St Louis

Reiter AM, Lewis JR and Okuda A (2005a) Update on the etiology of tooth resorption in domestic cats. *Veterinary Clinics of North America: Small Animal Practice* **35**, 913–942

Reiter AM, Lyon KF, Nachreiner RF *et al.* (2005b) Evaluation of calciotropic hormones in cats with odontoclastic resorptive lesions. *American Journal of Veterinary Research* **66**, 1446–1452

Reiter AM and Mendoza KA (2002) Feline odontoclastic resorptive lesions. An unsolved enigma in veterinary dentistry. *Veterinary Clinics of North America: Small Animal Practice* **32**, 791–837

Reiter AM and Schwarz T (2007) Computed tomographic appearance of masticatory myositis in dogs: seven cases (1999–2006). *Journal of the American Veterinary Medical Association* **231**, 924–930

Riehl J, Bell CM, Constantaras ME *et al.* (2014) Clinicopathologic characterization of oral pyogenic granuloma in 8 cats. *Journal of Veterinary Dentistry* **31**, 80–86

Riggio MP, Lennon A, Taylor DJ *et al.* (2011) Molecular identification of bacteria associated with canine periodontal disease. *Veterinary Microbiology* **150**, 394–400

Robinson W, Shales C and White RN (2014) The use of rigid endoscopy in the management of acute oropharyngeal stick injuries. *Journal of Small Animal Practice* **55**, 609–614

Rosselli DD, Platt SR, Freeman C *et al.* (2017) Cranioplasty using titanium mesh after skull tumor resection in five dogs. *Veterinary Surgery* **46**, 67–74

Roux P, Stich H and Schawalder P (2011) Multiple tooth resorption in an Italian greyhound. *Schweizer Archiv fuer Tierheilkunde* **153**, 281–286

Rybnícek J and Hill PB (2007) Suspected polymyxin B-induced pemphigus vulgaris in a dog. *Veterinary Dermatology* **18**, 165–170

Sakai H, Mori T, Iida T *et al.* (2008) Immunohistochemical features of proliferative marker and basement membrane components of two feline inductive odontogenic tumours. *Journal of Feline Medicine and Surgery* **10**, 296–299

Sancak A, Favrot C, Geisseler MD *et al.* (2015) Antibody titres against canine papillomavirus 1 peak around clinical regression in naturally occurring oral papillomatosis. *Veterinary Dermatology* **26**, 57–59

Sarowitz BN, Davis GJ and Kim S (2017) Outcome and prognostic factors following curative-intent surgery for oral tumours in dogs: 234 cases (2004 to 2014). *Journal of Small Animal Practice* **58**, 146–153

Scherl DS, Bork K, Coffman L *et al.* (2009) Application of the gingival contour plaque index: six-month plaque and gingivitis study. *Journal of Veterinary Dentistry* **26**, 23–27

Senhorinho GN, Nakano V, Liu C et al. (2011) Detection of Porphyromonas gulae from subgingival biofilms of dogs with and without periodontitis. Anaerobe 17, 257–258

Shetty V and Freymiller E (1989) Teeth in the line of fracture: a review. Journal of Oral and Maxillofacial Surgery 47, 1303–1306

Silver JG, Martin L and McBride BC (1975) Recovery and clearance of oral micro-organisms following experimental bacteremia in dogs. Archives of Oral Biology 20, 675–679

Smith MM and Reiter AM (2015) Salivary gland disorders. In: Clinical Veterinary Advisor, 3rd edn, ed. E Cote, pp. 916–919. Mosby, St Louis

Smithson CW, Smith MM, Tappe J et al. (2012) Multicentric oral plasmacytoma in three dogs. Journal of Veterinary Dentistry 29, 96–110

Spangler WL and Culbertson MR (1991) Salivary gland disease in dogs and cats: 245 cases (1985–1988). Journal of the American Veterinary Medical Association 198, 465–469

Strøm PC, Arzi B, Cissell DD et al. (2016) Ankylosis and pseudoankylosis of the temporomandibular joint in 10 dogs (1993–2015). Veterinary and Comparative Orthopaedics and Traumatology 29, 409–415

Supsavhad W, Dirksen WP, Martin CK et al. (2016) Animal models of head and neck squamous cell carcinoma. Veterinary Journal 210, 7–16

Suzuki S, Uchida K, Harada T et al. (2015) The origin and role of autophagy in the formation of cytoplasmic granules in canine lingual granular cell tumors. Veterinary Pathology 52, 456–464

Tafti AK, Hanna P and Bourque AC (2005) Calcinosis circumscripta in the dog: a retrospective pathological study. Journal of Veterinary Medicine A, Physiology, Pathology, Clinical Medicine 52, 13–17

Thaller SR and Mabourakh S (1994) Teeth located in the line of mandibular fracture. Journal of Craniofacial Surgery 5, 16–19

Thatcher G (2017) Oral Surgery: Treatment of a dentigerous cyst in a dog. Canadian Veterinary Journal 58, 195–199

Thomason JD, Fallow TL, Carmichael KP et al. (2009) Gingival hyperplasia associated with the administration of amlodipine to dogs with degenerative valvular diease (2004–2008). Journal of Veterinary Internal Medicine 23, 39–42

Tremolada G, Milovancev M, Culp WT et al. (2015) Surgical management of canine refractory retrobulbar abscesses: six cases. Journal of Small Animal Practice 56, 667–670

Trevejo RT, Lefevers SL, Yang M et al. (2018) Survival analysis to evaluate associations between periodontal disease and the risk of development of chronic azotaemic kidney disease evaluated at primary care veterinary hospitals. Journal of the American Veterinary Association 252, 710–720

Ulbricht RD, Manfra Marretta S and Klippert LS (2004) Mandibular canine tooth luxation injury in a dog. Journal of Veterinary Dentistry 21, 77–83

Valdez M, Haines R, Riviere KH et al. (2000) Isolation of oral spirochetes from dogs and cats and provisional identification using polymerase chain reaction (PCR) analysis specific for human plaque Treponema spp. Journal of Veterinary Dentistry 17, 23–26

Verhaert L (2007) Developmental oral and dental conditions. In: BSAVA Manual of Canine and Feline Dentistry, 3rd edn, ed. C Tutt, J Deeprose and D Crossley, pp. 77–95. BSAVA Publications, Gloucester

Verstraete FJ, Zin BP, Kass PH et al. (2011) Clinical signs and histologic findings in dogs with odontogenic cysts: 41 cases (1995–2010). Journal of the American Veterinary Medical Association 239, 1470–1476

Villamizar-Martinez LA, Reiter AM, Sanchez MD et al. (2016) Benign cementoblastoma (true cementoma) in a cat. Journal of Feline Medicine and Surgery Open Reports doi: 10.1177/2055116915626847

Voelter-Ratson K, Hagen R, Grundmann S et al. (2015) Dacryocystitis following a nasolacrimal duct obstruction caused by an ectopic intranasal tooth in a dog. Veterinary Ophthalmology 18, 433–436

Volmer C, Benal Y, Caplier L et al. (2009) Atypical vimentin expression in a feline salivary gland adenocarcinoma with widespread metastases. Journal of Veterinary Medical Science 71, 1681–1684

White TL (2010) Lip avulsion and mandibular symphyseal separation repair in an immature cat. Journal of Veterinary Dentistry 27, 228–233

Wildermuth BE, Griffin CE and Rosenkrantz WS (2012) Response of feline eosinophilic plaques and lip ulcers to amoxicillin trihydrate-clavulanate potassium therapy: a randomized, double-blind placebo-controlled prospective study. Veterinary Dermatology 23, 110–118

Wolf HF, Rateitschak EM, Rateitschak KH et al. (2005) Color Atlas of Dental Medicine – Periodontology, 3rd edn, p. 64. Thieme, Stuttgart

Yamasaki Y, Nomura R, Nakano K et al. (2012) Distribution of periodontopathic bacterial species in dogs and their owners. Archives of Oral Biology 57, 1183–1188

Chapter 6

Anaesthetic and analgesic considerations in dentistry and oral surgery

Norman Johnston and M. Paula Larenza Menzies

Dental and oral surgical procedures present the clinician with unique challenges in terms of anaesthetic techniques and skills. It is necessary to have good access to the oral cavity throughout the dental or surgical procedure, despite the presence of the endotracheal tube, pharyngeal packing and monitoring apparatus. Dental and oral surgical procedures are notoriously difficult to plan in terms of time and analgesic needs because pathology is frequently not apparent preoperatively. Case planning must allow for increased surgical time and include the possibility that a higher plane of intraoperative analgesia might be necessary than was first considered. Patient health status can be challenging in cats and aged small dog breeds, which provide proportionately higher patient numbers for dental and oral surgical procedures than the general companion animal population. Finally, patient comfort and safety must be paramount at all times.

A full examination of the head and oral cavity is an essential part of any clinical examination. In some cases, a more detailed oral examination under sedation or anaesthesia may be indicated if the patient is uncooperative or if lesions are very painful. If a patient strongly resists an awake examination of the oral cavity, chemical restraint may be indicated, both to ensure lesions are not missed and to protect the clinician. Although sedation will allow for an improved clinical examination of the oral cavity and performance of some minor non-painful procedures, the time limits imposed are unlikely to permit detailed radiological examination or definitive treatment. Most importantly, airway control is not present during sedation. Therefore, sedation cannot be considered a realistic option for anything other than preliminary diagnostic examination, or as premedication before the administration of a general anaesthetic.

This chapter is intended to provide information on anaesthetic techniques and skills within the confines of dental and oral surgical treatment. For further information on anaesthesia, including theory, drugs, techniques and equipment, the reader is directed elsewhere (Duke-Novakovski, 2007).

General considerations

The anaesthetic technique should be chosen according to the patient's physical status, the planned procedure, and available drugs and equipment. Patients for dentistry and oral surgery are frequently of a small breed, aged and may have suffered subacute to chronic disease for some time previously. Dentistry and oral surgery can prove to be a lengthy procedure. The anaesthetic technique should aim to provide an unconscious, immobile, relaxed patient with appropriate analgesia or anti-nociception. Since the perfect anaesthetic agent that provides all of these conditions without side effects does not exist, a balanced anaesthetic technique (i.e. combination of the minimal effective doses of multiple drugs with synergistic or complementary properties) is used to minimize side effects.

For each anaesthetic procedure performed, a written record should be completed in real time. This should include signalment containing patient identity, species, breed, gender and age. The weight of the patient should be recorded to allow accurate calculation of drug doses. The anaesthetic record should also include a minimum database along with a summary of the relevant recent history pertinent to the anaesthetic episode and dental or oral surgical procedure. Pre-, intra- and immediate postoperative anaesthetic/analgesic agents should be recorded with the time, dose and route of administration. The patient's vital signs should be monitored every 5 minutes and recorded at least every 10 minutes. The duration of anaesthesia, dental/oral surgical and/or radiological procedures, complications and corrective measures should also be recorded (Figure 6.1).

Patient evaluation

With the exception of aggressive or uncooperative animals, a thorough clinical examination should be carried out before administering sedative or anaesthetic agents. The medical history of the patient should be reviewed and any disease processes or abnormal parameters recorded in the anaesthetic record. The pre-anaesthetic health assessment should aim to establish whether the patient can receive anaesthesia safely. If a condition potentially affecting the outcome of anaesthesia is recognized, it may be advisable to defer any elective dental and oral surgical procedure until the patient is stable.

When performing the clinical examination, particular attention should be given to the cardiovascular and respiratory systems, primarily because sedatives and anaesthetics alter normal cardiorespiratory function; in addition, the cardiorespiratory system is involved in the uptake, distribution and elimination of many anaesthetic drugs.

6.1 An example of an anaesthetic record sheet.
(Courtesy of the University of Helsinki)

Thoracic radiographs are indicated for patients with signs of cardiac or pulmonary disease and for patients with tumours in which pulmonary metastasis may be suspected. If heart murmurs and/or arrhythmias are detected, a thorough cardiac work-up is indicated.

For senior patients (i.e. dogs >8–10 years and cats >12 years of age), attention should also be paid to renal and hepatic function, as drug elimination could be compromised. Kidney function should be evaluated when long-term treatment with non-steroidal anti-inflammatory drugs (NSAIDs) is considered. Temperament should be assessed to anticipate and prevent episodes of anxiety, particularly during recovery from anaesthesia. Current medical treatment should be reviewed to anticipate potential drug interactions with agents planned for use. For information regarding specific conditions (e.g. cardiac disease, diabetes) the reader is directed to the *BSAVA Manual of Canine and Feline Anaesthesia and Analgesia*.

Preoperative laboratory tests, including haematology, serum biochemistry, blood coagulation and possibly blood gas tests, may be indicated in some patients. Patients that present with acute anaemia, electrolyte imbalances, coagulopathies and ventilation/oxygenation abnormalities should have their procedure rescheduled once their condition is stable. For patients in which bleeding may be a potential surgical complication after tooth extraction or other oral surgical procedure, blood typing or cross-matching tests should be performed. Once the history has been gathered and the clinical examination completed, the anaesthetic risk is evaluated and recorded using the American Society of Anesthesiologists (ASA) physical status classification system (Figure 6.2).

ASA class	Description	Clinical examples
I	Patient with no organic disease or in whom the disease is localized and is causing no systemic disturbance	Healthy animal
II	Patient with mild systemic disturbance that may or may not be associated with the surgical complaint	Controlled diabetes, obesity, geriatric patient, asymptomatic mitral valve insufficiency
III	Patient with moderate systemic disturbance that may or may not be associated with the surgical complaint and that usually interferes with normal activity, but is not incapacitating	Mitral valve insufficiency which is controlled with treatment, anaemia, moderate hypovolaemia, dehydration, renal insufficiency
IV	Patient with extreme systemic disturbance that is incapacitating, is a constant threat to life and seriously interferes with the animal's normal function	Decompensated mitral valve insufficiency, severe pneumothorax from lacerated lung, shock, uraemia, severe hypovolaemia
V	Patient presented in a moribund condition and not expected to survive 24 hours with or without surgery. The term moribund implies that medical treatment cannot improve the animal's condition. Surgery is usually required immediately to alleviate pain	Major trauma, multi-organ dysfunction, end-stage cancer, advanced renal and cardiac disease
E	An emergency operation in a patient falling in any of the classifications I–V. These patients are at greater risk than non-emergency patients of similar status	Avulsed tooth, acute pulp exposure, jaw fracture, uncontrolled oral bleeding

6.2 American Society of Anesthesiologists (ASA) physical status classification system.

Animals considered to be 'healthy' (i.e. ASA physical status I–II) will cope well with most anaesthetic agents and techniques. 'Sick' patients (i.e. ASA physical status III–V) may not tolerate some agents that alter cardio-vascular function or are poorly eliminated. A UK study of 98,036 dogs and 79,178 cats concluded the risk of anaesthetic and sedation-related death was 0.05% and 0.17%, respectively, for ASA physical status I and II (Brodbelt *et al.*, 2008). Deaths increased significantly to 1.33% and 1.40%, respectively, for ASA physical status III–V, hence the importance of thoroughly assessing health preoperatively.

Preparation for anaesthesia

Equipment preparation

Anaesthesia and sedation may carry higher than normal risk if performed without adequate preparation. All anaesthesia-related equipment should be checked before commencing premedication. Using a checklist has been shown to reduce the risk of accidents related to human error and speed up the setting-up process (Figures 6.3 and 6.4).

Airway management

Dentistry and oral surgery demand good airway management to prevent accidental aspiration of fluids (e.g. coolant water, blood, saliva) and solids (calculus, instruments, parts of teeth). Well fitting, secured, cuffed endotracheal tubes are mandatory in addition to pharyngeal packing (Lamata *et al.*, 2012).

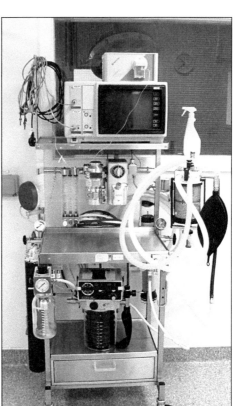

6.4
Anaesthetic trolley ready for use.

Intubation equipment
• Endotracheal tubes (various) of appropriate sizes
• Reliability of cuff checked (i.e. inflating cuff for 1–2 minutes)
• Tube lubricant
• Laryngoscope
• Endotracheal tube ties
• Gauze
• Lidocaine spray (for cats)

Anaesthetic machine
• Anaesthetic machine connected to O_2 source
• Availability of O_2 checked
• Flowmeter working at 200 ml/min and at 2 l/min
• Vaporizer: inhaled agent filled, working
• O_2 flush valve tested
• Fresh gas outlet: attached to machine and breathing system
• CO_2 absorber canister(s) filled, no purple soda-lime, fitting well to prevent leaks
• Breathing system of appropriate size attached
• Reservoir bag attached
• Scavenge hose attached to pop-off valve and to passive/active scavenging system
• Pop-off valve working
• One-way valves in place
• Perform leak-test

Other equipment
• Monitoring equipment prepared and electronic monitoring equipment turned on
• Connected cables and probes
• Warming devices prepared/turned on
• Fluids, pumps, extension lines prepared
• Intravenous catheterization set prepared

6.3 Checklist for use when setting up equipment prior to general anaesthesia.

Endotracheal tubes

Cuffed tubes are preferred, as they seal the space between the trachea and the endotracheal tube. This, in addition to the pharyngeal pack, will help prevent aspiration of foreign material and leakage of volatile anaesthetic agents into the operating room. For prolonged anaesthesia (>2 hours), high-volume, low-pressure cuffs are preferred over low-volume, high-pressure cuffs, as they allow for better perfusion of tracheal mucosa, thus reducing the risk of tissue damage. Care must be taken not to overinflate the cuff, particularly in smaller patients. Overinflating an endotracheal tube cuff may result in tracheal rupture in cats (Hardie *et al.*, 1999; Mitchell *et al.*, 2000). The volume of air needed in the cuff to obtain an airtight seal ranges from approximately 1 to 2 ml in most intubated healthy cats. The integrity of the cuff can be tested prior to induction by test-inflating it for 2 minutes. Usually, 3, 5 and 10 ml syringes are used to inflate the endotracheal tube cuffs of patients <5 kg, 5–15 kg and >15 kg, respectively. After endotracheal intubation and cuff inflation the intracuff pressure can be checked with a manometer via the pilot balloon of the tube. Intracuff pressures above 30 mmHg should be avoided to minimize hypoperfusion of the tracheal mucosa.

Patients should receive the widest tube that fits in their trachea. This can be estimated by palpating the trachea or by extrapolating the diameter of the trachea from the weight of the patient (Figure 6.5). The length of the tube can be determined by measuring the distance between the incisor teeth and the thoracic inlet. However, also consider where the pilot line inserts, as the tube tie that will be level with the lip commissures will be just rostral or caudal to it (depending on patient size). Longer tubes can either be inserted too deeply in the endobronchial tree

Bodyweight (kg)	Internal diameter (mm)
Cats	
2	3
4	4
6	4.5–5
Dogs	
2	5
4	6
7	7
9	7–8
12	8
14	9–10
16–20	10–11
30	12
40–50	14–16

6.5 Typical endotracheal tube sizes.

and accidentally insufflate only one lung or stick out of the mouth adding dead space. Conventional endotracheal tubes have a gentle radius of curvature. Preformed tubes with a more pronounced bend or the use of angled plastic connections may be preferred in certain procedures facilitating the connection to the breathing system from behind.

Endotracheal tubes must be well secured in dental and oral surgical patients. Frequent turning of the head and neck during these procedures can easily lead to movement of the tube and tracheal irritation. Inadvertent dislodging of the endotracheal tube from the trachea or from the anaesthetic tubing is not uncommon. A minimum of one (and possibly two) tracheal ties are necessary to secure the tube, one being placed behind the ears and perhaps another around either the upper or lower jaw. Coloured plastic ties are preferable to bandages or gauze because they are highly visible, do not cling to hair and do not soak up saliva or blood. They are also disposable, cleaner, and hold on to the tube, thus preventing the potential damage that can occur to the trachea if the tube accidentally moves (Figure 6.6).

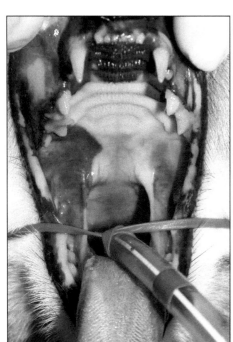

6.6 Endotracheal tube secured with a coloured plastic tie (Trinity Trach-Tube Ties; www.trachtubeties.com) in a 5-year-old female spayed European Domestic Shorthaired cat that showed difficulty closing the mouth due to a fractured and displaced right maxillary fourth premolar tooth.

To prevent tracheal tears and ruptures, the clinician should be aware of head and neck positioning and move the head with the tube to avoid counter-rotation of the tube. When turning the patient, it is also wise to detach the endotracheal tube from the anaesthetic machine for the same reason.

The patient should be placed in such a way that will allow fluids to run out of the mouth. If in lateral recumbency, padding under the neck will allow this. In dorsal recumbency, a pad extending the neck will achieve the same result.

Alternatives to transoral intubation

In some cases the surgical procedure may require the endotracheal tube to bypass the oral cavity; for example, surgery for craniomaxillofacial trauma or oral neoplasia and any procedure where the surgeon needs to establish a functional occlusion intraoperatively without the need to constantly extubate and re-intubate. Other circumstances that may require an alternative technique would exist if access to the pharynx is not possible (e.g. large pharyngeal mass) or the patient is unable to open the mouth (e.g. masticatory muscle myositis or temporomandibular joint ankylosis).

Pharyngotomy intubation: Intubation via a pharyngotomy is the most common alternative to transoral intubation. Pharyngotomy refers to making an incision into the pharynx through which an endotracheal tube is inserted for anaesthesia. The incision sites described vary in the literature, but if the primary purpose is to place an endotracheal tube, the incision should be made rostral to the epihyoid bone and rostroventral to the angular process of the mandible. This rostral site is not suited to the placement of a feeding tube, as there is risk of trapping the epiglottis and closing off the airway.

Anaesthesia should be established first, with transoral intubation if possible. The side chosen will depend on how the patient is positioned for surgery; either side is possible for pharyngotomy intubation. The hair is clipped and skin prepared for aseptic surgery. The clinician should be familiar with the important structures of the area and palpate the landmarks prior to incision (Figure 6.7). With sterile, curved tissue forceps in the mouth creating lateral pressure against the pharyngeal wall, an incision is made in the skin near the unnamed ventral notch immediately rostral to the angular process of the mandible. The tissue forceps are pushed through the incision. The distal end of a wire-reinforced endotracheal tube is placed between the jaws of the tissue forceps and withdrawn through the incision into the oral cavity. The transorally placed endotracheal tube is removed, and the wire-reinforced tube is turned and inserted into the trachea. The tube is secured to the skin with a Chinese finger trap suture or skin sutures secured to tape wrapped around the tube at its exit site. Wire-reinforced tubes (i.e. tubes that contain an embedded metal spiral) should be used to prevent kinking and airway obstruction (Figure 6.8).

Transmylohyoid intubation: An alternative to pharyngotomy intubation for the surgical management of maxillofacial fractures in the dog is transmylohyoid intubation, where an endotracheal tube is inserted through a stoma created by an incision through the skin, subcutaneous tissue, mylohyoid muscle and sublingual mucosa immediately medial to the lingual mandibular cortex at the level of the mandibular first molar tooth (Soukup and Snyder, 2015).

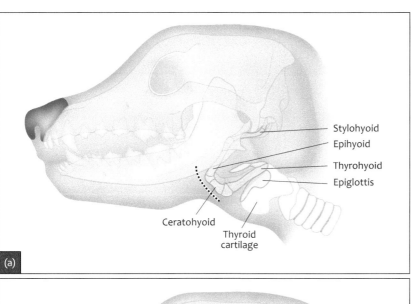

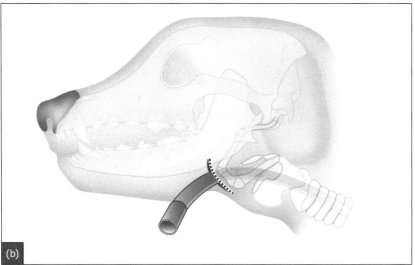

6.7 Pharyngotomy intubation. (a) Anatomical location of incision. (b) Diagram of tube placement through the pharyngotomy site.

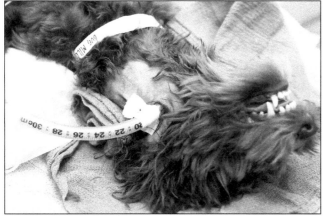

6.8 Wire-reinforced pharyngotomy tube in place. (Courtesy of Dr J. Yee)

Tracheotomy intubation: Intubation via a tracheotomy is indicated if the operator is unable to open the patient's mouth sufficiently to allow transoral intubation. The hair must be clipped and the skin prepared for aseptic surgery in the area of the cervical trachea. With the patient in dorsal recumbency (support under the patient's neck and the forelegs secured caudally along either side of the thorax), the larynx and trachea are palpated, and a skin incision is made in the ventral midline from the cricoid cartilage extending 3–4 cm caudally. The sternohyoid muscles are separated and pulled laterally. The trachea is visualized. Stay sutures are placed just cranial and caudal to the proposed annular ligament incision, allowing for stabilization of the trachea when inserting or changing the tube. The incision is made in one of the annular ligaments between the third and fifth tracheal rings and should not extend more than 50% of the diameter of the trachea. Blood and mucus are suctioned from the lumen, and a cuffed sterile tube is placed. The sternohyoid muscles, subcutaneous tissue and skin cranial and caudal to the tube are apposed. The tube is secured to gauze tied around the neck. Following removal of the tube after anaesthesia, the tracheotomy site is left to heal by second intention. If postoperative respiratory distress (swelling, oedema) is likely, a tracheostomy tube (made of nylon, PVC or metal) can be kept temporarily in place until the patient is stable enough to have it removed.

Pharyngeal pack

The purpose of a pharyngeal pack is to prevent fluids or solids passing from the oral cavity into the pharynx/larynx/oesophagus/trachea. The pack must be absorbent, well fitting and capable of being removed quickly in an emergency. Sponge butterfly packs with long plastic leads are recommended in preference to swabs, which can easily become saturated and dislodged (Figure 6.9). Alternative methods may include using gauze swabs tied in bundles with white open wove (WOW) bandage (2.5 cm width) or human throat packs. These throat packs are cotton wool wrapped in cotton gauze with a removal cord. The disadvantage of using bundles of gauze swabs is possible loss of swabs from the bundle. For this reason swabs must be counted both in and out of the pharynx. Over-packing the pharynx is rare, but too many swabs can disrupt lymph drainage causing swelling of the tissue rostral to the pack.

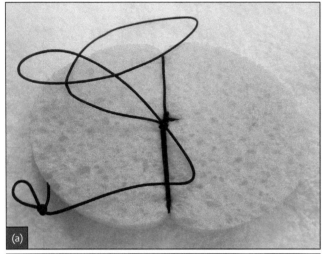

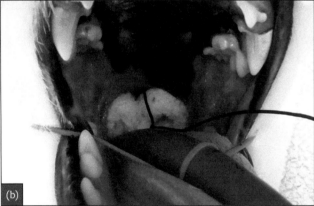

6.9   (a) Sponge flange mouthpack. (b) Pack placed to occlude the pharynx around the endotracheal tube.

Patient preparation and fluid therapy

Patients should have solid food withdrawn a minimum of 8 hours before premedication (Bednarski *et al.*, 2011). A longer fasting period than this can promote regurgitation of stomach contents (Posner, 2007). Access to water can be allowed up to 1 hour before premedication. Some opioids may also increase the risk of regurgitation and aspiration during anaesthesia.

Without exception, all patients should receive an intravenous catheter after premedication. Administration of anaesthetics without patent intravenous access is a dangerous practice and must be avoided. For healthy patients undergoing routine dental and oral surgical procedures, a balanced crystalloid solution of isotonic fluids at 5–10 ml/kg/hour is sufficient. Dehydrated patients require additional fluids to correct the deficit over a period of 6–12 hours. In rare cases where extensive blood loss is anticipated or occurs, a higher rate and/or synthetic colloids or blood replacement should be considered. It should be

recognized that patients undergoing dental and oral surgery may not voluntarily use their mouths for a period postoperatively, necessitating the continuation of fluid therapy.

Fluid overload may accidentally occur in small-sized patients. Signs of fluid overload include watery nasal discharge, increased lung sounds and pulmonary oedema. Furosemide (2 mg/kg i.v.) should be administered if accidental fluid overload is suspected. To avoid this complication, the use of infusion pumps, syringe drivers or burettes that accurately measure the delivery of fluids is advised (Figure 6.10). The cost of infusion pumps is now relatively low, and their use provides accurate dosing and peace of mind. Fluid restriction should be applied to patients at risk of pulmonary oedema due to underlying conditions (e.g. cardiac disease, anuria). In these patients, balanced crystalloid solutions should be administered at lower rates of 2–3 ml/kg/hour.

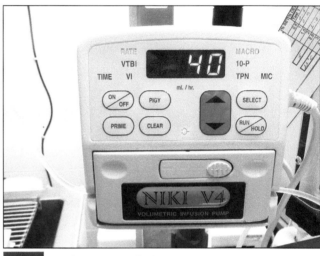

6.10   Simple intravenous fluid pump.

Body temperature maintenance

Hypothermia intraoperatively and postoperatively is a very real concern for dental and oral surgical patients. Heat is lost during anaesthesia by four mechanisms: conduction, radiation, convection and evaporation. Immobility during long procedures combined with an open mouth plus copious cold fluid irrigation reduces core body temperature very quickly. Small-sized patients are at higher risk of hypothermia because of their increased ratio of body surface area to bodyweight. Perioperative hypothermia is associated with cardiovascular, metabolic, immunological, renal and neurological complications (Armstrong *et al.*, 2005). Thermoregulation is impaired during anaesthesia due to vasodilatation, lack of muscle activity and decreased metabolic rate. Measures to prevent hypothermia should be taken as soon as the patient is intubated and continued well into recovery.

Mild hypothermia (32–37°C) can cause catecholamine release, an increase in heart rate, vasoconstriction, prolonged platelet aggregation, arrhythmias and increased blood loss during surgery. Moderate hypothermia (28–32°C) causes severe arrhythmias including ventricular fibrillation. Severe hypothermia (below 28°C) is associated with depression, coma, hypoxia, acute respiratory distress syndrome, decreased glomerular filtration rate, acute tubular necrosis and cardiac arrest.

Core body temperature, continuously measured by an oesophageal probe, can show an alarming drop in body temperature in the first few minutes of general anaesthesia, even when warming devices are employed. Hypothermia must be prevented in all dental and oral surgical cases by using a combination of passive warming devices to diminish heat loss (e.g. blankets or mats) and active warming devices to increase the body temperature of the patient (e.g. circulating warm-water heating mattresses, forced-air warming blankets) (Figure 6.11). The use of hot water bottles or 'hot hands' is not advised because severe thermal burns can occur from contact of the skin with hot objects in anaesthetized animals.

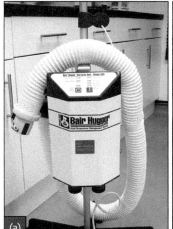
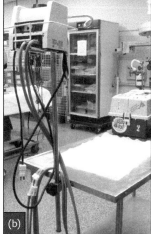
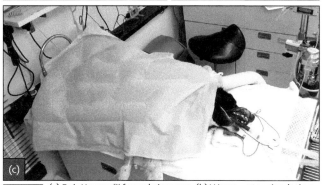

6.11 (a) Bair Hugger™ forced air pump. (b) Warm water circulating under-blanket. (c) Darvall over-blanket for use with a Bair Hugger™ warming unit.

Mouth gags

Spring-loaded gags must be used with great care. Holding the mouth fully open for long periods of time can cause injury to the temporomandibular joints and masticatory muscles. Post-anaesthetic cortical blindness has been reported in cats anaesthetized for oral and other procedures. Gags were identified as a potential risk factor for cerebral ischaemia and blindness in cats (Stiles *et al.*, 2012). Maxillary arterial blood flow has been shown to be reduced in anaesthetized cats when the mouth is kept fully open (Barton-Lamb *et al.*, 2013). Use of gags with spring-limiting devices is an improvement. Rubber mouth props are much more tooth and joint friendly (Figure 6.12). Gags must be removed every 5 to 10 minutes and the jaws manipulated.

Ocular protection

During dental and oral surgical procedures, the corneas should be protected from desiccation due to the lack of a blink reflex using an appropriate liquid gel. Contamination

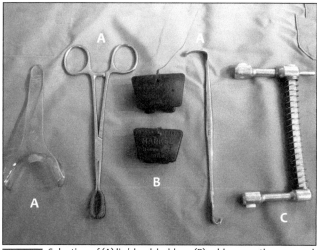

6.12 Selection of (A) lip/cheek holders, (B) rubber mouth props and (C) a spring-loaded gag. Use of a spring-loaded gag should be avoided.

from bacteria-laden aerosols when using water-cooled power equipment is another risk. The pupils may also be dilated by opioids or other drugs. If so, the retinas must be protected from overexposure to bright operating lights by hand towels, a mask or hood.

Anaesthetic techniques

A properly planned anaesthesia includes planning of the agents for premedication, induction, maintenance and recovery for each individual patient depending on its health status and the procedures anticipated.

Premedication

The purpose of premedication is to calm the patient, reduce anxiety and provide pre-emptive analgesia. The most reliable and common route of administration of premedication is intramuscular; however, intravenous, subcutaneous and even oral administration of sedatives and/or analgesics may also be considered.

Many premedication protocols include the use of a sedative or a tranquillizer plus an opioid (Figures 6.13 and 6.14). Anticholinergic agents may be added to prevent the severe bradycardia that can result from the use of large doses of opioids. Care must be taken in debilitated patients, as they may experience excessive central nervous system depression after the administration of a sedative. Patients undergoing dental charting, dental radiography and professional dental cleaning may not require high-level opioid analgesics. However, it is common for routine dental procedures to expand into oral surgery, and so the advantages and disadvantages of administering opioid analgesics as part of the premedication protocol should be weighed against the inability to increase the level of analgesia during the procedure if a partial agonist is chosen.

Acepromazine

Acepromazine is one of the most commonly used tranquillizers in veterinary medicine. Onset of action is approximately 30 minutes after intramuscular injection. It is considered to be a safe tranquillizer, as it provides anti-emetic and anti-histamine actions and may prevent re-entry arrhythmias. Despite this, it does have some effects

Drug combination and doses	Indications	Expected effects and comments
Acepromazine (0.01–0.02 mg/kg i.m.) + butorphanol (0.2 mg/kg i.m.)	Sedation for dental charting of ASA I or II patients	Moderate to poor sedation; not suitable as a sole analgesic for surgery
Acepromazine (0.01–0.02 mg/kg i.m.) + methadone or morphine (0.2–0.5 mg/kg i.m.)	Sedation and preventive analgesia for ASA II patients undergoing tooth extraction/oral surgery	Mild to moderate sedation; vomiting may occur (less common with methadone)
Butorphanol (0.01 mg/kg i.m.) + medetomidine (0.01 mg/kg i.m.)	Premedication or sedation of ASA I or II patients undergoing routine procedures	Excellent sedation for induction, but low-level analgesia if extractions needed
Medetomidine (0.005–0.01 mg/kg i.m.) or dexmedetomidine (0.0025–0.005 mg/kg i.m.) + morphine or methadone (0.5 mg/kg i.m.)	Sedation and preventive analgesia for excitable/ nervous ASA II patients undergoing tooth extraction/oral surgery	Moderate to deep sedation; bradycardia and hypertension are common side effects; vomiting may occur (less common with methadone)
Hydromorphone (0.1 mg/kg i.m.) or morphine or methadone (0.3 mg/kg i.m.) + midazolam (0.2 mg/kg i.m.) ± atropine (0.01 mg/kg i.m.)	Sedation and preventive analgesia for ASA III patients undergoing tooth extraction/oral surgery	Mild to moderate sedation; vomiting may occur (less common with methadone); administer atropine if bradycardia occurs
Fentanyl (0.002 mg/kg i.v.) or methadone or morphine (0.1 mg/kg i.v.)	Preventive analgesia for ASA IV E patients undergoing emergency oral surgery	Minimal sedation; usually administered to depressed patients; fentanyl is metabolized quickly, thus continue with a CRI during surgery

6.13 Examples of premedication protocols for dogs. ASA = American Society of Anesthesiologists; CRI = continuous rate infusion.

Drug combination and doses	Indications	Expected effects and comments
Acepromazine (0.01–0.02 mg/kg i.m.) + butorphanol (0.2 mg/kg i.m.)	Dental charting and professional dental cleaning of ASA I or II patients	Mild to moderate sedation; not suitable as a sole analgesic for surgery
Medetomidine (0.005–0.01 mg/kg i.m.) or dexmedetomidine (0.0025–0.005 mg/kg i.m.) + oxymorphone (0.1 mg/kg i.m.) or methadone (0.2 mg/kg i.m.)	Dental charting, professional dental cleaning and tooth extractions/oral surgery of fractious ASA II patients	Moderate to deep sedation; vomiting, bradycardia and hypertension are common side effects; hyperthermia may occur
Medetomidine (0.005–0.01 mg/kg i.m.) or dexmedetomidine (0.0025–0.005 mg/kg i.m.) + ketamine (3–5 mg/kg i.m.)	Dental charting, professional dental cleaning and tooth extractions/oral surgery of fractious/ aggressive ASA II patients	Deep sedation or even anaesthesia; vomiting, bradycardia and hypertension are common side effects; hyperthermia may occur
Midazolam (0.2 mg/kg i.m.) + oxymorphone (0.1 mg/kg i.m.) or methadone (0.2 mg/kg i.m.)	Dental charting, professional dental cleaning and tooth extractions/oral surgery of ASA III patients	Mild to moderate sedation; hyperthermia may occur
Midazolam (0.2 mg/kg i.m.) + ketamine (5–6 mg/kg i.m.) + oxymorphone (0.05 mg/kg i.m.) or methadone (0.2 mg/kg i.m.)	Dental charting, professional dental cleaning and tooth extractions/oral surgery of fractious/ aggressive ASA III patients	Deep sedation or even anaesthesia; hyperthermia may occur
Fentanyl (0.002 mg/kg i.v.) or methadone (0.1 mg/kg i.v.) or oxymorphone (0.05 mg/kg i.v.)	Emergency oral surgery of ASA IV E patients	Minimal sedation; usually administered to depressed patients; fentanyl is metabolized quickly, thus continue with CRI during surgery

6.14 Examples of premedication protocols for cats. ASA = American Society of Anesthesiologists; CRI = continuous rate infusion.

that must be considered, such as vasodilation and hypotension, particularly when associated with general anaesthesia. Therefore, its use in patients with hypovolaemia, coagulopathies or shock should be avoided. Acepromazine may render the animal slightly more cooperative, but deep sedation is usually not observed, even after large doses. However, acepromazine has synergistic effects when associated with opioids (i.e. neuroleptanalgesia), and profound sedation and analgesia may be seen when combined with agents of this drug class.

Medetomidine and dexmedetomidine

Medetomidine and dexmedetomidine are alpha-2 adrenergic agonists with potent sedative and analgesic properties. They are commonly used in combination with opioids for premedication of dental and oral surgical patients, as these drugs work synergistically. In combination with butorphanol the patient is very compliant, but the level of analgesia is lower than would be the case with buprenorphine or a full agonist such as methadone or morphine. The effects of medetomidine and dexmedetomidine can be reversed with atipamezole, and this can significantly reduce the amount of time needed for recovery.

Due to their side effects on the cardiovascular system, the use of medetomidine and dexmedetomidine in sick, very young or old patients is not recommended. They should also be used with caution in patients with cardiac disease or haemodynamic complications. Medetomidine and dexmedetomidine will induce transient vasopressor effects, characterized by substantial increases in systemic vascular resistance and hypertension. Bradycardia (e.g. heart rate of 30–40 beats/min in dogs and 80–100 beats/min in cats) is often observed as a reflex mechanism to the hypertensive event, cardiac output is decreased, and atrioventricular blocks and escape beats may be observed.

Benzodiazepines

Benzodiazepines (e.g. diazepam and midazolam) are agents with anxiolytic and hypnotic properties. Their use is commonly limited to the very young, very old or debilitated canine and feline patient because they may cause paradoxical behavioural side effects (e.g. excitement, pacing, and dysphoria-like events) in young adult and middle-aged dogs and cats (Haskins et al., 1986; Ilkiw et al., 1996). At clinical doses they produce minimal cardiovascular depression and can be used in debilitated patients to enhance the sedative effects of opioids. As they prevent seizure-like episodes, they are usually used in patients with a history of epilepsy.

Opioids

A wide range of opioids is currently available for dogs and cats. They are mainly used for premedication of the dental and oral surgical patient due to their potent analgesic effects and because they enhance the sedative effects of tranquillizers and sedatives. Since opioids have sedative effects of their own, they may be used as the sole pre-anaesthetic agent in debilitated or old animals. However, opioids may cause dysphoria and hyperthermia in some animals, particularly in cats (Posner et al., 2010).

Opioids are relatively safe agents but have a wide range of known side effects, which can include respiratory depression, bradycardia, nausea, vomiting and regurgitation. Constipation, pruritus and urinary retention may also occur. Most of these complications can be easily treated and/or prevented with the use of anticholinergics, anti-emetic agents and means to support ventilation, particularly when high doses of opioids are anticipated. In addition, specific opioid antagonists such as naloxone or methylnaltrexone may be used to reverse undesired side effects. The most commonly used opioids in feline and canine dentistry are described in the analgesia section of this chapter.

Other analgesics

NSAIDs and other analgesics such as tramadol may be administered with anaesthetic premedication. These drugs are discussed in more detail in the analgesia section below.

Induction of anaesthesia

Intravenous anaesthetic agents are usually used to induce anaesthesia because they cause a rapid loss of consciousness. They can also be used as the sole drug for very short procedures, to provide sedation, or to maintain anaesthesia for longer procedures by intravenous infusion. The most common drugs currently in use include propofol, thiopental, etomidate, alfaxalone, ketamine and tiletamine/zolazepam (Figure 6.15).

Drugs	Dose
Alfaxalone	Dogs: 1–3 mg/kg i.v. Cats: 2–5 mg/kg i.v.
Etomidate + midazolam or diazepam	0.5–2 mg/kg i.v. (etomidate) + 0.2 mg/kg i.v. (midazolam or diazepam)
Ketamine + midazolam or diazepam	2–5 mg/kg i.v. (ketamine) + 0.2 mg/kg i.v. (midazolam or diazepam)
Propofol	2–4 mg/kg i.v.
Thiopental	4–7 mg/kg i.v.
Tiletamine/zolazepam	2 mg/kg i.v.

6.15 Doses of induction agents.

Propofol

Propofol is very commonly used in practice as an induction agent. It is a short-acting general anaesthetic with an onset of action of approximately 30 seconds and a rapid and smooth recovery. Propofol is administered intravenously only. Due to rapid elimination, it is an ideal agent for total intravenous anaesthesia (TIVA). Propofol does cause significant respiratory depression, and apnoea is often observed after induction. It may also cause a significant fall in blood pressure after bolus administration due to systemic vasodilatation. These side effects are dose dependent and can be minimized by slow injection. Propofol should be used with caution in patients with shock. Traditional formulations of propofol support bacterial growth, so once the vial is opened it should be discarded within 6–12 hours. Newer forms of propofol have a shelf life of approximately 1 month; however, some have been associated with pain at injection (Minghella et al., 2010).

Sodium thiopental

Thiopental is less commonly used now. It is a barbiturate, most often employed at a concentration of 2.5%. It is given intravenously only, and accidental extravasation may cause local irritation and tissue necrosis. Induction doses of thiopental produce a rapid and smooth onset of hypnosis. Recovery after a single dose is rapid due to redistribution to fat, although metabolism is slow and occurs in the liver. Greyhound-type breeds, which may lack the enzyme systems responsible for the metabolism of barbiturates, can suffer a prolonged recovery. Thiopental depresses the respiratory system and may cause ventricular arrhythmias and hypotension. Its use should be reserved for patients with normal cardiovascular function.

Etomidate

Etomidate causes the least cardiovascular depression of the intravenous anaesthetic agents, with only a small reduction in cardiac output and blood pressure. Thus, it is the preferred induction agent for patients with reduced myocardial contractility (i.e. dilated cardiomyopathy). Induction of anaesthesia is fast, but can be accompanied by involuntary movements that may be mistaken for generalized seizure activity. Administering etomidate together with a benzodiazepine can minimize these involuntary movements. Etomidate is administered intravenously only. The respiratory depression caused by etomidate is similar to that seen with propofol and thiopental. Etomidate use has been reserved for induction of anaesthesia only, as it causes corticoadrenal suppression that may become severe if large doses are administered. In some countries, etomidate is formulated with propylene glycol, which may cause haematuria.

Alfaxalone

Alfaxalone has a short and rapid duration of action and minimal side effects. It can be used as an intravenous induction agent and also to maintain anaesthesia. It can be administered intramuscularly, although the dose required to induce anaesthesia by this route can be large. Intramuscular administration of sedative doses of alfaxalone may be advantageous in cats. Its clinical use and properties can be compared with propofol but with minimal cardiovascular effects. Therefore, alfaxalone may be used in cardiovascularly compromised patients.

Ketamine

Ketamine is a dissociative anaesthetic that has hypnotic, analgesic and local anaesthetic properties. The unique state provided by ketamine is typified by 'catalepsy' in which the eyes may stay open, and the corneal and light reflexes remain intact. It is a poor muscle relaxant and is often used with a benzodiazepine or an alpha-2 adrenergic agonist to prevent hypertonus. It is unique amongst induction drugs in that it can be administered intravenously, intramuscularly, orally, nasally and rectally. The onset is slower than that of other induction drugs, and the end point can be difficult to judge; the patient appears to be staring into the distance and keeps its swallowing reflex. Ketamine is usually associated with tachycardia, increased blood pressure and increased cardiac output and is useful in compensatory stages of shock. At clinically used doses, ketamine has a minimal effect on central respiratory drive. Therefore, it may be beneficial in the difficult-to-intubate patient because it is less likely to cause apnoea during induction of anaesthesia.

Tiletamine/zolazepam

Tiletamine is a phencyclidine derivate (like ketamine) available as a compound in combination with the benzodiazepine drug zolazepam as a 50:50 mixture. It can be used for induction or as the sole agent for short procedures in cats and is also an acceptable induction agent for sight hounds (such as Greyhounds). Recovery from tiletamine in dogs tends to be more agitated compared with recovery from ketamine/diazepam.

Maintenance of anaesthesia

Maintenance of general anaesthesia is best carried out using a balanced anaesthetic technique; this provides better cardiovascular support, minimizes fluctuations in anaesthetic drug requirements throughout the period and provides better intraoperative anti-nociception and postoperative analgesia than single-agent anaesthetic techniques.

Commonly used balanced anaesthetic protocols are based on the administration of an inhaled anaesthetic together with analgesic and/or sedative agents, although intravenous anaesthetics may also be used. Opioids, medetomidine, dexmedetomidine, ketamine, lidocaine and vasoactive agents such as dobutamine, dopamine, phenylephrine and noradrenaline (norepinephrine) are drugs that may be administered as a continuous rate infusion (CRI) as part of a balanced anaesthesia regime. CRIs are calculated from the pharmacokinetic profile of the agent and assume an initial 'loading-dose' bolus followed by a rate calculated per hour or per minute (Figure 6.16).

Drug	Loading dose	Intraoperative CRI dose
Dexmedetomidine	1–3 µg/kg i.v.	0.5–2 µg/kg/h
Fentanyl	3–5 µg/kg i.v.	5–10 µg/kg/h
Ketamine	0.5–2 mg/kg i.v.	2–100 µg/kg/min (0.12–6 mg/kg/h)
Lidocaine (dogs)	2 mg/kg i.v.	120 µg/kg/min (7 mg/kg/h)
Morphine	0.1–0.2 mg/kg i.m. or slowly i.v.	0.12–0.17 mg/kg/h
Propofol	2–4 mg/kg i.v.	0.1–0.4 mg/kg/min (6–24 mg/kg/h)
Remifentanil	4–10 µg/kg i.v.	6.0–15 µg/kg/h
Dobutamine	–	0.5–2 µg/kg/min
Dopamine	–	5–10 µg/kg/min
Noradrenaline	–	0.1–0.3 µg/kg/min

6.16 Recommended loading and intraoperative doses of drugs commonly administered as a continuous rate infusion (CRI).

Inhaled anaesthetics

Inhaled anaesthetics have the advantages of providing faster changes of anaesthetic depth than some injectable agents and being inexpensive. The most commonly used inhaled anaesthetics in small animal anaesthesia are isoflurane, sevoflurane and desflurane. The minimum alveolar concentration (MAC) of an inhaled anaesthetic is a parameter used to measure their potency and, for practical purposes, can be regarded as the 'dose'. In patients that receive no premedication or other associated drugs, 1.2–1.5 x MAC may be required to maintain anaesthesia for dentistry and oral surgery. If the inhaled anaesthetic is associated with other sedatives or analgesics (i.e. balanced technique), it is possible to reduce the concentration of the anaesthetic to values of 0.8–0.9 x MAC. The MAC of commonly used agents are as follows:

- Isoflurane: dogs 1.3%; cats 1.6%
- Sevoflurane: dogs 2.2%; cats 2.7%
- Desflurane: dogs 8%; cats 10%.

Desflurane and sevoflurane may offer some clinical advantages over isoflurane, such as faster recovery from anaesthesia after long procedures, with desflurane being even faster than sevoflurane. However, efficient use of isoflurane (e.g. reducing the concentration towards the end of the procedure) adds only a few minutes to the recovery. All three agents cause concentration-dependent cardiovascular depression, mainly as a result of vasodilation and a reduction in myocardial contractility. They all cause concentration-dependent respiratory depression, but isoflurane causes apnoea at lower MAC values compared with sevoflurane and desflurane.

All inhaled anaesthetics are vaporized in oxygen as the carrier gas. Medical air and/or nitrous oxide can be added to oxygen as well to improve analgesia (nitrous oxide) or to prevent lung atelectasis during prolonged procedures.

Total intravenous anaesthesia

Anaesthesia may also be maintained by means of repeated bolus administration or by using a CRI of injectable anaesthetics. Propofol and alfaxalone are the most commonly used injectable anaesthetic agents used for total intravenous anaesthesia (TIVA) because of their fast elimination. As with inhaled agents, they are combined with sedatives or analgesics to reduce their doses and improve cardiovascular function and support intraoperative nociception and postoperative analgesia. TIVA may be desirable when the endotracheal tube has to be removed from time to time to determine a functional occlusion (e.g. jaw fracture repair, prosthetic crown placement). Other indications for TIVA may include patients with head trauma or lung disorders. An example of a TIVA protocol for dogs and cats is propofol at 12–30 mg/kg/h + fentanyl at 0.002–0.01 mg/kg/h.

Monitoring of anaesthesia

Anaesthesia monitoring comprises the continuous evaluation of anaesthetic depth and vital signs, to anticipate complications and minimize anaesthetic morbidity. Monitoring includes evaluation of the cardiac rate and rhythm, oxygenation, ventilation, adequacy of anaesthetic depth, muscle relaxation, body temperature and analgesia. Detailed guidelines for anaesthesia monitoring are available at the website of the American College of Veterinary Anesthesia and Analgesia (www.acvaa.org) (Figure 6.17).

Parameter	Method(s)	Normally expected under anaesthesia	Common complication	Comment/treatment
Anaesthetic depth	Evaluation of jaw tone	Decreased tone	Light or deep anaesthetic plane	Increase or decrease anaesthetic delivery
	Eyeball positioning	Ventromedial rotation		
	Elicit eyelid reflex	Absent		
	Elicit corneal reflex	Present		
Capillary refill time (CRT)	Palpation of oral mucosa	1–2 seconds	Decreased CRT	Shock; administer fluids
			Increased CRT	Early stages of shock; administer fluids
Mucus membrane colour	Visual inspection of oral mucosa	Pink	Pale pink/white	Check for anaemia, shock
			Hyperaemic (red)	Early stages of shock, sepsis
Heart rate/ rhythm and pulse rate	Cardiac auscultation, electrocardiography, palpation of peripheral artery (e.g. femoral, metatarsal), Doppler ultrasonography, pulse oximetry	Heart/pulse rate: • Dogs: 60–150 beats/min • Cats: 150–200 beats/min Sinus arrhythmia may be normal in some breeds of dogs	Sinus bradycardia	Check anaesthetic depth (too deep?); administer anticholinergics (unless bradycardia is induced by alpha-2 agonist and patient is hypertensive)
			Sinus tachycardia	Check anaesthetic depth (too light?), analgesia (insufficient?), acute hypovolemia (haemorrhage)
			Ventricular tachycardia	Administer lidocaine at 2 mg/kg i.v.; check cause (e.g. myocardial disease, ischaemia, electrolyte imbalances and pain)
			Atrioventricular dissociation	Check anaesthetic depth (too deep?), vagal stimulation (e.g. pulling endotracheal tube); administer anticholinergics. Note that alpha-2 agonists may cause atrioventricular blocks
Blood pressure	Doppler ultrasonography and manometer, oscillometry, invasive with arterial catheter	60–140 mmHg	Hypotension	Check anaesthetic depth (too deep?), heart rate (bradycardia?); administer fluid bolus (unless patient has cardiac disease) and vasoactive drug (e.g. dopamine)
			Hypertension	Check anaesthetic depth (too light?), analgesia (insufficient?); may be related to alpha-2 agonist administration
Respiratory rate/ effort and ventilation	Visual inspection of chest excursions, rebreathing bag inflation–deflation, capnography and end-tidal carbon dioxide (ETCO₂), arterial blood gases, respirometer to measure tidal volume	Respiratory rate: 6–12 breaths/min; no effort ETCO₂: 35–45 mmHg (4.5–6% volume), normal capnographic waves Tidal volume: 10–15 ml/kg	Increased effort	Check for obstructions in the breathing system and endotracheal tube, check for pneumothorax
			Bradypnoea/apnoea	Check anaesthetic depth (too deep?); support ventilation (manually squeezing rebreathing bag or with mechanical ventilator)
			Tachypnoea	Check anaesthetic depth (too light?)
Oxygenation	Pulse oximetry (S$_p$O₂), arterial blood gas analysis	S$_p$O₂: 95–100%	Hypoxia/ hypoxaemia	Check for obstructions in the breathing system and endotracheal tube; oxygen source connected? Apnoea? (support ventilation); check for pneumothorax, aspiration of regurgitated stomach contents, blood and other fluids
Temperature	Rectal thermometer	37.8–39.2°C	Hypothermia	Apply external source of heating (e.g. forced warm air device, circulating warm water blankets)
			Hyperthermia	Check for fever, over-heating patient; may be caused by opioids in cats

6.17 Anaesthesia monitoring, complications and treatment.

Management of perioperative pain

Assessment of perioperative pain

Pain recognition is essential to anticipate and construct a successful analgesic plan for a given patient based on the procedure performed. Anaesthetic agents blunt the perception of pain during surgery, but nociceptive pathways are activated after noxious stimulation (i.e. tooth extraction), which may result in autonomic responses during surgery. Increases in heart rate and blood pressure are usually interpreted as intraoperative nociception, and the administration of analgesic drugs is indicated. If not treated, intraoperative nociception may lead to postoperative hyperalgesia and chronic pain. Therefore, painful or nociceptive events should not only be treated during and after surgery; they should be anticipated by the clinician and treated prior to their occurrence to optimize the success of the treatment.

Many dental and oral surgical procedures start with a long period of assessment – charting, dental radiography, scaling and polishing. If tooth extraction or other surgery is then performed, the analgesia given at the time of premedication may no longer be adequate for the treatment period. The use of pure mu opioid agonists for premedication allows for immediate upward titration intravenously whereas the use of partial agonists does not. Nerve blocks are also rapidly acting and indicated in these circumstances.

Systemic analgesic drug selection

The use and choice of analgesic agents are based on their pharmacological profile, patient health, procedure anticipated and assessment of the likely degree of pain. Patients likely to experience a low degree of pain may only require the administration of a single analgesic agent. Patients with moderate to severe pain or those that are to undergo extensive oral surgery require a multimodal approach to pain management. A multimodal approach (i.e. balanced analgesia) uses a combination of different analgesic agents, with different modes and sites of action to take advantage of their synergistic effects, and often utilizes lower doses to minimize side effects.

Commonly used analgesic protocols for dental and oral surgical procedures include an opioid given at the time of premedication in combination with a tranquillizer or sedative, to enhance both sedation and analgesia (e.g. methadone and medetomidine). A nerve block may be administered before starting the surgical procedure, and an NSAID given at/before premedication, at induction or after anaesthesia. Postoperative analgesia for home use generally includes an NSAID plus an opioid (e.g. tramadol). Other analgesics (such as infusions of opioids, ketamine, medetomidine or lidocaine) may be required for intraoperative and immediate postoperative analgesia. Tramadol, gabapentin and amantadine may be considered for long-term pain treatment in some patients.

Non-steroidal anti-inflammatory drugs

NSAIDs help decrease the actions of inflammatory mediators released during surgery (Figure 6.18). NSAIDs with preferential action on COX-2 are preferred over non-selective COX-inhibitors to minimize renal and gastrointestinal complications. This group of drugs has a wide range of contraindications, and their use should be carefully considered in unhealthy or elderly animals. NSAID use for dentistry and oral surgery tends not to be lengthy, but patients on prolonged NSAID therapy should be monitored periodically for changes in haematological or biochemical parameters. Owners often find home administration easy when palatable formulas are used.

Caution should be exercised when using NSAIDs in cats. Delayed hepatic biotransformation can lead to prolonged half-lives and the potential for toxicity. One of the few NSAIDs that appear to be well tolerated in cats is meloxicam. It is recommended that cats are monitored closely for adverse effects. In some countries meloxicam is authorized only for single use in cats.

Drug	Dose
Dogs	
Carprofen	4.4 mg/kg i.v., i.m., s.c. preoperatively or at time of anaesthetic induction, then 4.4 mg/kg orally q24h or 2.2 mg/kg orally q12h on subsequent days
Deracoxib	1–2 mg/kg orally q24h
Etodolac	10–15 mg/kg orally q24h
Meloxicam	0.2 mg/kg i.v., i.m., s.c., orally on day 1, then 0.1 mg/kg i.v., i.m., s.c., orally q24h on subsequent days
Tepoxalin	10 mg/kg orally q24h
Cats	
Meloxicam	0.05–0.1 mg/kg i.v., s.c., i.m., orally q24h for 3–5 days, then 0.025–0.05 mg/kg i.v., s.c., i.m., orally every 2–3 days for long-term treatment

6.18 Doses of non-steroidal anti-inflammatory drugs for dogs and cats.

Opioids

Opioids are very effective drugs in controlling dental and oral surgical pain in dogs and cats (Figure 6.19). The pure mu opioid agents allow an upward titration of the dose intraoperatively if the circumstances of the procedure change. They are also widely used to control postoperative pain, as they have minimal cardiovascular side effects. Pure mu opioid receptor agonists are generally very safe and effective but do have the potential to produce side effects. They are all Schedule 2 Controlled Drugs, and their use must be recorded to fulfil legal requirements (see the *BSAVA Guide to the Use of Veterinary Medicines* for further information).

Drug	Dose
Buprenorphine	0.01–0.03 mg/kg i.v., s.c., i.m. q6–8h
Butorphanol	0.1–0.3 mg/kg i.v q40min–2h or 0.2–0.5 mg/kg s.c., i.m. q1–4h
Fentanyl	0.002–0.005 mg/kg i.v. q15min; CRI: 0.002–0.02 mg/kg/h; patch: 0.002–0.004 mg/kg/h
Hydromorphone	0.1–0.2 mg/kg s.c., i.m. or 0.05–0.1 mg/kg i.v. q2–4h
Methadone	0.3–1 mg/kg s.c., i.m. or 0.1–0.3 mg/kg i.v. q2–4h
Morphine	0.3–1 mg/kg s.c., i.m. or 0.1–0.3 mg/kg i.v. q2–4h; CRI: 0.1–0.3 mg/kg/h
Oxymorphone	0.1–0.2 mg/kg s.c., i.m. or 0.05–0.1 mg/kg i.v. q2–4h
Pethidine (meperidine)	1–5 mg/kg s.c., i.m. q1–2h
Tramadol	Dogs: 2–5 mg/kg orally q8–12h or q6h Cats: 2–4 mg/kg orally q12h
Naloxone	Opioid antagonist dose: 0.01–0.04 mg/kg s.c., i.m., i.v.

6.19 Doses of opioids for dogs and cats. CRI = continuous rate infusion.

Methadone and pethidine are authorized for use in dogs in the UK as Controlled Drugs. Other Schedule 2 opioids (e.g. morphine, hydromorphone and oxymorphone) are also used in veterinary practice under the cascade system. The cascade system provides legal flexibility for veterinary surgeons (veterinarians) to use authorized veterinary medicines where they are available and professional freedom to prescribe other products where they are not. It is for the individual practitioner to select opioids on this basis, depending on the circumstances of the case at the time.

Fentanyl is authorized for use in dogs as an injectable agent or a transdermal solution. The transdermal solution is applied topically to the skin of the dorsal scapular area using a special syringe; in this form its effect lasts for up to 4 days. The injectable formulation can be used as a CRI intraoperatively and postoperatively. Fentanyl patches are also available (although not authorized) in 25, 50, 75 and 100 μg/h strengths. They are normally replaced every 3 days. Patches must be protected from accidental ingestion by the patient or children in the household. To reduce the risk of harm, owners must be counselled in the correct handling of used patches; these should be folded in half with the sticky sides together and then returned to the veterinary surgeon for final disposal. The patches should not be placed in household bins where children or pets may find them, as they can be especially harmful, and possibly fatal, in a single dose. For this reason some practices hospitalize patients that have patches applied.

Buprenorphine is a partial mu receptor agonist, which means that it binds at mu receptors but only partially activates them. It is authorized for dogs and cats and produces few side effects and minimal sedation. Buprenorphine has a very high affinity for the mu receptors and will competitively inhibit pure mu agonists from binding. This property makes it useful for reversing the effects of mu agonists if adverse consequences arise. A ceiling effect on analgesia may exist with partial agonists making them less useful for severe pain (Cowan *et al.*, 1977). Newer studies suggest that there may not be such ceiling effects in regard to analgesia, but there are scarce data in dogs or cats. Buprenorphine is not available as a specific oral preparation, but the injectable form can be easily applied to the oral mucosa for at home treatment and is reported as being very successful in cats. A number of studies appear to indicate that oral transmucosal administration is also effective in dogs (Abbo *et al.*, 2008; McInnes *et al.*, 2008).

Butorphanol has a short-lived effect, with pain relief less optimal than other opioids. Mixed with medetomidine as a premedicant, it produces profound sedation.

Tramadol is commonly used to treat mild to moderate pain in the postoperative period. It can be used with or without NSAIDs. Side effects are rare and may include dysphoria, sedation and vomiting. Currently available tablet formulations (10 mg, 25 mg, 50 mg and 100 mg) are bitter and may cause salivation; tablets should not be broken. Generally, cats tolerate the bitterness poorly.

Other analgesic drugs and therapies

Lidocaine, ketamine, medetomidine and dexmedetomidine can be used as CRIs during anaesthesia when local blockade is not possible and severe pain is anticipated, or to reduce the concentration or dose of general anaesthetic agents. Their use can be extended into the postoperative period after extensive surgery has been performed (e.g. mandibulectomy) to improve postoperative analgesia.

Intravenous forms of lidocaine (adrenaline-free) can be used either alone or in combination with ketamine and morphine (MLK infusion) or fentanyl (FLK infusion). Caution should be exercised in cats, as lidocaine infusion may reduce the cardiovascular function in this species.

Ketamine at sub-anaesthetic doses prevents the development of chronic pain by inhibiting the wind-up phenomenon responsible for the amplification of pain intensity. It also increases opioid receptor sensitivity, reduces opioid tolerance and minimizes rebound hyperalgesia.

If sedation is required together with analgesia, infusions of medetomidine or dexmedetomidine are a valid option. They are potent analgesics, although they affect the cardiovascular system, causing bradycardia, vasoconstriction and reduction in cardiac output. To minimize these adverse side effects, small doses are usually infused (see Figures 6.16 and 6.20).

Other drugs used for treatment of chronic oral pain include amantadine and gabapentin. Amantadine is the most commonly used oral *N*-methyl-D-aspartate (NMDA) receptor antagonist. The dose for dogs and cats is 3–5 mg/kg orally q24h. It may be given on a continuous basis if required, although in most cases it can be given daily for 7–14 days and then discontinued until pain worsens again. Amantadine is available as 100 mg capsules and a 10 mg/ml liquid for oral use. Elimination is almost exclusively via the kidneys, so dose reduction should be considered in cases of severe renal insufficiency. Side effects are rare but can include agitation or diarrhoea.

Drug	Dog dose	Cat dose
Acepromazine	0.005–0.01 mg/kg i.v. 0.01–0.1 mg/kg i.m., s.c. 1–2 mg/kg orally	0.005–0.01 mg/kg i.v. 0.01–0.1 mg/kg i.m., s.c. 1–2 mg/kg orally
Atropine	0.02–0.04 mg/kg i.m., s.c. 0.01–0.02 mg/kg i.v.	0.02–0.04 mg/kg i.m., s.c. 0.01–0.02 mg/kg i.v.
Buprenorphine	0.01–0.03 mg/kg i.m., s.c., i.v., orally	0.01–0.03 mg/kg i.m., s.c., i.v., orally
Butorphanol	0.1–0.3 mg/kg i.v. 0.2–0.5 mg/kg i.m., s.c.	0.1–0.3 mg/kg i.v. 0.2–0.5 mg/kg i.m., s.c.
Dexmedetomidine	0.001–0.005 mg/kg i.v. CRI: 0.0005–0.002 mg/kg/h i.v. or 0.002–0.01 mg/kg i.m.	0.001–0.005 mg/kg i.v. CRI: 0.0005–0.002 mg/kg/h i.v. or 0.002–0.01 mg/kg i.m.
Diazepam	0.2–0.5 mg/kg i.v.	0.2–0.5 mg/kg i.v.
Etomidate	0.5–2 mg/kg i.v.	0.5–2 mg/kg i.v.
Fentanyl	0.002–0.005 mg/kg i.v. Transdermal patch: 0.002–0.004 mg/kg/h	0.002–0.005 mg/kg i.v. Transdermal patch: 0.002–0.004 mg/kg/h
Flumazenil	0.02–0.04 mg/kg i.v., i.m., s.c.	0.01–0.02 mg/kg i.v., i.m., s.c.
Glycopyrrolate	0.01–0.02 mg/kg i.m., s.c. 0.005–0.01 mg/kg i.v.	0.01–0.02 mg/kg i.m., s.c. 0.005–0.01 mg/kg i.v.
Hydromorphone	0.05–0.1 mg/kg i.v. 0.1–0.2 mg/kg i.m., s.c.	0.05–0.1 mg/kg i.v. 0.1–0.2 mg/kg i.m., s.c.
Ketamine	2–5 mg/kg i.v. 3–7 mg/kg i.m.	2–5 mg/kg i.v. 3–10 mg/kg i.m.
Lidocaine	1–2 mg/kg i.v. CRI: 3–6 mg/kg/h i.v.	–
Medetomidine	0.002–0.01 mg/kg i.v. 0.005–0.02 mg/kg i.m.	0.002–0.01 mg/kg i.v. 0.005–0.02 mg/kg i.m.
Methadone	0.1–0.3 mg/kg i.v. 0.2–1 mg/kg i.m., s.c.	0.1–0.2 mg/kg i.v. 0.1–0.3 mg/kg i.m, s.c.
Midazolam	0.2–0.5 mg/kg i.v., i.m., s.c.	0.2–0.5 mg/kg i.v., i.m., s.c.
Morphine	0.1–0.3 mg/kg i.v. 0.2–1 mg/kg i.m., s.c. CRI: 0.1–0.3 mg/kg/h i.v.	0.1–0.2 mg/kg i.v. 0.1–0.3 mg/kg i.m., s.c.
Naloxone	0.005–0.02 mg/kg i.v. 0.01–0.04 mg/kg i.m., s.c.	0.005–0.02 mg/kg i.v. 0.01–0.04 mg/kg i.m., s.c.
Oxymorphone	0.05–0.1 mg/kg i.v. 0.1–0.2 mg/kg i.m., s.c.	0.05–0.1 mg/kg i.v. 0.1 mg/kg i.m., s.c.
Propofol	1–4 mg/kg i.v.	1–4 mg/kg i.v.
Thiopental	2–4 mg/kg i.v.	2–4 mg/kg i.v.
Tiletamine/zolazepam	2 mg/kg i.v. 4 mg/kg i.m.	2 mg/kg i.v. 4 mg/kg i.m.

6.20 Doses of commonly used anaesthetic and analgesic drugs. CRI = continuous rate infusion.

Gabapentin is an anticonvulsant medication with adjunctive analgesic action. Its mechanism of action is unclear, although it may provide inhibition of postsynaptic neuron firing. Gabapentin has been used for many forms of chronic oral pain, particularly neuropathic pain in cats with feline orofacial pain syndrome (FOPS). The dose may vary significantly among individuals and may have to be adjusted according to the desired effect (5–35 mg/kg orally q12h or q8h). The normal recommendation is to start at the low end of the dose range. If there is no effect in 4 weeks, the dose should be increased. Potential side effects include sedation and weight gain.

Other adjunctive therapies include acupuncture and physiotherapy.

Local and regional anaesthesia and analgesia

The use of local anaesthetics to block the transmission of noxious stimuli before incision or to potentiate analgesia postoperatively is widely performed in human and veterinary dentistry and oral surgery. Local anaesthetics prevent nociceptive transmission by interacting with axonal Na$^+$ channels and inhibiting the depolarization of the nerve membrane and the propagation of the action potential. This means that they abolish the transmission of nociceptive stimuli to higher neurological centres.

Their use in veterinary dentistry and oral surgery can be as part of a planned multimodal approach or as a late adjunct if circumstances demand it. An example of this may be when patients undergoing procedures that increase in scope from the original plan need analgesia augmented intraoperatively.

One study in dogs (Snyder and Snyder, 2013) compared the MAC of isoflurane on a noxious stimulation of the dental pulp before and after an infraorbital nerve block with mepivacaine. A significant reduction in isoflurane MAC (23%) was seen after an infraorbital nerve block was given, compared with before its administration. It was concluded that the reduction in MAC of isoflurane supported the provision of regional anaesthesia for painful dental and oral surgical procedures. A survey of Diplomates of the American Veterinary Dental College (AVDC) in 2012 found that almost all responding specialists use nerve blocks in addition to other analgesics (unpublished data). Most respondents to the survey used bupivacaine as the main local anaesthetic agent.

Local anaesthesia refers to the application or injection of a local anaesthetic on to or into tissue at a surgical site. Although traditionally not commonly performed in veterinary dentistry and oral surgery, this method of anaesthesia is gaining in popularity. Topical anaesthetic gels (sometimes used for closed extractions of single-rooted teeth) may provide temporary relief from superficial pain, but their effects are extremely short-lived. Other examples include injection of a local anaesthetic along planned incisions (infiltration anaesthesia) or into the periodontal ligament (intraligamentous injection). A splash block (wound irrigation) refers to the dropping of a local anaesthetic directly into a wound at the end of surgery prior to closure of the surgical site.

Regional anaesthesia (nerve block) refers to injection of a local anaesthetic around a major nerve. Nerves that are frequently blocked in dentistry and oral surgery include the maxillary nerve, infraorbital nerve, major palatine nerve, inferior alveolar nerve, and middle mental nerve.

The main concerns for local and regional anaesthesia are damage to neurovascular tissues and/or haematoma with poor injection technique, and systemic toxic effects from the agent used. Information with regard to neurovascular damage in animals is scant, but one study in dogs concluded that use of fine needles and good operator skill will reduce the risk of iatrogenic damage to the neurovascular tissues (Anthony, 2008). It is recommended that 27 G needles are used when going through oral mucosa and into bony foramuria/canals (e.g. infraorbital foramina/canal), and 25 G needles are used when going through skin and injecting the solution around the nerve outside restricted bony structues (e.g. at the mandibular foramen). The needle should be inserted parallel to the nerve (rather than perpendicular), and back-and-forth or side-to-side movement of the needle is to be avoided once inserted. Systemic toxic effects generally occur due to overdosing, especially in small dogs and cats, and inadvertent administration into arteries or veins. Dental aspirating syringes have a thumb ring on the plunger that makes initial drawback to check for accidental venepuncture easier (Figure 6.21). All local anaesthetics cause vasodilatation, which can lead to more rapid absorption from the site. Vasoconstrictors (mainly adrenaline) can be added to counteract this for the shorter-acting agents.

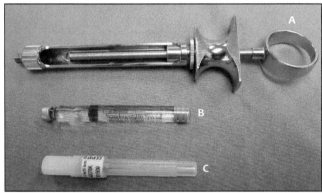

6.21 (A) Dental aspirating syringe with thumb ring. (B) Glass vial containing mepivacaine. (C) Needle.

Local anaesthetics

Local anaesthetics exert their effects at the site of administration, and their effectiveness is related to their ability to spread along the target nerve or nerves (Beckman and Legendre, 2002; Lantz, 2003; Rochette, 2005; Lemke, 2007). For this reason, the administration of local anaesthetics differs from that of systemically administered drugs. Instead of dosing them by concentration of drug per bodyweight of the patient (e.g. mg/kg), they are dosed in total volume per anatomical area (e.g. total ml required to desensitize a region of the body) or in volume per bodyweight (e.g. ml/kg). In addition, because local anaesthetic uptake by venous capillaries and subsequent systemic distribution may cause some undesired side effects (that can potentially be lethal), a maximal dose in mg/kg of bodyweight is usually calculated in order to avoid such complications (Figure 6.22). Aspiration is required before delivery to ensure the needle has not entered a blood vessel.

The presence of infected or inflamed tissues at the site can make a local anaesthetic agent ineffective because such tissues have a low pH, which decreases the effect of the agent. If large volumes of local anaesthetics are required, commercially available solutions may be diluted with saline solution. However, the effectiveness of local anaesthetics is also related to the concentration of the solution.

Mepivacaine and bupivacaine are among the most commonly used local anaesthetics for regional analgesia in veterinary dentistry and oral surgery. Although it has a relatively rapid time of onset (1–2 minutes), lidocaine is less useful, as it only lasts for up to 2 hours. Mepivacaine also has a reported onset of 1.5 to 2 minutes and lasts around 30 minutes to 2 hours. Bupivacaine has the longest onset at 6–10 minutes but provides the longest analgesic effects (lasting between 4 and 6 hours) (Beckman, 2013). One study demonstrated the anaesthetic effect of bupivacaine lasting longer than previously described, possibly more than 24 hours when used during acute dental/oral surgical pain (Snyder and Snyder, 2016). In the same study, the authors were not able to prove in a statistically significant

Drug	Maximum total dose per patient	Onset of action (in minutes)	Duration of action (in hours)	Maximum volume per site
Lidocaine (2%)	Dogs: 5 mg/kg Cats: 3 mg/kg	1–2 min	0.5–2 h	Cats: 0.1–0.3 ml Dogs <6 kg: 0.1–0.3 ml Dogs 6–25 kg: 0.3–0.6 ml Dogs 26–40 kg: 0.6–0.8 ml Dogs >40 kg: 0.8–1 ml
Mepivacaine (2%)	Dogs: 5 mg/kg Cats: 2.5 mg/kg	1.5–2 min	2–3 h Pulp: 0.5–1 h	
Bupivacaine (0.5%)	Dogs: 2.5 mg/kg Cats: 1.5 mg/kg	6–10 min	4–6 h Pulp: 1.5–3 h Foramen: 6–8 h	
Lidocaine (2%) + bupivacaine (0.5%)	1 mg/kg of each agent in the same syringe	2–10 min	4–6 h Pulp: 1.5–3 h Foramen: 6–8 h	

6.22 Dosages of commonly used local anaesthetic and analgesic drugs.
(Liu *et al.*, 1983; Avery *et al.*, 1984; Kasten and Martin, 1985; Oka *et al.*, 1997; Pascoe, 1997; Duke, 2000)

manner that the duration of the combined bupivacaine/buprenorphine blocks was extended. However, this combination remains a theory worthy of further investigation, as there are numerous anecdotal reports of the benefit of adding an opiate to a local anaesthetic agent. The total volume of local anaesthetic in any one site depends mostly on patient size (more volume in large patients) and injection site (whether it is injected near a foramen or inside a canal). However, a maximum volume of 0.8–1 ml in any one site for dogs weighing >40 kg, 0.6–0.8 ml for dogs weighing 26–40 kg, 0.3–0.6 ml for dogs weighing 6–25 kg and 0.1–0.3 ml for cats and small dogs (weighing <6 kg) is usual.

Mepivacaine is available as a 2% solution (i.e. 20 mg/ml) in prefilled glass vials that fit aspirating dental syringes. These syringes will take long length (35 mm) and fine bore (27 G) needles for ease of insertion into foramina.

Bupivacaine is available commercially at 0.75% (7.5 mg/ml), 0.5% (5 mg/ml) and 0.25% (2.5 mg/ml) solutions in 10 ml ampoules. Analgesic effects have also been reported at concentrations as low as 0.125% (1.25 mg/ml). The maximum dose for dogs is reported to be 2 mg/kg and for cats 1.5–2 mg/kg, even though toxic doses are much higher.

Specific nerve blocks

Infraorbital nerve block: The infraorbital canal runs from the maxillary foramen in the orbit, rostrally immediately dorsal to the maxillary molar teeth and fourth premolar tooth, and ends at the infraorbital foramen, dorsal to the maxillary third premolar tooth (see Chapter 2). It contains the infraorbital neurovascular bundle. The nerve is sensory to the ipsilateral bones, teeth and soft tissues of the face. Placement of the infraorbital nerve block is best performed intraorally, even though a transcutaneous approach may be preferred in cats (Gracis, 2013). The needle is inserted into the mucosa or the skin overlying the maxilla just rostral to the foramen (at the level of the mesial root of the third premolar tooth) and advanced caudally for a very short distance into the canal, parallel to the course of the nerve and hard palate (Figure 6.23). It must be noted that sensory nerves to the maxillary molar teeth leave the main nerve trunk of the maxillary branch of the trigeminal nerve before it enters the maxillary foramen. However, deep insertion of the needle in the infraorbital canal should be avoided due to the risk of iatrogenic damage to the vessels and nerve, and a

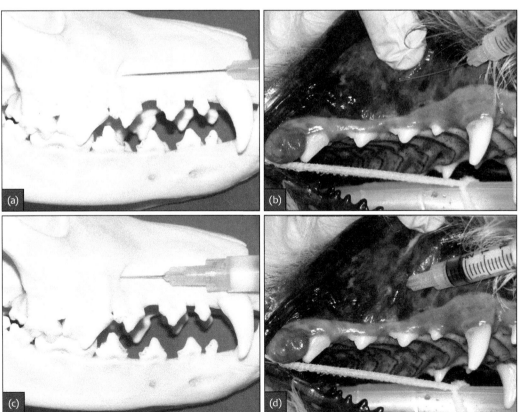

6.23 Right infraorbital nerve block in a dog. (a and c) Skull demonstration. (b and d) Clinical case. The needle has been inserted into the infraorbital canal to provide analgesia to the maxillary fourth premolar tooth and surrounding tissues. To be effective it only needs to be placed just past the infraorbital foramen, decreasing the risk of iatrogenic trauma to the neurovascular bundle.
(© Dr Alexander M. Reiter)

maxillary nerve block should be performed to anaesthetize the maxillary molar teeth. It should also be noted that the infraorbital nerve block may be inconsistently efficacious in blocking the maxilliary fourth premolar tooth (Pascoe, 2016).

In cats and brachycephalic dogs the infraorbital canal is very short. Therefore, the needle should always be inserted for a very short distance and angled ventrally, otherwise puncture of the eye is possible.

Maxillary nerve block: This block desensitizes similar tissues to the infraorbital nerve block, as well as the ipsilateral soft palate, hard palate, bone and mucosa, ventral nasal meatus and the maxillary recess. It is performed when the infraorbital approach is not possible or to avoid unnecessarily deep insertion of the needle into the canal when trying to reach the maxillary nerve and anaesthetize the maxillary fourth premolar tooth and molar teeth.

There are three approaches to the nerve within the pterygopalatine fossa. One approach is to insert the needle through the oral mucosa perpendicularly to the hard palate, immediately caudomedial to the last maxillary molar tooth and advancing it for a very short distance to avoid eye globe puncture (maxillary tuberosity approach) (Figure 6.24) (Gracis, 2013). A second approach is to insert the needle through skin into the space between the rostroventral border of the zygomatic arch, the caudal margin of the maxilla and the rostral aspect of the coronoid process of the mandible (subzygomatic approach) (Gracis, 2013). The needle direction should be slightly rostral and parallel to the hard palate. Thirdly, the needle can be inserted through the conjunctiva of the eye and advanced ventrally until the operator assesses the needle tip to be close to the maxillary foramen (the entrance to the infraorbital canal) (Dugdale, 2010).

Major palatine nerve block: The major palatine nerve block desensitizes the tissues of the hard palate and is of use in procedures such as palate surgery, maxillectomy, and closure of oronasal or oroantral fistulae. The nerve is a branch of the maxillary nerve and is sensory, along with the accessory palatine nerve, to the mucosa of the hard palate. It may be accessed either at the entrance or at the exit of the palatine canal. With the first approach (also called the caudal major palatine nerve block) the local anaesthetic solution is injected in the pterygopalatine fossa, using the same approaches indicated for the maxillary nerve block (Gracis, 2013). With this block the minor palatine nerve is also likely to be affected, and the soft palate anaesthetized.

The rostral major palatine nerve block is achieved by injecting the anaesthetic solution at the major palatine foramen, located at the maxillopalatine suture below the palatal mucosa (Gracis, 2013). The foramen is located half way between the distal root of the maxillary fourth premolar tooth and the midline and usually cannot be palpated. For the rostral technique in dogs, the needle should enter the mucosa of the hard palate at the level of the distal root of the maxillary third premolar tooth or the mesial roots of the maxillary fourth premolar tooth, and be directed caudally towards the nerve exit at the major palatine foramen (Figure 6.25). In cats, the foramen is located slightly more rostrally.

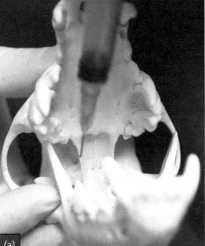

6.24 Right maxillary nerve block in a dog. (a) Skull demonstration. (b) Clinical case.
(© Dr John Lewis)

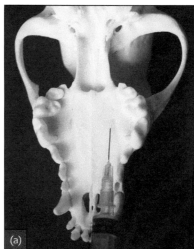

6.25 Right major palatine nerve block (rostral approach) in a dog. (a) Skull demonstration. (b) Clinical case.
(© Dr John Lewis)

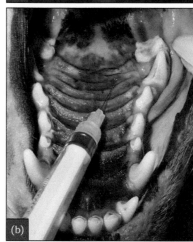

Inferior alveolar nerve block: The mandibular branch of the trigeminal nerve becomes the inferior alveolar nerve just before entering the mandibular foramen, runs within the mandibular canal and exits at the mental foramina in the rostral portion of the mandible. It provides sensory innervation to the soft and hard tissues of the mandible.

Neurotransmission can be blocked at the mandibular foramen, which is located on the medial surface of the ramus of the mandible. The foramen may be palpated from inside the mouth half way between the last mandibular molar tooth and the angular process of the mandible. The needle is introduced intraorally under the mucosa medial to the last mandibular molar tooth and directed ventrocaudally as close to the bone as possible towards the finger of the operator, which is placed over the foramen (Figure 6.26). This block can also be performed percutaneously by inserting the needle medial to the mandible, at the level of an unnamed notch at the ventral mandibular border immediately rostral to the angular process, and directing it dorsally towards a finger, which is inserted into the mouth and used to palpate the foramen.

With the inferior alveolar nerve block there is the possibility that the local anaesthetic is injected close to the lingual nerve, infrequently resulting in temporary desensitization of the tongue. This complication can be avoided by guiding the needle as close to the bone as possible and not injecting unnecessarily large volumes of local anaesthetic.

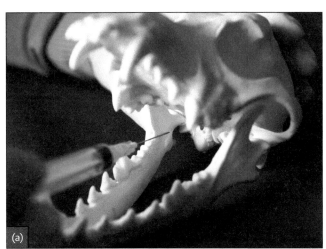
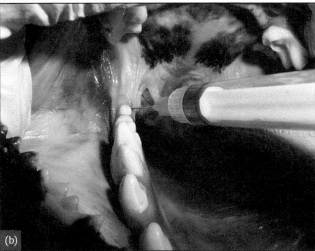

6.26 Intraoral right inferior alveolar nerve block in a dog. (a) Skull demonstration. (b) Clinical case.
(© Dr John Lewis)

Middle mental nerve block: The mental nerves are the terminal branches of the inferior alveolar nerve. They innervate only the rostral part of the mandible, lower lip and chin. The block can be performed by introducing the needle through the oral mucosa at the level of the middle mental foramen, ventral to the mandibular second premolar tooth (Figure 6.27). The needle may be introduced either rostral or caudal to the unnamed lip frenulum. One author suggested that entry of even small bore needles (27 G) into the middle mental foramen (performed to desensitize the final portion of the inferior alveolar nerve and the mandibular canine and incisor teeth) causes iatrogenic damage to the neurovascular structures on every occasion during the study (Anthony, 2008). The rostral and caudal mental foramina are even smaller. For that reason, needle entry into the mental foramina is not advised, as regional anaesthesia can be achieved more reliably and with less iatrogenic damage by means of an inferior alveolar nerve block.

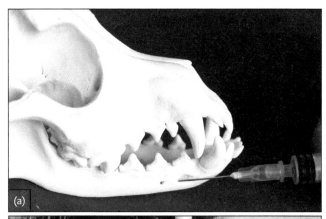
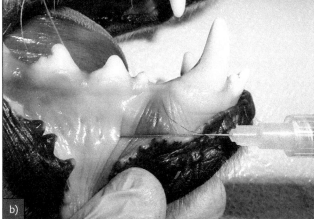

6.27 Right middle mental nerve block in a dog. (a) Skull demonstration. In this case the needle was inserted into the middle mental foramen, but this should be performed with caution as damage to the vessels and nerve is possible. (b) Clinical case. The tip of the needle was placed near the middle mental foramen to anaesthetize the rostral mandibular soft tissues.
(© Dr John Lewis)

References and further reading

Abbo LA, Ko JC, Maxwell LK *et al.* (2008) Pharmacokinetics of buprenorphine following intravenous and oral transmucosal administration in dogs. *Veterinary Therapeutics: Research in Applied Veterinary Medicine* **9**, 83–93

Anthony JA (2008) Direct iatrogenic effects of oral nerve blocks in dogs. *Proceedings of the 17th European Congress of Veterinary Dentistry, Uppsala, Sweden*, p. 8

Armstrong SR, Roberts BK and Aronsohn M (2005) Perioperative hypothermia. *Journal of Veterinary Emergency and Critical Care* **15**, 32–37

Avery P, Redon D, Schaenzer G and Rusy B (1984) The influence of serum potassium on the cerebral and cardiac toxicity of bupivacaine and lidocaine. *Anesthesiology* **61**, 134–138

Barton-Lamb AL, Martin-Flores M, Scrivani PV *et al.* (2013) Evaluation of maxillary arterial blood flow in anesthetized cats with the mouth closed and open. *Veterinary Journal* **196**, 325–331

Beckman B (2013) Anesthesia and pain management for small animals. *Veterinary Clinics of North America: Small Animal Practice* **43**, 669–688

Beckman B and Legendre L (2002) Regional nerve blocks for oral surgery in companion animals. *Compendium on Continuing Education for the Practicing Veterinarian* **24**, 439–444

Bednarski R, Grimm K, Harvey R *et al.* (2011) AAHA anesthesia guidelines for dogs and cats. *Journal of the American Animal Hospital Association* **47**, 377–385

Brodbelt DC, Blissit KJ, Hammond RA *et al.* (2008) The risk of death: the confidential enquiry into perioperative small animal fatalities. *Veterinary Anaesthesia and Analgesia* **35**, 365–373

Cowan A, Doxey JC and Harry EJ (1977) The animal pharmacology of buprenorphine, an oripavine analgesic agent. *British Journal of Pharmacology* **60**, 547–554

Dugdale A (2010) *Veterinary Anaesthesia: Principles to Practice.* Wiley-Blackwell, Oxford

Duke T (2000) Local and regional anesthetic and analgesic techniques in the dog and cat: part II – infiltration and nerve blocks. *Canadian Veterinary Journal* **41**, 949–952

Duke-Novakovski T (2007) Dental and oral surgery. In: *BSAVA Manual of Canine and Feline Anaesthesia and Analgesia, 2nd edn*, ed. C Seymour and T Duke-Novakovski, pp. 194–199. BSAVA Publications, Gloucester

Duke-Novakozski T, de Vries M and Seymour C (2016) *BSAVA Manual of Canine Feline Anaesthesia and Analgesia, 3rd edn*. BSAVA Publications, Gloucester

Gracis M (2013) The oral cavity. In: *Small Animal Regional Anesthesia and Analgesia*, ed. L Campoy and MR Read, pp.119–140. Wiley-Blackwell, Oxford

Gross ME, Pope ER, O'Brien D *et al.* (1997) Regional anesthesia of the infraorbital and inferior alveolar nerves during noninvasive tooth pulp stimulation in halothane-anesthetized dogs. *Journal of the American Veterinary Medical Association* **211**, 1403–1405

Hardie EM, Spodnick GJ, Gilson SD *et al.* (1999) Tracheal rupture in cats: 16 cases (1983–1998). *Journal of the American Veterinary Medical Association* **214**, 508–512

Haskins SC, Farver TB and Patz JD (1986) Cardiovascular changes in dogs given diazepam and diazepam-ketamine. *American Journal of Veterinary Research* **47**, 795–798

Ilkiw JE, Suter CM, Farver TB *et al.* (1996) The behaviour of healthy awake cats following intravenous and intramuscular administration of midazolam. *Journal of Veterinary Pharmacology and Therapeutics* **19**, 205–216

Kasten GW and Martin ST (1985) Bupivacaine cardiovascular toxicity: comparison of treatment with bretylium and lidocaine. *Anesthesia and Analgesia* **64**, 911–916

Lamata C, Loughton V, Jones M *et al.* (2012) The risk of passive regurgitation during general anaesthesia in a population of referred dogs in the UK. *Veterinary Anaesthesia and Analgesia* **39**, 266–274

Lantz GC (2003) Regional anesthesia for dentistry and oral surgery. *Journal of Veterinary Dentistry* **20**, 181–186

Lemke KA (2007) Pain management 2: local and regional anaesthetic techniques. In: *BSAVA Manual of Canine and Feline Anaesthesia and Analgesia, 2nd edn*, ed. C Seymour and T Duke-Novakovski, pp. 104–114. BSAVA Publications, Gloucester

Lui PL, Feldman HS, Giasi R, Patterson MK and Covino BG (1983) Comparative CNS toxicity of lidocaine, eidocaine, bupivacaine and tetracaine in awake dogs following rapid intravenous administration. *Anesthesia and Analgesia* **62**, 375–379

McInnes F, Clear N, James G *et al.* (2008) Evaluation of the clearance of a sublingual buprenorphine spray in the beagle dog using gamma scintigraphy. *Pharmaceutical Research* **25**, 869–874

Minghella E, Benmansour P, Iff I *et al.* (2010) Pain after injection of a new formulation of propofol in six dogs. *Veterinary Record* **167**, 866–867

Mitchell SL, McCarthy R, Rudloff E *et al.* (2000) Tracheal rupture associated with intubation in cats: 20 cases (1996–1998). *Journal of the American Veterinary Medical Association* **216**, 1592–1595

Nind F and Mosedale P (2016) *BSAVA Guide to the Use of Veterinary Medicines.* BSAVA Publications, Gloucester. Available at: www.bsava.com/Resources/Veterinary-resources/Medicines-Guide

Oka S, Shimamoto C, Kyoda N and Misaki T (1997) Comparison of lidocaine with and without bupivacaine for local dental anesthesia. *Anesthesia Progress* **44**, 86–86

Pascoe PJ (1997) Local and regional anesthesia and analgesia. *Seminars in Veterinary Medicine and Surgery (Small Animal)* **12**, 94–105

Pascoe PJ (2012) Anesthesia and pain management. In: *Oral and Maxillofacial Surgery in Dogs and Cats*, ed FJ Verstraete and MJ Lommer, pp. 23–42. Saunders Elsevier, Philadelphia

Pascoe PJ (2016) The effects of lidocaine or lidocaine-bupivacine mixture administered into the infraorbital canal in dogs. *American Journal of Veterinary Research* **77**, 682–687

Posner LP (2007) Pre-anaesthetic assessment. In: *BSAVA Manual of Canine and Feline Anaesthesia and Analgesia, 2nd edn*, ed. C Seymour and T Duke-Novakovski, pp. 6–11. BSAVA Publications, Gloucester

Posner LP, Pavuk AA, Rokshar JL *et al.* (2010) Effects of opioids and anesthetic drugs on body temperature in cats. *Veterinary Anaesthesia and Analgesia* **37**, 35–43

Reiter AM (2012) Dental and oral diseases. In: *The Cat: Clinical Medicine and Management*, ed. SE Little, pp.329–370. Saunders, St Louis

Rochette J (2005) Regional anesthesia and analgesia for oral and dental procedures. *Veterinary Clinics of North America: Small Animal Practice* **35**, 1041–1058

Snyder CJ and Snyder LB (2013) Effect of mepivacaine in an infraorbital nerve block on minimum alveolar concentration of isoflurane in clinically normal anesthetized dogs undergoing a modified form of dental dolorimetry. *Journal of the American Veterinary Medical Association* **242**, 199–204

Snyder LBC and Snyder CJ (2016) Effects of buprenorphine added to bupivacaine infraorbital nerve blocks on isoflurane minimum alveolar concentration using a model for acute dental/oral surgical pain in dogs. *Journal of Veterinary Dentistry* **33**, 90–96

Soukup JW and Snyder CJ (2015) Transmylohyoid orotracheal intubation in surgical management of canine maxillofacial fractures: an alternative to pharyngotomy endotracheal intubation. *Veterinary Surgery* **44**, 432–436

Stiles J, Weil AB, Packer RA *et al.* (2012) Post-anaesthetic cortical blindness in cats: 20 cases. *Veterinary Journal* **193**, 367–373

Chapter 7

Management of periodontal disease

Peter Southerden and Alexander M. Reiter

Periodontal disease is the most common pathological condition occurring in adult dogs and cats. It refers to infection and inflammation of the periodontium (gingiva, periodontal ligament, alveolar bone and cementum) due to plaque bacteria and the host's response to the bacterial insult (Hoffmann and Gaengler, 1996; Lund *et al.*, 1999; Lommer and Verstraete, 2001; Kortegaard *et al.*, 2008; Girard *et al.*, 2009; Reiter *et al.*, 2012).

The two main presentations of periodontal disease are gingivitis and periodontitis. Inflammation can spread along the periodontal space towards the root apex and causes loss of alveolar bone as it progresses. If allowed to continue to develop, it can affect the periapical region of the tooth root, leading to retrograde pulpal infection. Thus, endodontic disease can occur as a result of severe periodontal disease (Marretta, 1987; Lobprise, 2000a; Nemec *et al.*, 2007; Reiter and Harvey, 2010), and *vice versa* (Marretta *et al.*, 1992). Severe periodontitis may also result in oronasal fistula formation and chronic nasal disease (Marretta, 1992), lead to pathological mandibular fracture (Niemiec, 2008) or cause organ disease and systemic effects (DeBowes *et al.*, 1996).

Diagnosis of periodontal disease requires a thorough periodontal examination by means of dental exploration and periodontal probing (Lewis and Miller, 2010), supported by full-mouth dental radiography (Tsugawa and Verstraete, 2000; Tsugawa *et al.*, 2003). Management of periodontal disease includes several different types of preventive and treatment procedures in the conscious and anaesthetized patient. Frequent home oral hygiene and professional dental cleaning are the primary procedures. Professional dental cleaning under anaesthesia is necessary when there is moderate accumulation of plaque and calculus. Gingivitis and mild or moderate periodontitis can be managed effectively by scaling and polishing followed by frequent (preferably daily) home oral hygiene in an otherwise healthy dog or cat (Harvey, 2005). Home oral hygiene and professional dental cleaning are not sufficient when there is extensive periodontitis or when complicating factors such as systemic illness are present. The most commonly indicated treatment for periodontal disease in dogs and cats is tooth extraction. However, even severely affected teeth can be successfully retained in the mouth by a combination of professional dental cleaning, closed and open periodontal therapy, and advanced periodontal surgery performed by a trained veterinary health care provider as well as conscientiously applied home oral hygiene executed daily by a committed pet owner (Reiter and Harvey, 2010).

Equipment, instruments and materials

Having the proper equipment, instruments and materials is paramount for the successful diagnosis and treatment of periodontal disease (Anthony, 2000a).

Power scalers

Power scalers enable the rapid removal of plaque and calculus. Ultrasonic and sonic scalers appear to achieve similar results to hand instruments. They may even be more effective than hand instruments in the furcation area, as they are slimmer and therefore facilitate better access. They need to be used carefully because they can cause damage to the tooth surface if not used properly. Power scalers should be held using the modified pen grasp technique (see 'Holding of instruments').

Ultrasonic scalers

Ultrasonic scalers are used more commonly in veterinary practice. They convert electrical energy into a mechanical vibration. The scaling tip oscillates at 18–50 kilohertz (kHz) (i.e. cycles per second) and is water-cooled. The tip oscillation is driven by a micromotor using either a magnetostrictive or piezoelectric mechanism. Magnetostrictive scalers operate between 10 and 45 kHz (Figure 7.1). The vibration is generated by the effect of a magnetic field on a metal stack or ferroceramic rod, and the tip movement may be elliptical (metal stack) or circular (ferroceramic rod). Piezoelectric scalers operate at 25–50 kHz (Figure 7.2). They have crystals within the handpiece, resulting in linear (back and forth) vibration of the tip when activated by an electric current (Holmstrom, 2000).

High energy is produced in the oscillation generator and delivered to the tip, causing vibration at amplitudes from 0.01 to 0.02 mm (magnetostrictive scaler) and 0.2 mm (piezoelectric scaler). Plaque and calculus are removed by three different mechanisms, including a mechanical chipping action of the oscillating tip, the cavitation effect of the coolant, comprising the formation and implosion of small bubbles within the coolant able to exert a disruptive force on dental deposits, and flow of the coolant irrigating the tooth surface (Holmstrom, 2000).

Ultrasonic scalers can be used to remove both supragingival and subgingival dental deposits. A large array of tips is available. A relatively wide scaler tip (beaver-tail

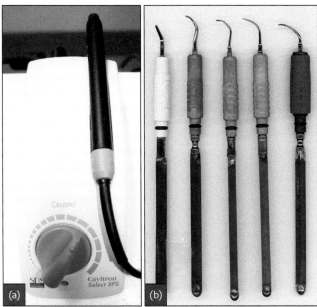

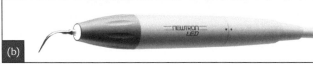

7.1 (a) Magnetostrictive scaler. (b) Metal stack inserts with various tips.
(© Dr Alexander M. Reiter)

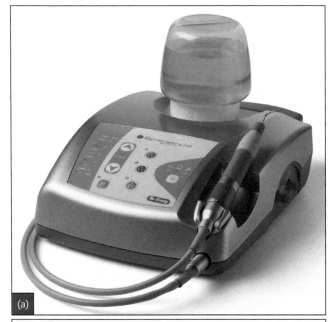

7.2 (a) Piezoelectric scaler and reservoir. (b) Piezoelectric scaler handpiece with LED light and universal tip.
(a, Courtesy of Accesia, Sweden; b, Courtesy of Satelec, France)

insert) should only be used supragingivally (if at all), while a thinner tip (periodontal insert) can be used for subgingival scaling as well. The power setting may be modified, with a higher power setting increasing the amplitude of tip oscillation and therefore effectiveness. However, there is considerable heat generation at the scaler tip which, if used carelessly, can cause iatrogenic injury to the pulp. It is therefore important to adjust to the lowest effective power, use the sides of the instrument tip only, apply light pressure, keep the scaler moving, and not scale any one tooth for

more than a few seconds (i.e. move from tooth to tooth and later return to a tooth not yet sufficiently scaled). The flow of coolant should be enough to keep the tip cool to touch. If this is not the case, the power of the scaler should be reduced or the flow of coolant increased. The flow should be adjusted so that a mist of microscopic droplets, rather than a flow of large droplets, forms at the tip. Ultrasonic scalers used at low to medium power cause less damage to the tooth surface than either sonic or hand scalers (Lewis and Miller, 2010).

It is advisable to direct the tip apically, with the last 2–3 mm of the tip in contact with the tooth and at an angle of less than 15 degrees to the tooth surface (Figures 7.3 and 7.4). As tips may wear with time, their length should be checked frequently using dedicated wear guides provided by the manufacturers, as 1 mm of shortening may correspond to up to 25% loss of efficiency.

Sonic scalers

Sonic scalers are air turbine units driven by compressed air. Their tips oscillate in an elliptical (figure-of-eight) or circular fashion at sonic frequencies of 3–8 kHz (Figure 7.5). They are less effective at removing calculus compared with ultrasonic scalers because of the reduced mechanical effect and minimal cavitation, but they generate less heat and are therefore safer to use (Holmstrom, 2000). They can be used to remove both supragingival and – with the appropriate tip – subgingival dental deposits. Given their amplitude of 0.5 mm, sonic scalers, to some extent, 'hammer' the tooth surface irrespective of the tip's alignment to the tooth.

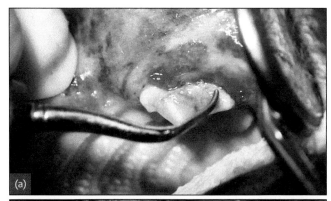

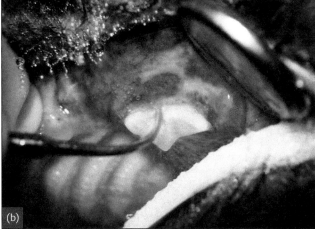

7.3 Ultrasonic scaling of the left maxillary fourth premolar tooth in a cat. (a) Lip retraction is performed with a dental mirror. (b) The scaler tip is directed apically, with its last 2–3 mm in contact with the tooth and at an angle of less than 15 degrees to the tooth surface.
(© Dr Alexander M. Reiter)

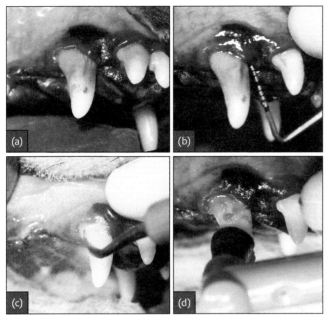

Most compressed air-driven dental units sold for veterinary use have outlets for one or two water-cooled high-speed handpieces, one low-speed handpiece, and an air/water syringe (Holmstrom, 2000). These units can be mounted on a cart or wall-mounted (Figure 7.6). They are powered by a compressor, which may be mounted on the cart or, in the case of wall-mounted units, be located away from the operating room. Compressors vary in both capacity and power, but they usually operate at about 30 psi. Oil-less compressors are advantageous for operative dentistry (e.g. provision of dental restorations), as they do not produce oil droplets in the air line, which can contaminate the restorative material. They are also less expensive and require less maintenance than oil-cooled compressors. The downside is that they are much noisier and thus may only be used when they can be placed out of the operating room.

7.4 Scaling and polishing of the right maxillary canine tooth in a dog. (a) There is severe plaque and calculus accumulation and gingivitis. (b) Probing reveals a 6 mm deep periodontal pocket at the mesiolabial aspect of the tooth. (c) The scaler tip is directed apically, with its last 2–3 mm in contact with the tooth and at an angle of less than 15 degrees to the tooth surface. (d) The surface of the tooth is polished.
(© Dr Alexander M. Reiter)

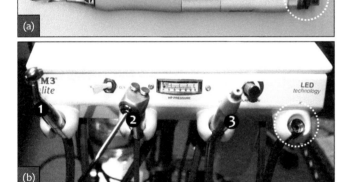

7.5 (a) Sonic scaler. (b) Dental unit. The dotted circles indicate the attachment of the sonic scaler handpiece to a high-speed handpiece tubing in order to receive water, which is required for cooling of its tip. 1 = high-speed handpiece; 2 = air/water syringe; 3 = low-speed handpiece.
(© Dr Alexander M. Reiter)

Rotary scalers

Rotary burs are used in the high-speed handpiece and rotate at about 300,000 revolutions per minute (rpm), which is equivalent to a frequency of about 30 kHz. They are not recommended due to considerable risk of iatrogenic tooth damage (Holmstrom, 2000).

Air-driven dental unit

Air-driven dental units consist of a compressor (or use compressed gas from a cylinder), control unit and handpieces. The control unit controls the supply of air and water to the handpieces. Water is usually supplied from pressurized bottles attached to the control unit.

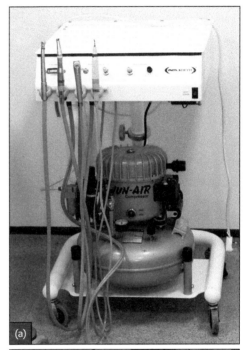

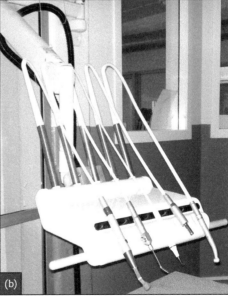

7.6 (a) Air-powered dental cart with compressor. (b) Wall-mounted dental unit.
(a, © Dr Peter Southerden; b, Courtesy of Accesia, Sweden)

Handpieces

All handpieces should be held using the modified pen grasp technique.

High-speed handpiece

The high-speed handpiece (Figure 7.7) has an air-driven turbine in its head. The chuck of the turbine holds friction-grip (FG) burs, which are used to section teeth, aid in defect and crown preparation, and remove bone. Burs are usually changed by depressing a push button on the back of the turbine (older versions use a chuck key). Coolant is delivered to the site of action of the bur, and many also have an integral fibreoptic light. The handpiece can work at up to 400,000 rpm (Holmstrom, 2000). The handpiece produces very low torque, which allows the bur to stall with relatively low pressure. Therefore, the handpiece and bur are used with a gentle brushing technique.

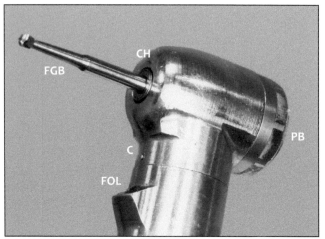

7.7 Head of a high-speed handpiece. C = coolant; CH = chuck; FGB = friction-grip bur; FOL = fibreoptic light; PB = push button.
(© Dr Peter Southerden)

High-speed handpieces are primarily used for cutting holes into teeth for endodontic access, preparing dental defects for restoration, preparing the crown in prosthodontic dentistry, sectioning multi-rooted teeth into single-rooted crown-root segments in preparation for extraction, removing and shaping alveolar bone, and making precise cuts into bony structures during mandibulectomy and maxillectomy procedures. Various shapes, sizes and lengths of burs are available. Round, cross-cut fissure, 12-fluted, diamond, and acrylic burs are most commonly used in dentistry and oral surgery (Holmstrom, 2000).

There are two different types of coupling that can be used to attach the handpiece to the dental unit. These are the four-hole mid-west fitting and the two- or three-hole Burden fitting. The mid-west is the most common fitting in the UK. Handpieces may also have a swivel fitting, allowing the handpiece to rotate independently of the hose and thus placing less stress on the hand of the operator (Figure 7.8).

Low-speed handpiece

The low-speed handpiece (Figure 7.9) can work in forward and reverse up to 30,000 rpm. It produces high torque, which means it takes greater pressure to make it stall. If used at maximum speed, thermal damage to the pulp of a tooth can occur if the working burs are uncooled for more than a few seconds. Geared handpieces can be used, which allow the speed to be increased or decreased. Low-speed handpieces generally give greater tactile sensitivity and are therefore often used for more precise finishing and polishing.

A nose cone attached to a low-speed handpiece engine can take long straight handpiece (HP) burs that are primarily used for reducing elongated teeth in pet lagomorphs and rodents and for trimming resin splints and stone models. Other attachments that can be secured to the nose cone are the prophy angle and contra-angle. The prophy angle allows the use of a prophy cup for polishing

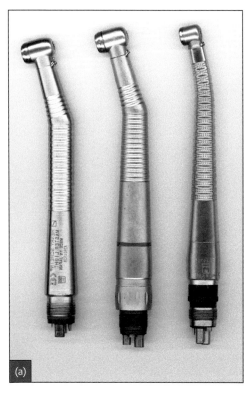

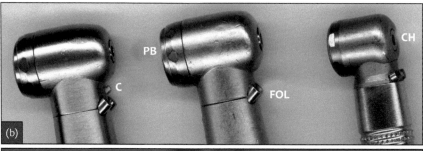

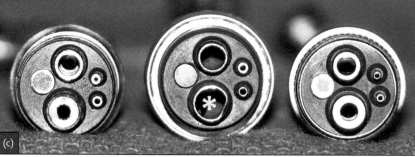

7.8 High-speed handpieces. (a) The handpieces in the middle and to the right have a swivel fitting. The one to the right has a mini head used to work in areas with limited space. (b) Close-up of the heads of the three handpieces. (c) The handpieces have four-hole mid-west fittings. Note the kinked air exhaust hole (*) in the handpiece in the middle. C = coolant; CH = chuck; FOL = fibreoptic light; PB = push button.
(© Dr Alexander M. Reiter)

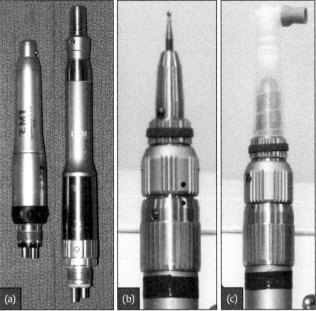

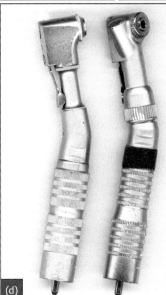

7.9 (a) Low-speed handpieces consisting of engine (or motor) and nose cone. (b) Low-speed handpiece with a long straight (HP) bur. (c) Low-speed handpiece with a disposable prophy angle. (d) Contra-angles. The one on the right has a 10:1 reduction gear.
(a, d © Dr Alexander M. Reiter; b, c © Dr Peter Southerden)

teeth after cleaning (single-use versions are also available). The contra-angle is used to change either the direction or speed of rotation and can accommodate latch-grip right angle (RA) burs for removal of bone, shaping defects for restorations, prepare natural crowns for receiving prosthodontic crowns and smoothing restorations (Holmstrom, 2000).

Air/water syringe

The air/water syringe is used for rinsing and drying (Holmstrom, 2000). The syringe can deliver a stream of water for gentle rinsing, water mixed with air for flushing (when both buttons are pushed at the same time), or air only for drying. The operator is advised not to blow air on to bleeding surfaces or into the root canal in order to avoid the risk of embolism.

Micromotor unit

A micromotor unit can be used to activate a low-speed handpiece for sectioning teeth, removing bone, and polishing dental surfaces and restorations. The electric motor is attached directly to the handpiece by an 'e' fitting. It works

at 0–40,000 rpm, has a very high torque and can be put in forward and reverse (Holmstrom, 2000). While it is less expensive than air-driven units, it is also less efficient and much slower. Geared handpieces can be used to increase the working speed to 400,000 rpm. An external source of coolant must be provided for both cooling and lubrication. While micromotors usually do not have water cooling, some versions used in oral surgery may have a built-in lactated Ringer's irrigation system. A battery-powered unit may also be useful (Terpak and Verstraete, 2012).

Burs

All burs have a head, neck and shank. There are three shank types: a long straight shank ('HP'), which fits into the nose cone of a straight low-speed handpiece; a latch-type shank ('RA'), which fits into the latch of a contra-angle on a low-speed handpiece; and a short, straight shank friction-grip ('FG'), which fits into the chuck of a high-speed handpiece. Burs with a round, elongated (fissure), pear-shaped or inverted-cone head are most commonly used, but many different shapes are available. Long versions are also available, which are good for working on teeth and bone where a long reach is required (Holmstrom, 2000). Tungsten carbide burs are commonly used for tooth sectioning during extraction, perforating the tooth surface during endodontic procedures and performing more aggressive bone work, while diamond burs are mainly used for fine bone remodelling and for crown preparation in prosthodontic procedures. Special tungsten, carbide and diamond burs may also be used on gingival tissues during gingivectomy and gingivoplasty procedures. Stainless steel and composite burs are available but less commonly utilized. See Figure 12.4 for a selection of FG burs.

Tungsten carbide burs

Round burs: The cutting tip of the bur is round. These burs are numbered ¼, ½, and from 1 to 8. They can be used for removal of bone, sectioning of smaller teeth, accessing the pulp chamber, and preparing dental defects (Holmstrom, 2000).

Fissure burs: Fissure burs with cross-cuts are numbered in the 500s and 700s. Their cutting surface is on the sides, and to a lesser extent on their tips. They are primarily used for sectioning teeth. They may also be used for preparing dental defects (Holmstrom, 2000).

Pear-shaped and inverted-cone burs: Pear-shaped burs are numbered in the 320s and 330s. They have a round cutting tip, cutting sides and a slight taper for undercutting. They may be used similarly to round burs and for sectioning teeth. Inverted-cone burs are numbered in the 30s. They are used for undercutting in dental defect preparation.

Finishing burs: Finishing burs are either made of stone or have multiple flutes. They are used for finishing restorations (Holmstrom, 2000).

Diamond burs

These are burs covered with diamond grit of various degrees of coarseness. Round versions are used for smoothing sharp bony edges and bevelling the enamel during dental defect preparations. Long, tapered versions with various tip shapes are used for crown preparations (Holmstrom, 2000).

Hand instruments

Dental explorer

The dental explorer has a slender working end that tapers to a sharp-pointed tip. It is designed to give maximum tactile sensitivity and is used in sedated or anaesthetized patients to:

* Detect softened enamel and/or dentine, which may indicate caries
* Explore the structural integrity of the tooth surface (e.g. tooth fractures, tooth resorption, enamel hypoplasia)
* Feel for the presence of subgingival and supragingival dental deposits
* Evaluate the margins of restorations and prosthodontic crowns
* Determine the presence of pulp exposure.

The dental explorer (Figure 7.10) is held with the modi-fied pen grasp technique and is only used on hard tissue. The 'shepherd's hook' or No. 23 dental explorer is the most commonly known in veterinary practice and is often paired with a periodontal probe to form a double-ended instrument. However, it is bulky, inflexible and less adapt-able to subgingival use when compared with other explorers (Lewis and Miller, 2010; Reiter, 2012). The Orban explorer has a 2 mm tip that is bent at a 90-degree angle from the shank, allowing it to be used subgingivally with little tissue distention (stretching of the gingiva away from the tooth) or trauma to the epithelial lining of the sulcus. The curved and long-shanked working end of the 11/12 ODU dental explorer makes it adaptable to use on rostral and caudal teeth, supragingivally and subgingi-vally, and its slender and pointed tip allows for detection of subtle hard tissue defects (Figure 7.11) (Lewis and Miller, 2010).

Periodontal probe

The periodontal probe is a graduated miniature ruler used to obtain measurements (Lewis and Miller, 2010). It has a pointed round or rectangular flat working end whose tip has a diameter of 0.5–0.6 mm. The blunt instrument tip reduces

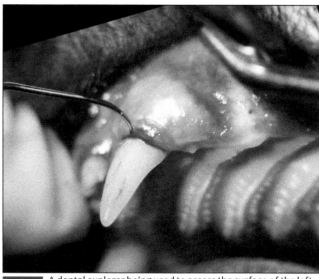

7.11 A dental explorer being used to assess the surface of the left maxillary canine tooth in a cat for any irregularities.
(© Dr Alexander M. Reiter)

the possibility of tissue trauma when inserted into the gin-gival sulcus or periodontal pocket. The periodontal probe is used to:

* Measure the depth of the gingival sulcus, gingival pockets or periodontal pockets
* Assess the extent of gingival recession or gingival enlargement
* Assess the severity of gingival inflammation and gingival bleeding
* Evaluate the extent of furcation involvement or exposure in multi-rooted teeth
* Measure the severity of tooth mobility
* Feel for the presence of subgingival and supragingival dental deposits
* Explore sinus tracts (often located near the mucogingival junction), which may indicate endodontic/ periapical disease or neoplasia
* Create bleeding points on the outer gingival surface prior to gingivectomy
* Measure the size of oral lesions.

The blunt tip of the probe is usually calibrated in milli-metres. Some probes have a small 0.5 mm ball on the end to minimize tissue trauma; however, these probes typically have markings at 3.5, 5.5, 8.5 and 11.5 mm, resulting in inexact determination of periodontal pocket depth. While many probes exist, a probe with markings beginning at 1 mm is necessary for assessing subtle periodontal pocket depths in cats (Lewis and Miller, 2010). The CP-15 UNC probe is marked every millimetre, with a black band at 5, 10 and 15 mm; it is very useful for large dogs or patients with deep periodontal pockets (Figure 7.12). Another common probe used in veterinary practice has circumfer-ential Williams markings at 1, 2, 3, 5, 7, 8, 9 and 10 mm. The Michigan-O probe with Williams markings is best suited for use in cats because the working end of the probe is the narrowest in diameter (Figure 7.13). Other styles of probes contain colour-coded bands for easier viewing of calibra-tions. A Nabers probe is a curved furcation probe that is used to assess the extent of bone loss in the furcation area of multi-rooted teeth (Lewis and Miller, 2010; Reiter, 2012).

The periodontal probe is held with the modified pen grasp technique (Figures 7.14 and 7.15). The use of the periodontal probe during periodontal examination is

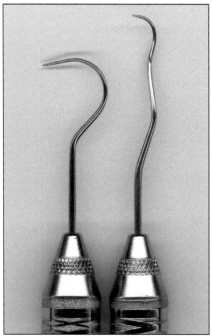

7.10 Shepherd's hook (or No. 23) dental explorer (left) and 11/12 ODU dental explorer (right).
(© Dr Alexander M. Reiter)

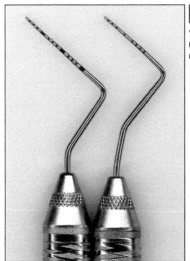

7.12 CP-15 UNC probe (left) and a probe with Williams markings (right).
(© Dr Alexander M. Reiter)

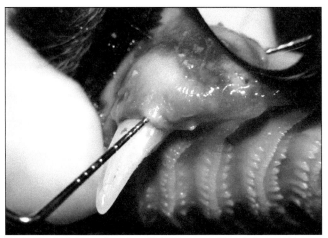

7.13 A Michigan-O probe with Williams markings being used to measure the depth of the gingival sulcus of the left maxillary canine tooth in a cat.
(© Dr Alexander M. Reiter)

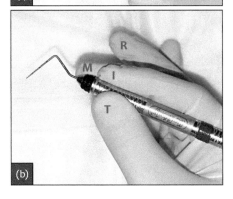

7.14 Modified pen grasp. (a) The instrument is first grasped between the thumb (T) and index finger (I), and then (b) the middle finger (M) is brought towards the shank of the probe. R = ring finger.
(© Dr Alexander M. Reiter)

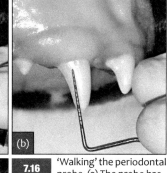

7.15 The modified pen grasp is shown during probing of a right maxillary canine tooth. The instrument is held with the thumb (T) and index (I) and middle (M) fingers, while the hand is supported with the ring finger (R) on an incisor tooth.
(© Dr Alexander M. Reiter)

explained in Chapter 3. Briefly, for sulcus or pocket depth measurement, the probe is gently inserted between the tooth and gingiva down to the bottom of the gingival sulcus or periodontal pocket with light pressure until slight resistance is felt (Reiter *et al.*, 2012). The probe should be 'walked' around the circumference of the tooth with short up-and-down strokes every few millimetres (Figure 7.16). The recommended probing force is 0.1–0.2 Newton (about 10–20 gram-force). Care should be taken not to probe too forcefully, as this may cause the tip of the probe to be forced through the bottom of the gingival sulcus or periodontal pocket. The depth of the gingival sulcus or periodontal pocket should be measured in at least six sites around each tooth. The gingival sulcus should not be deeper than 0.5 mm in cats and 3 mm in dogs. Greater measurements indicate the presence of a periodontal pocket or, in the case of gingival enlargement, a gingival pocket (pseudopocket) (Reiter *et al.*, 2012).

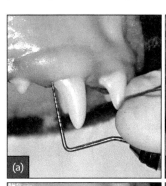

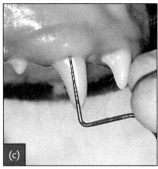

7.16 'Walking' the periodontal probe. (a) The probe has been inserted at the distolabial aspect of the right maxillary canine tooth. (b) The probe is removed and then (c) reinserted at the labial aspect of the tooth. Note that this alternative approach differs slightly from that described in Chapter 3 where the instrument is not completely removed during walking of the probe.
(© Dr Alexander M. Reiter)

Dental mirror

Dental mirrors come in a variety of sizes and may be plain or magnifying (Wolf *et al.*, 2005). Practice is required in order to visualize the reflected image. Condensation can be prevented by applying special anti-fogging solutions or by wiping the mirror across the oral mucosa before use (Figure 7.17). If single-ended, the opposite blunt end of the instrument handle can also be used to evaluate for tooth mobility (by holding the tooth between an index finger and the instrument end) or for gentle percussion of teeth to assess for discomfort in the conscious patient. A dental mirror is held with the modified pen grasp technique and used to:

- Allow indirect visualization of lesions and areas of interest that are not approachable at the front or side of the mouth (e.g. the palatal/lingual/distal surfaces of teeth, particularly of the maxillary and mandibular molars in dogs)
- Reflect light on to and magnify areas of interest
- Retract the cheeks to the side, push the tongue medially or ventrally, and lift the soft palate dorsally or pull it rostroventrally
- Protect oral soft tissues (e.g. by placing the mirror as a barrier between the sublingual area and the mandibular cheek teeth when using power equipment on those teeth).

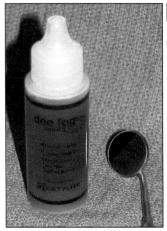

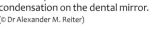 Anti-fogging solution for prevention of condensation on the dental mirror.
(© Dr Alexander M. Reiter)

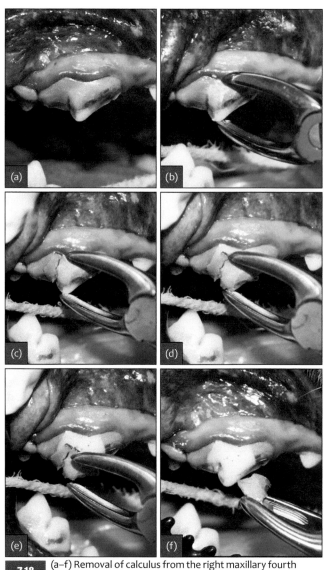

7.18 (a–f) Removal of calculus from the right maxillary fourth premolar tooth in a dog using extraction forceps.
(© Dr Alexander M. Reiter)

Calculus-removing forceps

Calculus-removing forceps are similar to extraction forceps except that one beak is straight and longer and the other curved and shorter. The straight beak is placed on top and slightly behind the tooth, and the curved beak is placed to engage the calculus at or above the gingival margin. The handles of the forceps are gently squeezed, and the beaks are brought together, thereby removing large pieces of calculus at the beginning of a professional dental cleaning procedure (Holmstrom, 2000). Extraction forceps may – with adequate practice and proper, gentle technique – also be used to remove gross calculus attached to the crown of a tooth (Figure 7.18).

Scaling instruments

In general, dental hand instruments consist of three parts: the handle, the shank, and the working end. The handle contains the instrument's identification, its description with abbreviations that include the name or school of the designer, the manufacturer, the classification type and the design number. Classifications are determined by the design of the working ends and the instrument's intended purpose (Lewis and Miller, 2010). Scaling instruments include scalers, curettes, files and hoes. Hollow, lightweight handle designs are more efficient in transmitting vibrations detected through tactile sensitivity. Use of wider handle sizes minimizes finger pinching and hand fatigue, and various patterns of surface texture on the handle prevent fingers from slipping (Lewis and Miller, 2010).

The (functional) shank connects the handle with the working end. The curvature and length of the shank determines the best suited location within the mouth for use of the instrument. The terminal shank is that portion of the instrument between the working end and the first bend on the functional shank. An instrument may have one single working end (SE) or it may be double-ended (DE). The working end of a scaler and curette (Figure 7.19) is called the blade and has two lateral sides, a face, a back, a heel, and a rounded toe or pointed tip. The face and lateral surfaces meet to form a cutting edge. The back is formed by the convergence of the two lateral surfaces. The angulation of the face of the blade in relation to the terminal shank will classify the instrument as being either universal or area-specific (Lewis and Miller, 2010). Scalers and curettes should be held with the modified pen grasp technique.

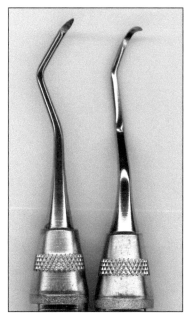

7.19 Scaler with pointed tip (left) and curette with rounded toe (right).
(© Dr Alexander M. Reiter)

Hand scalers: Hand scalers have straight lateral surfaces that converge and, together with the straight or curved face, form a pointed back and sharp tip. The blade has two cutting edges, and either may be used depending on how the handle is tipped. In fact, even if scalers with a bent shank have the face of the working end at a 90-degree angle to the lower shank, only one cutting edge may be applied with the appropriate angle to the working tooth surface. The working end is triangular in cross-section with 70–80-degree internal angles between the face and lateral surfaces (Lewis and Miller, 2010). Hand scalers must not be used subgingivally to avoid iatrogenic soft tissue trauma by their sharp tips. When placing the blade against the tooth, the face should be at an angle of 60–80 degrees to the tooth surface. The cutting edge is directed to the apical edge of the calculus, and lateral pressure is applied against the tooth. Hand scalers are used with a pulling motion away from the gingival margin to remove supragingival plaque and calculus (Lewis and Miller, 2010). A commonly used instrument is a straight double-ended sickle scaler. The sharp tip of the scaler may be used to scale thin developmental grooves on the crown of canine teeth in cats and premolar and molar teeth in cats and dogs (Figure 7.20).

Hand curettes: Hand curettes either have two cutting edges, which are arranged perpendicular to the terminal shank (Universal curette), or a single cutting edge with the working blade at an angle of 70 degrees to the terminal shank (Gracey curette) (Figure 7.21a). The face is curved lengthwise from the heel to the rounded toe, meeting the lateral surfaces to create a cutting edge that extends around the toe. The lateral surfaces of the curette are rounded, creating a round back that is easier to insert into a sulcus or pocket. The cross-section of the curette is semi-circular with internal angles of 70–80 degrees between the face and lateral surfaces (Lewis and Miller, 2010). The terminal 2–3 mm of the blade should be used in contact with the tooth.

Hand curettes have mirror images on opposite ends. From the midline of each tooth the toe of the instrument should be pointed towards the proximal surface, which means both ends of the curette will be used for the buccal and lingual surfaces of each tooth. Universal curettes are designed to adapt to all tooth surfaces. They have straight shanks that are used with the handle parallel to the working surface of the tooth. Gracey curettes are area-specific instruments designed for use on different tooth surfaces in the human dentition. They have shanks attached to the instrument handle at varying angles to allow scaling of different tooth surfaces of various teeth. Generally the low-numbered curettes (1–4), which are used for the anterior teeth in people (rostral in animals), are most useful in veterinary dentistry. Gracey curettes are used effectively when the terminal shank, not the handle, is held

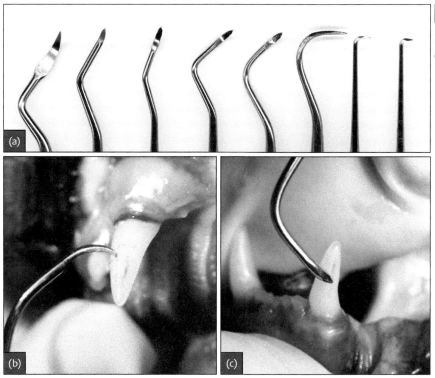

7.20 (a) Working ends of various hand scalers. (b, c) Scalers are often used to scale supragingival grooves such as those in the crowns of maxillary and mandibular canine teeth in cats.
(© Dr Alexander M. Reiter)

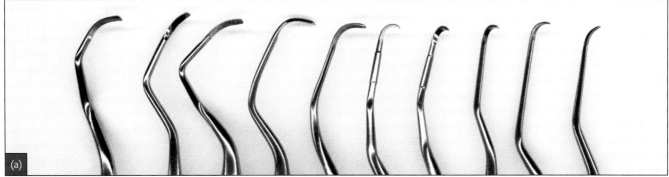

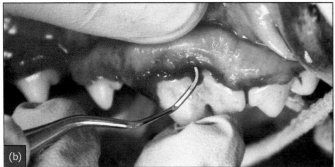

7.21 (a) Working ends of various hand curettes. (b) A curette being used to scale and plane the subgingival surface of the roots of a left maxillary fourth premolar tooth in a dog.
(© Dr Alexander M. Reiter)

parallel to the working surface of the tooth. Only the lower cutting edge of the 70-degree angled blade can be utilized for scaling. If the wrong cutting edge is placed on the tooth surface, and the terminal shank is held parallel to the working surface of the tooth, the face of the instrument will be facing the operator, and the side or the back of the working end will be sliding on the tooth, impeding effective removal of plaque and calculus.

Langer curettes have a combination of universal curette qualities (face perpendicular to terminal shank) with the Gracey curvature of shanks and may be used by holding the handle parallel to the working surface of the tooth. The so-called After Five® curettes have 3 mm longer shanks, and may be used to clean deep pockets in large animals. Mini hand curettes (Langers and Graceys) have long shanks and shorter blades and are useful for cleaning narrow pockets on small dogs and cats (Lewis and Miller, 2010).

Hand curettes are used for removing supragingival and subgingival plaque and calculus and for planing smooth the root surfaces. They are used with a pull stroke, in a coronal, lateral oblique or lateral direction (Figure 7.21b). When used subgingivally, the blade is carefully inserted in the periodontal pocket with the back towards the inner gingival surface and the face towards the tooth surface. The instrument is gently advanced apically until resistance is felt (i.e. to the bottom of the sulcus or pocket), then the handle is tilted away from the tooth until the blade is at 60–80 degrees to the tooth surface, engaging the cutting edge on the tooth surface with a pulling action to remove subgingival plaque and calculus. Hand curettes may also be used for gingival curettage, using the sharp edge against the inner surface of the gingiva and gently removing inflamed and infected pocket epithelium and connective tissue.

Hoes, chisels, surgical curettes and files

Hoes are designed to remove supragingival and subgingival plaque and calculus. They have a very small blade, which in time is lost due to repeated re-sharpening of the instrument. There is a fixed angle of 99 degrees between the shank and blade. Hoes have a cutting edge bevelled at 45 degrees. They are used by means of a

pulling technique for scaling of ledges or rings of calculus. Different types are designed to fit the anatomy of the tooth (Wolf *et al*., 2005). Chisels are used on interproximal surfaces of teeth with a pushing technique (Figure 7.22). Surgical curettes are used for removal of debris and granulation tissue from a soft tissue wound, a bone surface or defect, or an alveolar socket after tooth extraction. Various shapes and sizes are available, including Spratt (single-ended with round cups), Volkmann (double-ended with round or oval cups) and Miller (with spoon-shaped working tips) curettes (Reiter, 2013). Files have a series of blades on a base and are used to fracture or remove large solid pieces of calculus. They are relatively aggressive instruments that can gouge and roughen the tooth surfaces (Wolf *et al*., 2005). Several of these instruments may also be used for alveolectomy and alveoloplasty procedures.

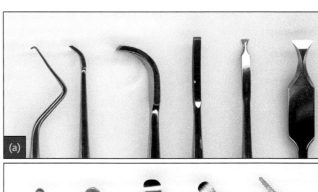

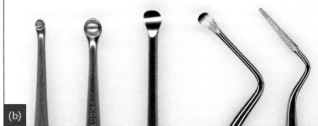

7.22 Assortment of periodontal surgical instruments. (a) Hoes and chisels. (b) Surgical curettes and files.
(© Dr Alexander M. Reiter)

Prophy angles, polishing cups, brushes and pastes

Smoothing of tooth surfaces is achieved by using polishing paste and a prophy cup (or occasionally a soft brush) screwed to or snapped on a prophy angle (depending on the design) or latched on to a contra-angle attached to a low-speed handpiece (Figure 7.23). To reduce friction, the prophy cup should be filled with polishing paste, used for a few seconds on each tooth, moved continuously on the tooth surface and rotated at very low speed (less than 3000 rpm) (Wolf *et al.*, 2005). The rotating cup is pressed gently against the surface of the tooth, causing the edge of the cup to flare out and polish the tooth surface above and below the gingival margin. Disposable plastic prophy angle attachments are available for single use and are designed to aid in infection control.

Polishing pastes (including pumice and specific pastes for surface treatment of restorations) are used with a prophy cup or brush to remove plaque and stains and smooth the tooth surfaces (Figure 7.24). These pastes contain abrasives such as aluminium oxide and zirconium silicate (Wolf *et al.*, 2005). They are often graded as coarse, medium and fine. Coarse pumice may deliberately be used to create scratches in the tooth surfaces in an attempt to increase retention of temporary bis-acryl composite devices (such as splints for non-invasive jaw fracture repair or direct inclined plane fabrication). Small containers with polishing paste can comfortably be held in one hand during polishing of the teeth (Figures 7.25 and 7.26).

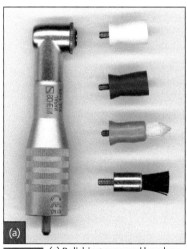
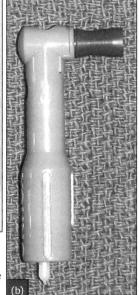

7.23 (a) Polishing cups and brushes that can be screwed on to a prophy angle. (b) Disposable plastic prophy angle with polishing cup for single use.
(© Dr Alexander M. Reiter)

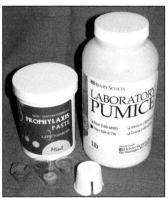

7.24 Various polishing pastes in small and large containers. Note also the white dappen dish containing some pumice.
(© Dr Alexander M. Reiter)

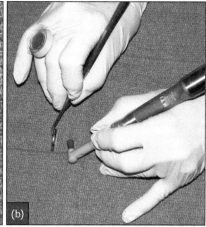
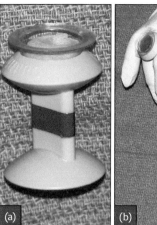

7.25 (a) Small container with polishing paste snapped into a chalice-like device. (b) The device is held between the middle and ring fingers.
(© Dr Alexander M. Reiter)

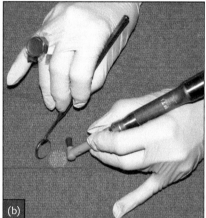
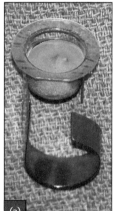

7.26 (a) Small container with polishing paste snapped into a ring-like device. (b) This device is worn on the ring finger.
(© Dr Alexander M. Reiter)

Air-powder polishing

Air-powder polishing is used with a specially designed handpiece, delivering an air-powder slurry of warm water and sodium bicarbonate to the tooth surface. It is very effective for the removal of extrinsic stains and soft deposits (Pattison *et al.*, 2002). The flow rate of abrasive cleansing powder can be adjusted to increase the amount of powder for heavier stain removal. The abrasive effect of the air-powder polishing device can result in loss of cementum and dentine and roughen the surface of restorations. It is contraindicated in patients with respiratory illness, hypertension or a weakened immune system and those receiving haemodialysis.

Gingival knives

Gingival knives are designed for the excision of excess gingiva (i.e. gingivectomy). They are hand-held instruments with a handle, an angled shaft, and a sharp-pointed cutting blade at the distal end (Lipscomb and Reiter, 2005). The Orban knife is spear-shaped with cutting edges on both sides of the blade. Its double-ended or single-ended blades are used for delicate procedures, such as the removal of gingival tissue in interdental areas. The Kirkland knife is kidney-shaped. Its double-ended or single-ended blades are used for removal of large amounts of firm tissue, as the entire periphery is the cutting edge (Figure 7.27). The blades of both knives must

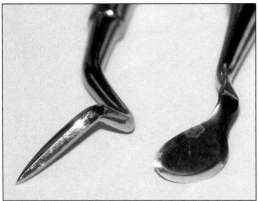

7.27 Orban gingival knife (left) and Kirkland gingival knife (right).
(© Dr Alexander M. Reiter)

be kept sharp to be effective. Gingivectomy knives have largely been replaced by other means of gingivectomy and gingivoplasty (such as cold scalpel blade, electrosurgery and radiosurgery, laser, and 12-fluted burs) (Reiter, 2013).

Periosteal elevators

Periosteal elevators come in various sizes and blade shapes (Figure 7.28). These are sharp instruments used to separate soft tissue from bone when raising a flap. Periosteal elevators are often double-ended instruments with one end rounded and flat, and the other end pointed or square. The blade portion is used with the flat side against the bone and the convex side against the soft tissue, reducing the chances of tearing or puncturing the elevated soft tissue (Lipscomb and Reiter, 2005).

The Molt No. 9 periosteal elevator is commonly used in oral surgery in veterinary patients. The broad rounded blade is used to raise mucoperiosteal flaps with a pushing stroke, while the more pointed end is used to raise the more delicate gingival part of a flap, utilizing a prising motion. Sharp and narrow-tipped (2–6 mm) periosteal elevators (such as Mead No. 3 or Periosteal No. EX-9M for middle-sized and larger dogs, and Glickman No. 24G or Periosteal No. EX-9 for small dogs and cats) are also very useful in reflecting the mucoperiosteum during periodontal flap procedures, mandibulectomies, maxillectomies and hard palate surgery (Reiter, 2013).

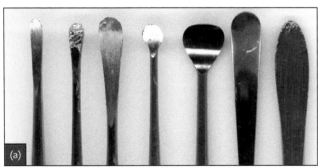
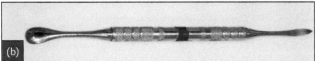

7.28 (a) Working ends of various periosteal elevators. Note the bur mark scratches in the metal surface that are acquired when the instrument is used for tissue retraction. When the blade is damaged, the instrument should no longer be used for flap elevation. (b) Molt No. 9 periosteal elevator.
(a, © Dr Alexander M. Reiter; b, © Dr Peter Southerden)

Pocket-marking forceps

Pocket-marking forceps have two different tips. The blunt tip, which is sometimes marked in millimetres, is inserted into the pocket (Figure 7.29). The forceps are then closed, causing the right-angled, pointed tip to create a bleeding point on the labial or buccal side of the gingiva at the level of the base of the pocket (Figure 7.30), thus indicating the proposed line of incision for gingivectomy (Reiter, 2013).

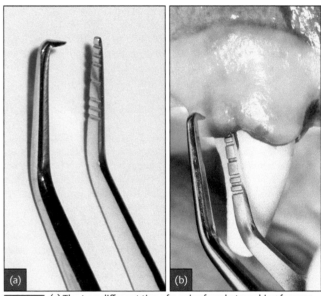

7.29 (a) The two different tips of a pair of pocket-marking forceps. (b) The blunt tip with millimetre markings is inserted down to the bottom of the gingival pocket at the labial aspect of the right maxillary canine tooth in a dog.
(© Dr Alexander M. Reiter)

7.30 Same case as in Figure 7.29. (a) The pocket-marking forceps are closed, causing the right-angled, pointed tip to create a bleeding point on the labial or buccal side of the gingiva at the level of the base of the pocket. (b, c) This process is repeated at several points around the tooth, thus indicating (d) the proposed line of incision for gingivectomy.
(© Dr Alexander M. Reiter)

Scalpel handles and blades

Oral surgery often requires precise control of instruments, especially when sulcular incisions are made in and around teeth. For this reason scalpel handles are often held using a pen or modified pen grasp. Rounded scalpel handles allow easy rotation of the scalpel handle, which facilitates curved incisions around teeth. Longer handles are useful when operating in the caudal oral cavity (Lipscomb and Reiter, 2005).

The No. 3 handle (with metric ruler markings) is most commonly used in oral surgery (Figure 7.31). The rounded No. 5 is perhaps better suited to the pen or modified pen grasp, and the longer No. 7 is useful when making incisions deep within the oropharynx in larger patients. Surgical blades No. 15 and the finer No. 15C are most frequently used, which have short rounded cutting edges, ideal for making precise incisions. Some dentists and oral surgeons also prefer No. 11 blades. Others prefer finer instruments such as Beaver® blades and handles, which give excellent precision and control in more delicate procedures (especially in cats) (Reiter, 2013).

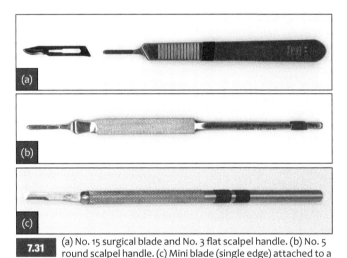

7.31 (a) No. 15 surgical blade and No. 3 flat scalpel handle. (b) No. 5 round scalpel handle. (c) Mini blade (single edge) attached to a round Beaver® handle.
(a, b, © Dr Alexander M. Reiter; c, © Dr Peter Southerden)

Thumb forceps

Thumb forceps are used to grasp and stabilize tissue during a surgical procedure, especially during dissection and suturing. They should be able to grasp delicate tissue securely without traumatizing it. Thumb forceps should not be used to grasp needles as this may damage their tips (Reiter, 2013). They are held between the thumb and two or three additional fingers of the same hand. The tips should meet, and any intermeshing striations or teeth should align perfectly. There are many different patterns and sizes available, but atraumatic forceps such as a delicate Adson 1 x 2 with a fine rat-toothed grip are particularly suited to periodontal surgery, causing minimal trauma to mucosal and submucosal tissue (Figure 7.32). They are preferred over DeBakey and other thumb forceps in dentistry and oral surgery (Lipscomb and Reiter, 2005).

Scissors

Various tissue scissors are used for cutting or blunt dissection in periodontal surgery. Metzenbaums are blunt-nosed scissors used for fine cutting, blunt dissection and undermining of periodontal tissues (Figure 7.33). These scissors come in several types, shapes and lengths. Smaller sized,

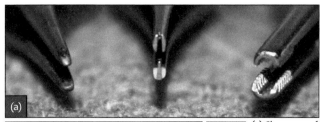
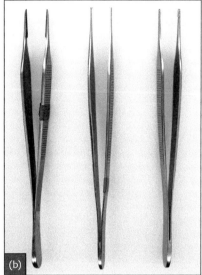

7.32 (a) Close-ups of the tips and (b) full views of three types of thumb forceps: Adson plain (left), Adson 1 x 2 (middle) and Adson-Brown (right).
(© Dr Alexander M. Reiter)

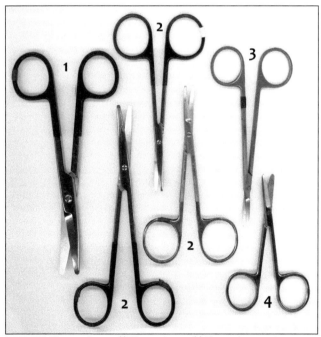

7.33 Tissue scissors. (1) Mayo scissors. (2) Metzenbaum scissors. (3) Iris scissors. (4) Suture scissors.
(© Dr Alexander M. Reiter)

curved and blunt-ended versions with serrated blades are most useful in oral surgery (Reiter, 2013). Straight or curved Iris and LaGrange scissors, which have narrower blades with pointed ends, are used primarily for removing excess gingival tissue or to make very precise cuts into oral mucosa. Tissue scissors should be kept sharp. Scissors with tungsten carbide cutting edges stay sharp for longer; they can be identified by their gold-coloured handle rings.

It is important not to use tissue scissors for cutting sutures, as this will rapidly blunt the blades. In the absence of specific suture scissors, it is appropriate to use more robust scissors such as a designated pair of Mayo operating scissors for this purpose. These are either curved or straight and come in a variety of sizes (Lipscomb and Reiter, 2005).

Suture material

The ideal suture material for oral surgery is swaged on to a needle, rapidly absorbed, pliable, knots securely, has low capillarity, and is minimally plaque retentive. Poliglecaprone 25 (Monocryl®) is the material of choice for many dentists and oral surgeons, as it displays all of these characteristics (Figure 7.34). It is absorbed by hydrolysis, loses 20–30% of its tensile strength after 2–3 weeks and is completely absorbed at 90 days (Lipscomb and Reiter, 2005). An antibiotic (triclosan) coated version of poliglecaprone 25 (Monocryl® Plus) is also available. Other suture materials used in the oral cavity may contain polyglycolic acid and polyglactin 910. Polydioxanone should only be used where prolonged suture strength is required, such as for palate surgery and ligation of larger vessels, persisting in the oral cavity for about 6–8 weeks. Nylon with a swaged-on, reverse cutting needle is preferred for skin sutures (Reiter, 2013).

Suture sizes 2 metric (3/0 USP), 1.5 metric (4/0 USP) and 1 metric (5/0 USP) (depending on the size of the patient and type of procedure performed) are commonly used in dentistry and oral surgery in dogs and cats. Taper-point round, non-cutting needles are preferred by many dentists and oral surgeons for wound closure in the oral cavity and oropharynx, particularly when suturing delicate or friable soft tissue (Lipscomb and Reiter, 2005). Reverse cutting needles are also commonly used in periodontal surgery, as they are flat on the inner surface of the needle, which reduces the risk of the needle cutting through tissue ('cut out'). Commonly utilized needles are ⅜-circle needles. In less accessible areas, ½-circle and ⅝-circle needles may be used. Square or surgeon's knots should be followed by at least three more throws to ensure knot security (Reiter, 2013).

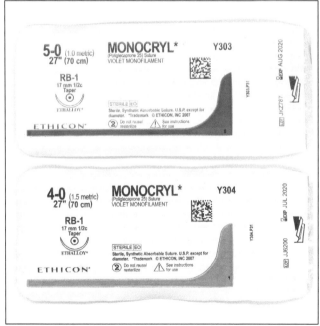

7.34 Poliglecaprone 25 is a commonly used suture material in the mouths of dogs and cats.
(© Dr Alexander M. Reiter)

Needle holders

Many different sizes and shapes of needle holders are available (Figure 7.35). Needle holders should be matched to the size of needles used in oral surgery. They are used for grasping and manipulating curved needles during suturing and preferably have a ratchet mechanism, which allows the needle to be held securely while driving it through soft tissue. Halsey (more sturdy) and DeBakey (more delicate) needle holders with serrated jaws are often used in periodontal surgery (Lipscomb and Reiter, 2005). Castroviejo needle holders may be suitable for very fine and delicate procedures. Olsen-Hegar needle holders also allow cutting sutures.

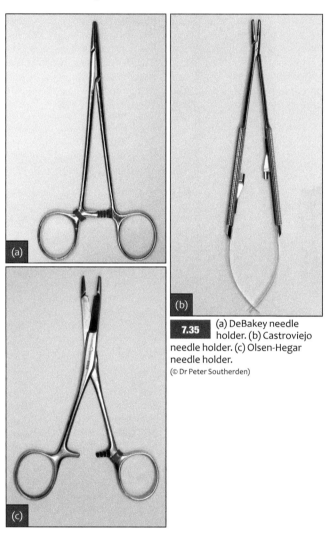

7.35 (a) DeBakey needle holder. (b) Castroviejo needle holder. (c) Olsen-Hegar needle holder.
(© Dr Peter Southerden)

Cotton-tipped applicators

These have long wooden or plastic handles with a cotton bud tip on one end and are useful for absorbing blood from delicate tissue or for applying a topical haemostatic agent (such as aluminium chloride) or tissue protectant (such as tincture of myrrh and benzoin) to the cut gingival surfaces (Figure 7.36).

Swabs

Gauze swabs and small sponges are used to absorb blood from bleeding surfaces. They can also be useful for temporary packing of the pharynx of large dogs during oral procedures to provide protection against aspiration of

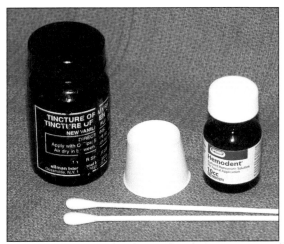

7.36 Cotton-tipped applicators (front), tissue protectant (left), dappen dish (middle), and topical haemostatic agent (right).
(© Dr Alexander M. Reiter)

foreign material, in addition to an endotracheal tube with an inflatable cuff. Gauze swabs may need to be frequently replaced during procedures causing oral bleeding or requiring mechanical instruments with coolant. It is wise to count the number of swabs placed into the throat to ensure none is remaining at the time of extubation. Size 7.6 x 7.6 cm (3 x 3 inches) gauze swabs (Figure 7.37) are commonly used in dentistry and oral surgery (Lipscomb and Reiter, 2005).

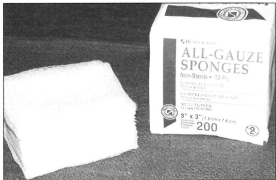

7.37 Size 7.6 x 7.6 cm (3 x 3 inches) gauze swabs.
(© Dr Alexander M. Reiter)

Bone replacement materials

A bone graft is bone (or a bone graft substitute) used to take the place of a removed piece of bone or fill a bony defect (Reiter, 2013). Particulate grafting materials can also be used to fill a bony defect as a barrier to prevent the rapid downgrowth of gingival epithelial and connective tissue cells and to provide a framework for ingrowth of adjacent bone (osteoconduction) or to stimulate bone production by mesenchymal cells that differentiate into osteoblasts (osteoinduction). Osteoinductive materials have the potential for the creation of new bone, while osteoconductive materials only serve as a space maintainer or stabilizer of the blood clot. The defect needs to be cleaned (debrided and rinsed) prior to introduction of the bone graft.

Autogenous bone grafts are collected from the patient itself. It is somewhat questionable whether they can be considered the best material to use, as research indicates this graft to be resorbed more than other types (Araujo and Lindhe, 2010). They are the only truly osteogenic

graft, containing vital osteoblasts, and may be harvested from local (close to the defect), regional (other areas of the mouth, such as edentulous dental arch segments) or distant sites (proximal humerus, wing of the ilium) (Smith et al., 1993). Rongeurs with narrow jaws to collect marginal and septal alveolar bone, manual trephines or trephine burs that retrieve larger blocks of cortical and cancellous bone, and sharp periodontal or surgical curettes, back-action chisels, or cortical bone collectors whose blades are scraped along an exposed bone surface can be used (Figure 7.38). The harvested autogenous bone is collected in a sterile dappen dish and reduced to chips as needed (Reiter, 2013).

Alloplasts are synthetic and bioactive materials, which are primarily designed to act as a barrier material. Bioglass materials (Figure 7.39) contain salts of calcium, sodium, phosphorus and silica, stimulating both collagen and new bone formation (DeForge, 1997).

Allografts are freeze-dried or frozen, natural, real bone grafts taken from an animal of the same species. Demineralization of freeze-dried bone exposes the underlying collagen and other active substances such as bone morphogenetic protein, and it is thus considered osteoinductive (Figure 7.40). Non-demineralized freeze-dried bone (often called cancellous bone chips) is considered to be osteoconductive.

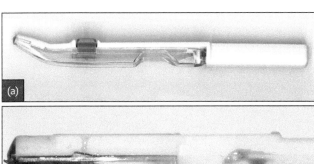
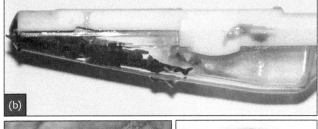
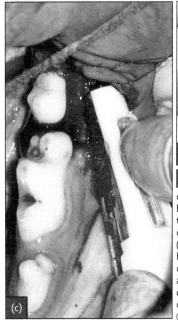
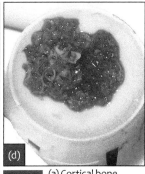

7.38 (a) Cortical bone collector. (b) Side view of frontal aspect of the cortical bone collector, showing transparent chamber filled with cortical bone chips. (c) Autogenous bone being harvested using the cortical bone collector at the caudobuccal aspect of the left mandible in a dog. (d) Dappen dish filled with cortical bone chips.
(© Dr Alexander M. Reiter)

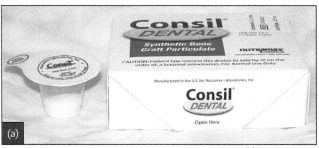

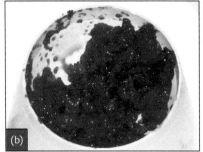

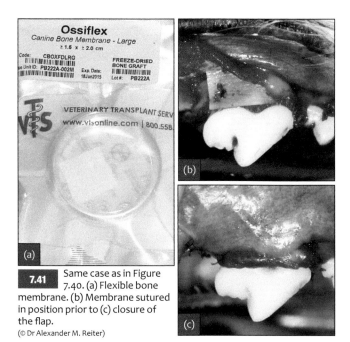

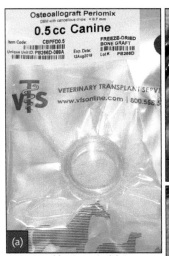

7.39 (a) Bioglass. (b) Bioglass mixed with fresh blood.
(© Dr Alexander M. Reiter)

7.41 Same case as in Figure 7.40. (a) Flexible bone membrane. (b) Membrane sutured in position prior to (c) closure of the flap.
(© Dr Alexander M. Reiter)

better suited to veterinary use, as they do not need a second procedure under general anaesthesia for their removal (Bianucci *et al.*, 1998; Terpak and Verstraete, 2012).

Rinsing solutions and fluoride products

A concentration of 0.12% chlorhexidine gluconate is recommended for irrigating the teeth and mucosal surfaces prior to oral procedures. Higher concentrations of this antimicrobial agent are to be avoided, as they may elicit epithelial desquamation and wound healing complications (Lipscomb and Reiter, 2005). The use of chlorhexidine and isotonic saline for lavage of wounds prior to their closure is discouraged, as cytotoxic effects on connective tissue cells can occur. Lactated Ringer's solution is better suited for this purpose (Buffa *et al.*, 1997).

Sodium fluoride (1.23%) foam may be applied at the end of a dental cleaning procedure on to teeth with exposed root surfaces, in cats with tooth resorption or in dogs with caries. Fluoride becomes incorporated into the dental hard tissues, making them harder and more resistant to various insults. The owner may also apply stannous fluoride (0.4%) once a week on to sensitive teeth (Figure 7.42).

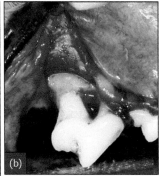

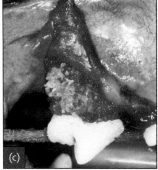

7.40 (a) Allograft. (b) Open periodontal therapy (creation of flap, root planing and bone contouring) was performed at the buccocaudal aspect of the right maxillary fourth premolar tooth in a dog. (c) Allograft has been placed over the denuded root surfaces.
(© Dr Alexander M. Reiter)

Xenografts are grafts taken from other species. Bovine cancellous bone is occasionally used in veterinary dentistry. To prevent infection or graft rejection, the bone is heated to 1,100°C, and the material is considered to be osteoconductive only.

Barrier membranes

Membranes are an integral part of guided tissue regeneration. This technique is utilized to regenerate lost periodontal tissues such as alveolar bone, periodontal ligament and cementum. Membranes are placed to avoid the rapid downgrowth of gingival epithelial and connective tissue cells into a defect, which would prevent the regeneration of the slower growing components of the periodontium. They can be used with or without a bone graft or bone substitute. Both absorbable and non-absorbable membranes are available (Figure 7.41). Absorbable membranes are

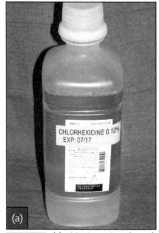

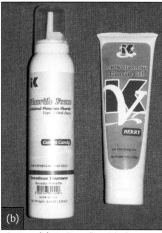

7.42 (a) Chlorhexidine (0.12%) solution. (b) Sodium fluoride foam (left; to be applied by the veterinary dentist) and stannous fluoride gel (right; to be applied by the client).
(© Dr Alexander M. Reiter)

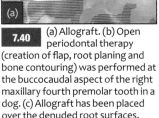

Holding of instruments

The palm grip and modified pen grasp (Figure 7.43) are effective ways to hold most dental instruments. With the palm grip an instrument is held in the palm at the base of the fingers. The index finger may be placed on top of the instrument to give additional stability and to increase the sensitivity of this grip. The thumb may be rested in the patient's mouth acting as a fulcrum. This is a strong grip but has less tactile sensitivity in comparison with the modified pen grasp. The palm grip is commonly used for periosteal elevators. A modification of this grip is the palm and thumb grip where the thumb is placed on the back of the shaft. This is used for dental elevators and luxators.

For the modified pen grasp, the instrument handle is held between the thumb and the index finger, and the pad of the middle finger rests against the side of the junction of the shank and handle of the instrument while the fingers are bent. The ring finger and little finger are used for control or as a fulcrum within the patient's mouth (e.g. on a tooth close to the tooth being worked on, or on another firm surface), thus giving the instrument stability. Poorly controlled instrumentation, using no finger rest or a rest that is too far away from the tooth being worked on, will cause injury of the soft tissues of the periodontium. This grasp is used for handpieces, scalers, curettes, probes and mirrors (Lewis and Miller, 2010). Some dentists and oral surgeons also use it for periosteal elevators and dental elevators and luxators. The required movements can be obtained with the fingers, small movements of the wrist and lower arm, and, when necessary, by small movements of the upper arm.

Periodontal therapy

The goal of periodontal therapy is the removal of supra- and subgingival plaque and calculus, and the reduction or elimination of periodontal pockets, preferably accomplished by means of mechanical techniques (Figure 7.44). Associated aims include the prevention of disease progression and provision of a situation that allows the pet owner to maintain oral health through home oral hygiene (Grove, 1990, 1998). Supragingival and subgingival dental cleaning is an important part of the procedure, creating biologically acceptable tooth surfaces that will delay accumulation of dental deposits.

Professional dental cleaning is initially performed with power scalers, followed by the use of hand scalers to remove residual calculus in pits, fissures and developmental grooves of the crowns supragingivally. Hand curettes are then used to clean and plane exposed root surfaces subgingivally and remove the inflamed and infected soft tissue lining of the periodontal pocket (Niemiec, 2003). Once scaling is complete, the tooth surfaces are polished with fine polishing paste and a rubber cup on a prophy angle that is attached to a low-speed handpiece (Cleland, 2000). Some dentists then apply special barriers in the form of sealants, adhesives or gels to the cleaned tooth surface and gingiva in an attempt to delay plaque accumulation (Gengler et al., 2005; Bonello and Squarzoni, 2008; Bellows et al., 2012). However, such agents must not cover exposed root surfaces within the periodontal pockets, as they may inhibit reattachment of the gingiva to the tooth when the goal should be pocket reduction.

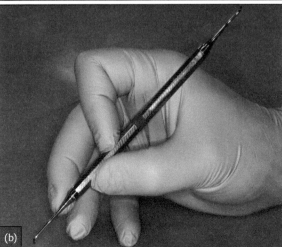
7.43 (a) Palm grip. (b) Modified pen grasp.
(© Dr Peter Southerden)

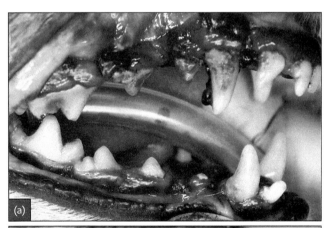
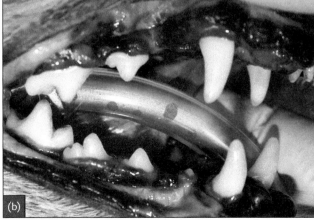
7.44 (a) Before and (b) after professional dental cleaning, closed periodontal therapy and extraction of selected teeth in a dog.
(© Dr Alexander M. Reiter)

Professional dental cleaning

Supragingival and subgingival plaque and calculus are removed using a combination of power scaling and hand scaling, followed by polishing of the cleaned tooth surfaces (Operative Technique 7.1). Because of their higher frequency of operation, ultrasonic scalers work faster than sonic scalers, but both are faster than hand scaling, which takes considerable time and particular skill to perform. All methods have been shown to be effective in removing plaque and calculus from tooth surfaces, thereby reducing the bacterial load in periodontal pockets. However, smoother root surfaces (which are less plaque retentive) are obtained with curettes than with power instruments.

Power scaling is used in most cases for initial plaque and calculus removal (Niemiec, 2003). The scaler tip should point in an apical direction, with the last 2–3 mm in contact with the tooth. The long axis of the scaler tip is used at an angle of less than 15 degrees to the tooth surface. It is important to keep the scaler moving, apply light pressure and use copious volumes of water to cool the tip (Figure 7.45). The flow rate should be at least 20–30 ml/min in the application region. The tip of the scaler should not be used perpendicular to the tooth surface because of the concentration of energy (risk of structural damage to the dental hard tissues) and heat (risk of pulp injury). It should also not point in a coronal direction, as the uncooled part of the scaler could make contact with oral mucosa or skin (Figure 7.46). No more than 15 seconds should be spent on a tooth continuously before moving to another one. It would seem sensible to reduce this time for small teeth (e.g. in cats) and teeth where the pulp is likely to be closer to the tooth surface (worn teeth and those with uncomplicated fractures). Power scalers should be used cautiously in subgingival areas because the coolant may not cool the scaler tip sufficiently, risking thermal damage to the gingiva (Niemiec, 2003). Thus, the scaler should be kept moving and used for as short a time as possible. Special slimline periodontal inserts are available, allowing the coolant to reach the tip through a groove on the instrument head.

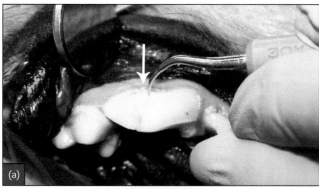

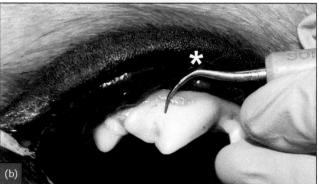

7.46 Inappropriate use of an ultrasonic scaler. (a) Tip perpendicular (arrowed) to the tooth surface risks structural damage to dental hard tissue and heat injury to the pulp. (b) Tip pointing in a coronal direction risks the uncooled part of the scaler (*) making contact with and causing burn injury to the oral mucosa or skin.
(© Dr Alexander M. Reiter)

Once power scaling is completed, hand scalers and curettes can be used to remove any remaining supragingival and subgingival plaque and calculus in areas that are not accessible to a power scaler. After irrigation of the area to remove any debris, the tooth surfaces should be evaluated with a dental explorer for detection of any remaining calculus. 'Adaptation' of a hand scaler or curette refers to the application of the cutting edge against the tooth (Lewis and Miller, 2010). Approximately one-third of the cutting edge of the working end should remain in contact with the tooth surface. The instrument handle can be rolled between the thumb and forefinger so that contact of the cutting edge with the tooth is maintained when its surface curves. 'Angulation' refers to the relationship of the face of the instrument to the tooth (Lewis and Miller, 2010). When inserting a hand curette into a periodontal pocket, the face should be parallel with the root surface and the back positioned against the soft tissue lining of the pocket. Once the blade has reached the bottom of the pocket, the handle is tilted away from the tooth so that the face and root surface create an angle of 60–80 degrees. The exploratory stroke is used for initial assessment of the topography of the tooth surface by very lightly feeling for irregularities. The working stroke is performed by applying pressure against the tooth and pulling the blade vertically (in a coronal direction), horizontally or obliquely in a short controlled motion. A root planing stroke is longer in length, and light pressure is used to avoid removal of excessive amounts of cementum (which could expose sensitive dentine). The minimum number of strokes should be applied to accomplish the task (Lewis and Miller, 2010).

The cleaned tooth surfaces are polished to remove any remaining plaque and smooth minor scratches and irregularities. Polishing is usually performed using a rubber

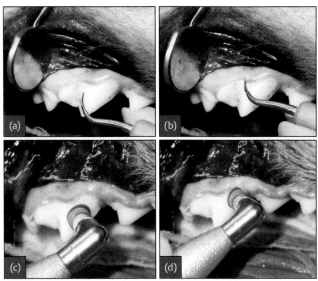

7.45 Proper lip retraction with a mirror during (a) supragingival and (b) subgingival ultrasonic scaling. Copious water irrigation should be used to cool the tip (not shown). (c) As the crown is polished, the prophy cup should be flared underneath the gingival margin to polish (d) the subgingival crown and exposed root surfaces.
(© Dr Alexander M. Reiter)

prophy cup and polishing paste. It is important to use gentle pressure at a speed of less than 3000 rpm and short contact times to avoid thermal or structural damage (Fichtel *et al.*, 2008). The prophy cup should be flared underneath the gingival margin to polish subgingival crown and exposed root surfaces. Finally, residual polishing paste is removed by means of rinsing or spraying with the air/water syringe.

Closed periodontal therapy

Closed treatment is indicated when periodontal pocket depth is shallow, i.e. not exceeding 4–5 mm in dogs and 1–2 mm in cats. However, these measurements are only approximate, as they may have different clinical significance based on animal and tooth size (e.g. a 5 mm pocket on a first premolar tooth of a Chihuahua dog may be considered severe, while a maxillary canine tooth of a large-breed dog may show a nearly normal gingival sulcus of 5 mm). Adequate access for debridement becomes more difficult with increasing pocket probing depth. The teeth are first scaled with power scalers. Hand scalers are used to remove residual plaque and calculus in pits, fissures and developmental grooves of the crowns. Complete removal of dental deposits in deep pockets is unlikely to be successful when using hand instruments only, due to the difficulty in achieving suitable access, and slimline power scalers may be more effective in these situations.

A study of periodontally compromised teeth in 40 mongrel dogs demonstrated a recovery rate of approximately 38% by means of scaling, root planing and home care, a 49% recovery rate by means of scaling, root planing, gingival curettage and home care, and an 85% recovery rate by means of open periodontal therapy (Shoukry *et al.*, 2007).

Subgingival scaling

This procedure is part of a professional dental cleaning with power or hand instruments, and relates to the removal of adherent and non-adherent plaque and calculus on subgingival tooth surfaces. When using a hand curette, it is placed into the depth of the periodontal pocket. The blade is angled so that it engages the root surface and then pulled coronally. A series of overlapping strokes are performed until the root surface is clean (Lewis and Miller, 2010).

Root planing

This procedure involves the smoothing of root surfaces and removal of endotoxin-containing layers of cementum by means of hand curettes (Figure 7.47). Complete removal of cementum should not be a primary goal of root planing, as sensitive dentine will be exposed. Studies have established that endotoxin is weakly adsorbed to the root surface and can also be removed with light, overlapping strokes using a power scaler (Lewis and Miller, 2010).

Gingival curettage

Following scaling and root planing, subgingival debridement is completed by gingival curettage. This procedure involves the removal of the infected and inflamed pocket epithelium and subepithelial connective tissue using a hand curette (Figure 7.48). The curette is inserted into the periodontal pocket with the face facing the pocket wall. A finger can be used to apply pressure against the gingiva

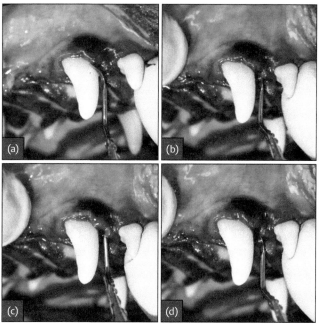

7.47 Same case as in Figure 7.4. (a) Removal of subgingival plaque and calculus with a hand curette. (b) The blade is inserted in the periodontal pocket with the back towards the inner gingival surface and the face towards the tooth surface. (c) The instrument is gently advanced apically until resistance is felt (i.e. to the bottom of the sulcus or pocket). (d) The handle is then tilted away from the tooth until the blade is at 60–80 degrees to the tooth surface, engaging the cutting edge on the tooth surface with a pulling action to remove subgingival plaque and calculus.
(© Dr Alexander M. Reiter)

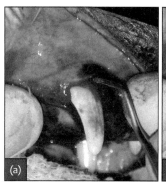
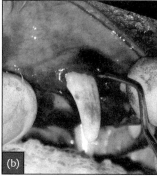
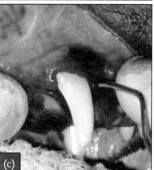

7.48 Same case as in Figure 7.4. (a) Gingival curettage with a hand curette. (b, c) The sharp edge of the curette is pressed against the inner surface of the gingiva to gently remove inflamed and infected pocket epithelium and connective tissue.
(© Dr Alexander M. Reiter)

while the curette is slightly angled towards the tooth surface and gently engaged in removing diseased soft tissue with a pull stroke. The goal is to not leave any inflamed granulation tissue attached to the pocket wall, particularly when dentine is exposed, as this may result in external root resorption rather than reattachment of the periodontal tissues. Excessive tissue damage should be avoided. Regional anaesthesia may be performed to reduce postoperative discomfort (Lewis and Miller, 2010).

Lavage

After scaling, root planing, gingival curettage and polishing are completed, the teeth and subgingival areas are rinsed with water from the air/water syringe to remove any remaining debris (Lewis and Miller, 2010). Then the tooth surfaces are dried with the air/water syringe, looking for any remaining calculus, which, once dried, will show as a chalky material. The tooth surfaces are also evaluated with a periodontal probe for smoothness. If any irregularity is found, the area is scaled and polished again. Finally, the gingival sulcus/periodontal pocket and the mouth are rinsed with 0.12% chlorhexidine.

Local antimicrobial therapy

Low-dose doxycycline gel (e.g. Doxirobe® Gel) may be inserted into cleaned periodontal pockets greater than 4–5 mm (exact value depends on the size of the tooth) after root planing and gingival curettage (Harvey, 1998; Zetner and Rothmueller, 2002; Harvey, 2005). Once the gel has been mixed following the manufacturer's instructions (Figure 7.49), it is applied via a syringe into cleaned periodontal pockets and exposed furcation areas. Adding a few drops of cold water makes the gel more pliable, and it can then be gently packed deeper into areas of interest using a beaver-tail hand instrument so that the hardened gel is positioned subgingivally (Figure 7.50). Doxycycline and similar compounds have antimicrobial, anti-inflammatory, anti-collagenolytic and immunomodulatory effects. They have a high affinity for hydroxyapatite in bone and dental hard tissues, thus the delivery of the drug into the tissues surrounding the periodontal pocket is long-term (for weeks to months following application) (Hayashi et al., 1998; Hirasawa et al., 2000; Dennis et al., 2012). Control of periodontal disease was also accomplished after application of a clindamycin hydrochloride gel into cleaned periodontal pockets of teeth in dogs (Johnston et al., 2011).

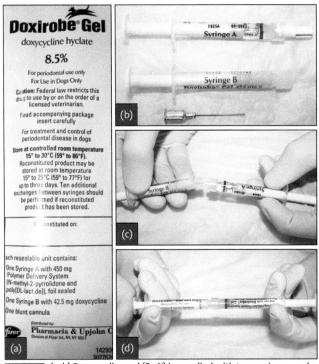

7.49 (a, b) Doxycycline gel (8.5%) is supplied with two syringes and a cannula. (c, d) Syringe A (containing liquid polymer) is attached to syringe B (containing doxycycline powder) to mix the contents.

(© Dr Alexander M. Reiter)

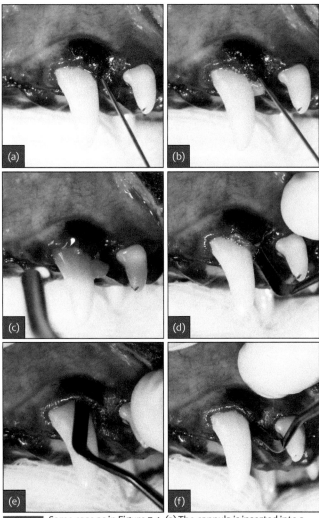

7.50 Same case as in Figure 7.4. (a) The cannula is inserted into a cleaned periodontal pocket for (b) injection of doxycycline gel. (c) A few drops of cold water are added to make the gel more pliable. (d–f) A beaver-tail composite instrument is used to gently pack the hardened gel deeper into areas of interest so that it is positioned subgingivally.

(© Dr Alexander M. Reiter)

Open periodontal therapy

Open periodontal therapy is indicated when periodontal pocket depths exceed 5–6 mm in dogs and 2–3 mm in cats (greatly depending on the size of the tooth). It is performed following reflection of a gingival or mucoperiosteal flap. First, professional dental cleaning is performed. The modified Widman flap procedure utilizes a partially mobilized envelope flap with an internal bevel incision slightly apical to the gingival margin and down to the alveolar bone; no vertical incisions are made, and the gingival flap is not reflected beyond the mucogingival junction (Wolf et al., 2005).

More visibility to the surgical site is achieved by elevation of a mucoperiosteal flap beyond the mucogingival junction (Operative Technique 7.2). This usually requires one or two vertical (slightly diverging) releasing incisions to be made into the gingiva, extending beyond the mucogingival junction into the alveolar mucosa (Figure 7.51). A vertical incision should preferably be made at the line angle (which is the junction of two surfaces of the crown of a tooth), rather than over a root, furcation or interdental papilla (Smith, 2003). Osseous surgery, placement of bone grafts and implants, and guided tissue regeneration

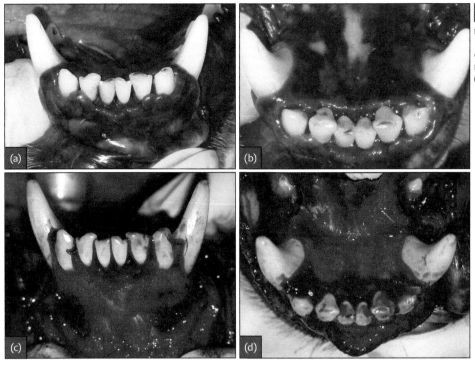

7.51 (a) Front and (b) occlusal views of the mandibular incisor teeth with moderate periodontal disease in a dog. (c) Front and (d) occlusal views after creating labial and lingual flaps with releasing incisions.
(© Dr Alexander M. Reiter)

are possible with this flap design (Smith, 1995; Stapleton, 1995; Wiggs *et al.*, 1998; Anthony, 2000b; Lobprise, 2000b; Niemiec, 2001; Beckman, 2004; Barthel, 2006; Beebe and Gengler, 2007; Greenfield, 2010; Klima and Goldstein, 2010). Inflamed and infected soft tissue can be removed with power scalers, dental burs and hand instruments, followed by planing of exposed root surfaces and recontouring of the alveolar margin with hand curettes. Exposed tooth surfaces are polished, the wound is rinsed with lactated Ringer's solution, and the flap is apposed and sutured at varying locations (original, coronal or apical) (Figure 7.52) (Beckman, 2003; Holmstrom *et al.*, 2004).

Gingivectomy and gingivoplasty

Gingivectomy refers to removal of excess gingiva surrounding a tooth. An example is excision of marginal (free) gingiva to eliminate pseudopockets in patients with gingival enlargement (Figure 7.53). It can also be performed for crown lengthening procedures and exposure of subgingival dental defects. Gingivoplasty is a form of gingivectomy performed to restore physiological contours of the gingiva. Gingivectomy and gingivoplasty are contraindicated when there is less than 2 mm of attached gingiva and when horizontal or vertical bone loss extends beyond the mucogingival junction (Lewis and Reiter, 2005).

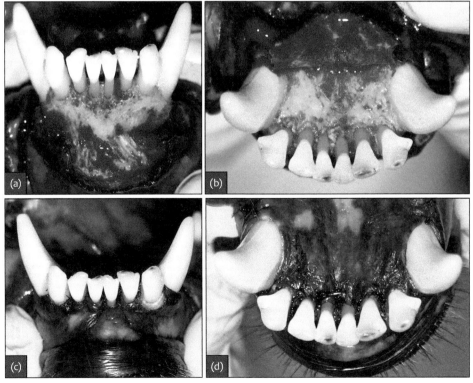

7.52 Same case as in Figure 7.51. (a) Front and (b) occlusal views after removal of inflamed and infected soft tissue, planing of exposed root surfaces and recontouring the alveolar margin. (c) Front and (d) occlusal views after apposition of the flaps towards the alveolar bone and teeth in a slightly apical position.
(© Dr Alexander M. Reiter)

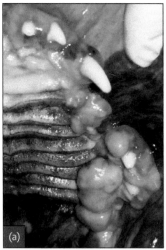
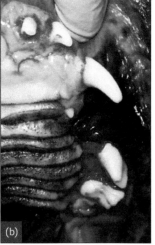
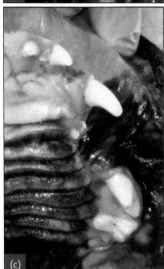

7.53 Left maxillary jaw quadrant in a dog (a) prior to and (b) immediately after gingivectomy and gingivoplasty. (c) Same area 3 months later.
(© Dr Alexander M. Reiter)

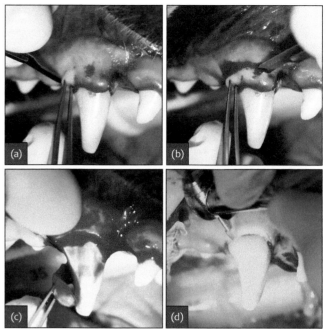
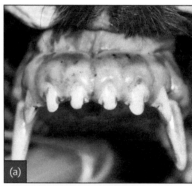

7.54 Same case as in Figure 7.29. (a, b) An external bevel incision is made (slightly apical to the bleeding points) with the blade held at a 45-degree angle. (c) The excess gingiva is removed. (d) A bullet-shaped 12-fluted bur on a high-speed handpiece with water cooling provides instant haemostasis while fine-contouring the cut gingival surface.
(© Dr Alexander M. Reiter)

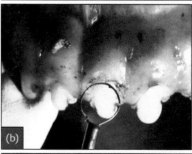
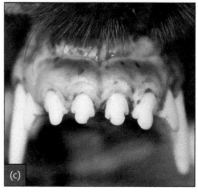

7.55 (a) Maxillary incisor teeth with gingival enlargement in a dog. (b) The excess gingiva is removed with an electrosurgical loop. (c) Front view following gingivectomy and gingivoplasty. The activated loop should never come into contact with the tooth and bony surfaces.
(© Dr Alexander M. Reiter)

The depth of the pocket is marked on the outer gingival surface using a periodontal probe or a pocket marker to create bleeding points (Operative Technique 7.3). An external bevel incision is made, starting slightly apical to the bleeding points with the blade held at a 45-degree angle to completely remove the pseudopocket and achieve a natural gingival contour; haemostasis and fine-contouring can then be accomplished with a bullet-shaped 12-fluted bur on a high-speed handpiece with water cooling (Figure 7.54). Gingivectomy and gingivoplasty can also be performed using electrosurgical loops (Figure 7.55). At least 2 mm of attached gingival tissue must be preserved after the procedure is completed. The freshly exposed tooth surface is scaled and polished. Bleeding from the cut gingival surface is controlled with gauze sponges. An astringent can also be applied, followed by coating with a layer of surface protectant (Figure 7.56).

Frenuloplasty

The mucosa may create folds (frenula) between the lips and the gingiva. Unlike the lower lip where no definite median mucosal fold is present, a median frenulum can often be noted between the upper lip and the gingiva in cats and dogs. A much more distinct, but unnamed frenulum attaches the lower lip to the gingiva on either side of the lower jaw in the space between the mandibular canine and the first premolar tooth (dog) or third premolar tooth (cat).

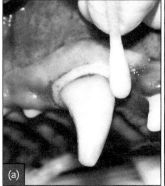
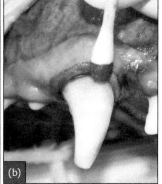
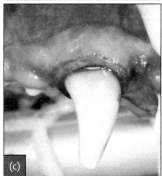

7.56 Same case as in Figure 7.29. (a) Cotton-tipped applicators are used to apply an astringent to the cut gingival surface. (b, c) They are then used to coat the astringent with a layer of surface protectant.
(© Dr Alexander M. Reiter)

A frenulum sometimes exerts an excessive pull upon the gingival margin and interdental gingival papilla, thus resulting in local gingival recession. For this reason, a frenulum that splays far towards the gingival margin should be eliminated by means of simple surgical separation (frenulotomy) or by partial or total removal of the frenulum (frenulectomy). The triangular or rhomboid wound that exists after frenulotomy or frenulectomy may be left open to granulate and epithelialize on its own, be resutured away from the gingival margin, or be covered with a free gingival graft (Holmstrom *et al.*, 2004).

Advanced periodontal surgery

While there are certain limitations in the cat due its delicate and small oral soft and hard tissues, a variety of advanced periodontal surgeries can be performed in the dog. These surgeries include laterally positioned flaps for repair of gingival defects, gingival and connective tissue grafting to halt or cover gingival recession, apically positioned flaps for crown lengthening and periodontal pocket reduction procedures, guided tissue regeneration with or without bone grafting, and partial tooth resection for teeth with severe focal alveolar bone loss. Even though it can prolong the presence of the dentition (DuPont, 1995), the authors do not recommend splinting of periodontally affected teeth, as the splint's surface is plaque retentive, and effective home oral hygiene for splinted teeth is difficult to perform.

Guided tissue regeneration

After periodontal debridement, four tissues compete to enter the cleaned periodontal pocket space: oral epithelium, gingival connective tissue, alveolar bone and periodontal ligament. The guided tissue regeneration (GTR) procedure involves the placement of a physical barrier to separate the oral epithelium and gingival connective tissue from the tooth surface, periodontal ligament and alveolar bone. This allows undisturbed regeneration of the periodontal ligament and alveolar bone. GTR is often utilized in conjunction with a bone graft or bone graft substitute (Reiter, 2013).

The custom-fitted barrier membrane can be non-absorbable or absorbable and solid or liquid (the latter type hardens once placed). It is placed between the prepared and treated bone defect (which may be filled with a bone graft) and the covering mucoperiosteal flap, thus inhibiting the growth of gingival epithelium and gingival connective tissue into the defect and allowing time for the more slowly growing tissues (periodontal ligament, cementum and alveolar bone) to occupy the defect and reestablish normal periodontal architecture (Gingerich and Stepaniuk, 2011; Rice *et al.*, 2012; Reiter, 2013). The periodontal flap is sutured over the barrier membrane at the end of the procedure (Figures 7.57 and 7.58).

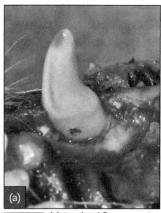
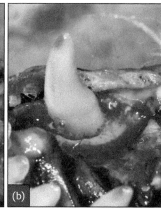

7.57 (a) A palatal flap was raised to expose a palatal pocket at the left maxillary canine tooth in a dog. Note the vertical bone loss and the brownish lesion in the root surface (inflamed and infected soft tissue has already been removed). (b) Same view after planing of the exposed root surface and recontouring the alveolar margin.
(© Dr Alexander M. Reiter)

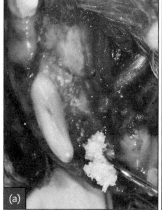
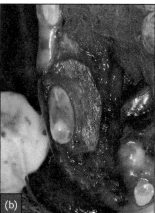
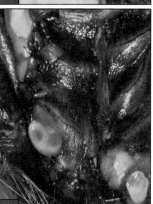

7.58 Same case as in Figure 7.57. (a) A graft material was placed into the bone defect. (b) A custom-fitted, absorbable barrier membrane was secured over the site. (c) The palatal flap was sutured closed. The releasing incision allowing the flap to adapt to the tooth is left to granulate and epithelialize.
(© Dr Alexander M. Reiter)

Partial tooth resection

Resection of a portion of a tooth can be a useful treatment option for periodontally and/or endodontically involved carnassial teeth affected individually or in the line of a jaw fracture. Indications for partial tooth resection include inoperable root or crown-root fracture, external root resorption involving one root, impaired endodontic treatment of a particular root, advanced periodontitis affecting only one root, severe furcation involvement, and teeth in the line of a jaw fracture (Reiter *et al.*, 2005).

Root resection is the removal of a root with maintenance of the entire crown. Its indications are restricted to multi-rooted teeth where one or more roots cannot be saved. Hemisection is the splitting of a tooth into two separate portions. Trisection is the splitting of a tooth into three separate portions. After sectioning of the tooth, all tooth portions are either retained or one or more tooth portions are extracted. If a tooth portion that includes part of the crown is extracted, this procedure then differs from root resection in that it removes the corresponding crown of the resected root. Any retained crown-root segment must be treated endodontically. Traumatic hemisection refers to complete fracture through a furcation, resulting in severance of a fragment from the tooth. If crown-root segments with adequate bone support can be retained near jaw fracture sites, they may act as anchorage structures for interdental wiring and provide surface areas for intraoral splints (Reiter *et al.*, 2005).

The procedure begins with a periodontal flap on the buccal/labial side with one releasing incision along the line angle of the part of the tooth to be resected. A small envelope flap is made on the lingual/palatal side. The buccal/labial flap is raised up to the furcation of that tooth to permit sectioning without trauma to the gingiva. Sectioning of the tooth is performed, and the crown-root segment in question is extracted with minimal alveolectomy. Vital pulp therapy or standard root canal therapy is performed on the remaining portion of the tooth (Figure 7.59). The extraction site is debrided, followed by alveoloplasty, rounding of the acute corners of the cut surface of the remainder of the tooth, polishing of the tooth surface, and suturing of the flap tightly around the tooth. It is imperative that the remainder of the tooth is surrounded by a band of gingiva at the end of the procedure (Reiter *et al.*, 2005).

Laterally positioned flap

Laterally positioned flaps are moved distally or mesially to their original location along the dental arch to repair a localized area of gingival recession (e.g. a gingival cleft)

(Figure 7.60) associated with a solitary root adjacent to either an edentulous region or a region where ample gingival tissue can be harvested without affecting the periodontal health of adjacent teeth (Rawlinson and Reiter, 2005). Whether the flap is harvested distal or mesial to the gingival defect depends on the amount of gingiva available at the donor site; i.e. the thicker the band of gingiva, the less likely is it that the donor site will be compromised negatively following surgery. The flap should always be harvested from mesial in the case of a mandibular canine tooth because the unnamed frenulum-like attachment distal to it prevents proper execution of the procedure (Startup, 2012).

The procedure involves elevation of a pedicle flap adjacent to the gingival defect, periodontal debridement (root planing, removal of inflamed and infected soft tissue, and alveoloplasty), advancement of the flap horizontally (mesiodistally or distomesially), and attachment of the flap over the region of the gingival defect (Beckman, 2005). The goals are to cover the denuded root, reestablish a 3 mm minimum width of gingiva, ensure gingival attachment, maintain height of the underlying alveolar bone, and separate the tooth surface from the thin, sensitive alveolar mucosa that is less able to resist trauma from masticatory forces (Rawlinson and Reiter, 2005).

Free gingival or connective tissue graft

There are two indications for employment of this procedure:

- Widening the band of attached gingiva and thus halting the progression of gingival recession by replacing or enhancing the mobile, non-keratinized alveolar mucosa with keratinized or connective tissue
- Covering (repairing) an area of gingival recession by placing keratinized or connective tissue over the recession area.

The free gingival graft is usually obtained from hard palate mucosa, preferably from an area that does not contain palatine rugae, or an area of oral mucosa that has plenty of attached gingiva to harvest from. This can be accomplished by means of a hand mucotome, motor-driven mucotome, gingivectomy knife, or scalpel blade. The graft needs to be thinned and trimmed prior to attaching it to the prepared recipient bed. An alternative is to use a connective tissue graft, which is also obtained from the hard palate and partially, or in some areas completely, covered with gingiva or alveolar mucosa at the recipient bed (Takei and Azzi, 2002; Wolf *et al.*, 2005).

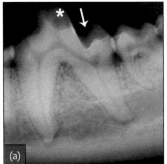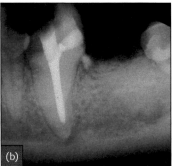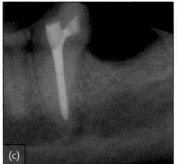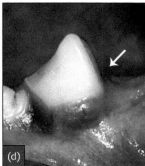

7.59 Partial tooth resection. (a) The main cusp of the left mandibular first molar tooth in a dog is fractured (∗). In addition, there is an axial fracture affecting the distal crown-root segment of the tooth (arrowed). (b) Resection of the distal crown-root segment was performed, followed by root canal therapy of the mesial crown-root segment and grafting of the extraction site with bioglass. (c) Radiograph and (d) clinical photograph of the tooth at the 6-month recheck examination. Note the height of the alveolar bone at the extraction site and the band of gingiva (arrowed) at the distal aspect of the remainder of the tooth.

(© Dr Alexander M. Reiter, reproduced from Reiter *et al.* (2005) with permission from the *Journal of Veterinary Dentistry*)

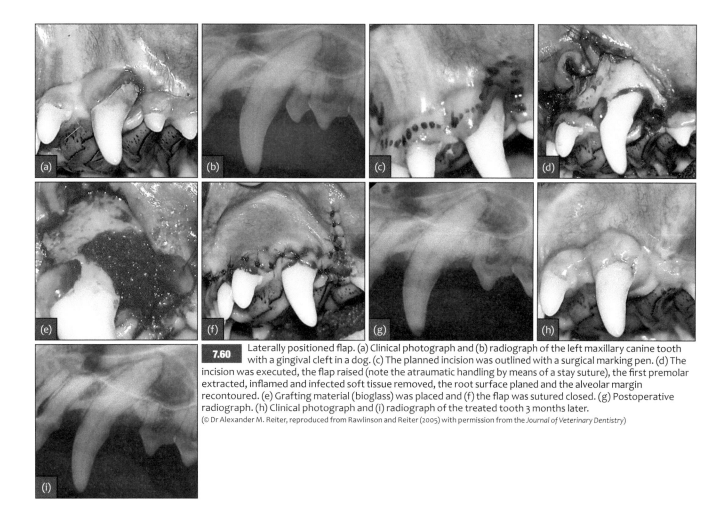

7.60 Laterally positioned flap. (a) Clinical photograph and (b) radiograph of the left maxillary canine tooth with a gingival cleft in a dog. (c) The planned incision was outlined with a surgical marking pen. (d) The incision was executed, the flap raised (note the atraumatic handling by means of a stay suture), the first premolar extracted, inflamed and infected soft tissue removed, the root surface planed and the alveolar margin recontoured. (e) Grafting material (bioglass) was placed and (f) the flap was sutured closed. (g) Postoperative radiograph. (h) Clinical photograph and (i) radiograph of the treated tooth 3 months later.

(© Dr Alexander M. Reiter, reproduced from Rawlinson and Reiter (2005) with permission from the *Journal of Veterinary Dentistry*)

Apically positioned flap

Apically positioned flaps are periodontal flaps with releasing incisions and accompanied by alveolectomy and alveoloplasty, thus exposing more of the tooth surface and allowing the flap to move apically. These flaps are utilized for various procedures, including crown lengthening of teeth with little clinical crown available for placement of prosthodontic crowns, periodontal pocket reduction, and periodontal pocket prevention after restoration of defects at the cervical portion of the tooth (Reiter and Lewis, 2008).

The surgical technique usually includes creation of mucoperiosteal flaps with one or more releasing incision(s), extraction of adjacent teeth if indicated, removal of tooth-supporting alveolar bone (alveolectomy) followed by recontouring of the alveolar margin (alveoloplasty), debridement of granulation tissue, restoration if indicated, root planing, polishing of the tooth surface, rinsing with lactated Ringer's solution, and apical positioning and suturing of the flaps (Figures 7.61 to 7.63). A gingival collar expansion technique has also been described (Reiter and Lewis, 2008).

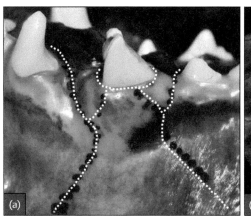
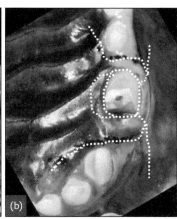

7.61 Apically positioned flap ('summer dress' technique, Alexander M. Reiter). (a) Lateral and (b) occlusal views of the fractured right maxillary canine tooth in a dog. The fracture involves both the crown and root of the tooth (crown-root fracture). The white dotted lines indicate planned incisions (staying about 1 mm away from the adjacent teeth). The yellow dotted line borders the extra piece of palatal tissue removed prior to suturing the flap closed.

(© Dr Alexander M. Reiter)

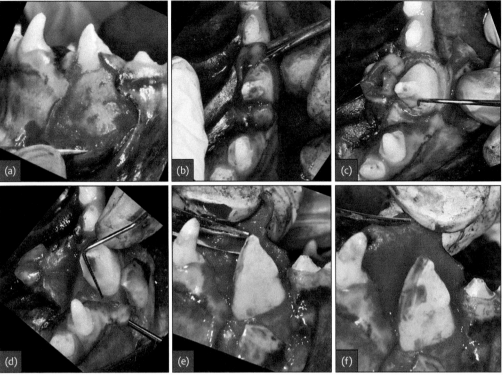

7.62 Same case as in Figure 7.61. (a) Labial and (b) palatal flaps are elevated. Bone is reduced until (c) the end of the fracture has been found and (d) there is sufficient clinical crown height. (e) The flaps are slightly thinned at their connective tissue side and (f) a half-moon-shaped piece of tissue is removed from the edge of the palatal flap.
(© Dr Alexander M. Reiter)

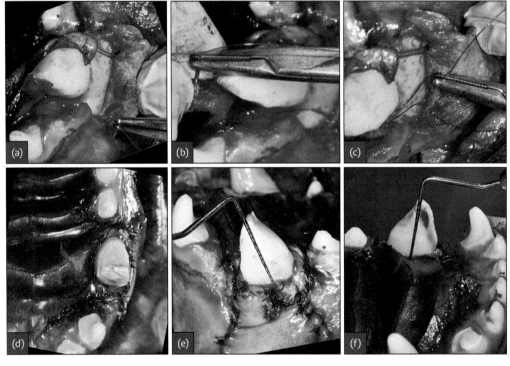

7.63 Same case as in Figure 7.61. (a–c) The fingers of the palatal flap are sutured to periosteum at the base of the labial flap, thus avoiding unwanted coronal pulling on that flap. (d) The labial flap is then sutured closed. Note the resulting clinical crown height (e) labially and (f) palatally at the end of the procedure.
(© Dr Alexander M. Reiter)

References and further reading

Anthony JM (2000a) Periodontal surgery equipment. *Clinical Techniques in Small Animal Practice* **15**, 232–236

Anthony JM (2000b) Advanced periodontic techniques. *Clinical Techniques in Small Animal Practice* **15**, 237–242

Araujo MG and Lindhe J (2010) Socket grafting with the use of autologous bone: an experimental study in the dog. *Clinical Oral Implants Research* **22**, 9–13

Barthel RE (2006) Treatment of vertical bone loss in a dog. *Journal of Veterinary Dentistry* **23**, 237–242

Beckman BW (2003) Mandibular incisor apically repositioned flap in the dog. *Journal of Veterinary Dentistry* **20**, 245–249

Beckman BW (2004) Treatment of an infrabony pocket in an American Eskimo dog. *Journal of Veterinary Dentistry* **21**, 159–163

Beckman BW (2005) Lateral sliding pedicle flap for gingival cleft at the maxillary canine tooth. *Journal of Veterinary Dentistry* **22**, 282–285

Beebe DE and Gengler WR (2007) Osseous surgery to augment treatment of chronic periodontitis of canine teeth in a cat. *Journal of Veterinary Dentistry* **24**, 30–38

Bellows J, Carithers DS and Gross SJ (2012) Efficacy of a barrier gel for reducing the development of plaque, calculus, and gingivitis in cats. *Journal of Veterinary Dentistry* **29**, 89–94

Bianucci HC, Smith MM, Saunders GK *et al.* (1998) Periodontal healing of canine experimental grade-III furcation defects treated with autologous fibrinogen and absorbable barrier membrane. *American Journal of Veterinary Research* **59**, 1329–1338

Bonello D and Squarzoni P (2008) Effect of a mucoadhesive gel and dental scaling on gingivitis in dogs. *Journal of Veterinary Dentistry* **25**, 28–32

Buffa EA, Lubbe AM, Verstraete FJ *et al.* (1997) The effects of wound lavage solutions on canine fibroblasts: an *in vitro* study. *Veterinary Surgery* **26**, 460–466

Cleland WP (2000) Nonsurgical periodontal therapy. *Clinical Techniques in Small Animal Practice* **15**, 221–225

DeBowes LJ, Mosier D, Logan E *et al.* (1996) Association of periodontal disease and histologic lesions in multiple organs from 45 dogs. *Journal of Veterinary Dentistry* **13**, 57–60

DeForge DH (1997) Evaluation of Bioglass/PerioGlas (Consil) synthetic bone graft particulate in the dog and cat. *Journal of Veterinary Dentistry* **14**, 141–145

Dennis M, Wilson T and Woodward T (2012) Retention of antimicrobial activity after reconstitution of doxycycline gel. *Journal of Veterinary Dentistry* **29**, 84–87

DuPont G (1995) Tooth splinting for severely mobile mandibular incisor teeth in a dog. *Journal of Veterinary Dentistry* **12**, 93–95

Fichtel T, Crha M, Langerova E *et al.* (2008) Observations on the effects of scaling and polishing methods on enamel. *Journal of Veterinary Dentistry* **25**, 231–235

Gengler WR, Kunkle BN, Romano D *et al.* (2005) Evaluation of a barrier dental sealant in dogs. *Journal of Veterinary Dentistry* **22**, 157–159

Gingerich W and Stepaniuk K (2011) Guided tissue regeneration for infrabony pocket treatment in dogs. *Journal of Veterinary Dentistry* **28**, 282–288

Girard N, Servet E, Biourge V *et al.* (2009) Periodontal health status in a colony of 109 cats. *Journal of Veterinary Dentistry* **26**, 147–155

Greenfield BA (2010) Open root planing for a periodontal pocket of a maxillary canine tooth. *Journal of Veterinary Dentistry* **27**, 34–39

Grove TK (1990) Problems associated with the management of periodontal disease in clinical practice. *Problems in Veterinary Medicine* **2**, 110–136

Grove TK (1998) Treatment of periodontal disease. *Veterinary Clinics of North America: Small Animal Practice* **28**, 1147–1164

Harvey CE (1998) Periodontal disease in dogs. Etiopathogenesis, prevalence, and significance. *Veterinary Clinics of North America: Small Animal Practice* **28**, 1111–1128

Harvey CE (2005) Management of periodontal disease: understanding the options. *Veterinary Clinics of North America: Small Animal Practice* **31**, 819–836

Hayashi K, Takada K and Hirasawa M (1998) Clinical and microbiological effects of controlled-release local delivery of minocycline on periodontitis in dogs. *American Journal of Veterinary Research* **59**, 464–467

Hirasawa M, Hayashi K and Takada K (2000) Measurement of peptidase activity and evaluation of effectiveness of administration of minocycline for treatment of dogs with periodontitis. *American Journal of Veterinary Research* **61**, 1349–1352

Hoffmann T and Gaengler P (1996) Epidemiology of periodontal disease in poodles. *Journal of Small Animal Practice* **37**, 309–316

Holmstrom SE (2000) Dental instruments and equipment. In: *Veterinary Dentistry for the Technician and Office Staff, 1st edn*, ed. SE Holmstrom, pp. 65–95. Saunders, Philadelphia

Holmstrom SE, Frost Fitch P and Eisner ER (2004) *Veterinary Dental Techniques for the Small Animal Practitioner, 3rd edn*, pp. 246–248, 254–264. Saunders, Philadelphia

Johnston TP, Mondal P, Pal D *et al.* (2011) Canine periodontal disease control using a clindamycin hydrochloride gel. *Journal of Veterinary Dentistry* **28**, 224–229

Klima LJ and Goldstein GS (2010) Modified distal wedge excision for access and treatment of an infrabony pocket in a dog. *Journal of Veterinary Dentistry* **27**, 16–23

Kortegaard HE, Eriksen T and Baelum V (2008) Periodontal disease in research beagle dogs – an epidemiological study. *Journal of Small Animal Practice* **49**, 610–616

Lewis JR and Miller BR (2010) Dentistry and oral surgery. In: *McCurnin's Clinical Textbook for Veterinary Technicians, 7th edn*, ed. JM Bassert and DM McCurnin, pp. 1093–1148. Saunders, Philadelphia

Lewis JR and Reiter AM (2005) Management of generalized gingival enlargement in a dog – case report and review of the literature. *Journal of Veterinary Dentistry* **22**, 160–169

Lipscomb V and Reiter AM (2005) Surgical materials and instrumentation. In: *BSAVA Manual of Canine and Feline Head, Neck and Thoracic Surgery, 1st edn*, ed. DJ Brockman and DE Holt, pp. 16–24. BSAVA Publications, Gloucester

Lobprise HB (2000a) Treatment planning based on examination results. *Clinical Techniques in Small Animal Practice* **15**, 211–220

Lobprise HB (2000b) Complicated periodontal disease. *Clinical Techniques in Small Animal Practice* **15**, 197–203

Lommer MJ and Verstraete FJM (2001) Radiographic patterns of periodontitis in cats: 147 cases (1998–1999). *Journal of the American Veterinary Medical Association* **218**, 230–234

Lund EM, Armstrong PJ, Kirk CA *et al.* (1999) Health status and population characteristics of dogs and cats examined at private veterinary practices in the United States. *Journal of the American Veterinary Medical Association* **214**, 1336–1341

Marretta SM (1987) The common and uncommon clinical presentations and treatment of periodontal disease in the dog and cat. *Seminars in Veterinary Medicine and Surgery Small Animals* **2**, 230–240

Marretta SM (1992) Chronic rhinitis and dental disease. *Veterinary Clinics of North America: Small Animal Practice* **22**, 1101–1117

Marretta SM, Schloss AJ and Klippert LS (1992) Classification and prognostic factors of endodontic-periodontic lesions in the dog. *Journal of Veterinary Dentistry* **9**, 27–30

Nemec A, Pavlica Z, Stiblar-Martincic D *et al.* (2007) Histological evaluation of the pulp in teeth from dogs with naturally occurring periodontal disease. *Journal of Veterinary Dentistry* **24**, 212–223

Niemiec BA (2001) Treatment of mandibular first molar teeth with endodontic-periodontal lesions in a dog. *Journal of Veterinary Dentistry* **18**, 21–25

Niemiec BA (2003) Professional teeth cleaning. *Journal of Veterinary Dentistry* **20**, 175–180

Niemiec BA (2008) Periodontal disease. *Topics in Companion Animal Medicine* **23**, 72–80

Pattison AM, Pattison GL and Takei HH (2002) The periodontal instrumentarium. In: *Carranza's Clinical Periodontology, 9th edn*, ed. MG Newman, HH Takei and FA Carranza, pp. 567–593. WB Saunders, Philadelphia

Rawlinson JE and Reiter AM (2005) Repair of a gingival cleft associated with a maxillary canine tooth in a dog. *Journal of Veterinary Dentistry* **22**, 234–242

Reiter AM (2012) Dental and oral diseases. In: *The Cat: Clinical Medicine and Management, 1st edn*, ed. SE Little, pp. 329–370. Saunders, St. Louis

Reiter AM (2013) Equipment for oral surgery in small animals. *Veterinary Clinics of North America: Small Animal Practice* **43**, 587–608

Reiter AM and Harvey CE (2010) Periodontal and endodontic disease. In: *Mechanisms of Disease in Small Animal Surgery, 3rd edn*, ed. MJ Bojrab and E Monnet, pp. 125–128. Teton NewMedia, Jackson

Reiter AM and Lewis JR (2008) Dental bulge restoration and gingival collar expansion after endodontic treatment of a complicated maxillary fourth premolar crown-root fracture in a dog. *Journal of Veterinary Dentistry* **25**, 34–45

Reiter AM, Lewis JR and Harvey CE (2012) Dentistry for the surgeon. In: *Veterinary Surgery: Small Animal, 1st edn*, ed. KM Tobias and SA Johnston, pp. 1037–1053. Elsevier, St. Louis

Reiter AM, Lewis JR, Rawlinson JE *et al.* (2005) A case series study on hemisection of carnassial teeth in client-owned dogs. *Journal of Veterinary Dentistry* **22**, 216–226

Rice CA, Snyder CJ and Soukup JW (2012) Use of an autogenous cortical graft in combination with guided tissue regeneration for treatment of an infrabony defect. *Journal of Veterinary Dentistry* **29**, 166–171

Shoukry M, Ben Ali L, Abdel Naby M *et al.* (2007) Repair of experimental plaque-induced periodontal disease in dogs. *Journal of Veterinary Dentistry* **24**, 152–165

Smith MM (1995) Treatment of a mandibular periodontal interproximal defect with a bone graft in a dog. *Journal of Veterinary Dentistry* **12**, 59–62

Smith MM (2003) Line angle incisions. *Journal of Veterinary Dentistry* **20**, 241–244

Smith MM, Saunders GK, Moon ML *et al.* (1993) Evaluation of the caudoventral portion of the mandible as a donor site for corticocancellous bone for periodontal surgery in dogs. *American Journal of Veterinary Research* **54**, 481–486

Stapleton BL (1995) Endodontic therapy and management of grade II furcation periodontal disease in a mandibular first molar tooth of a dog. *Journal of Veterinary Dentistry* **12**, 63–67

Startup SL (2012) Lateral sliding pedicle flap for gingival cleft at the mandibular canine tooth. *Journal of Veterinary Dentistry* **29**, 60–66

Takei HH and Azzi RA (2002) Periodontal plastic and esthetic surgery. In: *Carranza's Clinical Periodontology, 9th edn*, ed. MG Newman, HH Takei and FA Carranza, pp. 851–875. Saunders, Philadelphia

Terpak CH and Verstraete FJM (2012) Instrumentation, patient positioning and aseptic technique. In: *Oral and Maxillofacial Surgery in Dogs and Cats, 1st edn*, ed. FJM Verstraete and MJ Lommer, pp. 55–68. Saunders, Philadelphia

Tsugawa AJ and Verstraete FJ (2000) How to obtain and interpret periodontal radiographs in dogs. *Clinical Techniques in Small Animal Practice* **15**, 204–210

Tsugawa AJ, Verstraete FJ, Kass PH *et al.* (2003) Diagnostic value of the use of lateral and occlusal radiographic views in comparison with periodontal probing for the assessment of periodontal attachment of the canine teeth in dogs. *American Journal of Veterinary Research* **64**, 255–261

Wiggs RB, Lobprise H and Mitchell PQ (1998) Oral and periodontal tissue. Maintenance, augmentation, rejuvenation, and regeneration. *Veterinary Clinics of North America: Small Animal Practice* **28**, 1165–1188

Wolf HF, Rateitschak EM, Rateitschak KH *et al.* (2005) *Color Atlas of Dental Medicine – Periodontology, 3rd edn*, pp. 64, 309–317 and 419–434. Thieme, Stuttgart

Zetner K and Rothmueller G (2002) Treatment of periodontal pockets with doxycycline in beagles. *Veterinary Therapeutics* **3**, 441–452

OPERATIVE TECHNIQUE 7.1

Professional dental cleaning and closed periodontal therapy

INDICATIONS

Calculus and plaque accumulation; teeth with mild to moderate periodontal disease (periodontal pockets not exceeding 4–5 mm in dogs and 1–2 mm in cats).

POSITIONING

Lateral recumbency.

ASSISTANT

Not required.

ADDITIONAL EQUIPMENT

Diluted chlorhexidine solution; calculus removal forceps (or extraction forceps); dental mirror; power scaler (ultrasonic or sonic); hand scalers; hand curettes; air-driven dental unit; low-speed handpiece with prophy angle and cup; polishing paste; air/water syringe; periodontal probe; dental explorer.

SURGICAL TECHNIQUE

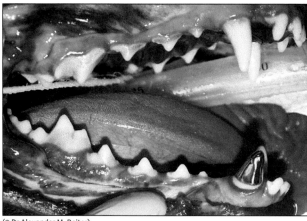

1   Assess the situation by performing a periodontal examination as well as taking photographs and radiographs.

2   Rinse the mouth with diluted chlorhexidine solution.

3   Remove large deposits of calculus with calculus removal forceps (or – with adequate practice and proper, gentle technique – extraction forceps).

4   Use a dental mirror to retract the lips and cheeks laterally and the tongue medially.

(© Dr Alexander M. Reiter)

5   Use a power scaler to remove supra- and subgingival plaque and calculus.
  • Direct the scaler tip apically (not coronally to avoid contact of the hot instrument with soft tissue), with the last 2–3 mm in contact with the tooth, and at an angle of less than 15 degrees (but never perpendicular) to the tooth surface.
  • Ensure that there is copious water flow, and keep the scaler tip moving continuously over the tooth surface (do not use for longer than 15 seconds continuously on any one tooth).

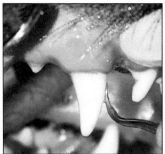
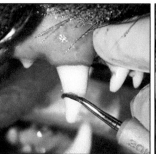
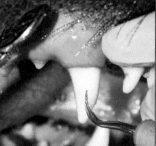
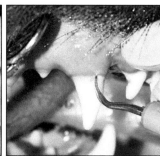

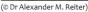
(© Dr Alexander M. Reiter)

→ **OPERATIVE TECHNIQUE 7.1 CONTINUED**

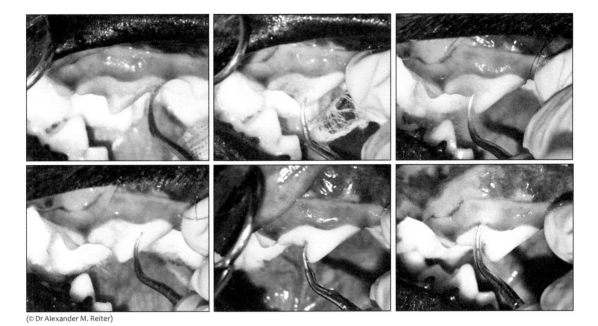

(© Dr Alexander M. Reiter)

6 Use hand scalers to remove any residual supragingival plaque and calculus. When placing the blade against the tooth, the face should be at an angle of 60–80 degrees to the tooth surface.

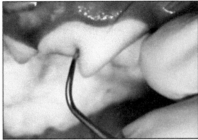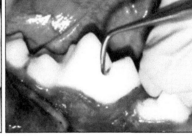

(© Dr Alexander M. Reiter)

   a. Direct the cutting edge to the apical edge of the calculus, and exert lateral pressure against the tooth.

   b. Employ a pulling motion away from the gingival margin to remove supragingival plaque and calculus.
   c. Use the sharp tip of the instrument to scale thin developmental grooves on the crowns.

7 Use hand curettes to remove any residual subgingival plaque and calculus, plane the root surface and perform gingival curettage. When placing the blade against the tooth, the face should be at an angle of 60–80 degrees to the tooth surface.

   a. Carefully insert the instrument in the gingival sulcus or periodontal pocket with the back towards the inner gingival surface and the face towards the tooth surface.
   b. Advance the instrument gently apically until resistance is felt (i.e. to the bottom of the sulcus or pocket).
   c. Engage the cutting edge on the tooth surface with a pulling action to remove subgingival plaque and calculus.
      – Exploratory stroke: Initial assessment of the topography of the tooth surface by very lightly feeling for irregularities.
      – Working stroke: Applying pressure against the tooth and pulling the blade vertically, horizontally or obliquely in a short, controlled motion.
      – Root planing stroke: Longer in length with light pressure to avoid removal of excessive amounts of cementum.
   d. Insert the tip of the curette into the periodontal pocket with the face directed against the pocket wall, and use the sharp blade against the inner gingival surface to remove inflamed and infected granulation tissue.

8 Polish all tooth surfaces.

   a. Attach a prophy angle and cup to a nose cone secured on a low-speed handpiece engine.
   b. Fill the polishing cup with polishing paste.
   c. Use gentle pressure with the cup on the tooth surface at low speed and with short contact times.
   d. Carefully flare out the edge of the cup underneath the gingival margin to polish subgingival crown and exposed root surfaces.

→ **OPERATIVE TECHNIQUE 7.1 CONTINUED**

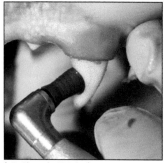 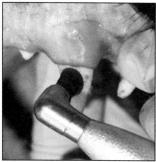 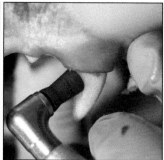 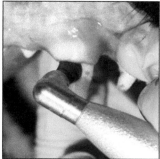

(© Dr Alexander M. Reiter)

9 Rinse debris and residual polishing paste from the gingival sulcus or periodontal pocket with the air/water syringe.

10 Dry the tooth surfaces with the air/water syringe and evaluate the root surface with a periodontal probe and crown surface with a dental explorer for smoothness and complete removal of dental deposits.

11 Place low-dose doxycycline gel (when available) into cleaned periodontal pockets deeper than 4–5 mm.

12 Rinse the mouth with diluted chlorhexidine solution.

13 Document your work by taking photographs.

14 Provide instructions for home oral hygiene.

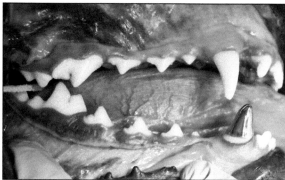

(© Dr Alexander M. Reiter)

PRACTICAL TIPS

- It is important to keep the power scaler moving, apply light pressure and use copious volumes of water to cool its tip
- The blades of hand scalers and hand curettes must be kept sharp to be effective
- Avoid:
  - Holding the tip of a power scaler perpendicular to the tooth surface
  - Directing the tip of a power scaler coronally (otherwise there is a greater chance for the less cooled part of the scaler to inadvertently contact oral mucosa)
  - Spending more than 15 seconds on a tooth continuously with a power scaler
  - Using a power scaler on teeth with prosthodontic crowns and in areas of restorations (use hand instruments instead)
  - Injuring the gingival attachment to the tooth when performing subgingival work
  - Spending more than 3 seconds on a tooth continuously with a rotating polishing cup

OPERATIVE TECHNIQUE 7.2

Open periodontal therapy

INDICATIONS

Calculus and plaque accumulation; teeth with moderate to severe periodontal disease (periodontal pocket depths exceeding 5–6 mm in dogs and 2–3 mm in cats).

POSITIONING

Lateral recumbency.

ASSISTANT

Preferable.

ADDITIONAL EQUIPMENT

In addition to that listed in Operative Technique 7.1: scalpel handle and blade; swabs; periosteal elevator; thumb forceps; tissue scissors; assortment of burs; cotton-tipped applicators; agents for root surface treatment; bone replacement material; barrier membrane; needle holder; suture material; suture scissors.

SURGICAL TECHNIQUE

Following professional dental cleaning and closed periodontal therapy:

1   Assess the situation by performing a periodontal examination as well as taking photographs and radiographs.

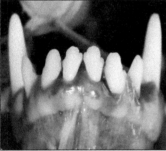
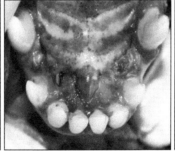
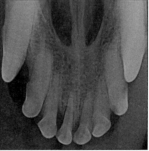

(© Dr Alexander M. Reiter)

2   Make an internal bevel incison slightly apical to the gingival margin and down to the alveolar bone.

3   Create mucoperiosteal flaps:

a. Modified Widman flap: Partially mobilized envelope flap; no vertical incisions are made and the gingival flap is not reflected beyond the mucogingival junction; or

b. Flap beyond the mucogingival junction: Requires one or two vertical (or slightly diverging) releasing incisions into gingiva and alveolar mucosa preferably to be made at the line angle (which is the junction of two surfaces of the crown of a tooth), rather than over a root, furcation or interdental papilla.

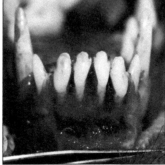
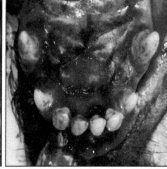

(© Dr Alexander M. Reiter)

→ **OPERATIVE TECHNIQUE 7.2 CONTINUED**

4 Use a power scaler to scale the exposed tooth surfaces; continue with hand curettes to remove inflamed and infected soft tissue and residual plaque and calculus; plane the root surface.

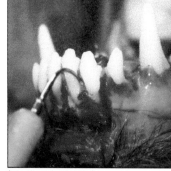
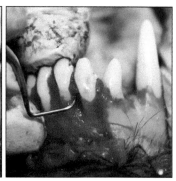

(© Dr Alexander M. Reiter)

5 Perform alveoloplasty (recontouring of the alveolar margin to obtain a knife-edge finish) using round diamond burs and hand curettes. Avoid reducing bone height.

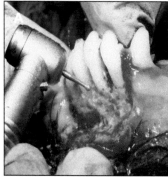
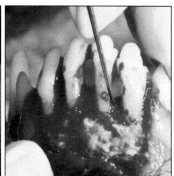

(© Dr Alexander M. Reiter)

6 Polish exposed tooth surfaces with fine pumice and rinse the wound with lactated Ringer's solution; then proceed with removing inflamed and infected soft tissue from the inside (connective tissue side) of the flaps.

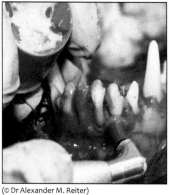
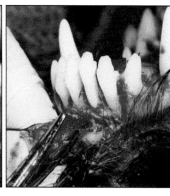

(© Dr Alexander M. Reiter)

7 Rinse the tissues one more time.

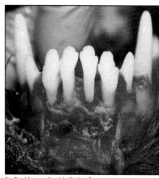
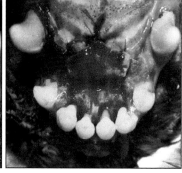

(© Dr Alexander M. Reiter)

→ **OPERATIVE TECHNIQUE 7.2 CONTINUED**

8 Optional:

 a. Utilize agents for root surface treatment (e.g. citric acid, ethylenediamine tetra-acetic acid, fluoride).

 b. Place bone replacement materials in bone defects with or without the use of a barrier membrane.

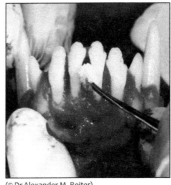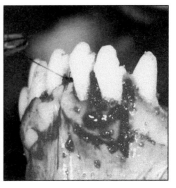

(© Dr Alexander M. Reiter)

9 Suture the flaps closed to their original, or in a slightly apical, position and document your work by taking photographs and radiographs.

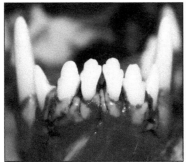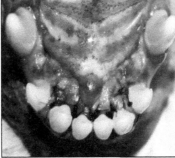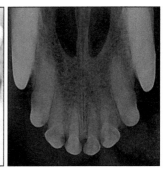

(© Dr Alexander M. Reiter)

PRACTICAL TIPS

- Always use fresh scalpel blades when performing periodontal surgery
- Use stay sutures attached to the inside (connective tissue side) of the flap when manipulating or retracting it
- Plan a periodontal and radiographic re-examination under anaesthesia about 3 months following treatment
- Avoid:
  - Excessively removing cementum from root surfaces with hand curettes, as this will expose sensitive dentine and possibly compromise soft tissue reattachment
  - Removing healthy tooth-supporting bone during alveoloplasty procedures
  - Letting inflamed granulation tissue on the inside (connective tissue side) of the flaps come into contact with exposed dentine surfaces, as this could result in root resorption

OPERATIVE TECHNIQUE 7.3

Gingivectomy and gingivoplasty

INDICATIONS

Benign gingival enlargement.

POSITIONING

Lateral recumbency.

ASSISTANT

Optional.

ADDITIONAL EQUIPMENT

In addition to that listed in Operative Technique 7.1: pocket-marking forceps; scalpel handle and blade; gingival knives; bullet-shaped 12-fluted bur; electrosurgical wire loops; swabs; cotton-tipped applicators; aluminium chloride; tincture of myrrh and benzoin.

SURGICAL TECHNIQUE

1 Make a series of bleeding points on the outer gingival surface to mark the base of any pseudopockets:

- Insert the blunt tip of a pocket-marking forceps into the pocket and close the forceps; the right-angled, pointed tip of the forceps will create a bleeding point; or
- Insert a periodontal probe down to the base of the pocket and measure its depth. Remove the probe and hold it on the outer gingival surface at the measured pocket depth. Then poke the blunt tip of the probe perpendicularly into the gingiva to create a bleeding point.

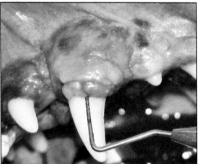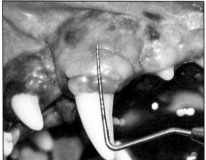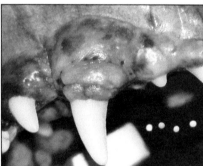

(© Dr Alexander M. Reiter, reproduced from Lewis and Reiter (2005) with permission from the *Journal of Veterinary Dentistry*)

2 Make an external bevel incision slightly (1–2 mm) apical to the bleeding points with a scalpel blade held at a 45-degree angle to remove a band of excess gingiva, thus eliminating the pocket and establishing a natural gingival contour; it is also possible to use loop, needle or diamond-shaped electrodes in a fully rectified mode (cutting and coagulating) or a bullet-shaped 12-fluted bur on a high-speed handpiece with water-cooling to shave off excess free gingiva while contouring the remaining attached gingiva.

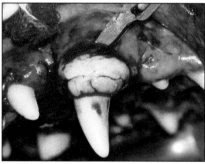

(© Dr Alexander M. Reiter, reproduced from Lewis and Reiter (2005) with permission from the *Journal of Veterinary Dentistry*)

→ **OPERATIVE TECHNIQUE 7.3 CONTINUED**

3   Scale and polish the freshly exposed tooth surface.

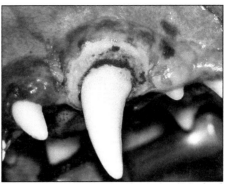

(© Dr Alexander M. Reiter, reproduced from Lewis and Reiter (2005) with permission from the *Journal of Veterinary Dentistry*)

4   Control bleeding from the cut gingiva digitally with gauze sponges or apply a topical haemostatic agent (aluminium chloride) using a cotton-tipped applicator.

5   Coat the cut gingival surface with a tissue protectant (tincture of myrrh and benzoin) using a cotton-tipped applicator.

PRACTICAL TIPS

- Remove the bulk of excess gingiva with a scalpel blade (gingivectomy) and then recontour the gingiva (gingivoplasty) with a 12-fluted bur or an electrode
- Ensure that at least 2 mm of attached gingiva is preserved after completion of the procedure
- Avoid:
  - Contact of the 12-fluted bur with the crown, as enamel damage will occur
  - Contact of the electrode with the crown, root or alveolar bone, as thermal tissue damage and delayed wound healing can occur

Management of selected non-periodontal inflammatory, infectious and reactive conditions

Margherita Gracis, Alexander M. Reiter and Laura Ordeix

Conditions of the oral mucosa

The most common inflammatory condition of the oral cavity in dogs and cats is periodontal disease, which is caused by plaque bacteria and mainly affects the periodontal tissues (e.g. gingiva, periodontal ligament, cementum and alveolar bone) (see Chapter 5). Oral mucosal linings other than gingiva may also be affected by inflammatory disorders of infectious, reactive or immunological origin. Stomatitis is defined as inflammation of the oral mucosal linings; however, stomatitis is a broad term rather than a specific disease, and it includes different pathological conditions. In clinical use the term should be reserved to describe widespread oral inflammation, beyond gingivitis and periodontitis (AVDC, 2013). If only certain anatomical areas in the mouth are involved, specific terms should be used, such as glossitis or palatitis. Oral inflammation is a common feature of certain systemic diseases and neoplastic disorders. Thus, it is necessary to consider a list of differential diagnoses for each affected patient, evaluating the particular pattern and distribution of lesions.

The clinical presentation, pattern and distribution of lesions are particularly important, as they may vary based on aetiological factors. In certain instances, the skin and mucocutaneous areas are involved, and systemic clinical signs may be present. Possible oral inflammatory lesions include vesicles, bullae, ulcers, plaques and nodules. Typically, vesicles and bullae affecting canine and feline oral mucosa rarely persist long enough to be observed, due to constant trauma from chewing, playing and grooming (Lommer, 2013a). Therefore, secondary ulcerative lesions in the oral cavity are relatively more common.

To narrow the list of differential diagnoses, oral inflammatory conditions are described here primarily according to the type of lesion they produce (i.e. ulcerative *versus* nodular lesions) rather than according to their aetiology.

Ulcerative lesions

Ulcers are deep, secondary lesions characterized by loss of tissue, and affecting both the epithelium and underlying connective tissue.

Feline chronic stomatitis

Feline chronic stomatitis is a persistent inflammatory disease of the oral mucosal tissues that causes significant discomfort and distress for the affected patient. Cats of any age, sex and breed may be affected, although a predilection for young adults (less than 8 years old) has been

reported (Farcas *et al.*, 2014). The gingiva, alveolar, labial and buccal mucosa are always involved (Figure 8.1a), while the lingual and sublingual mucosa and mucocutaneous junction are involved less frequently, and the pharyngeal and palatal mucosa are rarely affected. Gingivitis and oral mucositis may be generalized or localized. In the latter case, the premolar/molar tooth area is more commonly involved than the rostral portion of the mouth. Caudal stomatitis (inflammation of caudal oral mucosa lateral to the palatoglossal folds) is a typical feature of refractory cases (Figure 8.1b). For this reason, the authors suggest that two different conditions be distinguished:

* Feline chronic stomatitis with caudal involvement (ST/CS)
* Feline chronic stomatitis without caudal involvement (ST).

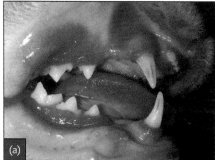

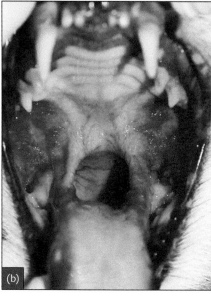

8.1
(a) Ulcerative gingivitis and alveolar, labial and buccal mucositis in a 1-year-old Domestic Shorthaired cat.
(b) Chronic stomatitis (ST/CS) with the typical bilateral caudal inflammation in a 12-year-old Domestic Shorthaired cat.
(© Dr Margherita Gracis)

The focus is on the discussion of ST/CS, and differences between ST/CS and ST are described when present and of interest. In this chapter, the term 'stomatitis' is used as a synonym for ST/CS.

Prevalence and clinical signs: The prevalence of the disease in the general cat population is unknown, with only a few studies reporting values from 0.7–12%. Distribution seems to vary from country to country, but no specific data are available.

Clinical signs are those typical of a very painful oral condition, characterized by depression or aggressiveness, social withdrawal, dysphagia, and anorexia. Halitosis, weight loss, dehydration, poor hair coat due to limited grooming activity, mandibular lymphadenopathy, pawing at the face and mouth, restricted mouth opening during yawning, vocalization during feeding and grooming, oral bleeding, and ptyalism and drooling are also common. Saliva is usually thick and malodorous due to bacterial infection.

Great care should be taken when manipulating the head in these patients during the clinical examination. Animals are usually head shy, and palpation of the perioral region and mandibular lymph nodes may elicit hyperalgesia (i.e. an exaggerated pain sensation in response to a light stimulus). Gentle elevation of the upper lip allows evaluation of the oral vestibule to locate any soft tissue lesions. Opening of the mouth for evaluation of the oral cavity proper can be achieved by gently grasping the head of the patient with one hand and slightly extending it dorsally. The lower jaw often drops when executing this manoeuvre and can be further pushed ventrally by cautiously placing an index finger on the mandibular incisors, avoiding contact with inflamed tissues. Excessive mouth opening should be avoided, as stretching of affected oral mucosa may cause pain and stimulate an aggressive reaction. Chemical restraint may be necessary for a thorough oral examination.

Location and character of lesions: Oral lesions may be primarily ulcerative or ulcero-proliferative, the latter possibly developing from long-standing ulcers in chronic stages of the disease (Figure 8.2). In affected areas, gingivitis is usually diffuse (i.e. the entire height of tissue being involved), except at the maxillary canine teeth where gingiva is more abundant and gingivitis may assume a more geographical pattern (i.e. irregular areas of tissue involved) (see Figure 8.1a). Mucositis generally affects (but may not be limited to) areas of the alveolar and labial/buccal mucosa facing plaque-laden teeth, developing so-called contact ulcers or 'kissing lesions' (see Figure 8.1a). The involvement of the palatoglossal folds and the mucosa lateral to them (i.e. caudal stomatitis) is a key feature of the disease (see Figure 8.1b), and its absence in certain individuals may actually be a good prognostic factor, possibly indicating a different disease entity. The gingiva on the palatal aspect of the teeth may be affected as well, but not the other areas of the palatal mucosa. Often, chronic inflammation involving the periodontal tissues leads to gingival recession, periodontal pocket formation, horizontal and vertical alveolar bone loss, furcation exposure and external inflammatory tooth resorption (Farcas *et al.*, 2014). Periodontal lesions are exacerbated by the undisturbed accumulation of plaque and calculus, due to minimal chewing activity as a result of severe oral pain. Sometimes, perioral cutaneous ulceration and ulceration of the labial philtrum are also present (Figures 8.3 and 8.4).

Aetiology: The aetiology of ST/CS is unclear, but it is believed to be multifactorial, involving viruses, bacteria and possibly other exogenous factors. Affected individuals may also have an altered, exaggerated immune response to antigens of infectious or non-infectious agents.

Feline immunodeficiency virus and feline leukaemia virus: Despite chronic oral inflammation being a common clinical feature in cats with long-standing feline immunodeficiency

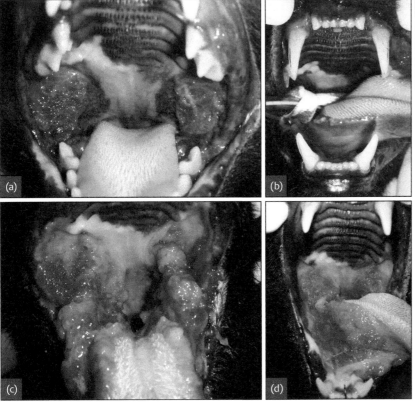

8.2 (a, b) A 4-year-old Domestic Shorthaired cat with bilateral caudal ulcerative stomatitis. (c, d) A year later, the same patient is unresponsive to partial-mouth tooth extraction (i.e. premolar and molar teeth) and different medical treatments. Note the severe bilateral ulcero-proliferative stomatitis, involving the caudolateral and ventrolateral surface of the tongue. (© Dr Margherita Gracis)

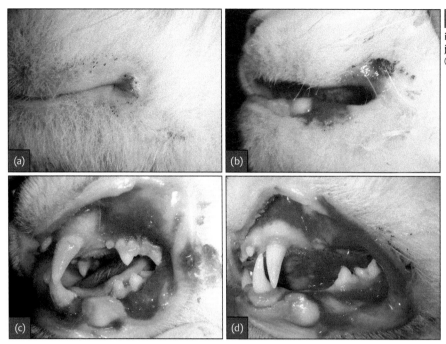

8.3 (a–d) Four different cats with stomatitis, showing progressively severe inflammation and ulceration of the mucocutaneous junctions.
(© Dr Margherita Gracis)

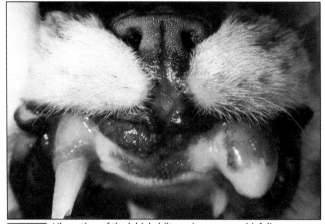

8.4 Ulceration of the labial philtrum in a 12-year-old, feline calcivirus (FCV)-positive and feline herpesvirus (FHV), feline immunodeficiency virus (FIV) and feline leukaemia virus (FeLV)-negative cat with stomatitis (ST/CS).
(© Dr Margherita Gracis)

virus (FIV) infection and frequently seen in feline leukaemia virus (FeLV)-infected cats, the prevalence of FIV and FeLV among cats with stomatitis is not significantly different from that of the general population (Belgard et al., 2010). Immunosuppression caused by these infectious agents may indirectly favour the development of stomatitis in infected cats, but it is unlikely that FIV and FeLV have any other role. Often, co-infection with feline calicivirus (FCV) is diagnosed in FIV- or FeLV-positive cats with stomatitis, which makes the determination of the exact role of each virus difficult.

Feline calicivirus: A history of recent or past upper respiratory disease is commonly reported in cats with ST/CS. FCV can be isolated from 85 to 100% of cats affected by ST/CS, *versus* a prevalence of up to 20–30% in the general population. However, its exact role in the disease process remains unclear, and experimental reproduction of chronic stomatitis or chronic carrier status have never been demonstrated (Radford et al., 2009). Therefore, FCV could be an opportunistic agent rather than the cause of

the disease. The theory that FCV may play an important role in the pathogenesis of the disease is supported by a recent study that shows a positive correlation between clinical disease severity and the presence of FCV (Dolieslager et al., 2013). The detection of FCV is also significantly correlated with the presence of caudal stomatitis compared with cats with oral inflammation that lack caudal stomatitis (Hennet and Boucrault-Baralones, 2005), supporting the view that caudal stomatitis may be an FCV-associated lesion (Reubel et al., 1992). Two case reports described cessation of FCV shedding following the resolution of clinical signs in two cats with stomatitis treated by different medical protocols (Addie et al., 2003; Southerden and Gorrel, 2007). However, the FCV load does not seem to be correlated with the severity of the oral lesions (or with the outcome following dental extractions) (Druet and Hennet, 2017).

The most common oral features of acute FCV infection are short-term, transient palatal ulcers and the development of lingual vesicles and ulceration, particularly on the rostro-dorsal aspect of the tongue (Radford et al., 2009). Interestingly, in chronic stomatitis cases, the ventral surface of the tongue, the sublingual mucosa, and the tongue's caudolateral portions at the base of the palatoglossal folds are more commonly involved (see Figure 8.2d). In contrast with cats with acute calicivirus infection that may have hard and soft palate lesions, the majority of the palate in cats with chronic stomatitis is usually unaffected by inflammation. The gingiva on the palatal aspect of maxillary teeth is occasionally involved, or inflammation may slightly extend from caudal mucosal lesions into the palate (Figure 8.5).

Feline herpesvirus: The role of feline herpesvirus (FHV) in the disease process is still controversial, with a single study showing a prevalence of 92% in stomatitis cases compared with 25% of controls (periodontally affected cats) (Lommer and Verstraete, 2003). Other studies have shown a much lower prevalence, similar in both ST/CS and ST cats (Hennet and Boucrault-Barolones, 2005). FHV carriage was also not correlated with the presence of caudal stomatitis neither in ST/CS cats co-infected with FCV nor in FCV-negative ST cats (Hennet and Boucrault-Baralones,

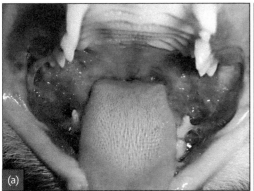
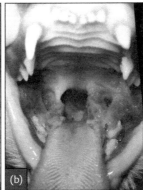

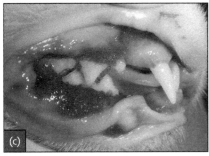
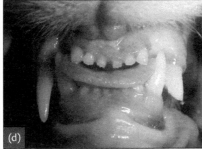
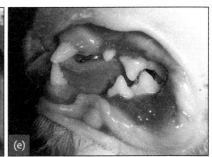

8.5 A 4-year-old, feline calcivirus (FCV) and feline immunodeficiency virus (FIV)-positive, feline herpesvirus (FHV) and feline leukaemia virus (FeLV)-negative cat with stomatitis. (a, b) Bilateral caudal stomatitis, inflammation of the palatal mucosa adjacent to the dental arch and slightly asymmetrical proliferation of the palatoglossal folds. (c–e) Gingivitis and mucositis along the upper and lower dental arches.
(© Dr Margherita Gracis)

2005). It is important to consider, however, that FHV is shed intermittently, when carriers are stressed or immuno-suppressed, and may be difficult to detect.

Dental plaque: Bacteria are considered to play an important role in the disease process, and plaque control is a key point in the treatment of both ST/CS and ST cats. Bacteria may act as complicating or causative factors, as is suggested by the resolution of clinical signs following tooth extraction in a large proportion of cats with caudal stomatitis and in almost all cats without caudal involvement (Hennet, 1997). Importantly, the degree of inflammation is independent of the amount of plaque and calculus accumulation.

A number of Gram-negative anaerobic bacteria have been identified in the oral cavity of cats affected by chronic stomatitis, including *Bacteroides* spp., *Fusobacterium* spp., *Porphyromonas* spp. and *Pseudomonas* spp. (Dolieslager *et al.*, 2011). *Pasteurella multocida* subsp. *multocida* is most commonly isolated. Interestingly, the microbial diversity of the oral flora of cats with stomatitis is significantly decreased compared with unaffected cats, possibly due to competition for nutrients. The presence of *Tannerella forsythia*, an obligate anaerobic bacterium considered to be a strong periodontopathogen in humans and shown to be very common in plaque samples from both healthy cats and cats with periodontal disease (Booij-Vrieling *et al.*, 2010), has recently been shown in cats with stomatitis to be correlated with an increase in some cytokines and Toll-like receptors as well as worsening of clinical disease severity (Dolieslager *et al.*, 2013). It may, therefore, play an important role in the pathogenesis of the disease.

Bartonella henselae: Bartonella henselae is a Gram-negative haemotropic Alphaproteobacterium transmitted by fleas and ticks. It has been implicated in the disease process of stomatitis (Ueno *et al.*, 1996; Glaus *et al.*, 1997), but a cause–effect relationship has never been proven. Given the wide distribution of the infection in the healthy population, the role of *Bartonella* in the development of stomatitis remains speculative (Quimby *et al.*, 2007; Dowers *et al.*, 2009; Belgard *et al.*, 2010).

Immune system: Although the exact immunological abnormality remains to be identified, the likelihood of an immunological basis for the disease is supported by the fact that cats affected by chronic stomatitis show hyperproteinaemia and polyclonal hypergammaglobulinaemia, with altered levels of serum and salivary IgG, IgM and IgA immunoglobulins (Harley *et al.*, 2003). Furthermore, it has been demonstrated that in healthy cats the cell population of the oral mucosa shows a predominantly Th1 profile of gene expression, and that in individuals with inflammation of the oral mucosa the immunological response switches to a mixed type 1 and type 2 cytokine response as the lesions progress, with higher levels of mRNA for interleukins and interferon gamma (Harley *et al.*, 1999). Generally, elevated levels of the pro-inflammatory serum cytokines TNF-α, IL-1β and IFN-γ and very low IL-6 have been reported in cats with stomatitis (Arzi *et al.*, 2016).

The histological findings on tissue samples obtained from cats with stomatitis also suggest an immune response to chronic antigenic stimulation or an immune dysregulation. On the other hand, it has been demonstrated that neutrophilic function in these cats is normal, and that there is adequate B cell responsiveness, normal absolute counts and ratio of CD4 (helper) and CD8 (cytotoxic) T lymphocytes, or increased levels of CD8 T lymphocytes, supporting the theory that affected cats are not immunosuppressed (Harley *et al.*, 2011; Arzi *et al.*, 2016). A cytotoxic cell-mediated response could be consistent with a viral aetiology (Harley *et al.*, 2011).

Diagnostic evaluation and differential diagnosis: In particularly fractious animals, sedation or general anaesthesia may be necessary to permit a complete oral examination. A diagnosis of stomatitis is usually suspected based on clinical presentation and distribution of the soft tissue lesions involving the gingiva, alveolar mucosa, labial/buccal mucosa and caudal oral mucosa. Typically, inflammation is bilateral and relatively symmetrical (see Figures 8.2 and 8.5). However, a confirmatory biopsy may be indicated in some cases to exclude the presence of autoimmune conditions (e.g. subepithelial blistering diseases with oral involvement) and, particularly if lesions are unilateral, neoplastic disease. The development of malignant oral neoplasms in areas of inflammation has also been reported in chronically affected cats (Anderson, 1996), possibly indicating that stomatitis represents a pre-neoplastic condition. Other differential diagnoses for ST/CS and ST include erythema multiforme, uraemic stomatitis, and, in localized forms, eosinophilic granuloma complex.

Complete blood count, serum chemistry profile, urinalysis and FIV and FeLV serological testing should be performed to evaluate the general condition of the patient and exclude distant organ diseases. Protein electrophoresis may also be indicated. In the majority of cases, neutrophilia with or without a left shift, hyperproteinaemia and hypergammaglobulinaemia are identified. Azotaemia, with elevated urea and creatinine levels, is also frequent. FCV and FHV testing may be performed by polymerase chain reaction (PCR) on samples obtained with a swab or a cytobrush run over the inflamed oral mucosa to collect blood, cells and saliva. To decrease discomfort, the procedure may be performed in the sedated or anaesthetized patient at the time of tooth extraction.

If deemed necessary, a tissue sample is obtained and submitted for histopathological examination. Histologically, acute and chronic inflammatory cells, with a non-specific diffuse submucosal infiltrate of lymphocytes, plasma cells, neutrophils, occasional Mott cells and histiocytes, are normally present, often accompanied by superficial ulceration and a suppurative process (Arzi et al., 2016). An increase in mast cell numbers has also been demonstrated in oral tissues of cats with stomatitis (Arzi et al., 2010, 2016). Interestingly, a recent histological and immunohistochemical study on samples of oral mucosa of specific pathogen-free cats demonstrated regional differences in the distribution of immune cells (Arzi et al., 2011). It remains to be determined if this could have any influence on the development of different inflammatory lesions in stomatitis with and without caudal involvement. Different levels of CD3[+] T cells (in the epithelium and subepithelial stroma) and CD20[+] B cells (in the subepithelial stroma only) have been demonstrated by immunohistochemistry in biopsy samples taken from the oral cavity of cats with stomatitis (Arzi et al., 2016). In cases of clinical remission, these cells appear to be cleared from affected tissues (Arzi et al., 2016).

Treatment: Protocols described in the literature may be difficult to compare with each other and should be evaluated with caution, as cases with oral inflammation but without caudal stomatitis are often included in the study population and/or the lesion distribution and inclusion criteria are not described. Therefore, it is possible that patients with inflammatory diseases other than ST/CS are incorrectly included under the same definition. Indeed, the prognosis in the presence or absence of caudal stomatitis differs significantly, with the former cases being difficult to cure. An effective treatment for all stomatitis cases is currently unavailable. A thorough systematic review of the literature on therapeutic management of the disease has recently been published (Winer et al., 2016). Management of these patients should always aim to:

- Modulate immunological response
- Decrease inflammation and eliminate any inflammatory factors from the oral cavity
- Control plaque bacteria and treat any secondary infections
- Control oral pain and discomfort.

Tooth extraction: In the initial approach to stomatitis, the main goal should be the elimination of any potentially inflammatory stimulus from the oral cavity. It is therefore mandatory to perform a thorough oral examination under general anaesthesia, including dental exploration, periodontal probing, and intraoral radiography of all teeth to detect dental and periodontal disease (tooth resorption, retained roots, alveolar bone loss, endodontic/periapical disease). Complete (i.e. all portions of a tooth) and selective (i.e. diseased teeth) tooth extraction should be performed, accompanied by professional dental cleaning (i.e. supragingival and subgingival plaque and calculus removal, gingival curettage, and polishing) of any remaining teeth. Postoperative adjunctive medical treatment may be prescribed based on the clinical situation of each patient. Home oral hygiene measures should always be recommended to control or prevent plaque and calculus accumulation, but in many stomatitis cases tooth brushing is difficult or impossible to perform. Anti-inflammatory and antimicrobial treatment may be attempted before tooth brushing is established to decrease tissue inflammation and oral discomfort. If home care is not possible or is ineffective, frequent professional dental cleaning may be required.

A conservative approach is rarely effective in ST/CS cats. Without thorough plaque control, the effectiveness of any medical treatment will be significantly decreased or totally impaired, and recurrence will rapidly occur. If so, a more aggressive surgical approach may be necessary. Extraction of (diseased and healthy) teeth that are in contact with soft tissue lesions should therefore be performed. Full-mouth (FME) or partial-mouth (i.e. all premolar and molar teeth) (PME) tooth extraction is recommended in severe and refractory cases and should be performed early in the disease process rather than as the last treatment option after numerous and possibly confounding medical treatments. No other treatment regimen has been shown to provide beneficial results comparable to those achieved with FME or PME, with 30–60% of cases in clinical remission and about 20% of cases significantly improved at the time of follow-up (Hennet, 1997; Druet and Hennet, 2017) (see Figures 8.5, 8.6 and 8.7). Another study found complete resolution (28.4%), substantial clinical improvement (39%), little improvement (26.3%) and no improvement (6.3%) in cats with stomatitis following FME or PME (Jennings et al., 2015). After tooth extraction, the need for medical treatment has also been demonstrated to decrease significantly (Girard and Hennet, 2005). Thus, tooth extraction is a critical and essential step in the treatment of ST/CS. The clinical improvement seen in cats treated by FME or PME is supposedly due to significant reduction of plaque bacteria, removal of diseased teeth causing discomfort and inflammation, and possibly removal of contact between the hard dental surface and the ulcero-proliferative soft tissues. However, a small set of animals may show only little or no improvement (see Figure 8.2), and it is important to discuss this possibility with the pet owner before surgery is performed. Extraction of teeth in contact with mucosal lesions in cases affected by stomatitis without caudal involvement is normally curative, although some cases may require medical treatment for a certain period of time following extraction.

FME may be performed in one stage by an expert veterinary dentist or oral surgeon. Otherwise, it is recommended to first extract diseased teeth and those located near the most severe soft tissue lesions, which in the majority of cases include the premolar and molar teeth.

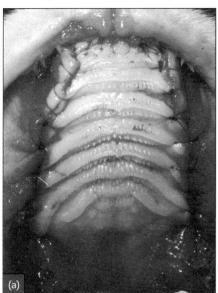
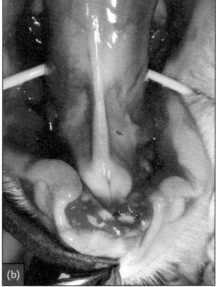

8.6 (a, b) The same patient as in Figure 8.5 immediately following full-mouth tooth extraction. Adjunctive postoperative medical treatment included a short course of oral co-amoxiclav and topical application of 0.12% chlorhexidine gel. Two months after extraction, submucosal inoculation of recombinant feline interferon omega (rFeIFN-ω) was performed, followed by topical oromucosal administration for 3 months.
(© Dr Margherita Gracis)

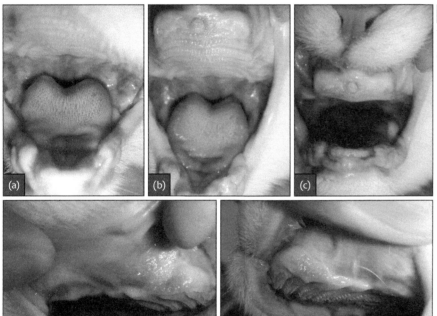

8.7 (a–e) The same patient as in Figures 8.5 and 8.6 at the 8-month postoperative follow-up visit, showing resolution of the inflammatory lesions.
(© Dr Margherita Gracis)

Extraction of canine and incisor teeth may be postponed to a later time. If the rostral alveolar and labial mucosa is not inflamed and extraction of caudal teeth leads to clinical improvement, healthy canine and incisor teeth may be maintained (Jennings et al., 2015; Druet and Hennet, 2017).

Extractions should be performed with an open technique, gently elevating mucoperiosteal flaps, and holding soft tissues with fine instruments or stay sutures. The use of envelope flaps, obtained with a single horizontal incision along the alveolar margin of either the lower or upper dental arch, maximizes blood supply to the tissues and provides sufficient exposure of bone and teeth. Each flap can be extended to include all teeth in a single quadrant or even all teeth in the same dental arch (Figure 8.6). Before suturing, any sharp bony edges are removed with a large round diamond bur, and the flap margins are excised to eliminate highly inflamed and torn tissues. The suture material should be monofilament, fine (1 metric, 5/0 USP) and absorbable (e.g. poliglecaprone 25). A continuous suture pattern is currently not recommended due to the risk of early material dissolution in a heavily inflamed environment. To minimize inflammation during the healing period, rather than waiting for suture dissolution some surgeons prefer to remove the stitches within 1–2 weeks of placement in the sedated patient.

Proliferative inflamed tissue may be excised surgically, using cold scalpel blades or laser technology. The goals of laser surgery are to resolve self-induced trauma and entrapment of food and debris in tissue pockets, stimulate fibrosis to make tissues less prone to inflammation and proliferation, and reduce the bacterial load in the abnormal tissues (Lewis et al., 2007). Multiple treatments may be necessary to achieve satisfactory results. However, very little information has been published on the use of laser surgery in cats with stomatitis, and definitive recommendations on its indications, modality of use and outcome cannot be made.

Perioperative multimodal analgesic treatment in patients undergoing FME or PME is imperative, using local and regional anaesthesia and systemic pain medications. At least one night's hospitalization is recommended before discharge to appropriately control pain and administer supportive care. Adjunctive postoperative medical treatment may be prescribed based on individual needs. If canine and incisor teeth are maintained, daily tooth brushing should be instituted as soon as possible to prevent or minimize plaque accumulation.

Antibiotics and antimicrobials: Antibiotics are only able to temporarily suppress rather than eliminate the resident oral flora and cannot disrupt or eliminate the bacteria of the dental plaque biofilm. Therefore, as a single treatment modality they may have limited effect, with quick and frequent relapses in both ST/CS and ST cats. However, they may be indicated as adjunctive treatment. Antibiotics with activity against Gram-negative and anaerobic bacteria, such as co-amoxiclav (amoxicillin/clavulanic acid), metronidazole (with or without spiramycin), and clindamycin may be used.

The topical use of 0.05–0.12% chlorhexidine digluconate solution or gel may be recommended. Chlorhexidine is a synthetic antimicrobial agent with a large spectrum and non-specific mechanism of action. It shows substantivity, being able to adhere to oral tissues and remain active for 8–12 hours. Unfortunately, cats rarely tolerate its long-term oral application. Zinc ascorbate gel may also be used as an oral antiseptic.

Anti-inflammatory, immunosuppressive and immunomodulatory drugs: The use of immunosuppressive drugs in FHV- and FCV-positive cats carries the risk of exacerbating the disease and should therefore be considered with caution. If glucocorticoids are utilized, anti-inflammatory doses of short-lasting formulations are preferable to immunosuppressive doses of long-lasting molecules. Tapering doses should be prescribed and frequent re-examinations performed, determining the lowest effective dose. Although in most patients the effect of glucocorticoids is immediate, with diminished inflammation and reduced pain, with long-term treatment a decrease in effectiveness is common. The use of these molecules should therefore be reserved for critical, anorexic patients and when other treatment protocols have failed. They should possibly be used for short periods of time but certainly not as an alternative to FME or PME. The value of a transdermal glucocorticoid-containing ointment has not been evaluated scientifically, but the authors have witnessed promising clinical results in some patients with refractory disease that are unwilling to receive oral medications. The ointment is produced by a compounding pharmacy and applied to the pinnae of the ears (the person applying it must wear gloves and alternate between pinnae with each application). Interestingly, a recent study evaluating ciclosporin treatment in cats with stomatitis has shown greater improvement in cats that have never received steroids prior to entering the study compared with cats that had previously been administered steroids (Lommer, 2013b).

There is increased evidence that, with appropriate precautions, some non-steroidal anti-inflammatory drugs (NSAIDs) may be used long term to treat chronic pain in cats (Sparkes *et al.*, 2010). Meloxicam, a COX-2 preferential NSAID, has been licensed in various countries for this use, and robenacoxib, a COX-2 selective NSAID, is authorized for treatment for up to 6 days. Titration to the lowest effective dose should also be recommended when using

NSAIDs. Some clinicians administer anti-inflammatory drugs in the preoperative period to decrease tissue inflammation and friability, thus facilitating handling of the flaps during FME or PME.

The use of oral microemulsified ciclosporin following tooth extraction has recently been reported in the treatment of chronic, refractory stomatitis in FIV/FeLV-negative cats (Lommer, 2013b). A significant difference in the activity level of the patient and the clinical findings was demonstrated between treated and placebo groups. An association between trough whole-blood ciclosporin level and improvement in oral inflammation was also shown (i.e. 72.3% of improvement in cats with trough whole-blood ciclosporin level >300 ng/ml as compared with 28.2% of improvement in cats with trough whole-blood ciclosporin level <300 ng/ml).

Thalidomide, an immunosuppressive agent with immunomodulatory, anti-inflammatory and antineoplastic activity, was used in one ST/CS cat in addition to lactoferrin, a glycoprotein with antimicrobial activity (Addie *et al.*, 2003). Although clinical signs resolved after 15 months of titrated treatment, definitive conclusions on the effectiveness of this treatment protocol cannot be drawn at this time.

Recombinant feline interferon omega (rFeIFN-ω) is a type I interferon with antiviral, antiproliferative, anti-inflammatory and immune regulatory functions. It has been shown to improve clinical signs (including oral ulcers/gingivitis and caudal stomatitis), reduce concurrent viral excretion in cats naturally infected with retrovirus (Gil *et al.*, 2012), and have beneficial effects in feline herpesvirus type 1 (FHV-1), feline coronavirus (FCoV), feline parvovirus (FPV) and feline calicivirus (FCV) infected or co-infected cats. Specific studies on rFeIFN-ω treatment of ST/CS populations are scarce, but promising. Subcutaneous, topical oromucosal, and perilesional or submucosal/subgingival routes of administration have been used and may all potentially be effective. Improvement or resolution of ST/CS has been reported in animals refractory to tooth extraction following rFeIFN-ω treatment (Southerden and Gorrel, 2007; Camy, 2010; Gracis *et al.*, 2010; Hennet *et al.*, 2011). A randomized, multi-centre, controlled, double-blind study showed significant improvement of clinical lesions (caudal stomatitis and alveolar/buccal mucositis) and decrease in pain level in cats treated by daily topical oromucosal administration of 0.1 MU of rFeIFN-ω for 90 days (Hennet *et al.*, 2011). The rFeIFN-ω treatment was found to be at least as good as short-term oral administration of a tapering anti-inflammatory dose of prednisolone. Topical oromucosal administration is achieved by slowly dispensing the solution under the cheek tissues, while maintaining the cat with its mouth closed for 30–60 seconds. Maximizing mucosal contact is important, as the beneficial effects of orally administered interferon are mediated via interactions with mucosal lymphoid tissues, and this cytokine is actually destroyed during transit through the digestive tract, if ingested. Adjunctive treatment with antibiotic and anti-inflammatory drugs may be necessary during the first couple of weeks of rFeIFN-ω treatment because of the slow onset of its clinical effect (Hennet *et al.*, 2011).

Mesenchymal stem cell therapy represents a new, promising, immunomodulatory treatment modality. A recent study described the use of fresh, autologous adipose-derived mesenchymal stem cells administered intravenously to seven cats with refractory stomatitis (Arzi *et al.*, 2016). Complete remission was shown in three cases, substantial clinical improvement was seen in two cases, and a lack of response was evident in two cases.

Interestingly, the study also demonstrated a different level of systemic immunomodulation between the patients that responded to the treatment (reduction in total circulating CD8$^+$ T cells, resolution of neutrophilia, reduction of IL-1β and IFN-γ, and an increase in serum IL-6 levels) and those which did not. More significantly, the blood level of cytotoxic CD8 T cells with low expression of CD8 (CD8^{lo}) was identified as a potential biomarker that could be used to predict the patient response to treatment, with cats with low levels of CD8^{lo} responding considerably better (Arzi et al., 2016).

Analgesics: Pain control in cats with stomatitis is paramount. Chronic pain can be very debilitating and has a negative impact on the patient's general wellbeing. A multimodal approach is recommended, with administration of NSAIDs as well as opioids (e.g. buprenorphine, tramadol, fentanyl) and/or other medications (e.g. gabapentin). Buprenorphine is a partial mu agonist and 100% bioavailable via the transmucosal route; sublingual or buccal administration is very effective in cats.

Palmitoylethanolamide (PEA), an endogenous fatty acid amide analogue of the endocannabinoid anandamide with anti-inflammatory and antinociceptive properties, has been shown to be effective in treating chronic pain in human patients and may represent an additional treatment modality in cats as well (Re et al., 2007; Gatti et al., 2012). Although clinical studies demonstrating the effectiveness of acupuncture and laser therapy in cats with stomatitis are lacking, these may also represent valid adjunctive modalities to control pain and/or promote tissue healing (Bellows, 2013; Fry et al., 2014).

Diet: The role of diet in the management of stomatitis is unknown, and there are no data showing specific benefits of any particular micronutrient. A recent study showed no influence of two diets with different omega-6/omega-3 polyunsaturated fatty acid ratios on inflammation or wound healing in affected cats following PME (Corbee et al., 2012).

A variety of high-quality foods should be offered to patients to stimulate appetite and food ingestion, aid healing following tooth extraction, and encourage an effective immunological response. Interestingly, many affected cats prefer eating dry kibble rather than soft, canned food.

Prognosis: Prognosis of ST/CS is always guarded, as it is currently impossible to predict treatment response for any single patient. Although specific scientific data are limited or unavailable, negative prognostic factors may include a long history of glucocorticoid treatment and the presence of severe, diffuse mucosal proliferations, possibly also denoting long duration of the inflammatory lesions. The later proper treatment is initiated, the more difficult the resolution of the clinical signs may become. It is therefore strongly recommended to avoid long and repeated attempts of various medical treatments before tooth extraction is finally performed. It must also be considered that although a certain degree of inflammation may last for variable periods of time following tooth extraction, most patients can live a relatively comfortable life when properly treated.

Prognosis for ST is more predictable. The lack of caudal stomatitis in cats with inflammation of the gingiva, alveolar and vestibular mucosa is a positive prognostic factor, with resolution of clinical signs in most cases following tooth extraction and appropriate medical treatment (Figure 8.8).

Monitoring disease progress: Owners should be advised to keep a daily journal to record treatments applied and any changes in behaviour and demeanour. This information may become of great importance in long-standing, refractory cases and possibly help recognize the best treatment modality for any single patient. The use of an evaluation form with a list of specific questions for the owner concerning activity level and perceived comfort of the cat, and the use of a predetermined evaluation scale for clinical signs are also helpful to obtain objective data on disease progress at each follow-up visit. Examples of important

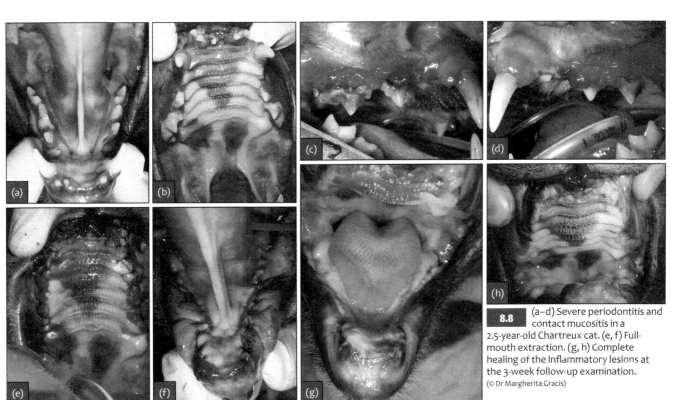

8.8 (a–d) Severe periodontitis and contact mucositis in a 2.5-year-old Chartreux cat. (e, f) Full-mouth extraction. (g, h) Complete healing of the Inflammatory lesions at the 3-week follow-up examination.
(© Dr Margherita Gracis)

clinical information to be collected include the weight of the patient, the size of regional lymph nodes, the presence of ptyalism, the degree of inflammation in specific areas of the oral cavity, and the ability to open the mouth without causing a pain reaction. Owners should be questioned about appetite and activity levels, grooming behaviour, ability to yawn, and social behaviour of the cat at home.

Canine chronic ulcerative stomatitis

Canine chronic ulcerative stomatitis (CCUS) and chronic ulcerative paradental stomatitis (CUPS) are inflammatory oral diseases of dogs that are sometimes classified separately (Caiafa, 2007). However, their clinical presentation, histological features, prognosis and treatment options are comparable. Aetiology, although still only partially known, is also probably similar. They may, therefore, just be expressions of the same disease, and they are discussed here as one pathological entity (Anderson *et al.*, 2017).

CCUS affects adult dogs of any breed and sex, although small to medium breeds such as Maltese, Cocker Spaniels and terriers seem to be over-represented (Anderson *et al.*, 2017). An allergic hypersensitivity or intolerance to dental plaque has long been thought to be a key factor in the development of the disease, possibly similar to ST in cats (Lommer, 2013). However, a recent study has shown common clinical and histopathological features to human oral lichen planus, a chronic inflammatory disorder considered to be a T-cell mediated auto-immune disease (Anderson *et al.*, 2017). In dogs it is characterized clinically by contact mucositis, comprising inflammation and ulceration of the mucosa in contact with the surface of teeth affected by periodontitis or even those just showing plaque and calculus accumulation (Figure 8.9). In fact, most patients only show mild periodontitis (Anderson *et al.*, 2017). The alveolar, labial and buccal mucosa, the palatal mucosa along the dental arches, and the lateral margins of the tongue adjacent to the teeth may be affected, with variable distribution of lesions that are, however, often bilateral and symmetrical (Figures 8.9 and 8.10). There may be localized vestibular contact ulcers (also called 'kissing lesions') facing a few teeth (Figure 8.11) or diffuse ulceration of the tissues, especially in the cheek area (Figure 8.12). The gingiva is also frequently involved (see Figure 8.9). Typically, the maxillary soft tissues (particularly next to the canine and carnassial teeth) are more commonly affected than the mandibular soft tissues, possibly because of a different degree of mucosa-to-tooth contact (see Figure 8.9). However, the mucosa and mucocutaneous junction labial to the mandibular canine teeth are also frequently affected. When involved, the mucocutaneous junction of the lips may initially lose its pigmentation. The lesions may then progress to frank tissue loss (i.e. loss of the labial papillae or even more severe lesions) (Figure 8.13). Intertrigo and dermatitis of the lower lip secondary to drooling (Figure 8.13) and regional lymphadenomegaly are also common findings. The lesions may appear as ulcers, erosions with a pseudomembranous change, or as lesions showing a reticular/lichenoid pattern (i.e. lace-like white lesions), and in some cases affect the mucosa at edentulous areas as well (Anderson *et al.*, 2017).

Clinical signs include depression, anorexia, inability to fully open the mouth, restricted yawning, drooling and severe halitosis. Signs of primary or secondary periodontitis are present in the majority of cases. In chronic cases, severe scarring of the mucosal tissues at the lip commissures may reduce the ability or willingness to open

the mouth, which in turns leads to decreased chewing activity and further plaque accumulation, thus creating a vicious cycle. In some instances, tissue necrosis may develop, with formation of ulcers that are covered by a yellowish to greyish pseudomembranous debris (Figure 8.14). A foul odour, drooling of ropy saliva and severe oral

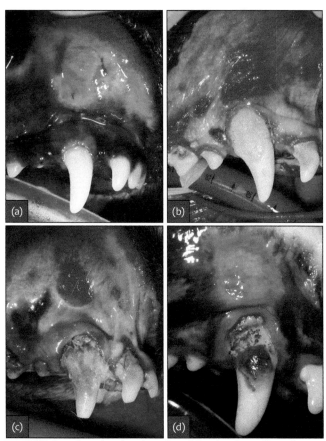

8.9 Four dogs showing ulceration of the alveolar and buccal mucosa facing the right maxillary canine tooth with different degrees of plaque and calculus accumulation as well as periodontitis: (a) mild, (b, c) moderate, (d) severe.
(© Dr Margherita Gracis)

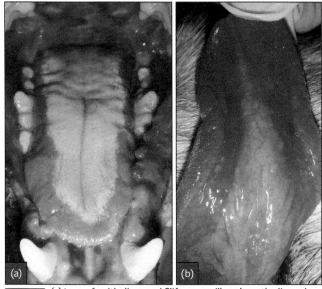

8.10 (a) Loss of epithelium and filiform papillae along the lingual margin in an 11-year-old crossbreed dog. (b) Ulceration of the ventral surface of the tongue in an 11-year-old Yorkshire Terrier.
(© Dr Margherita Gracis)

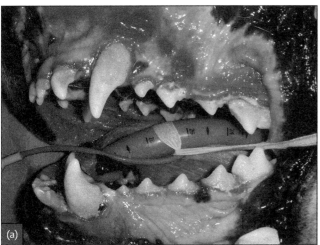
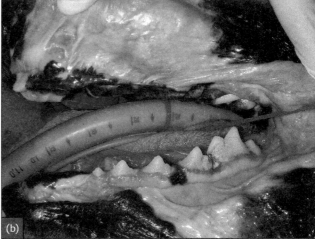

8.11 (a) Severe periodontitis and contact ulcerations in an 11-year-old Basset Hound. (b) At the 1-year follow-up examination, showing complete healing of the ulcerative lesions following selective tooth extraction.
(© Dr Margherita Gracis)

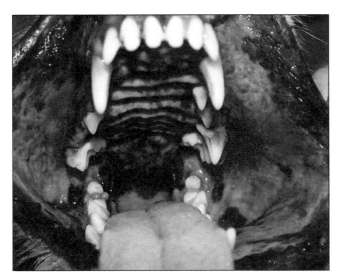

8.12 A 9-year-old Cocker Spaniel with bilateral generalized ulceration of the buccal mucosa.
(© Dr Margherita Gracis)

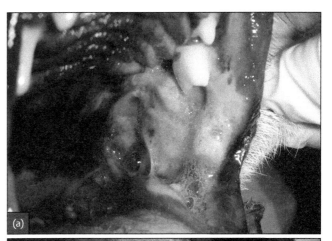
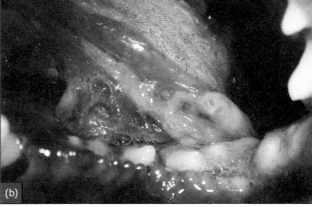

8.14 A 12-year-old Miniature Pinscher with chronic plaque-associated ulcerative gingivostomatitis complicated by necrosis. (a) Left buccal mucosa. (b) Left side of the tongue.
(© Dr Margherita Gracis)

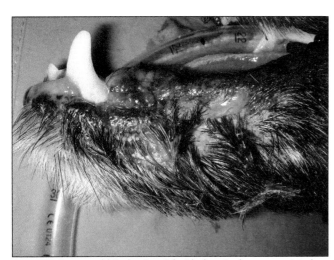

8.13 A 9-year-old Cocker Spaniel with chronic plaque-associated ulcerative stomatitis, showing dermatitis of the lower lip and loss of the mucocutaneous junction adjacent to the left mandibular canine tooth.
(© Dr Margherita Gracis)

pain are typical in these cases. It is unknown if involvement of the jaw bones (osteomyelitis and osteonecrosis) seen in certain stomatitis cases (particularly in the Cocker Spaniel) is a complicating factor of chronic plaque-associated ulcerative stomatitis or if it represents a different disease entity.

Diagnosis: Differential diagnoses include uraemic ulcers and ulcers secondary to leptospirosis, mucositis secondary to contact with various irritants (e.g. toxins, chemicals and plants), epidermal necrolysis secondary to medication and adverse drug reaction, stomatitis secondary to chemo-therapy, radiation therapy or chrysotherapy, autoimmune diseases, epitheliotropic T-cell lymphoma (mycosis fungoides), eosinophilic granuloma (in localized cases), traumatic mucositis, and electrical and thermal burns.

Diagnosis is based on detailed history, complete physical examination, clinical appearance and distribution of lesions, laboratory test results (complete blood count, serum chemistry profile and urinalysis), histopathological examination of tissue samples and treatment outcome. Histopathological and immunohistochemical features have recently been described and support the hypothesis of an immune-mediated pathogenesis (Anderson et al., 2017). Findings included a dense lichenoid lymphocytic-plasma-cytic infiltrate at the interface between the mucosal epithe-lium and subepithelial connective tissue, represented by B cells, plasma cells, T cells, T regulatory cells and IL-17-producing non-T cells (interface mucositis). Histologically, saw tooth rete ridge hyperplasia, basal cell vacuolization and apoptosis, cell degeneration/spongiosis, erosion and ulceration were common in the epithelium. Granulomatous changes, perivascular inflammation, suppurative inflamma-tion, necrosis and pseudomembrane formation, lymphoid nodules and mast cells were common in the subepithelium (Anderson et al., 2017).

Treatment: In mild cases, extraction of diseased teeth and periodic professional periodontal treatments (supra-gingival and subgingival plaque and calculus removal followed by polishing of teeth), accompanied by thorough and meticulous home oral hygiene (i.e. daily tooth brush-ing using antiseptics such as chlorhexidine gels or solu-tions, use of dental diets and specific treats/chews/toys) may favour healing of existing lesions and prevent devel-opment of new lesions. Compliance with home care is a key point, as in predisposed individuals even a mild accu-mulation of dental plaque may induce the development of contact ulcers. Adjunctive medical treatment may be necessary in some cases, including broad-spectrum anti-biotics, immunosuppressive or anti-inflammatory drugs and analgesics. There is evidence that the use of tapering doses of ciclosporin in adjunct to daily tooth brushing may be effective in some cases.

If conservative treatment is ineffective and in advanced cases, selective (i.e. diseased teeth and teeth next to the contact lesions) or full-mouth tooth extraction may be nec-essary to achieve healing and long-term control of the disease. Prognosis following tooth extraction is generally good to excellent. If any teeth are preserved, then home care measures should be implemented as described above. Frequent follow-up examinations should be planned to evaluate brushing efficiency and owner's com-pliance. Adjunctive and supportive medical treatments are normally indicated in the postoperative period until resolu-tion of clinical signs.

If osteomyelitis is present, thorough surgical curettage of necrotic tissues must be performed, and the surgical site closed with mucoperiosteal flaps. Aerobic and anaer-obic culture and antibiotic sensitivity testing may be indicated, although specific pathogens have not been identified in these patients; empirical use of antibiotics effi-cacious against Gram-negative anaerobic bacteria may therefore be acceptable. Co-amoxiclav, metronidazole (with or without spiramycin), clindamycin, cephalosporins and tetracyclines are possible choices. However, medical management of CCUS may also be considered. Two differ-ent regimens that focus on immune modulation and con-trolling inflammation are proposed. A recent clinical trial utilizing ciclosporin at 5 mg/kg q24h and metronidazole at 15 mg/kg q24h in 10 dogs with CCUS has resulted in clinical remissions (personal communication Drs K Ford, B Stapleton and J Anderson). Alternatively, a therapeutic regimen made up of pentoxifylline (20 mg/kg), doxycycline (5 mg/kg) and niacinamide (at 200–250 mg) given twice daily following a comprehensive oral health assessment and treatment, including extraction of hopeless teeth, has also been used successfully (personal communication, Dr J Anderson). Ongoing immunohistochemical and immuno-fluorescence research supports the positive response that these regimens may have in CCUS pathogenesis.

Erythema multiforme and toxic epidermal necrolysis

Erythema multiforme (EM) is an uncommon to rare mucosal and/or mucocutaneous disorder. It is probably an immune-mediated disease (Nemec et al., 2012), which may result from a host-specific cytotoxic T-lymphocyte attack on keratinocytes expressing non-self antigens that are typi-cally derived from drugs (Voie et al., 2012), microbes (Woldemeskel et al., 2011) or neoplasia (Tepper et al., 2011).

Clinically, EM manifests as a vesiculo-ulcerative disease of skin and/or mucous membranes, including the oral mucosal linings. It may display a wide spectrum of clinical manifestations, ranging from a mild ulcerative disease which might resolve spontaneously, particularly if the incit-ing cause is identified and treated (e.g. drug withdrawal), to a more aggressive ulcerative form known as toxic epider-mal necrolysis (TEN), affecting the skin and most of the mucus membranes with systemic clinical signs such as haemorrhagic diarrhoea or sepsis (Figure 8.15). Involvement of the oral cavity is described in approximately one-third of EM-TEN cases. Dysphagia and/or drooling secondary to oral ulceration may be the primary complaint at presen-tation. Lesions restricted to the oral cavity seem to be very rare in dogs compared with human beings (Nemec et al., 2012).

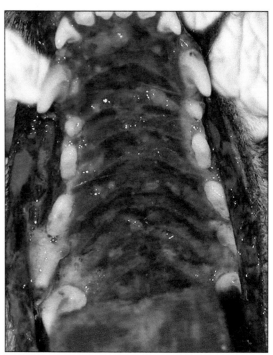

8.15 Ulcerative glossitis and stomatitis in an adult male crossbreed dog with toxic epidermal necrolysis associated with drug reaction to trimethoprim-sulfamethoxazole.
(© Dr Fabia Scarampella)

Diagnosis should be based on histopathological findings (Gross *et al.*, 2005; Yager, 2014). In some cases, it may be difficult to distinguish EM from epitheliotropic T-cell lymphoma (ETCL). Immunohistochemistry allows the identification of more abundant intraepithelial and mucosal lymphocytes (CD[3]-positive T cells) in ETCL cases (Nemec *et al.*, 2012). Proper diagnosis is crucial because mild cases of EM may resolve once the triggering factor is removed. Conversely, the prognosis for ETCL is poor, and TEN may be a life-threatening disease. These cases are a therapeutic challenge, and the response to immunosuppressive drugs such as glucocorticoids is often poor. Administration of human intravenous immunoglobulins may comprise part of the treatment plan for severe EM cases (Nuttall and Malham, 2004).

Subepithelial blistering diseases

Subepithelial blistering diseases (SBD) are a group of very rare mucosal and/or mucocutaneous conditions in dogs and cats, resulting from the disruption of the complex interaction between intra- and extracellular molecules in the epidermis or mucosal epithelial–dermal junction (Olivry *et al.*, 2010). This disruption may be the consequence of mutations of genes encoding many basement membrane proteins, resulting in hereditary epidermolysis bullosa (HEB). The same epidermal basement membrane proteins may also be targeted by autoantibodies in several distinct autoimmune subepithelial blistering diseases (AISBDs) (Olivry *et al.*, 2010). In humans and animals, the most common AISBDs include bullous pemphigoid (BP; main target is collagen XVII) and epidermolysis bullosa acquisita (EBA; target is collagen VII). Additionally, mucus membrane pemphigoid (MMP) is a clinically distinctive AISBD of humans, dogs and cats in which the autoimmune response is heterogeneous, with several basement membrane proteins (e.g. collagen XVII, collagen VII, integrin alpha-6/beta-4, laminin isoforms) targeted by autoantibodies.

SBDs are clinically characterized by the presence of tense vesicles that rapidly evolve to form extensive erosions and ulcers. Lesions may develop in the skin and/or mucocutaneous junctions, also involving the mucosa of the oral cavity (palate, gingiva and tongue) in approximately 50–60% of patients.

The distribution of the lesions is an important differential factor. In particular, MMP is a symmetrical mucosa-dominated disease that often spares the foot pads, whereas involvement of cutaneous areas exposed to friction and trauma (ear pinnae, foot pads and sometimes the skin of the axillae, groin and abdomen) is more common in EBA. In BP, skin lesions are predominant and do not tend to develop in areas of friction or those prone to trauma. Lesions restricted to the oral cavity only have not been reported with any subepithelial blistering disease.

Diagnosis is achieved by combining clinical signs and results of histopathological examination. It is not always possible to histologically diagnose individual AISBDs (Gross *et al.*, 2005). However, historical information, such as early age of onset, may suggest HEB. Moreover, many of the autoimmune blistering skin diseases exhibit a strong breed predisposition (e.g. Great Dane and EBA, German Shepherd and MMP) (Bizikova *et al.*, 2015). Immunological studies for detection of *in situ* or circulating autoantibodies directed against basement membrane components are needed for an accurate diagnosis of AISBDs.

There is no specific treatment for HEB. Treatment response and outcome of AISBDs to immunosuppressive protocols, such as systemic glucocorticoids alone (2.2 mg/kg daily of prednisolone or prednisone orally for induction) or in combination with azathioprine (2 mg/kg daily induction dose), tetracycline and niacinamide or doxycycline, appear to be heterogeneous, and generalizations cannot be made. Even though the prognosis for this group of diseases is not well known in dogs and cats, these diseases are considered severe and difficult to treat.

Pemphigus

Pemphigus is a group of acquired autoimmune pustular diseases of the skin and mucus membranes reported in both dogs and cats. It is thought that autoreactive IgG against the extracellular domains of desmosomal cell–cell adhesion molecules, expressed predominantly in stratified squamous epithelia, disrupts intercellular adhesion and leads to the development of intraepithelial pustules in the skin and mucus membranes (Nishifuji *et al.*, 2007).

Classically, pemphigus is divided into two major subtypes, according to the depth of the lesions in the epithelium: a superficial form, pemphigus foliaceus (PF), and a deeper form, pemphigus vulgaris (PV). Another uncommon subtype named paraneoplastic pemphigus (PNP) has been described in dogs (Gross *et al.*, 2005). A major autoantigen in canine PF has recently been identified as desmocollin-1 (Bizikova *et al.*, 2012), whereas anti-desmoglein-3 IgG antibodies capable of dissociating keratinocytes are found in dogs with PV and PNP (Nishifuji *et al.*, 2007). Moreover, autoantibodies to members of the plakin family have been identified in two PNP cases. Although naturally occurring pemphigus is associated with autoreactive IgG, drug-induced PV and PF have also been described in dogs and cats (Horvath *et al.*, 2007; Rybnicek and Hill, 2007).

Clinically, PF is a pustulo-crusting cutaneous disease affecting mainly facial and foot pad skin. Mucosal lesions in PF are rare, being reported in approximately 2% of dogs with this condition (Mueller *et al.*, 2006). However, drug-triggered PF manifests unusual features, such as more severe oral lesions.

PV and PNP are clinically more severe and are characterized by an ulcerative dermatitis affecting concave pinnae and auditory orifices, nasal planum, periocular skin, lip margins, genitalia, anus and haired skin. Most affected dogs and cats have lesions affecting the oral cavity (tongue, palate and gingiva) at the time of diagnosis. Although rare, lesions of PV may first develop in the oral cavity or at mucocutaneous junctions and then progress to haired skin. Thick, ropy, tenacious, odorous saliva is an additional feature. Definitive diagnosis is achieved by means of histopathological examination of cutaneous or oral tissue samples.

The prognosis for PF is generally good because patients usually respond to immunosuppressive protocols of prednisone (prednisolone) or methylprednisolone (2–6 mg/kg administered orally once or twice daily) alone or in combination with azathioprine (1.5–2.5 mg/kg daily) or clorambucil (0.1–0.2 mg/kg daily). Once control is achieved, both drugs are tapered, with the desired maintenance regime of alternate-day administration. Despite aggressive therapy with a combination of glucocorticoids and azathioprine or chlorambucil, the prognosis for PV is poor. PNP carries a very poor prognosis.

Other ulcerative oral conditions

Other less common conditions may cause oral ulceration. Most of these conditions are not restricted to the oral cavity, and oral signs are usually not the primary complaint. In fact, oral lesions may represent incidental findings in patients displaying other systemic and/or cutaneous clinical signs.

Cutaneous vasculitis: This is a disease where blood vessel walls are the targets of an inflammatory response. Oral ulcerative lesions in cases of cutaneous vasculitis are rare, and when present may cause the animal to salivate, become anorexic, or to be reluctant to open its mouth (Innerå, 2013).

Focal necrotic, crusty and desquamative areas on the tips of the ears, tail and distal extremities clinically characterize cutaneous vasculitis. Moreover, a multifocal alopecia with non-inflamed, atrophic and shiny skin and/or small circular cutaneous ulcers may be observed without any particular distribution. Occasionally, immune-mediated polyarthritis, uveitis and glomerulonephritis are also present and musculoskeletal, cardiovascular, gastrointestinal and neurological signs may be associated. When cutaneous vasculitis is clinically suspected, diseases or conditions causing circulating immune complexes (e.g. vector-borne infectious diseases including leishmaniosis, ehrlichiosis/anaplasmosis, rickettsiosis, babesiosis; systemic lupus erythematosus; adverse drug or vaccine reactions) need to be excluded before performing histopathological examination of skin and oral tissue samples. Due to the fact that inflammatory damage of vessels is transient, cutaneous vasculitis is rarely confirmed histologically.

Chemotherapy: Chemotherapy-associated oral ulceration may be quite severe in humans, and many chemotherapeutic regimes have been implicated. In animals, several anticancer drugs (e.g. methotrexate and 5-fluorouracil) can produce ulcerative stomatitis and enteritis together with diarrhoea and vomiting (Coppoc, 2009). However, chemotherapeutic drug toxicity appears to be less prevalent in animals than in humans.

Radiation therapy: Mucositis is a common acute side effect of radiation therapy that includes the oral and perioral regions in the radiation field (Pruitt and Thrall, 2011). Treatment includes gentle local cleansing and rinsing and the prescription of antibiotic, anti-inflammatory and analgesic medications. The use of compounded mouth washes containing various percentages of local anaesthetic gels (e.g. 2% lidocaine), antacids and protectants of the mucosa, and antihistamine drugs may also be recommended. Osteoradionecrosis, periodontal disease and xerostomia (dry mouth) may develop as late radiation effects.

Uraemic stomatitis: This is a disorder associated with uraemia in animals affected by renal failure. As with other manifestations of uraemia, it may be considered to be an intoxication secondary to the combined effects of metabolites retained as a result of loss of renal function. The oral lesions include erosions and ulcers of the oral mucosa and tongue that may progress to tissue necrosis, mucosal sloughing and haemorrhage. Clinical signs result from increased excretion of urea in the oral cavity, metabolism of urea to ammonia compounds by bacterial urease, and consequent tissue damage. Xerostomia and clotting deficiencies related to uraemia also contribute to the development of oral lesions. It is necessary to control renal disease to achieve resolution of uraemic stomatitis. Supportive treatment, including antibiotic, anti-inflammatory and analgesic medications, may be administered to control secondary infections and oral pain.

Candidiasis: This is a rare opportunistic fungal infection reported in dogs and cats secondary to immunosuppressive treatment and debilitating systemic diseases. Many drugs acting systemically can alter the ecosystem of the oral cavity (e.g. prolonged broad-spectrum antibiotic therapy) or depress the immune system of the animal (e.g. immunosuppressive agents), thus increasing susceptibility to oral infections. The oral mucosa, mucocutaneous junctions and distal extremities are commonly involved, but other cutaneous locations are also possible. Clinically, oral candidiasis manifests as a non-healing ulcer or erosion, covered by a whitish to greyish adherent, foul-smelling exudate (Jadhav and Pal, 2006).

Epitheliotropic T-cell lymphoma (ETCL): This is an uncommon, cutaneous neoplastic disease of dogs and cats, usually of T-lymphocyte origin (see Chapter 11). It is not an inflammatory disease, but should be considered in the differential diagnosis of ulcerative oral conditions because mucosal and mucocutaneous erythema, depigmentation and ulceration may develop in about 40% of cases. It can be misdiagnosed as chronic inflammatory mucocutaneous dermatitis or stomatitis of immune-mediated origin (Figure 8.16). Diagnosis is based on histopathological findings and demonstration of clonal T-cell receptor (TCR) rearrangement. Another important

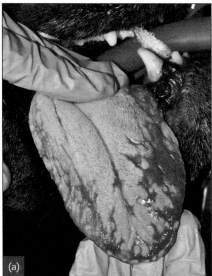
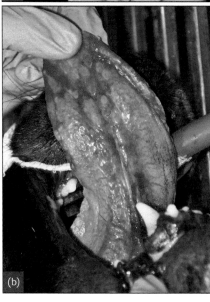

8.16 (a) Dorsal and (b) ventral views of ulcerative lesions on the tongue of a 9-year-old male Labrador Retriever affected by epitheliotropic T-cell lymphoma. (© Dr Laura Ordeix)

differential diagnosis is erythema multiforme. Immuno-histochemistry and clonality testing may be necessary but are sometimes not sufficient to reach a definitive diagnosis in these cases (Nemec *et al.*, 2012).

Other causes of oral ulceration: Other unusual causative factors of oral erythema, ulceration and erosion include the ingestion of harlequin (Asian) ladybirds (*Harmonia axyrids*) (Stocks and Lindsey, 2008); contact and ingestion of fox tails and burdock (Thiverge, 1973); contact with the hairs of certain caterpillars (Niza *et al.*, 2012); wood poisoning caused by shavings of the plant *Simarouba amara* (Declerq, 2004); the use of pancreatic enzyme supplementation (Snead, 2006); chemical exposure; thermal injury (Mackenzie *et al.*, 2012); electrical burns; and trauma. Treatment is directed towards the removal of the aetiological factor.

Nodular lesions
Traumatic mucogingival proliferative lesions

Ulcero-proliferative lesions of the mucosa may develop following occlusal contact with the teeth of the opposite arch (Figure 8.17). In cats, most frequently these develop in the alveolar or buccal mucosa buccal or distobuccal to the mandibular first molar tooth, from repeated trauma by the maxillary fourth premolar tooth and/or the first molar tooth (Collados Soto, 2009; Lyon and Okuda, 2009; Bellows, 2010; Gracis *et al.*, 2013; Riehl *et al.*, 2014). Other locations are also possible (Gracis *et al.*, 2013). These lesions have characteristics in common with reactive oral pyogenic granuloma in humans (Riehl *et al.*, 2014). Despite a clinically indistinguishable appearance, two different microscopic patterns, one dominated by a lymphoplasmacytic inflammatory component and one by a fibrovascular proliferation, have been described (Gracis *et al.*, 2013). Surgical excision of the lesion is not usually sufficient to avoid recurrence. After surgical excision of the lesion, blunting of the pointed cusps of involved teeth may give a better prognosis, while extraction of these teeth has been reported to be 100% effective (Gracis *et al.*, 2013).

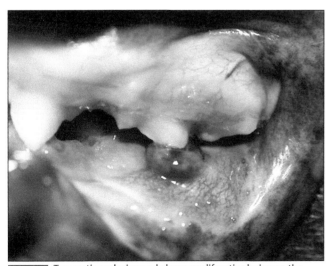

8.17 Traumatic occlusion and ulcero-proliferative lesion on the mucosa buccal to the left mandibular first molar tooth, in contact with the cusp of the maxillary fourth premolar tooth, in a 5-month-old male Chartreux cat.
(© Dr Margherita Gracis)

Feline oral eosinophilic granuloma

Oral eosinophilic granuloma (OEG) is traditionally considered to be a lesion of the feline eosinophilic granuloma complex (FeEGC). Variably eroded or ulcerated nodules with a white to orange/yellow surface clinically characterize OEG. The nodules may be localized on the tongue, hard or soft palate, and/or palatoglossal folds (Figure 8.18). OEG can be the only clinical sign, or may be associated with other FeEGC lesions and/or other dermatological manifestations of hypersensitivity skin reactions (e.g. auto-induced alopecia).

Importantly, FeEGC does not represent a specific dermatological diagnosis, and numerous aetiological factors have been proposed as potential causes (Buckley and Nuttall, 2012). It is suggested to be a non-specific mucosal and mucocutanous reactive condition associated with hypersensitivities, principally to arthropods, environmental allergens or foods, or of idiopathic origin.

Diagnosis of OEG is based on the clinical appearance and cytological and/or histopathological examination. Histopathological features are similar to other FeEGC lesions, namely an eosinophil-rich infiltrate. Deeply embedded hair shafts or insect parts within the inflammatory infiltrate have been described in some OEG (Gross *et al.*, 2005; Bloom, 2006) (Figure 8.19). These findings may suggest a local host reaction to foreign antigens (i.e. hair fragments or arthropod particles) possibly introduced via superficial tissue breakdown following trauma. Assessment and management of potential underlying aetiological factors is indicated. Idiopathic cases may require long-term symptomatic treatment with glucocorticoids or ciclosporin (Buckley and Nuttall, 2012).

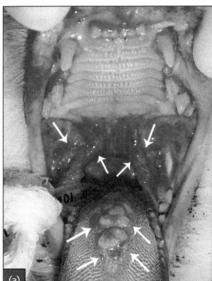

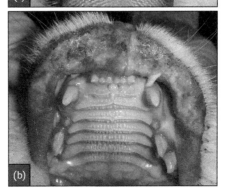

8.18 Oral eosinophilic granuloma in a 7.5-year-old neutered female Domestic Shorthaired cat. (a) Several nodular lesions are present on the tongue and palatoglossal folds (arrowed). (b) An extensive ulcerated plaque is also present on the upper lip.
(© Dr Margherita Gracis)

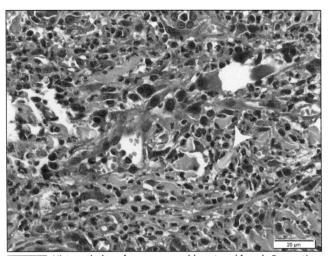

8.19 Histopathology from a 3-year-old neutered female Domestic Shorthaired cat with an eosinophilic granuloma on the tongue, showing an eosinophil-rich mucosal infiltrate with granulomatous reaction and deeply embedded material suggestive of an insect part (arrowhead).
(© Dr Laura Ordeix)

Canine oral eosinophilic granuloma

Oral eosinophilic granuloma is an uncommon disease in dogs. As described for its feline counterpart, canine OEG should be thought of as a reaction pattern to a variety of different stimuli rather than a disease. A genetic basis is suspected in the Siberian Husky, German Shepherd and Cavalier King Charles Spaniel (van Duijn, 1995; Bredal *et al.*, 1996). In non-genetically predisposed breeds, OEG is thought to occur as the result of local reaction or trauma with consequent foreign body entrapment (e.g. biting at bees, wasps or hornets).

Dogs may be presented with signs of clearing the throat, difficulty eating and swallowing, or coughing during and after eating (Lommer, 2013a). The disease is characterized by single or multiple ulcerated plaques or nodules that are located on the lateral or ventral surface of the tongue, soft or hard palate, and palatoglossal folds (Figure 8.20). Canine OEG has a similar histopathological appearance to its feline counterpart. It has been reported to be responsive to glucocorticoid therapy or to resolve spontaneously. Seasonal or chronic recurrence of lesions has been described (Bredal *et al.*, 1996).

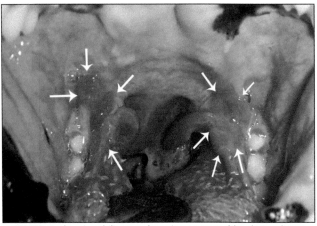

8.20 Oral eosinophilic granuloma in a 1.5-year-old male Cavalier King Charles Spaniel, showing ulcerative nodules and plaques on the oral mucosa and palatoglossal folds with the characteristic whitish and yellowish surface (arrowed).
(© Dr Margherita Gracis)

Canine oral papillomatosis

Canine papillomaviruses (CPVs) can infect epithelia and induce proliferative disorders (Lange and Favrot, 2011). Several clinical entities have been described, and different variants of CPVs have been found to be associated with distinct diseases. Oral papillomatosis is caused by canine papillomavirus 1 (CPV1).

Oral papillomatosis mainly affects young dogs. It is clinically characterized by cauliflower-like exophytic warts, located on the gingiva, alveolar, labial, buccal and sublingual mucosa and mucocutaneous junctions. The mucosa of the tongue, soft and hard palate, pharynx and oesophagus are occasionally affected (Figure 8.21). In some cases, lesions may occur concurrently on haired skin. Often oral papillomas are in small numbers, but occasionally severe manifestations of oral papillomatosis are seen with consequent difficulty prehending, chewing and swallowing, and oral bleeding secondary to mastication of large warts (Figure 8.22). Immunosuppression

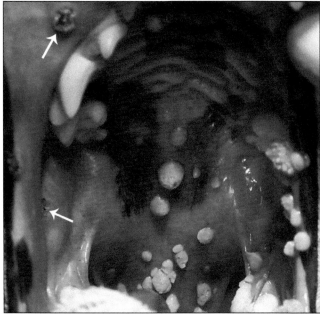

8.21 Multiple oral papillomas in a 1-year-old male Jack Russell Terrier. Some warts were excised using a CO_2 laser surgery unit (arrowed).
(© Dr Laura Ordeix)

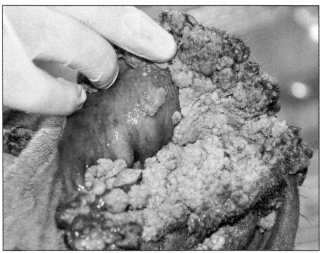

8.22 Severe oral papillomatosis in a 2-year-old male Shar-Pei.
(© Dr Laura Ordeix)

may be involved in the development of severe oral papillomatosis in older dogs, and possible causes (e.g. malignant lymphoma) should be evaluated. Canine oral papillomatosis in young dogs is clinically distinctive and may therefore be diagnosed based on clinical appearance. Otherwise, histopathological examination should be performed.

Most oral papillomas will spontaneously regress within 4 to 8 weeks. The treatment of choice for papillomas that do not regress and cause problems due to their size or location is surgery (conventional, laser or cryosurgery). It should be borne in mind that surgical excision has been reported to be associated with latent infection and increased recurrence (Lange and Favrot, 2011). Medical treatment with immune modulators, such as interferon or recombinant canine oral papillomavirus vaccine, has also been suggested (Kuntsi-Vaattovaara et al., 2003). Unfortunately, no controlled studies on their effectiveness in canine papillomatoses have been published. Although preventative vaccination is possible in dogs (Bell et al., 1994), commercial vaccines against canine PVs are not available.

Canine leishmaniosis

Canine leishmaniosis (CanL) is an infectious vector-borne disease caused by the protozoan *Leishmania infantum*, transmitted in Europe by a sandfly. CanL is endemic in the Mediterranean basin. However, it represents an emerging disease in many non-endemic regions including northern parts of Europe.

Skin lesions are the most common clinical manifestation, being described in 81–89% of sick dogs. The typical cutaneous clinical signs include scaly dermatitis (mainly on the face and/or trunk), ulcerative dermatitis affecting bony prominences, papular dermatitis and onychogryphosis. Papular dermatitis due to *Leishmania* is commonly described in areas without hair in shorthaired dogs (e.g. external surface of the mucocutaneous junction of the lips). These papules may ulcerate in the centre, acquiring a crateriform morphology (Ordeix et al., 2005) described as typical of human cutaneous leishmaniasis (the 'sign of the volcano'). Nevertheless, some atypical dermatological forms have been described. Rarely, plaque-like to nodular lesions are noted in mucocutaneous junctions and in oral (Figure 8.23), mainly lingual, or genital mucosa (Font et al., 1996; Viegas et al., 2012). It has been hypothesized that the lingual nodules are the result of parasite penetration

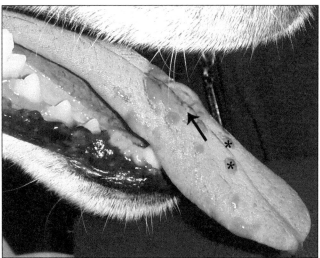

8.23 Papules (∗) and a plaque (arrowed) on the tongue of an adult male crossbreed dog with leishmaniosis.
(Courtesy of the Ophthalmology Service of Clinica Ars Veterinaria, Barcelona, Spain)

immediately after 'chewing' sandflies containing *Leishmania* (Foglia Manzillo et al., 2005). Moreover, CanL can occasionally cause erosive and ulcerative lesions of mucocutaneous junctions (Koutinas et al., 1992).

When leishmaniosis is clinically suspected, a cytological examination of material obtained by fine-needle aspiration from papules, plaques or nodules or by impression from ulcerated surfaces is recommended. Concurrently, testing for the presence of anti-*Leishmania* serum antibodies, as well as haematological, biochemical (including serum proteins) and urinary testing should be performed. Occasionally the parasite is not identified by cytological examination, and blood work-up may not reveal any changes, in which case a histological examination of skin and oral biopsy samples may be necessary. When clinical and histopathological lesions are suggestive of leishmaniosis and samples stained with haematoxylin and eosin do not show the presence of amastigotes, it is necessary to confirm or discard the diagnosis through more sensitive techniques such as immunohistochemistry and/or PCR testing.

Treatment of CanL is based on combined therapy with meglumine antimoniate and allopurinol or the use of oral miltefosine. Prognosis is variable, mainly based on the canine immune response. In particular, papular dermatitis is associated with a strong cell-mediated specific immune response and therefore with a favourable prognosis (Ordeix et al., 2005).

Other oral nodular conditions

In addition to the more common diseases previously described, a few other non-neoplastic disorders can result in nodular lesions in the oral cavity. These diseases may be of infectious origin (e.g. deep fungal infections) or sterile in nature (e.g. calcinosis circumscripta, amyloidosis, histiocytosis).

Fungal infections: Deep fungal infections such as cryptococcosis, sporotrichosis, histoplasmosis and conidiobolomycosis can occasionally result in ulcerated plaques or nodules in the oral cavity of dogs and cats (Brömel and Greene, 2012; Grooters and Foil, 2012; Pacheco Schubach et al., 2012; Sykes and Malik, 2012). However, the most common presenting complaints include skin nodules and ulcers, and signs of systemic dissemination such as weight loss, inappetence, fever, and signs of respiratory, gastrointestinal and/or neurological involvement.

Although clinical signs, patient history and epidemiological data can suggest a deep fungal infection, diagnosis may require cytological and histopathological examination. Special stains or immunohistochemical testing will support the diagnosis. Systemic fungal infections are generally treated with oral administration of azole derivates (e.g. ketoconazole, itraconazole or fluconazole). However, selection of the appropriate antifungal drug and dosage will depend on the specific disease (Grooters and Foil, 2012).

Calcinosis circumscripta: Deposition of calcium salts in soft tissues may cause the development of whitish nodules in the oral cavity. Lesions are usually solitary and occur most commonly at the tip of the tongue (Collados et al., 2002; Tafti et al., 2005) (Figure 8.24). Diagnosis is made by histopathological examination of biopsy samples, and the treatment of choice is conservative excision.

Amyloidosis: This can occasionally manifest as variably ulcerated, solitary or grouped pale papules and plaque-like lesions localized on the tongue and other oral mucosae.

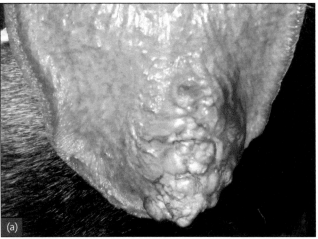

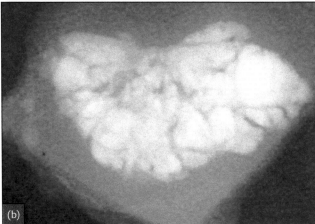

8.24 (a) Lingual calcinosis circumscripta in a dog. (b) A radiograph was taken of the excised tissue, showing a circumscribed lesion containing material with bone density that is arranged in lobules. (Reproduced from the BSAVA Manual of Canine and Feline Head, Neck and Thoracic Surgery)

Histopathological examination of biopsy samples will confirm an abnormal accumulation and deposition of pathological fibrillar protein surrounded by an inflammatory infiltrate composed mainly of plasma cells (Gross *et al.*, 2005).

Histiocytosis: A case of reactive histiocytosis in a dog with an unusual presentation characterized by a sublingual mass has been described (Cornegliani *et al.*, 2011). Treatment included oral administration of tetracycline and niacinamide.

Conditions of the jaws, masticatory muscles and salivary glands

Idiopathic osteomyelitis and osteonecrosis

Osteomyelitis is defined as inflammation of bone and bone marrow. There are anecdotal reports of idiopathic osteomyelitis and osteonecrosis in dogs, but very little is known about the aetiology, presentation, diagnosis and treatment of this condition (Marretta *et al.*, 1997; Reiter, 2001; Boutoille and Hennet, 2011; Zacher and Marretta, 2013; Peralta *et al.*, 2015). The below description of osteomyelitis and osteonecrosis does not relate to osteonecrosis of the jaws in previously irradiated fields, which is considered to be a separate pathological entity found in patients with oral tumours treated with radiation therapy (Nemec *et al.*, 2015).

Signalment, history, clinical signs and clinical laboratory findings

Breeds predisposed include the Cocker Spaniel, Labrador Retriever, Standard Poodle, Scottish Terrier and Dachshund, with young adult to middle-aged dogs being more often affected. They present with a history of lethargy, decreased activity and appetite, halitosis and oral pain. Increased rectal temperature, visible and firm mandibular or maxillofacial swellings, otitis externa, lip fold dermatitis, pododermatitis, oral, ocular and nasal discharge, atrophy of temporal and masseter muscles, and mandibular lymphadenomegaly are common clinical signs. Serum chemistry often reveals increased total protein due to hyperglobulinaemia, while haematological abnormalities typically include an increased white blood cell count, neutrophilia, presence of banded neutrophils, lymphopenia, monocytosis and thrombocytosis.

Oral examination

A conscious oral examination may be difficult to perform if soft tissues adjacent to affected bones are also infected and inflamed causing discomfort to the patient upon lip retraction and mouth opening. Findings obtained under general anaesthesia often include plaque and calculus accumulation, periodontal disease, missing teeth in or adjacent to areas of bone lesions, tonsillar enlargement, ulceration of alveolar, labial, buccal, sublingual and lingual mucosa. Two or more jaw quadrants are often involved, showing exposure of tooth roots and inflamed/necrotic bone, ulceration and necrosis of adjacent soft tissue, and contamination with hair, debris and pus (Figure 8.25a). Lesions are often centred at the mandibular first and second molars and maxillary fourth premolars and first molars. Large bone sequestra, some of which contain teeth, may be elevated from underlying tissues.

Radiographic findings

Radiographic findings include destruction of cortical outlines at the alveolar margin and lamina dura, widening of the periodontal space around tooth roots, and lamellated periosteal new bone formation along the ventral mandibular border. Multiple radiolucent areas of variable size with irregular and poorly defined borders in between islands of more opaque sequestra may create a moth-eaten or mottled bone appearance. Destruction of cortical bone may be present, with periosteal new bone formation showing a spiculated rather than lamellated pattern (Figure 8.25b).

Biopsy and culture findings

Fine-needle aspirates from mandibular lymph nodes may reveal reactive lymphoid hyperplasia. Histopathology of affected bone will show bacterial osteomyelitis, and – depending on the site of biopsy – varying degrees of osteonecrosis. Sampled soft tissues may indicate ulceration, necrosis and cellulitis. Identification of a specific infectious agent (particularly in chronic osteomyelitis) is usually difficult both microscopically and microbiologically. Sampling error is significant, either because of small, difficult-to-reach bacterial foci or because of contamination of the lesion by resident flora. Previous antibiotic use also reduces the chances of culturing the causative organism. Skin (including ear, nail and footpad) lesions, if present, should be biopsied and cultured.

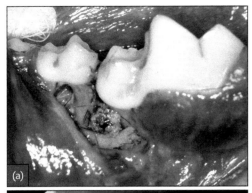

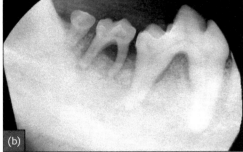

8.25 (a) Clinical image and (b) radiograph of the caudal aspect of the body of the right mandible in a 5-year-old entire male Labrador Retriever affected by multi-quadrant osteomyelitis and osteonecrosis.
(© Dr Alexander M. Reiter)

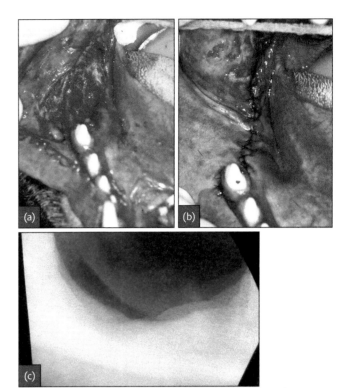

8.26 Same dog as in Figure 8.25. (a) Tooth extraction and debridement down to bleeding bone and (b) suturing of the wound were performed. (c) Postoperative radiograph.
(© Dr Alexander M. Reiter)

Treatment

Treatment consists of surgical debridement followed by prolonged antimicrobial therapy. Diseased teeth must be extracted. Bone sequestra must be removed and bone lesions surgically debrided down to bleeding bone (Figure 8.26a). Ulcerated and necrotic soft tissue may be excised if enough tissue is left for tension-free closure of wounds. Surgical debridement may result in exposure of the mandibular canal or infraorbital canal, and viable neurovascular structures may no longer be present when entering these spaces. The surgical sites are thoroughly rinsed with sterile Ringer's lactate solution prior to being sutured closed with a synthetic absorbable monofilament (such as poliglecaprone 25), and a postoperative radiograph should be obtained (Figure 8.26bc). Professional dental cleaning and periodontal therapy are performed for the remainder of the dentition. Skin lesions should be treated from a dermatological point of view (clipping of hair, washing with an antiseptic solution, use of ear cleansing solution, etc.). Postoperative management includes pain control and – depending on the severity of lesions – a 30- to 60-day course of antimicrobial therapy (initially empirical, then adjusted according to culture results). Commonly used oral antibiotics include clindamycin (11 mg/kg q12h), metronidazole (30 mg/kg q24h for 2 weeks and then tapered to 10 mg/kg q24h for 2 weeks), co-amoxiclav (12.5 mg/kg q12h), enrofloxacin (10 mg/kg q24h) and marbofloxacin (5 mg/kg q24h). Meticulous home oral hygiene must be followed (daily tooth brushing and oral application of a 0.12% chlorhexidine digluconate gel).

Prognosis

Signs of improvement include increased energy, activity and appetite, weight gain, resolution of halitosis, oral pain and discharge from the mouth, nose and eyes, gradual decrease of facial swellings and mandibular lymphadenomegaly, normal rectal temperature, and a gradual return of

masticatory muscle volume upon visual and palpatory evaluation. Frequent follow-up examinations should be performed, with radiographic evaluation of the surgical sites and professional dental cleaning as needed (Figure 8.27). The prognosis is cautious, as other jaw quadrants may become involved months or years after initial presentation.

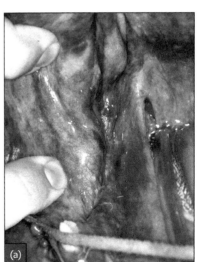

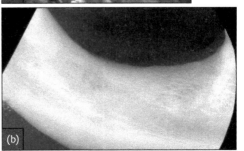

8.27 Same dog as in Figure 8.25 at the 8-month recheck examination. The previous surgery site was (a) inspected and (b) radiographed, showing healing.
(© Dr Alexander M. Reiter)

Masticatory muscle myositis

Masticatory muscle myositis (MMM) is an autoimmune disease affecting the temporal, masseter, and medial and lateral pterygoid muscles in dogs (and rarely in cats). It may also be called masticatory myositis, as myositis is already defined as muscle inflammation. Other synonyms used include eosinophilic myositis and atrophic myositis, but these terms should be avoided because they probably represent acute and chronic stages of a single disease, respectively.

Signalment

Dogs of any age, breed and sex can be affected. However, large-breed, young adult to middle-aged dogs appear to be most commonly affected (Gilmour *et al.*, 1992; Barone and Reiter, 2011), with the German Shepherd, Rottweiler, Samoyed, Dobermann, and Labrador Retriever over-represented.

Forms

An acute stage (painful muscle swelling/inflammation) may be followed by a latent stage (apparently healthy animal) which is then followed by a chronic stage (muscle atrophy) or a recurrent acute stage. Untreated acute episodes last 2 to 3 weeks, and relapses can occur in weeks or months. The chronic form may develop without the owner having observed acute signs (Barone and Reiter, 2011).

History and presenting complaint

Dogs with acute MMM have a history of decreased activity, lethargy, dysphagia, reluctance to eat, weight loss, drooling, change in bark, and pain on yawning or when prehending treats and toys. Dogs with chronic MMM are usually bright and alert, but they show progressive atrophy of masticatory muscles (Barone and Reiter, 2011).

Clinical signs

The acutely affected dog may show fever, regional lymphadenomegaly, swelling of temporal and masseter muscles, exophthalmos due to swelling of temporal and pterygoid muscles, inability to blink properly, ocular discharge, conjunctivitis and keratitis (Figure 8.28a). Blindness may rarely be present due to optic nerve compression by enlarged muscles. Pain may be elicited on palpation of the temporal and masseter muscles and regional lymph nodes. The dog may resist or is unable to open the mouth fully. The chronically affected dog may show decreased volume of the masticatory muscles, enophthalmos due to atrophy of the temporal and pterygoid muscles, and inability to open the mouth fully (Barone and Reiter, 2011) (Figure 8.28b). It is important to note that muscle swelling/atrophy can be asymmetrical.

Aetiology and pathogenesis

The temporal, masseter, and medial and lateral pterygoid muscles (but not the digastric muscles; thus they are not affected) possess 2M muscle fibres that differ from the common type 2C muscle fibres of other skeletal muscles. It is not known what causes autoantibodies to develop, but it has been hypothesized that they are generated in response to an infectious agent cross-reacting with endogenous antigens (Melmed *et al.*, 2004) or that early myofibre damage is initiated by CD8+ cytotoxic T cells,

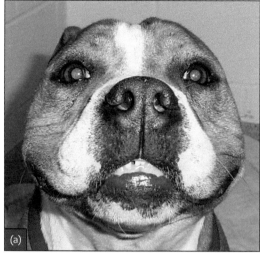
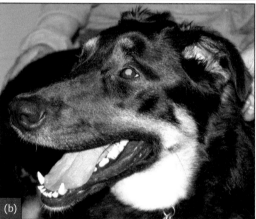

8.28 Dogs with masticatory muscle myositis (MMM). (a) A 3.5-year-old neutered female crossbreed dog presenting with acute swelling of masticatory muscles, exophthalmos and inability to open the mouth. (b) A 2-year-old, neutered female crossbreed dog presenting with chronic atrophy of masticatory muscles and enophthalmos. The dog's muscle atrophy is exacerbated by the catabolic effect of glucocorticoid therapy.
(© Dr Alexander M. Reiter)

which then leads to production of antibodies against muscle fibre protein (Neumann and Bilzer, 2006). The autoantibodies target the unique myosin component of type 2M fibres, resulting in muscle inflammation, necrosis and phagocytosis (Shelton *et al.*, 1985).

Differential diagnoses

Several other conditions can make a dog unwilling or unable to open its mouth. They include maxillofacial trauma, temporomandibular joint disease, neoplasia, foreign body penetration, ocular disease and space-occupying orbital/retrobulbar lesions, ear disease, other inflammatory muscle disorders (polymyositis, extraocular myositis, dermatomyositis and laryngeal myositis), tetanus, chronic exposure to glucocorticoids (which are catabolic to muscle), and craniomandibular osteopathy (Barone and Reiter, 2011).

Diagnosis

A definitive diagnosis of MMM can be made if inflammation is limited to the temporal, masseter, and medial and lateral pterygoid muscles, together with detection of antibodies against type 2M fibres in serum or immune complexes in muscle biopsy samples (Reiter and Schwarz, 2007). A complete blood count occasionally reveals leucocytosis and eosinophilia. Serum total protein, globulin and hepatic enzymes are occasionally increased. In contrast to polymyositis, serum creatine kinase is usually normal or only slightly elevated. A serum type 2M fibre antibody titre of <1:100 is negative, 1:100 is borderline, and >1:100 is positive (Barone and Reiter, 2011).

General anaesthesia allows for accurate assessment of the range of mouth opening. If the mouth cannot be opened enough to allow for transoral insertion of an endotracheal tube, temporary tracheostomy is required for intubation. Head radiographs are of limited use; they may simply aid in ruling out skeletal abnormalities. The gold standard in diagnostic imaging is computed tomography (CT) (Figure 8.29), which aids in ruling out most differentials of MMM, allows guided fine-needle aspiration of surgically inaccessible pterygoid muscles, shows changes in muscle size (larger due to oedema or inflammation; smaller due to atrophy, necrosis or fibrosis), pre-contrast tissue attenuation (hypoattenuated due to oedema) and contrast enhancement (heterogeneously enhanced due to inflammation) in affected muscles, and the presence of regional lymphadenomegaly (Reiter and Schwarz, 2007). Magnetic resonance imaging (MRI) may provide superior characterization of early muscle lesions compared with CT, but its cost, availability, length of executing the procedure, and insufficient bone evaluation are limiting factors. Electromyography may demonstrate spontaneous electrical activity, differentiate MMM from neuropathy (denervation atrophy) or polymyositis, and facilitate selection of sites for muscle biopsy (though it is less helpful than CT) (Barone and Reiter, 2011).

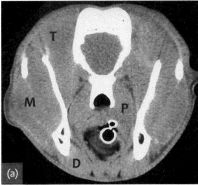

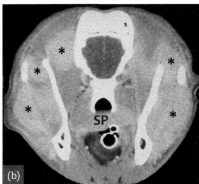

8.29 Transverse computed tomographic images in soft tissue algorithm of the head of the dog shown in Figure 8.28(a) obtained at the level of the mandibular ramus. (a) This image was obtained prior to intravenous administration of contrast medium. (b) This image was obtained after intravenous administration of contrast medium. Note the marked inhomogeneous contrast enhancement in multiple masticatory muscles suggestive of inflammatory oedema and increased vascularity (∗). The soft palate and blood vessels are normal. D = digastric muscle; M = masseter muscle; P = pterygoid muscle; SP = soft palate; T = temporal muscle.
(© Dr Alexander M. Reiter)

Muscle biopsy

Muscle biopsy samples are taken from areas of temporal or masseter muscles that show the most obvious contrast enhancement on CT. Temporary ptosis of the upper eyelid (lasting for several weeks) may occasionally be present after temporal muscle biopsy and trauma to the rostral auricular plexus. Injury to the dorsal and ventral buccal branches of the facial nerve may result in motor deficits of the muscles of the cheek and lips. Laceration of the parotid duct could cause formation of a sialocele.

Using the zygomatic arch as an anatomical landmark, a rostrocaudal skin incision is made either dorsal to it over the temporal muscle or ventral to it over the masseter muscle. Blunt or sharp dissection through the frontal muscle (overlying the temporal muscle) or platysma (overlying the masseter muscle) is performed, taking care to avoid damage to adjacent nerves or the parotid duct. Self-retaining retractors may be used to retract the skin and superficial muscles, exposing the white and shiny aponeurosis of the masticatory muscles. A semilunar incision is made into the aponeurosis, which is carefully released from underlying muscle tissue (Fink et al., 2013).

A 0.5 x 0.5 x 1 cm piece of muscle tissue is excised, wrapped in a dry or minimally moistened gauze sponge, and placed into a watertight container (e.g. a 10 ml red top tube). The sample is kept cool and shipped overnight (Comparative Neuromuscular Laboratory, University of California, San Diego, USA or Institut fuer Neuropathologie, Universitaet Duesseldorf, Duesseldorf Germany) (Fink et al., 3013). Because results from serum 2M fibre antibody testing and immunohistochemical tissue analysis may take 1–2 weeks to return, an additional smaller muscle sample should be obtained and placed into 10% neutral buffered formalin to be submitted for haematoxylin and eosin histopathological examination. A diagnosis of non-specific myositis in the absence of infection may further strengthen a presumptive diagnosis of MMM and thus justify the use of high doses of oral glucocorticoids, which – depending on the severity of clinical signs – can be initiated immediately after sampling or started once serum titre and immunohistochemical results are received.

Haemorrhage is controlled with digital pressure or use of an absorbable haemostatic gelatin sponge. Particular attention should be paid to wound closure, as glucocorticoids will delay connective tissue healing. The following layers are closed: muscle, aponeurosis, frontal muscle or platysma, subcutaneous tissues, and skin (continuous subcuticular pattern followed by cruciate or simple interrupted sutures).

Therapy

The goal of therapy is to alleviate pain, decrease inflammation, prevent muscle fibrosis, and restore normal opening and closing of the mouth. Glucocorticoid therapy should not be started prior to blood collection and muscle sampling. A dexamethasone injection (0.4 mg/kg i.v. once, after muscle biopsy) is helpful in the immediate reduction of inflammation in dogs with acute MMM. The patient is discharged with prednisone (1–2 mg/kg orally q12h) (Barone and Reiter, 2011), usually resulting in rapid (within days) improvement of clinical signs. After 2 to 3 weeks, the dose can be decreased to 1 mg/kg orally q24h for another 3 to 4 weeks before it is slowly tapered to the lowest possible alternate-day effective dose over a period of 8–12 months. Dogs that are unable to receive glucocorticoids, non-responsive to glucocorticoids alone, or showing unacceptable side effects in response to glucocorticoids may benefit from administration of azathioprine (1–2 mg/kg orally q24h) (Barone and Reiter, 2011).

Monitoring and prognosis

Follow-up examinations should take place 2 weeks and 1, 2, 6, 9 and 12 months after initiation of glucocorticoid therapy and once every 6 to 12 months thereafter, focusing on bodyweight, degree of muscle atrophy, pain on head palpation, and range of opening of the mouth (which is measured with a ruler between the incisal edges of the maxillary and mandibular incisors). Serum type 2M fibre antibody titres should be repeated 2, 6, 9 and 12 months after initiation of prednisone therapy and once every 6 to 12 months thereafter. Determining antibody titre is particularly important prior to decreasing prednisone doses when they are already very low (e.g. below 0.1–0.2 mg/kg every other day) (Barone and Reiter, 2011). The prognosis for acute MMM is good if therapy is instituted promptly and maintained indefinitely. Dogs with relapses should be reinstituted at the maximum prednisone dose and slowly tapered to the lowest possible alternate-day effective dosage. Dogs with chronic MMM and extensive atrophy and fibrosis of affected muscles may show a progressive inability to open the mouth.

Sialadenitis, sialadenosis and necrotizing sialometaplasia

Sialadenitis, sialadenosis and necrotizing sialometaplasia must be differentiated from salivary neoplasia. All may to a certain degree present with a similar history or produce similar clinical signs.

Sialadenitis

Sialadenitis is defined as inflammation of a salivary gland. Sialadenitis is typically seen in middle-aged to older dogs (Cannon et al., 2011). The patient may present with a painful swelling (dependent on location) along the vertical ear canal (parotid gland), caudal to the mandible (mandibular and/or sublingual gland), or orbital/retrobulbar area with exophthalmos (zygomatic gland). Other clinical signs include malaise, inappetence, lymphadenomegaly, fever, pain on palpation of the affected gland, on gentle retropulsion of the eye through closed eyelids, and on opening the mouth, and dysphagia secondary to pain or the enlarged inflamed gland that physically inhibits mouth opening. Mucopurulent discharge may be noted at the duct opening in the oral cavity. The soft palate may have an asymmetrical appearance from an enlarged, inflamed zygomatic gland, which seems to be most commonly affected (Smith and Reiter, 2011).

It is not clear what causes sialadenitis, but sialoliths (concretions of calcium phosphate or calcium carbonate) may be a contributing factor, since they can occur in dogs and are reported commonly in humans with sialadenitis. The associated ductal obstruction may then lead to inflammation of the glandular tissue. Differential diagnoses include oedema, cyst, seroma, haematoma, abscess, trauma, foreign body, sialolith, lymphadenitis, and neoplasia affecting the gland, lymph nodes, ear and eye. Advanced diagnostic imaging modalities, such as CT and MRI, may need to be considered (Cannon et al., 2011). Fine-needle aspiration and cytological evaluation of the

affected gland (zygomatic salivary gland may require aspiration through oral mucosa) and regional lymph nodes, bacterial culture and sensitivity testing (if infection is suspected), and three-view thoracic radiographs (if neoplasia is suspected) may be performed. However, a definitive diagnosis of sialadenitis requires an incisional biopsy and histopathological evaluation (Spangler and Culbertson, 1991; Smith and Reiter, 2011).

If needle aspiration yielded mucopurulent fluid, intraoral or percutaneous drainage to alleviate mucopurulent fluid accumulation and associated pressure causing discomfort may be attempted. Medical treatment includes management of pain (if present) and use of antibiotics (based on culture and sensitivity results of the fluid/tissue aspirate), NSAIDs, and anti-inflammatory doses of glucocorticoids. Depending on identification of the initiating cause and response to treatment, the prognosis is usually good (Smith and Reiter, 2011).

Sialadenosis and necrotizing sialometaplasia

Sialadenosis is defined as a non-inflammatory, non-neoplastic enlargement of a salivary gland. There are no obvious cytological or histological abnormalities (Sozmen et al., 2000). Necrotizing sialometaplasia (salivary gland necrosis or infarction) is defined as squamous metaplasia of the salivary gland ducts and lobules, with ischaemic necrosis of the salivary gland lobules (Spangler and Culbertson, 1991). Sialadenosis and necrotizing sialometaplasia can occur in dogs of all ages (but young adult to middle-aged dogs seem to be most often affected). Both occur more commonly in small breeds (e.g. terriers). Although both disorders may have similar history and clinical presentations, it is a matter of speculation whether sialadenosis can progress to necrotizing sialometaplasia (Smith and Reiter, 2011).

History in sialadenosis includes weight loss, reluctance to exercise, snorting, lip smacking, nasal discharge, hypersalivation, inappetence and depression. The affected patient may be presented with a regional swelling (location dependent on the gland affected), which is usually bilateral (mandibular gland most commonly affected), exophthalmos (if zygomatic gland affected), but without apparent pain. Clinical signs include retching and gulping elicited by mild excitement and occurring several times a day (Boydell et al., 2000).

Owners of patients with necrotizing sialometaplasia often report retching, gagging, regurgitation, chronic vomiting, weight loss, coughing, tachypnoea, dyspnoea, reverse sneezing, and abdominal respiration. Dogs will present with a painful and firm swelling caudal to the mandible (mandibular gland most commonly affected), will be very sensitive on palpation of the pharyngeal region, show pain associated with opening the mouth, and are usually depressed, nauseous and anorexic. Other clinical signs are ptyalism, persistent swallowing and lip smacking (Brooks et al., 1995; Schroeder and Berry, 1998).

Excessive saliva production in dogs with sialadenosis may be associated with increased parasympathetic activity or changes in sympathetic innervation. In contrast to necrotizing sialometaplasia, there are usually no abnormalities noted on oesophageal endoscopy (Smith and Reiter, 2011). A neurogenic pathogenesis is suspected to correlate with abnormalities of the vagal nerve in dogs with necrotizing sialometaplasia, and associated conditions and disorders include Spirocerca lupi infestation (oesophageal granulomas), megaoesophagus, oesophageal foreign body, oesophagitis, oesophageal diverticulum, giardiasis, and autoimmune sialadenitis (Schroeder and Berry, 1998; Smith and Reiter, 2011; van der Merwe et al., 2012).

Differential diagnoses include oedema, cyst, seroma, haematoma, abscess, trauma, foreign body, sialolith, lymphadenitis, and neoplasia affecting the gland, lymph nodes, ear and eye (Smith and Reiter, 2011). Advanced diagnostic imaging modalities, such as CT and MRI, should be considered. Fine-needle aspiration and cytological evaluation of the affected gland (zygomatic salivary gland may require aspiration through oral mucosa) and regional lymph nodes, bacterial culture and sensitivity testing (if infection is suspected), and three-view thoracic radiographs (if neoplasia is suspected) may be performed (Smith and Reiter, 2011). However, a definitive diagnosis of sialadenosis and necrotizing sialometaplasia requires an incisional biopsy and histopathological evaluation.

Surgical removal of the affected salivary gland produces minimal if any improvement. Medical treatment includes management of pain (if present), NSAIDs, anti-inflammatory doses of glucocorticoids, and control of internal parasites (*Spirocerca lupi* and *Giardia*). Oral phenobarbital administration (1–2 mg/kg orally q12h) has resulted in dramatic improvement in some cases, providing more support for a neurogenic pathogenesis in these salivary gland disorders (Boydell et al., 2000; Gilor et al., 2010). The prognosis is good for sialadenosis when treated with phenobarbital, but more guarded for necrotizing sialometaplasia.

References and further reading

Addie DD, Radford A, Yam PS et al. (2003) Cessation of feline calicivirus shedding coincident with resolution of chronic gingivostomatitis in a cat. *Journal of Small Animal Practice* **44**, 172–176

Anderson JG (1996) Periodontal and radiographic findings in cats with chronic lymphocytic plasmacytic gingivitis stomatitis complex: a review of 22 cases. *Proceedings of the Annual Veterinary Dental Forum* **10**, 106–108

Anderson JG, Peralta S, Kol A et al. (2017) Clinical and histopathologic characterization of canine chronic ulcerative stomatitis. *Veterinary Pathology* **54**, 511–519

Arzi B, Mills-Ko E, Verstraete FJM et al. (2016) Therapeutic efficacy of fresh, autologous mesenchymal stem cells for severe refractory gingivostomatitis in cats. *Stem Cells in Translational Medicine* **5**, 75–86

Arzi B, Murphy B, Baumgarth N et al. (2011) Analysis of immune cells within the healthy oral mucosa of specific pathogen-free cats. *Anatomica, Histologica, Embryologica* **40**, 1–10

Arzi B, Murphy B, Cox DP et al. (2010) Presence and quantification of mast cells in the gingiva of cats with tooth resorption, periodontitis and chronic stomatitis. *Archives of Oral Biology* **55**, 148–154

AVDC (2013) Oral and oropharyngeal inflammation. Available at: http://www.avdc.org/nomenclature.html#OP

Barone G and Reiter AM (2011) Masticatory myositis. In: *Clinical Veterinary Advisor, 2nd edn*, ed. E Cote, pp. 704–705. Mosby, St Louis

Belgard S, Truyen U, Thibault JC et al. (2010) Relevance of feline calicivirus, feline immunodeficiency virus, feline leukemia virus, feline herpesvirus, and *Bartonella henselae* in cats with chronic gingiva-stomatitis. *Berliner und Münchener Tierärztliche Wochenschrift* **123**, 369–376

Bell JA, Sundberg JP, Ghim SJ et al. (1994) A formalin-inactivated vaccine protects against mucosal papillomavirus infection: a canine model. *Pathobiology* **62**, 194–198

Bellows J (2010) Treatment of periodontal disease. In: *Feline dentistry: oral assessment, treatment, and preventative care*, ed. J Bellows, pp. 181–195. Wiley-Blackwell, Ames

Bellows J (2013) Laser and radiosurgery in veterinary dentistry. *Veterinary Clinics of North America: Small Animal Practice* **43**, 651–668

Bizikova P, Dean GA, Hashimoto T et al. (2012) Cloning and establishment of canine desmocollin-1 as a major autoantigen in canine pemphigus foliaceus. *Veterinary Immunology and Immunopathology* **149**, 197–207

Bizikova P, Linder KE, Wofford JA et al. (2015) Canine epidermolysis bullosa acquisita: a retrospective study of 20 cases. *Veterinary Dermatology* **26**, 441–450

Bloom PB (2006) Canine and feline eosinophilic skin diseases. *Veterinary Clinics of North America Small Animal Practice* **36**, 141–160

Booij-Vrieling HE, van der Reijden WA, Houwers DJ et al. (2010) Comparison of periodontal pathogens between cats and their owners. *Veterinary Microbiology* **144**, 147–152

Boutoille F and Hennet P (2011) Maxillary osteomyelitis in two Scottish terrier dogs with chronic ulcerative paradental stomatitis. *Journal of Veterinary Dentistry* **28**, 96–100

Boydell P, Pike R, Crossley D et al. (2000) Sialadenosis in dogs. *Journal of the American Veterinary Medical Association* **216**, 872–874

Bredal WP, Gunnes G, Vollset I et al. (1996) Oral eosinophilic granuloma in three Cavalier King Charles Spaniels. *Journal of Small Animal Practice* **37**, 499–504

Brömel C and Greene CE (2012) Histoplasmosis. In: *Infectious Diseases of the Dog and Cat, 4th edn*, ed. CE Green, pp. 614–621. Elsevier Saunders, St Louis

Brooks DG, Hottinger HA and Dunstan RW (1995) Canine necrotizing sialometaplasia: a case report and review of the literature. *Journal of the American Animal Hospital Association* **31**, 21–55

Buckley L and Nuttall T (2012) Feline eosinophilic granuloma complex(ities): some clinical clarification. *Journal of Feline Medicine and Surgery* **14**, 471–481

Caiafa A (2007) Canine infectious, inflammatory and immune-mediated oral conditions. In: *BSAVA Manual of Canine and Feline Dentistry, 3rd edn*, ed. C Tutt, J Deeprose and D Crossley, pp. 96–125. BSAVA Publications, Gloucester

Camy G (2010) Results of a pilot study exploring the use of peri-lesional infiltration of recombinant feline interferon omega in refractory cases of feline gingivostomatitis. *Proceedings of the European Congress of Veterinary Dentistry* **19**, 187–191

Cannon MS, Paglia D, Zwingenberger AL et al. (2011) Clinical and diagnostic imaging findings in dogs with zygomatic sialadenitis: 11 cases (1990–2009). *Journal of the American Veterinary Medical Association* **239**, 1211–1218

Collados J, Rodríguez-Bertos A, Peña L et al. (2002) Lingual calcinosis circumscripta in a dog. *Journal of Veterinary Dentistry* **19**, 19–21

Collados Soto J (2009) Oclusion y maloclusion. In: *Atlas visual de patologías dentales y orales en pequeños animales y exóticos*, ed. J Collados Soto, pp. 271–284. Servet, Zaragoza.

Coppoc GL (2009) Chemotherapy of neoplastic diseases. In: *Veterinary Pharmacology and Therapeutics, 9th edn*, ed. JE Riviere and MG Papich, pp. 1205–1231. Wiley-Blackwell, Ames

Corbee RJ, Booij-Vrieling HE, van de Lest CHA et al. (2012) Inflammation and wound healing in cats with chronic gingivitis/stomatitis after extraction of all premolars and molars were not affected by feeding of two diets with different omega-6/omega-3 polyunsaturated fatty acid ratios. *Journal of Animal Physiology and Animal Nutrition* **96**, 761–680

Corneqliani L, Gracis M, Ferro S et al. (2011) Sublingual reactive histiocytosis in a dog. *Journal of Veterinary Dentistry* **28**, 164–170

Declerq J (2004) Suspected wood poisoning caused by *Simarouba amara* (marupa/caixeta) shavings in two dogs with erosive stomatitis and dermatitis. *Veterinary Dermatology* **15**, 188–193

Dolieslager SMJ, Lapin DF, Bennett D et al. (2013) The influence of oral bacteria on tissue levels of Toll-like receptor and cytokine mRNAs in feline chronic gingivostomatitis and oral health. *Veterinary Immunology and Immunopathology* **151**, 263–274

Dolieslager SMJ, Riggio MP, Lennon A et al. (2011) Identification of bacteria associated with feline chronic gingivostomatitis using culture-dependent and culture-independent methods. *Veterinary Microbiology* **148**, 93–98

Dowers KL, Hawley JR, Brewer MM et al. (2009) Association of *Bartonella* species, feline calicivirus, and feline herpesvirus 1 infection with gingivostomatitis in cats. *Journal of Feline Medicine and Surgery* **12**, 314–321

Druet I and Hennet P (2017) Relationship between feline calicivirus load, oral lesions, and outcome in feline chronic gingivostomatitis (caudal stomatitis): retrospective study in 104 cats. *Frontiers in Veterinary Science* **4**, 209. doi: 10.3389/fvets.2017.00209

Farcas N, Lommer MJ, Kass PH et al. (2014) Dental radiographic findings in cats with chronic gingivostomatitis (2002–2012). *Journal of the American Veterinary Medical Association* **244**, 339–345

Foglia Manzillo V, Pagano A, Paciello O et al. (2005) Papular-like glossitis in a dog with leishmaniosis. *Veterinary Record* **156**, 213–215

Font A, Roura X, Fondevila D et al. (1996) Canine mucosal leishmaniasis. *Journal of the American Animal Hospital Association* **32**, 131–137

Fry LM, Neary SM, Sharrock J and Rychel JK (2014) Acupuncture for analgesia in veterinary medicine. *Topics in Companion Animal Medicine* **29**, 35–42

Gatti A, Lazzari M, Gianfelice V et al. (2012) Palmitoylethanolamide in the treatment of chronic pain caused by different etiopathogenesis. *Pain Medicine* **13**, 1121–1130

Gil S, Leal RO, Duarte A et al. (2012) Relevance of feline interferon omega for clinical improvement and reduction of concurrent viral excretion in retrovirus infected cats from a rescue shelter. *Research in Veterinary Science* **94**, 753–763

Gilmour MA, Morgan RV and Moore FM (1992) Masticatory myopathy in the dog: a retrospective study of 18 cases. *Journal of the American Animal Hospital Association* **28**, 300–306

Gilor C, Gilor S and Graves TK (2010) Phenobarbital-responsive sialadenosis associated with an esophageal foreign body in a dog. *Journal of the American Animal Hospital Association* **46**, 115–120

Girard N and Hennet P (2005) Retrospective study of dental extraction for treatment of chronic caudal stomatitis in 60 calicivirus-positive cats. *Proceedings of the Annual Veterinary Dental Forum* **19**, 447

Glaus T, Hofmann-Lehmann R, Greene C et al. (1997) Seroprevalence of Bartonella henselae infection and correlation with disease status in cats in Switzerland. Journal of Clinical Microbiology 35, 2883–2885

Gracis M (2010) Controlled study using a modified 2x2 cross-over design to compare the efficacy of recombinant feline interferon omega and prednisolone in refractory feline chronic gingivostomatitis. Proceedings of the European Congress of Veterinary Dentistry 19, 192

Gracis M, Molinari E and Ferro S (2013) Macroscopic and microscopic characterization of caudal mucogingival lesions secondary to traumatic occlusion in cats: description, treatment and follow-up of 28 cases. Proceedings of the 22nd European Congress of Veterinary Dentistry and the 12th World Veterinary Dental Congress, Prague (Czech Republic), pp. 140–143

Grooters AM and Foil CS (2012) Miscellaneous fungal infections. In: Infectious Diseases of the Dog and Cat, 4th edn, ed. CE Green, pp. 675–688. Elsevier Saunders, St Louis

Gross TL, Ihrke P, Walder E et al. (2005) Skin Diseases of the Dog and Cat. Clinical and Histopathologic Diagnosis, 2nd edn, pp. 4–26, 27–45, 65, 355–360, 383–386. Blackwell Science Ltd, Oxford

Harley R, Gruffydd-Jones TJ and Day MJ (2003) Salivary and serum immunoglobulin levels in cats with chronic gingivostomatitis. Veterinary Record 152, 125–129

Harley R, Gruffydd-Jones TJ and Day MJ (2011) Immunohistochemical characterization of oral mucosal lesions in cats with chronic gingivostomatitis. Journal of Comparative Pathology 144, 239–250

Harley R, Helps CR, Harbour DA et al. (1999) Cytokine mRNA expression in lesions in cats with chronic gingivostomatitis. Clinical and Diagnostic Laboratory Immunology 6, 471–478

Hennet P (1997) Chronic gingivo-stomatitis in cats: long-term follow-up of 30 cases treated by dental extractions. Journal of Veterinary Dentistry 14, 15–21

Hennet P and Boucrault-Baralones C (2005) Relationship between oral calicivirus and herpesvirus carriage and 'palatoglossitis' lesions. Proceedings of the Annual Veterinary Dental Forum 19, 443

Hennet PR, Camy GA, McGahie DM et al. (2011) Comparative efficacy of recombinant feline interferon omega in refractory cases of calicivirus-positive cats with caudal stomatitis: a randomized, multi-centre, controlled, double-blind study in 39 cats. Journal of Feline Medicine and Surgery 13, 577–587

Horvath C, Neuber A and Litschauer B (2007) Pemphigus foliaceus-like drug reaction in a 3-month-old crossbreed dog treated for juvenile cellulitis. Veterinary Dermatology 18, 353–359

Innerå M (2013) Cutaneous vasculitis in small animals. Veterinary Clinics of North America Small Animal Practice 43, 113–134

Jadhav VJ and Pal M (2006) Canine mycotic stomatitis due to Candida albicans. Revista Iberoamericana de Micología 23, 233–234

Jennings MW, Lewis JR, Soltero-Rivera MM, Brown DC and Reiter AM (2015) Effect of tooth extraction on stomatitis in cats: 95 cases (2000–2015). Journal of the American Veterinary Association 246, 654–660

Koutinas AF, Scott DW, Kantos V et al. (1992) Skin lesions in canine leishmaniosis (Kala-Azar): A clinical and histopathological study on 22 spontaneous cases in Greece. Veterinary Dermatology 3, 121–130

Kuntsi-Vaattovaara H, Verstraete FJ, Newsome JT et al. (2003) Resolution of persistent oral papillomatosis in a dog after treatment with a recombinant canine oral papillomavirus vaccine. Veterinary Comparative Oncology 1, 57–63

Lange CE and Favrot C (2011) Canine papillomaviruses. Veterinary Clinics of North America Small Animal Practice 41, 1183–1195

Lewis JR, Tsugawa AJ and Reiter AM (2007) Use of CO$_2$ laser as an adjunctive treatment for caudal stomatitis in a cat. Journal of Veterinary Dentistry 24, 240–249

Lommer MJ (2013a) Oral inflammation in small animals. Veterinary Clinics of North America Small Animal Practice 43, 555–571

Lommer MJ (2013b) Efficacy of cyclosporine for chronic, refractory stomatitis in cats: a randomized, placebo-controlled, double-blinded clinical study. Journal of Veterinary Dentistry 30, 8–17

Lommer MJ and Verstraete FJM (2003) Concurrent oral shedding of feline calicivirus and feline herpesvirus 1 in cats with chronic gingivostomatitis. Oral Microbiology and Immunology 18, 131–134

Lyon KF and Okuda A (2009) Feline oral mucosal inflammatory polyps. Proceedings of the 23rd Annual Veterinary Dental Forum, Phoenix, USA, pp. 519–521

Mackenzie SD, Blois S, Hayes G et al. (2012) Oral thermal injury associated with puncture of a salbutamol metered-dose inhaler in a dog. Journal of Veterinary Emergency and Critical Care 22, 494–497

Marretta SM, Brine E, Smith CW et al. (1997) Idiopathic mandibular and maxillary osteomyelitis and bone sequestra in Cocker Spaniels. Proceedings of the Annual Veterinary Dental Forum 11, 119

Melmed C, Shelton GD, Bergman R et al. (2004) Masticatory muscle myositis: pathogenesis, diagnosis, and treatment. Compendium on Continuing Education for the Practicing Veterinarian 26, 590–604

Mueller RS, Krebs I, Power HT et al. (2006) Pemphigus foliaceus in 91 dogs. Journal of the American Animal Hospital Association 42, 189–196

Nemec A, Zavodovskaya R, Affolter VK et al. (2012) Erythema multiforme and epitheliotropic T-cell lymphoma in the oral cavity of dogs: 1989 to 2009. Journal of Small Animal Practice 53, 445–452

Nemec A, Arzi B, Hansen K et al. (2015) Osteonecrosis of the jaws in dogs in previously irradiated fields: 13 cases (1989–2014). Frontiers in Veterinary Science 2, 5

Neumann J and Bilzer T (2006) Evidence for MHC I-restricted CD8[+] T-cell-mediated immunopathology in canine masticatory muscle myositis and polymyositis. Muscle and Nerve 33, 215–224

Nishifuji K, Olivry T, Ishii K et al. (2007) IgG autoantibodies directed against desmoglein 3 cause dissociation of keratinocytes in canine pemphigus vulgaris and paraneoplastic pemphigus. Veterinary Immunology and Immunopathology 117, 209–221

Niza ME, Ferreira ML, Coimbra IV et al. (2012) Effects of pine processionary caterpillar Thaumetopoea pityocampa contact in dogs: 41 cases (2002–2006). Zoonoses and Public Health 59, 35–38

Nuttall TJ and Malham T (2004) Successful intravenous human immunoglobulin treatment of drug-induced Stevens-Johnson syndrome in a dog. Journal of Small Animal Practice 45, 357–361

Olivry T, Bizikova P, Dunston SM et al. (2010) Clinical and immunological heterogeneity of canine subepidermal blistering dermatoses with anti-laminin-332 (laminin-5) auto-antibodies. Veterinary Dermatology 21, 345–357

Ordeix L, Solano-Gallego L, Fondevila D et al. (2005) Papular dermatitis due to Leishmania spp. infection in dogs with parasite-specific cellular immune responses. Veterinary Dermatology 16, 187–191

Pacheco Schubach TM, Caldas Menezes R and Wanke B (2012) Sporotrichosis. In: Infectious Diseases of the Dog and Cat, 4th edn, ed. CE Green, pp. 645–650. Elsevier Saunders, St Louis

Peralta S, Arzi B, Nemec A, Lommer M and Verstraete FJM (2015) Non-radiation-related osteonecrosis of the jaws in dogs: 14 cases (1996–2014). Frontiers in Veterinary Science 2, 7

Pruitt AF and Thrall DE (2011) Principles of radiation therapy. In: BSAVA Manual of Canine and Feline Oncology, 3rd edn, ed. JM Dobson and BDX Lascelles, pp. 80–90. BSAVA Publications, Gloucester

Quimby JM, Elston T, Hawley J et al. (2007) Evaluation of the association of Bartonella species, feline herpesvirus 1, feline calicivirus, feline leukemia virus and feline immunodeficiency virus with chronic feline gingivostomatitis. Journal of Feline Medicine and Surgery 10, 66–72

Radford AD, Addie D, Belak S et al. (2009) Feline calicivirus infection. ABCD guidelines on prevention and management. Journal of Feline Medicine and Surgery 11, 556–564

Re G, Barbero R, Miolo A et al. (2007) Palmitoylethanolamide, endocannabinoids and related cannabimimetic compounds in protection against tissue inflammation and pain: potential use in companion animals. Veterinary Journal 173, 21–30

Reiter AM (2001) Idiopathic bilateral mandibular osteomyelitis in a Labrador retriever. Proceedings of the Annual Veterinary Dental Forum 15, 154–156

Reiter AM and Schwarz T (2007) Computed tomographic appearance of masticatory myositis in dogs: seven cases (1999–2006). Journal of the American Veterinary Medical Association 231, 924–930

Reiter AM and Smith MM (2005) The oral cavity and oropharynx. In: BSAVA Manual of Canine and Feline Head, Neck and Thoracic Surgery, ed. DJ Brockman and DE Holt, pp. 25–43. BSAVA Publications, Gloucester

Reubel GH, Hoffmann DE and Pedersen NC (1992) Acute and chronic faucitis of domestic cats. A feline calicivirus-induced disease. Veterinary Clinics of North America Small Animal Practice 22, 1347–1360

Riehl J, Bell CM, Constantaras ME, Synder CJ, Charlier CJ and Soukup JW (2014) Clinicopathologic characterization of oral pyogenic granuloma in eight cats. Journal of Veterinary Dentistry 31, 80–86

Rybnicek J and Hill PB (2007) Suspected polymyxin B-induced pemphigus vulgaris in a dog. Veterinary Dermatology 18, 165–170

Schroeder H and Berry WL (1998) Salivary gland necrosis in dogs: a retrospective study of 19 cases. Journal of Small Animal Practice 39, 121–125

Shelton GD, Cardinet GH, Bandman E et al. (1985). Fiber type-specific autoantibodies in a dog with eosinophilic myositis. Muscle and Nerve 8, 783–790

Smith MM and Reiter AM (2011) Salivary gland disorders. In: Clinical Veterinary Advisor, 2nd edn, ed. E Cote, pp. 998–1001. Mosby, St Louis

Snead E (2006) Oral ulceration and bleeding associated with pancreatic enzyme supplementation in a German Shepherd with pancreatic acinar atrophy. Canadian Veterinary Journal 47, 579–582

Southerden P and Gorrel C (2007) Treatment of a case of refractory feline chronic gingivostomatitis with feline recombinant interferon omega. Journal of Small Animal Practice 48, 104–106

Sozmen M, Brown PJ and Whitbread TJ (2000) Idiopathic salivary gland enlargement (sialadenosis) in dogs: a microscopic study. Journal of Small Animal Practice 41, 243–247

Spangler WL and Culbertson MR (1991) Salivary gland disease in dogs and cats: 245 cases (1985–1988). Journal of the American Veterinary Medical Association 198, 465–469

Sparkes AH, Heiene R, Lascelles BDX et al. (2010) ISFM and AAFP consensus guidelines. Long-term use of NSAIDs in cats. Journal of Feline Medicine and Surgery 12, 521–538

Stocks IC and Lindsey DE (2008) Acute corrosión of the oral mucosa in a dog due to ingestion of Multicolored Asian Lady Beetles (Harmonia axyridis: Coccinellidae). Toxicon 52, 389–391

Sykes JE and Malik R (2012) Cryptococcosis. In: Infectious Diseases of the Dog and Cat, 4th edn, ed. CE Green, pp. 621–633. Elsevier Saunders, St Louis

Tafti AK, Hanna P and Bourque AC (2005) Calcinosis circumscripta in the dog: a retrospective pathological study. Journal of Veterinary Medicine Series A 52, 13–17

Tepper LC, Spiegel IB and Davis GJ (2011) Diagnosis of erythema multiforme associated with thymoma in a dog and treated with thymectomy. *Journal of the American Animal Hospital Association* **47**, e19–25

Thiverge G (1973) Granular stomatitis in dogs due to Burdock. *Canadian Veterinary Journal* **14**, 96–97

Ueno H, Hohdatsu T, Muramatsu Y *et al.* (1996) Does coinfection of *Bartonella henselae* and FIV induce clinical disorders in cats? *Microbiology and Immunology* **40**, 617–620

Van der Merwe LL, Christie J, Clift SJ *et al.* (2012) Salivary gland enlargement and sialorrhoea in dogs with spirocercosis: a retrospective and prospective study of 298 cases. *Journal of the South African Veterinary Association* **83**, 920

Van Duijn HE (1995) [3 cases of an oral eosinophilic granuloma in Siberian huskies]. *Tijdschrift voor diergeneeskunde* **120**, 712–714

Viegas C, Requicha J, Albuquerque C *et al.* (2012) Tongue nodules in canine leishmaniosis – a case report. *Parasitic Vectors* **5**, 120

Voie KL, Campbell KL and Lavergne SN (2012) Drug hypersensitivity reactions targeting the skin in dogs and cats. *Journal of Veterinary Internal Medicine* **26**, 863–874

Winer JN, Arzi B and Verstraete FJM (2016) Therapeutic management of feline chronic gingivostomatitis: a systematic review of the literature. *Frontiers in Veterinary Science* **3**, 54. doi: 10.3389/fvets.2016.00054

Woldemeskel M, Liggett A, Ilha M *et al.* (2011) Canine parvovirus-2b-associated erythema multiforme in a litter of English Setter dogs. *Journal of Veterinary Diagnostic Investigation* **23**, 576–580

Yager JA (2014) Erythema multiforme, Stevens-Johnson syndrome and toxic epidermal necrolysis: a comparative review. *Veterinary Dermatology* **25**, 406–464

Zacher AM and Marretta SM (2013) Oral and maxillofacial surgery in dogs and cats. *Veterinary Clinics of North America Small Animal Practice* **43**, 609–649

Chapter 9

Management of dental and oral trauma

Alexander M. Reiter and Margherita Gracis

Endodontic treatment and operative dentistry

Endodontics is the branch of dentistry concerned with the aetiology, prevention, diagnosis and treatment of conditions that affect the tooth pulp, root and periapical tissues (Figure 9.1). New techniques, materials, instruments and equipment are produced continuously. Knowledge of their indications, contraindications, interactions, use and potential complications is necessary to successfully perform endodontic procedures. Understanding dental anatomy and physiology is also very important (Lyon, 1998). Procedures are very technique-and operator-sensitive and should only be performed by veterinary dental specialists or highly trained veterinary surgeons (veterinarians).

Indications for endodontic treatment include:

- Blunt dental trauma and aseptic irreversible pulpitis
- Pulp exposure and bacterial invasion following complicated tooth fracture
- Crown reduction for malocclusion or disarming procedures
- Deep carious lesions (in dogs)
- Tooth displacement injuries (i.e. luxation and avulsion)
- Periodontal disease with secondary endodontic involvement.

Term	Definition
Apexification	A procedure to promote apical closure of a non-vital tooth
Apexogenesis	Physiological formation of the apex of a vital tooth
Apicoectomy	Removal of the apex of a tooth; also called root end resection
Crown reduction	Partial removal of tooth substance to reduce the height or an abnormal extension of the clinical crown
Crown amputation	Total removal of clinical crown substance
Direct pulp capping	A procedure performed as part of vital pulp therapy and involving the placement of a medicated material over an area of pulp exposure
Endodontics	Specialty in dentistry and oral surgery concerned with the prevention, diagnosis and treatment of diseases of the pulp–dentine complex and their impact on associated tissues
Hemisection	Splitting of a tooth into two separate portions
Indirect pulp capping	A procedure involving the placement of a medicated material over an area of near pulp exposure
Partial pulpectomy	Partial removal of pulp tissue to remove inflamed and diseased tissue and create space for medicated and restorative materials
Partial tooth resection	Removal of a tooth (usually a crown-root segment) with endodontic treatment of the remainder of the tooth
Retrograde filling	Restoration placed in the apical portion of the root canal after apicoectomy
Root resection (or root amputation)	Removal of a root with maintenance of the entire crown and endodontic treatment of the remainder of the tooth
Standard (orthograde) root canal therapy	A procedure that involves accessing, debriding (including total pulpectomy), shaping, disinfecting and obturating the root canal and restoring the access and/or fracture sites
Surgical (retrograde) root canal therapy	A procedure that involves accessing the bone surface (through mucosa or skin), fenestration of the bone over the root apex, apicoectomy, and retrograde filling
Trisection	Splitting of a tooth into three separate portions
Tooth repositioning	Repositioning of a luxated tooth
Tooth reimplantation	Reimplantation of an avulsed tooth
Vital pulp therapy	A procedure performed on a vital tooth with pulp exposure, involving partial pulpectomy, direct pulp capping and access/fracture site restoration

9.1 Terminology related to endodontic treatment.

Some contraindications to endodontic treatment also exist. Extraction may be the preferable treatment for:

* Endodontically affected deciduous teeth
* Functionally unimportant permanent teeth
* Teeth that show complicated or uncomplicated crown-root fractures
* Teeth that have lost the majority or all of the crown structure
* Teeth concomitantly affected by other disorders (e.g. advanced root replacement resorption)
* Whenever the operator is not properly trained, the instruments and materials required for endodontic treatment are not available, and referral to a veterinary dental specialist is not possible.

The size of the tooth and its pulp cavity may also influence the choice of treatment. While all endodontic techniques described in this chapter may be used in cats as well, most feline teeth (with the exception of the canine teeth) are too small to be treated appropriately.

The application of ergonomic rules (e.g. working in a sitting position, using a good light source and magnifying devices) is particularly important when performing procedures that require a high level of precision. Any endodontic procedure should be performed aseptically (Figure 9.2). The mouth should be prepared with an antiseptic solution and draped with sterile surgical towels. Professional dental cleaning should be performed. The tooth being treated should be polished with glycerin-free polishing pastes, as glycerin can interfere with the setting of restorative materials. A dental dam may be applied to isolate the tooth and decrease the risk of operative field contamination. Sterile gloves, handpieces, burs, instruments and materials should be used to decrease the chances of iatrogenic contamination of the pulp cavity.

A preoperative radiographic examination of any affected tooth is paramount in order to evaluate root development, lack of complicating factors (e.g. root canal obliteration, pulp stones, root resorption, root fracture),

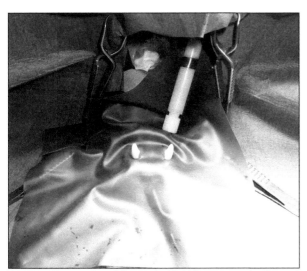

9.2 Preparation of the surgical field for crown reduction and endodontic treatment of the mandibular canine teeth in a dog. The patient was placed in sternal recumbency to enable concomitant work on both teeth. Sterile surgical drapes were used to delimit the oral cavity, and a rubber dam was placed to further isolate the teeth to be treated. A cuffed endotracheal tube and a pharyngeal pack are in place to decrease the chances of aspiration of fluids, debris, materials and small instruments. Excessive opening of the mouth is avoided using a short, not spring-held, mouth gag.
(© Dr Margherita Gracis)

presence of signs of pulp pathology (e.g. periapical radiolucency, lack of dentine deposition) and alveolar bone health (e.g. signs of periodontal disease, bone fracture). Any endodontically treated tooth should also be radiographically re-evaluated for some time after treatment, as many complications may only be noted upon radiographic examination. Owners should be made aware of the need for further re-examinations under sedation or general anaesthesia.

The choice of endodontic treatment depends upon the age of the affected tooth and patient, the presence, size and duration of pulp exposure, and the extent of infection and inflammation of the pulp (Figures 9.3 and 9.4). Recent enamel and uncomplicated crown fracture sites not nearing the pulp, may be smoothed of sharp edges with a water-cooled cone-shaped white stone bur followed by application of one or two layers of dental adhesive and periodic radiographic monitoring to ensure continued endodontic health. Commonly performed endodontic procedures and techniques are described in this chapter. The authors acknowledge that several modifications to these techniques are available.

Indirect pulp capping

Indirect pulp capping is defined as the placement of a dressing material over nearly exposed pulp to initiate the formation of tertiary dentine on the inner dentinal wall facing the site of injury (Dominguez *et al.*, 2003) (Figure 9.5). It is performed to decrease the risk of bacterial invasion of the pulp through exposed dentinal tubules and to reduce dentine sensitivity whenever a very thin layer of dentine covers vital pulp following tooth fracture, dental caries or restorative procedures. The main purpose of the procedure is to seal the dentinal tubules and cover the remaining dentine with appropriate materials.

If the layer of dentine is more than 0.5 mm thick, there may be less concern about irritation of the pulp, and the tooth can be restored with the restoration of choice (e.g. direct composite restoration). However, if the dentine thickness is ≤0.5 mm, a protective layer should be placed over the site of near pulp exposure and below the final restoration to seal the dentinal tubules and reduce the inflammatory reaction of the adjacent pulp tissue (Sigurdsson *et al.*, 2011). Varnishes, cavity liners and bases are pulp-protective agents. These materials provide different levels of electrical insulation, thermal and chemical protection against irritants released from restorative materials, mechanical support for the restoration and even some therapeutic benefit to the tooth.

Cavity varnishes are non-aqueous solvents that rely on evaporation for hardening. Most are based on copal or other resins dissolved in a volatile solvent. They are used as a very thin layer, mostly below amalgam restorations, which are rarely used these days. Some dentine-bonding agents may be used in shallow defect preparations below adhesive materials (i.e. glass ionomer cements and resin-based composites), as varnishes may be disrupted by monomers of these restorative materials. Varnishes have no significant mechanical strength and do not provide thermal insulation.

The most commonly used cavity liners (or suspension liners) are suspensions of calcium hydroxide (CaOH) in water or in an organic liquid, and eugenol containing biomaterials (e.g. zinc oxide–eugenol cements). They produce a thicker layer than varnishes. Because of its alkaline pH (i.e. pH >11), CaOH is irritating to the pulp, stimulates the formation of tertiary dentine and has antibacterial

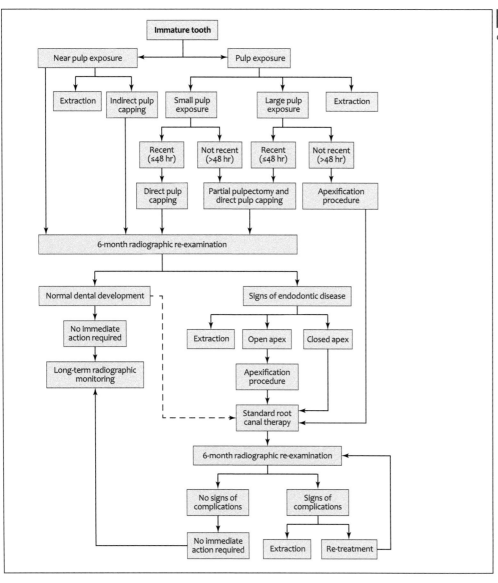

9.3 Algorithmic approach to the endodontic treatment of immature teeth.

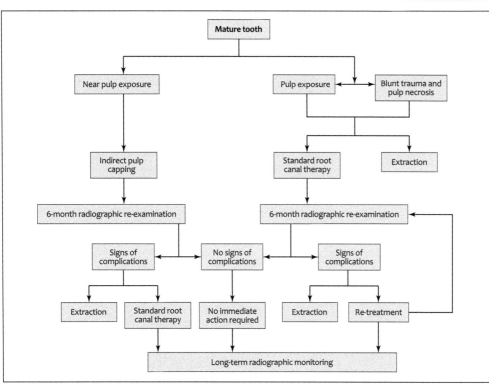

9.4 Algorithmic approach to endodontic treatment of mature teeth.

Type	Definition
Primary	Formed before completion of apex
Secondary	Formed after completion of apex (throughout the life of the animal)
Tertiary • Reparative • Reactionary	Formed as a result of injury: • Deposited by newly formed odontoblasts • Deposited by pre-existing odontoblasts

9.5 Types of dentine based on the timing of deposition.

(bactericidal and bacteriostatic) activity. Light-cured CaOH liners are available and easy to apply at the base of deep defect preparations before a base is placed. As it is soluble in oral fluids, CaOH should not be left on the margin of the prepared defect.

The most common cement bases include zinc oxide–eugenol (ZOE), CaOH, zinc phosphate and resin-modified glass ionomers (GI). They appropriately protect the pulp and, when applied in a relatively thick layer (>0.75 mm), are strong enough to withstand condensation forces during placement of restorations and to resist fracture under masticatory stress (Shen, 2003).

Indirect pulp capping is usually performed by first placing a 1 mm layer of CaOH liner, then adding a 1–2 mm GI base before the final composite restoration is placed. Follow-up radiographic examinations are recommended at least 6 and 12 months following treatment to assess continued vitality of the pulp.

Vital pulp therapy

Vital pulp therapy is performed to treat reversible pulpal injuries and maintain the vitality and function of the pulp in the case of acute pulp exposure following trauma, iatrogenic injury during restorative procedures or deliberate crown reduction. The treatment should create a tight seal above the healthy pulp. This procedure is normally warranted only in immature permanent teeth, which still have an open apex and very thin dentinal walls. Maintaining pulp vitality is necessary to allow for physiological root development, apical closure (i.e. apexogenesis) and continued dentine deposition.

The area and the duration of pulp exposure are important prognostic factors (Niemiec, 2001). The success rate in teeth treated within 48 hours of pulp exposure has been shown to be as high as 88.2%; however, the percentage of successful cases decreases significantly with duration of pulp exposure (41.4% and 23.5% of teeth treated within 1 week or 3 weeks of trauma, respectively) (Clarke, 2001). However, dentine production and apical closure can still happen for a certain period of time even in a tooth with irreversible pulpitis or focal pulp necrosis. Vital pulp therapy procedures have therefore been recommended even in severely affected immature teeth to stimulate apical closure, so that a standard root canal therapy can then be performed. It has been reported that vital pulp therapy can be successfully performed even after apical closure (Luotonen et al., 2014). However, whenever pulp exposure occurs in mature (with a closed apex) teeth, total pulpectomy and root canal therapy are preferred due to a more predictable outcome and lower risk of long-term complications.

Vital pulp therapy (Operative Technique 9.1) involves the removal of exposed, inflamed or infected pulp tissue (partial pulpectomy), direct pulp capping (placement of a dressing material over exposed pulp) and access or fracture site restoration. Preoperative periodontal and radiographic examinations should always be performed to confirm the lack of periodontal disease and endodontic or other complications. A bacteria-free operating environment should be created and aseptic techniques used. Varying opinions have been expressed about the use of perioperative systemic antibiotics, but their administration seems to be unnecessary if correct and strict aseptic techniques are applied (Luotonen et al., 2014).

Partial pulpectomy is performed using a sterile round or pear-shaped carbide or fine diamond bur on a sterile high-speed handpiece, cooled with sterile lactated Ringer's solution (Niemiec and Mulligan, 2001). The bur should be relatively large in diameter, as small burs are more likely to create irregular dentinal walls and deep defects in the pulp (increasing pulp injury and bleeding). Haemostasis is achieved by gently applying sterile paper points over the cut pulp stump. Restoring a tooth with a bleeding pulp will inevitably lead to increased pressure within the endodontic system, which in turn could lead to ischaemia and pulp death.

Once haemostasis is achieved, direct pulp capping is performed. An effective dressing material should enhance the formation of tertiary dentine without causing severe pulpal inflammation. Calcium hydroxide has been the material of choice for a long period of time. A small amount of pure CaOH powder is placed over the cut pulp; it can also be mixed to a thick paste with lactated Ringer's solution and gently placed against the pulp stump. Alternatively, a commercial hard-setting material may be used. Necrosis of the adjacent pulp tissue develops, and the contiguous tissue becomes inflamed. Dentine bridge formation occurs at the junction of the necrotic tissue and the inflamed vital pulp. Occasionally, however, in spite of successful bridge formation the pulp remains chronically inflamed or becomes necrotic. Tunnel defects in the dentine bridge (which may favour bacterial microleakage) have also been shown histologically in treated teeth.

Mineral trioxide aggregate (MTA) (ProRoot, Dentsply) is a relatively new material used as capping and retrofilling material to treat radicular perforations during standard root canal therapy and in apexification procedures. As a dressing material it is able to more frequently promote hard tissue formation, cause less pulp inflammation and provide superior bacteria-tight seals compared with CaOH (Galia Reston and de Souza Costa, 2009). It has a pH of 10.2 during manipulation and 12.5 during setting, which may impart some antimicrobial properties (although not against strict anaerobes). It has low solubility, does not shrink during setting and does not dissolve with time. Mixing the powder (which consists of fine hydrophilic particles of calcium silicate, bismuth oxide, calcium carbonate, calcium sulphate and calcium aluminate) with sterile water forms crystals of calcium oxide and results in a colloidal gel that hardens in approximately 3 hours in a moist environment. Once mixed it may be delivered with a small applicator or carrier and gently pressed into position. Irrigation of the area immediately after placement should be avoided as the material would be washed out. Finally, the restoration over calcium hydroxide or MTA is completed with an intermediate layer of glass ionomer and bonded composite resins or other restorative materials. Poor coronal restoration and marginal leakage greatly increase the risk for bacterial complications.

Follow-up

Teeth that have undergone vital pulp therapy should be re-evaluated radiographically at 3–6 months postoperatively,

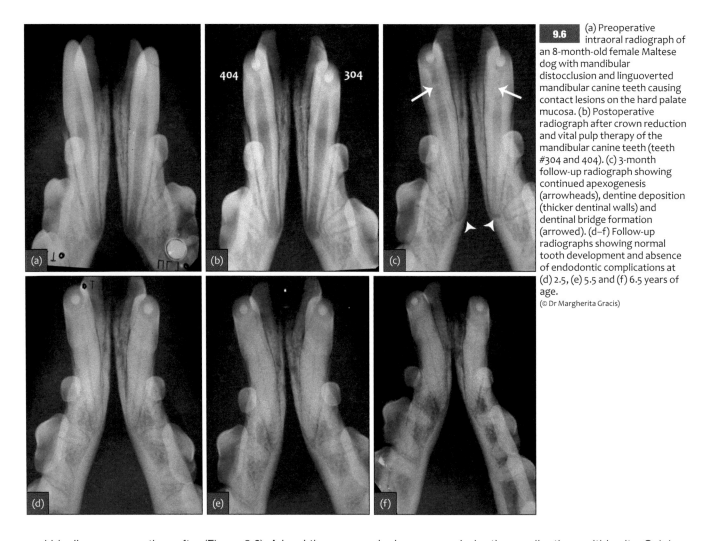

9.6 (a) Preoperative intraoral radiograph of an 8-month-old female Maltese dog with mandibular distocclusion and linguoverted mandibular canine teeth causing contact lesions on the hard palate mucosa. (b) Postoperative radiograph after crown reduction and vital pulp therapy of the mandibular canine teeth (teeth #304 and 404). (c) 3-month follow-up radiograph showing continued apexogenesis (arrowheads), dentine deposition (thicker dentinal walls) and dentinal bridge formation (arrowed). (d–f) Follow-up radiographs showing normal tooth development and absence of endodontic complications at (d) 2.5, (e) 5.5 and (f) 6.5 years of age.
(© Dr Margherita Gracis)

and ideally every year thereafter (Figure 9.6). A hard tissue barrier bridging the exposure site and overlying healthy pulp is expected to form within the first few months. Other desirable radiographic findings include a thickening of the dentinal walls (i.e. reduced width of the pulp cavity) and continued root development (root lengthening and apical closure). However, the radiographic presence of a more or less radiopaque dentinal bridge is not evidence for a tight seal or pulp vitality. Delayed tissue necrosis and persistent inflammation of the pulp tissue have been demonstrated in teeth apparently showing progressive dentine deposition. It is therefore important to monitor treated teeth for a long time after treatment. If signs of endodontic disease develop, either standard root canal therapy or extraction should be performed.

Apexification

Apexification is a procedure performed to promote apical closure of a non-vital, immature (with open apex and thin dentinal walls) or mature (open apex, for example due to apical resorption) permanent tooth to create an apical stop in preparation for standard root canal therapy. Because of the unpredictable outcome, length of time to achieve apical closure (it can take more than a year to happen), need for several anaesthetic procedures, and potential complications (e.g. fracture of the very thin-walled tooth during root canal therapy or because of trauma), apexification is not often performed in veterinary patients.

The technique involves total pulpectomy, debriding, shaping, disinfecting and drying of the pulp cavity, and placing an endodontic medication within it. Calcium hydroxide and MTA are both able to induce hard tissue formation, with MTA showing better results compared with CaOH. The material should be mixed to a creamy consistency and gently packed at the apex with a sterile coarse paper point or a sterile plugger to create a 3–5 mm plug, under strict radiographic control. After placing CaOH or MTA at the apex, the pulp cavity may be completely filled with CaOH paste with the aid of a spiral filler. A temporary coronal restoration is placed. A radiographic re-examination should be performed at intervals that may vary from 1 to 6 months. If necessary, the endodontic dressing (and temporary restoration) can be replaced. Once apical closure is evident, the remaining dressing is flushed out and root canal therapy completed with a standard technique, taking great care to avoid apical perforation and root fracture (Figure 9.7).

If MTA is used as the apical barrier, a moistened sterile paper point or cotton pellet is inserted within the root canal to enhance MTA setting, and a temporary restoration is placed over it. The tooth is re-entered (from 4 hours to a few days later), the portion of the root canal coronal to the plug is cleaned and obturated with standard techniques, and a permanent restoration is placed at the coronal access. A modified, one-visit apexification technique has recently been described in humans and cats (Juriga et al., 2008). It involves the immediate placement of an intermediate layer of dual-core glass ionomer over the MTA plug, followed by immediate obturation of the root canal and definitive tooth restoration.

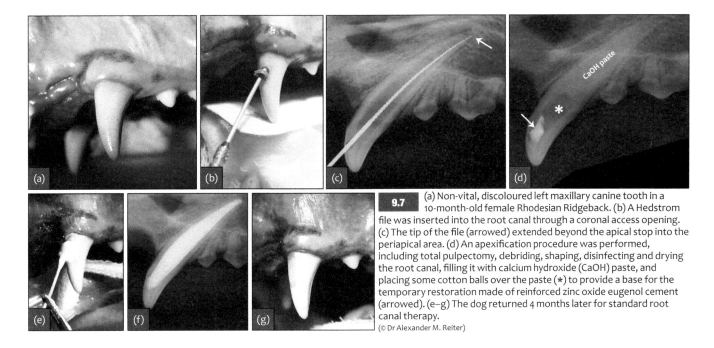

9.7 (a) Non-vital, discoloured left maxillary canine tooth in a 10-month-old female Rhodesian Ridgeback. (b) A Hedstrom file was inserted into the root canal through a coronal access opening. (c) The tip of the file (arrowed) extended beyond the apical stop into the periapical area. (d) An apexification procedure was performed, including total pulpectomy, debriding, shaping, disinfecting and drying the root canal, filling it with calcium hydroxide (CaOH) paste, and placing some cotton balls over the paste (*) to provide a base for the temporary restoration made of reinforced zinc oxide eugenol cement (arrowed). (e–g) The dog returned 4 months later for standard root canal therapy.

(© Dr Alexander M. Reiter)

Standard root canal therapy

A standard (or orthograde) root canal therapy is an endodontic procedure that involves accessing, debriding, shaping, disinfecting and obturating the root canal and restoring the access and/or fracture sites (Operative Technique 9.2). Indications include irreversible pulpitis (with or without pulp exposure), complicated crown (and sometimes crown-root) fractures, and partial tooth resection (Figure 9.8). When appropriately performed, it may permit the maintenance of strategically and functionally important teeth (or portions of teeth), with a low rate of treatment failure (Kuntsi-Vaatovaara *et al*., 2002).

Coronal access

When pulp exposure is present, the same exposure site may be used as access to the pulp cavity if it allows a direct and unrestricted path to the apex. Otherwise, a new access should be created (Figure 9.9) and preferably placed more than 2 mm coronal to the gingival margin to avoid soft tissue irritation following restoration. The access hole should be as small as possible to minimally affect coronal integrity but large enough to allow easy insertion of instruments. In teeth with large pulp cavities, a larger access hole may need to be made to allow for free movement of larger instruments. In multi-rooted teeth, all root canals should be accessed through one or more access holes. Knowledge of dental anatomy and morphology is therefore mandatory. Access sites for dog teeth have been described (Eisner, 1990; Marretta *et al*., 1993, 1994).

To avoid enamel chipping, the enamel is initially gouged with a small round carbide bur held perpendicular to the tooth surface. A larger bur is then used for actual perforation of the dentinal walls, directing it to the root apex until the pulp cavity is reached. In teeth with thin root canals it may be helpful to use a pathfinder to

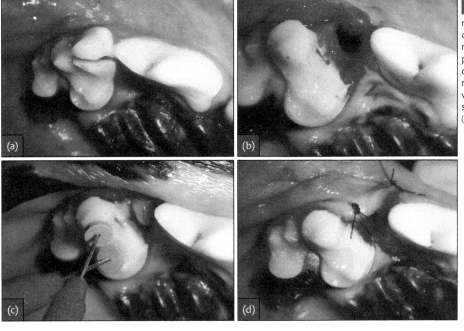

9.8 (a) Vertical fracture of the mesiobuccal crown-root of the right maxillary first molar tooth in a 15-month-old female Husky. (b) Resection of the mesiobuccal crown-root segment was performed, followed by (c) standard root canal therapy of the distobuccal and palatal roots. (d) The access and hemisection sites were restored, and a periodontal flap was sutured in position.

(© Dr Margherita Gracis)

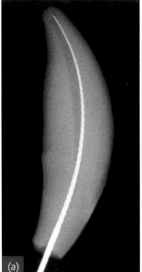
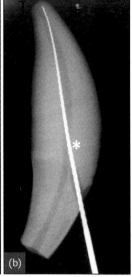
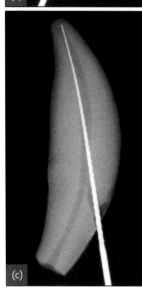

9.9 Radiographs of an extracted maxillary canine tooth of an adult dog. (a) A Hedstrom file has been inserted through the occlusal fracture site and bent to follow the curvature of the root canal. (b) An access hole has been created on the mesial surface of the tooth a few millimetres coronal to the imaginary gingival margin, and a file has been inserted into the root canal; note the bulge of dentine (∗) mesial to the file. (c) Flattening of the bulge of dentine by means of filing or burring allows for a more direct approach to the root apex.
(© Dr Margherita Gracis)

does not always allow the desired shape to be obtained. After widening of the coronal aspect of the pulp cavity and if the pulp is relatively intact, most of the soft tissue may initially be extirpated with barbed broaches that are inserted to the apical portion of the root canal until resistance is felt. Careful clockwise rotation of the broaches a few times before withdrawal will entangle the pulp at the barbs of the instrument (Figure 9.10). Broaches are very weak and delicate instruments, and breakage is possible if locked within the root canal while twisted. Therefore, the diameter of the broach should be significantly smaller than that of the root canal, to avoid contact of the barbed tips with the dentinal walls. For the same reason, lubrication of the canal with an irrigating solution or gel is also recommended.

Debriding and shaping of the root canal are performed concomitantly, using manual or mechanical instrumentation and appropriate irrigating solutions (Happasalo *et al.*, 2010). Various techniques may be used for debriding the root canal (Lyon, 1998; Niemiec, 2005), including the standardized technique (mainly using hand instruments), step-down technique (using either hand or rotary files), step-back technique (mainly using hand instruments) and hybrid techniques. The step-down technique (and the slightly different crown-down technique) entails the use of progressively smaller files, beginning with a relatively large instrument inserted to a short depth, continuing with progressively thinner instruments and ending with the instrument that is able to reach the apex. In the step-back technique, sufficiently fine instruments are initially inserted to the apex, and the procedure is continued with progressively larger files used at shorter working length, to taper the root canal (or a portion of it) in an apico-coronal direction.

The most common procedural errors during preparation of curved root canals are ledging, zipping, transportation, stripping and perforation. Ledging is the creation of a separate pathway at the outer curvature of

locate the pulp cavity. The access hole is then enlarged to the desired size, and the dentinal walls are flared with the use of progressively larger Gates Glidden drills, hand files or a bur with a non-cutting tip, removing any dentinal overhangs. After using each instrument, the area should be irrigated and the debris flushed out. Gates Glidden drills may also be used to prepare the coronal two-thirds of straight root canals using a step-back technique (i.e. tapering the canal in an apico-coronal direction using progressively larger drills).

Debriding, shaping and disinfecting

The main purposes of root canal therapy include the thorough debridement of the pulp cavity to completely remove infected, inflamed and necrotic tissues and the placement of a tight-seal obturation (Baugh and Wallace, 2005). It is still controversial if debridement of the entire pulp chamber is necessary or if entombing some coronal pulp after root canal obturation and coronal restoration is acceptable (e.g. in an intact canine tooth). If the tissue contained in the pulp chamber is to be removed, access holes should be modified accordingly.

Ideally, the root canal should be shaped to a uniform and continuous 10% taper, which is easier to clean and obturate. However, dental anatomy in dogs and cats

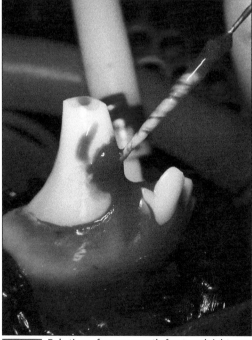

9.10 Pulp tissue from a recently fractured right mandibular canine tooth in a 20-month-old male Labrador Retriever is removed with a barbed broach.
(© Dr Margherita Gracis)

the canal due to not precurving the file or excessively forcing it into the canal. Zipping results from a flexible file that tends to straighten inside a curved canal, causing an over-enlargement of the canal along the outer side of the curvature and an under-preparation of the inner aspect of the curvature at the apical end point. Perforation into periapical tissues may happen due to persistent filing with too large an instrument or continual zipping. Transportation is the excessive removal of dentine from the outer wall of a curved canal in the apical segment. Stripping is a thinning of dentine at the inner curvature of the canal due to over-preparing and accidental straightening of the curved canal and can lead to perforation.

In the standardized technique for hand files, a thin file should be inserted to the apex and its position confirmed radiographically to determine working length (the distance from a reference point on the crown to the apical stop) (Figure 9.11). Every single instrument thereafter is used similarly, placing a rubber stop along the instrument shaft at the same distance from the tip, measuring with an endodontic ruler. Files of progressively larger sizes are used, up to the last file that is able to reach the apex (last file or master apical file). A radiograph is obtained to confirm the file fitting the apical portion of the root canal (Figure 9.11). After using each instrument, abundant irrigation of the root canal should be performed with 3–5 ml of full-strength (5.25%) or diluted sodium hypochlorite (NaOCl) through an endodontic needle that is positioned a few millimetres short of the apex and moved with an in-and-out motion. If resistance to the solution's flow is felt, the needle should be pulled out and a thinner needle used. Frequent recapitulation should also be performed to prevent blockage, using fine instruments after each file to ensure removal of all dentinal chips from the apical area. After each use, the files should be cleaned and disinfected in a 5.25% NaOCl bath. Filing and shaping is continued until the instruments collect clean white dentinal shavings. The apex should also be enlarged to a size that allows easy insertion of instruments and materials for obturation. Studies evaluating the minimum root canal size have not been performed in veterinary patients, but in humans it is recommended to enlarge the canal to a diameter of at least 0.35 mm (file #35) to facilitate debris removal and to allow adequate irrigation of the apical third (Baugh and Wallace, 2005). To simplify obturation in relatively thin root canals, the canal taper may be slightly increased using a step-back technique, with files larger than the master apical file set to decreasing working lengths.

Once the root canal has been debrided and shaped, it is abundantly irrigated with saline. Alternatively, 5–10 ml of NaOCl may be used, followed by 17% ethylenediamine tetra-acetic acid (EDTA) solution, which is left in place for about 1 minute to remove the smear layer (dentine debris produced during filing, coating the root canal walls and clogging the orifices of the dentinal tubules). NaOCl is then used as a final rinse or followed by a 95% ethanol rinse before obturation to favour drying of the root canal (Stevens et al., 2006). The root canal is also dried with the aid of paper points of appropriate sizes (Figure 9.12). The last paper point should be dry and white in colour. Any discoloration of the point's tip may indicate the presence of necrotic tissue or blood in the root canal or the apical delta, requiring further instrumentation or the application of a temporary dressing and restoration with delayed obturation. If necessary, a temporary CaOH dressing may be placed within the root canal with the aid of a spiral filler or a paper point and left in place for 2–4 weeks before proceeding with obturation.

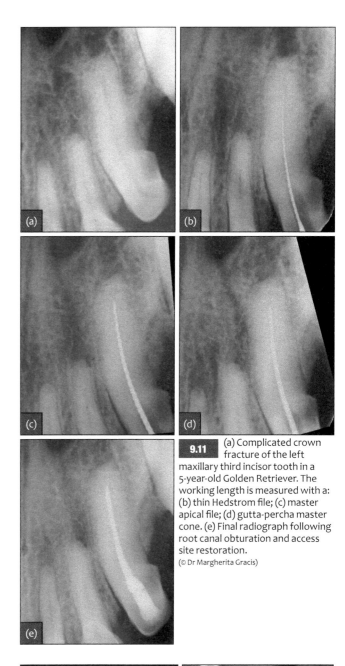

9.11 (a) Complicated crown fracture of the left maxillary third incisor tooth in a 5-year-old Golden Retriever. The working length is measured with a: (b) thin Hedstrom file; (c) master apical file; (d) gutta-percha master cone. (e) Final radiograph following root canal obturation and access site restoration.
(© Dr Margherita Gracis)

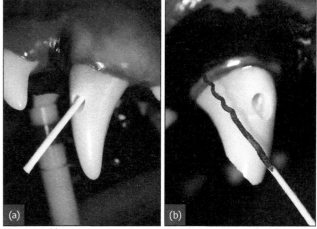

9.12 (a) A paper point is inserted into the root canal of a left maxillary canine tooth after debriding, shaping and disinfecting. (b) Discoloration of a paper point used to dry the root canal of the right maxillary canine tooth in a different patient indicates haemorrhage and the need for further instrumentation or placement of a temporary endodontic medication.
(© Dr Margherita Gracis)

Obturation

Uniform and dense obturation of the entire root canal is necessary to decrease the chances of bacterial microleakage and treatment failure (Girard *et al.*, 2006). The root canal should be sealed apically, laterally and coronally. Debridement, shaping, disinfecting and provision of a fluid-tight seal of the most apical 3 mm of the root canal are particularly important. The presence of small amounts of diseased pulp or blood in this location and the presence of voids that allow leakage from the periradicular tissues into the endodontic system are likely to lead to failure.

The material of choice for obturation is gutta-percha (GP), available as either cold points or thermoplastic materials. GP is a rubbery substance of vegetable origin. The material used in endodontics is a mixture of GP (the matrix, about 20%), zinc oxide (the filler, about 66%), heavy metal salts (the radiopacifers, about 11%) and wax or resins (the platicizers, about 3%).

Several root canal obturation techniques may be used, namely the cold lateral condensation technique, the warm vertical compaction or Schilder's technique (small portions of GP are softened with heat and condensed apically in incremental layers), the continuous wave compaction technique (the GP master cone is heated and compacted apically with the aid of an electric heat carrier designed as a plugger), and the warm lateral compaction technique (the cold GP master cone and accessory points are progressively condensed laterally with a heated tip) (Girard *et al.*, 2006). There are also a number of thermoplastic injection systems, which heat GP outside the tooth and then inject it into the root canal. Carrier-based systems use GP-coated plastic or titanium carriers to be inserted into the root canal. More recently manufactured carrier-based systems use soft-bonded resin in place of GP. Furthermore, thermomechanical compaction of GP uses an instrument (McSpadden compactor) run on a low-speed handpiece to soften GP by friction and move it apically. Finally, a cold flowable silicon-based sealer mixed with GP particles has recently been introduced. The sealer may be injected directly into root canals, followed by the placement of a single GP master cone. Some of these techniques may be used in combination.

Although the thermoplastic GP and carrier-based GP or resin systems may allow faster obturation and improve the apical seal, the cold lateral condensation is a very versatile technique. It entails the use of a master GP cone, which should correspond in diameter to the root canal diameter at working length (and therefore to the last file used to clean and shape the apical portion of the root canal) (see Figure 9.11). However, as there is a manufacturing size tolerance for files (±0.02 mm) and GP cones (±0.05 mm), the size of the master cone and that of the last file may not always match. GP cones of different sizes should therefore be tried before choosing the master cone. The cone should fit tightly at the apex, and when withdrawn from the root canal, it should provide a 'tug back' sensation (a small resistance to displacement). The position and size of the master cone should also be evaluated radiographically. It should appear to reach and completely fill the apical portion of the root canal, without visible voids around it. The master cone is then marked by grasping it with a pair of college pliers at a repeatable distance from the tip next to a reference point on the tooth crown. The measurement obtained should match the working length.

As GP may be unable to completely fill the root canal and bond to the dentinal walls, a small amount of endodontic sealer is used in conjunction with it. After choosing the master cone, the sealer is introduced in the empty root canal with the aid of a spiral filler run clockwise at very low speed, thus coating the dentinal walls. The diameter of the spiral filler should be smaller than that of the root canal, as spiral fillers are weak and prone to fracture if run at high speed or in the case of blockage within the root canal.

The master cone is coated with a thin layer of sealer, introduced into the canal at working length, and compacted apically and laterally with a spreader of appropriate length and diameter. To allow easier insertion of successive instruments and GP points, the excess GP may be removed slightly apical to the access hole with a heated instrument or with a bur on a low-speed or high-speed handpiece without water cooling, carefully avoiding pulling the master cone in a coronal direction. The eyes of the operator and patient should be protected when using rotary instruments, as small fragments of heated GP may be thrown some distance. Sealer-coated accessory GP points of decreasing sizes are consecutively added and placed in the space vacated by progressively thinner and shorter spreaders and pluggers, until the root canal appears completely obturated. The GP points are finally cut off at the coronal access, and the GP inside the pulp cavity is plugged apically.

Finally, appropriate obturation is confirmed radiographically, although it should be borne in mind that a two-dimensional radiographic evaluation may provide limited information (see Figure 9.11). Whenever possible, two orthogonal views should be obtained to maximize the possibility of detecting obturation defects (Figure 9.13). Cone-beam computed tomography (CBCT) has been shown to be superior to conventional radiography in detecting voids in the root filling of endodontically treated teeth (Liang *et al.*, 2011).

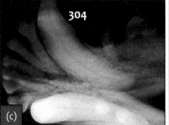
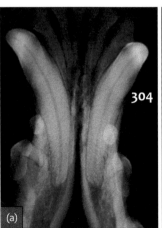
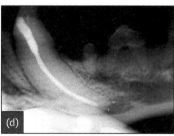
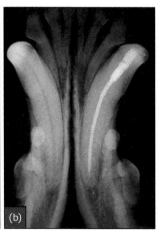

9.13 Radiographs of the left mandibular canine tooth (304) of a 4-year-old male Belgian Shepherd with irreversible chronic pulpitis of traumatic origin. Occlusal views (a) before and (b) after, and lateral views (c) before and (d) after standard root canal therapy; a small amount of extruded zinc oxide eugenol cement is visible periapically in the after images. The portion of the pulp chamber coronal to the access hole was not opened and treated and therefore appears radiolucent.
(© Dr Margherita Gracis)

Restorative materials and defect preparation

Any endodontic procedure should be completed with the placement of a well sealed restoration, which prevents bacterial invasion of the treated tooth. Coronal microleakage can be a reason for treatment failure (Figure 9.14). A direct composite restoration is normally utilized, unless crown integrity is severely compromised by the initial trauma and/or the animal is used for special activities (e.g. police dogs), potentially requiring reconstruction of the lost portion of the tooth. First, residual GP and sealer in the pulp chamber are removed with a heated excavator and a bur on a high-speed or low-speed handpiece, and then the restoration is applied. Numerous restorative materials are available (Colmery, 1998). The choice should be based on a number of factors, including the size and location (e.g. occlusal *versus* interproximal) of the defect, the need for aesthetics (tooth-coloured materials may be preferable in certain situations, even if the cosmetic result is less of a concern in animals than humans), the type of endodontic procedure performed and the type of endodontic material used for root canal obturation. The most common restorative material used in veterinary patients is compactable or flowable composite in combination with acid etching/dentine conditioning and adhesive bonding (Operative Technique 9.3).

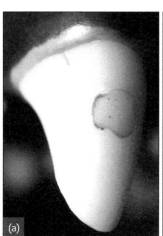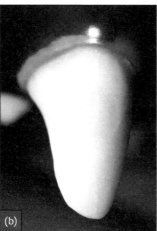

9.14 (a) An access restoration on the right maxillary canine tooth of a dog shows marginal leakage, evident as brownish discoloration of its margins; this restoration was also irregularly shaped and showed superficial porosity. (b) The restorative material was removed and replaced after radiographic confirmation of lack of endodontic complications.
(© Dr Margherita Gracis)

Crown preparation and placement of prosthodontic crowns

Metal crowns are primarily utilized to restore and protect fractured or weakened teeth of dogs that put their dentition at risk of trauma (e.g. police dogs, military dogs and prison dogs). Depending on how much of the natural crown of the tooth needs to be covered with metal, we distinguish a partial crown (only the tip and three sides of the tooth are covered in a so-called 'three-quarter crown') or a full crown (all sides of the root are covered) (Figure 9.15) (Visser, 1998; Luskin, 2001; Fink and Reiter, 2015). A crown margin preparation is performed to create space for a 1 mm thick metal crown to be seated on to the prepared tooth. Impressions of the prepared tooth (to make the metal crown) and impressions of all maxillary and mandibular teeth (to make stone models) are obtained, and a bite registration is made. The materials are submitted to a

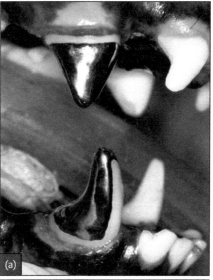

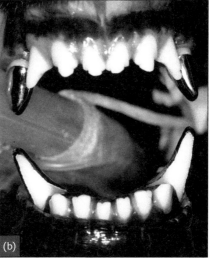

9.15 (a) Lateral view towards the mouth of a police dog showing a full crown at the right maxillary canine tooth and a partial crown at the right mandibular canine tooth; the opposite side has not yet undergone prosthodontic therapy. (b) Frontal view obtained in the same dog following completion of prosthodontic therapy.
(© Dr Alexander M. Reiter)

dental laboratory with instructions for how to fabricate the metal crown. Turn-around time is about 10–14 days, after which the metal crown is cemented in position (Visser, 1998; Coffman and Visser, 2007; Coffman *et al.*, 2007; Fink and Reiter, 2015).

Prognosis and follow-up of standard root canal therapy

A number of factors influence the prognosis of root canal therapy, including appropriate diagnosis, knowledge of dental anatomy and root morphology, thorough canal debridement and disinfection, fluid-tight seal obturation and coronal restoration. Most endodontic instruments, if used improperly, could break. If they break within the root canal, the successive steps may become complicated or impossible to perform, and extraction may also be necessary. Successfully treating very young (wide pulp cavity and thin dentinal walls) or old (very narrow pulp cavity and thick dentinal walls) teeth, or teeth with curved roots, may be particularly challenging. Complications of endodontic treatment are usually associated with pre-existing radiographic periapical lucency or pre-existing root resorption, with a failure rate of approximately 6% of treated roots (Kuntsi-Vaatovaara *et al.*, 2002). Failure may also be caused by defective preparation or obturation, use of inferior materials, or misuse of dental materials. Following the manufacturer's instructions is mandatory, and no changes in handling indications should ever be made. In humans, persistent intraradicular or extraradicular infection is the major cause of endodontic failure of both well treated and poorly treated teeth (Siqueira, 2001). Therefore, every effort should be made to achieve infection control and prevention (i.e. use of aseptic techniques, thorough debridement, use of appropriate irrigants, adequate obturation and restoration) (Siqueira, 2001).

Even for apparently well treated teeth, radiographic re-evaluation should be performed 3 months after root canal therapy, and ideally at 1 year and annually thereafter (especially if a pre-existing periapical radiolucency persists at follow-up) (Kuntsi-Vaatovaara *et al.*, 2002). Ideally, with time any preoperative periapical radiolucency should diminish and possibly resolve, the periodontal ligament space should be visible and be of normal width, and any pre-existing root resorption should have ceased. In human dentistry, CBCT has been increasingly utilized to diagnose early signs of endodontic failure, such as apical periodontitis and root resorption, because of its superior sensitivity compared with intraoral radiography (de Paula-Silva *et al.*, 2009; Garcia de Paula-Silva *et al.*, 2009; Patel, 2009).

Surgical root canal therapy

Surgical (retrograde) root canal therapy is a procedure that involves gaining access to the bone surface (through mucosa or skin), fenestration of the bone over the root apex, apicoectomy (the removal of the apex of the tooth), and retrograde filling (Hennet and Girard, 2005). Indications include unsuccessful standard root canal therapy, impossible orthograde treatment or re-treatment (e.g. root canal obliteration or presence of a pulp stone, post-and-core and/or prosthodontic crown in place, broken endodontic instrument that is impossible to remove or bypass) and fracture of the apical third of a root with pulp necrosis (Eisner, 2012a). Normally, even in the case of failed root canal therapy, a standard approach and re-treatment should be attempted first. Retrograde treatment should not be performed without prior or concurrent orthograde root canal therapy (Fulton *et al.*, 2012).

A full-thickness mucosal flap is initially raised on the labial/buccal side of the upper or lower jaw (Figure 9.16), except for the lower canine tooth, which is accessed through a percutaneous incision on the ventral aspect of the mandible (Eisner, 2012b). Access to the apex of the mesiopalatal root of the maxillary fourth premolar and palatal root of the molar teeth is not possible (extraction of the crown-root segments is performed instead). Bone is removed using a carbide round bur on a water-cooled high-speed handpiece, using a gentle, brushstroke technique, or a piezosurgery unit with an appropriate ostectomy tip. It may be wise to drill a small hole into the bone, place a radiopaque marker into it, and radiographically identify the apex before full osteotomy is performed. The bone is then removed for a distance of 1–2 mm apical to the root apex and exposing about 5–6 mm of the root end. Any diseased periapical tissues are removed with a bone curette. Depending on the size of the tooth the apical 3–4 mm of the root are resected at an 80–90-degree angle to the long axis of the root using a fissure bur and producing a smooth, flat root surface. Great care should be taken to

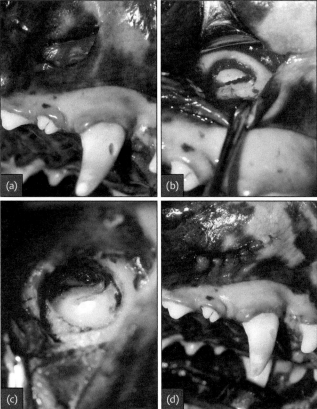

9.16 Discoloration and irreversible chronic pulpitis of traumatic origin affecting the right maxillary canine tooth in a dog. Orthograde access was performed, but the middle third of the root canal was obliterated. Surgical root canal therapy was therefore performed. (a) A semilunar flap was elevated in the alveolar mucosa over the apex of the tooth. (b) The apex and periapical areas were exposed following osteotomy, and about 3 mm of the apex was removed; cutting through the apex was performed at an angle of about 45 degrees to the long axis of the root, although an 80–90-degree angle would be preferable. (c) Following retrograde debriding, shaping, disinfecting and gutta-percha filling, a restoration was placed. (d) The mucosal flap was sutured and the coronal access site restored.
(© Dr Margherita Gracis)

avoid perforation of the palatally (or lingually) located alveolar bone plate during this procedure.

If orthograde root canal therapy is not possible, the procedure is performed through the retrograde access. Finally, the apical aspect of the root canal is prepared to a depth of 3–4 mm, using a small round or inverted-cone bur on a micro-handpiece or ultrasonic equipment with appropriate diamond-coated retrotips. The preparation should be made along the long axis of the tooth. Modified zinc oxide eugenol cements, glass ionomer cements and MTA are among the most common retrograde filling materials. MTA in particular is able to allow overgrowth of cementum and formation of bone and facilitate the regeneration of periodontal ligament fibres. The filling material is packed and condensed in the defect preparation, allowed to set and finally smoothed. The area is then curetted and irrigated to remove any debris. In humans, the use of grafting material is limited to cases of severe periapical bone loss with concomitant periodontal lesions. The depth and density of the retrograde filling is confirmed radiographically before the flap is sutured closed. Non-steroidal anti-inflammatory drugs and/or opioids should be administered for a few days to manage postoperative pain. A recent study has documented that retrograde root canal therapy is a reliable and effective procedure in dogs (Fulton *et al.*, 2012).

Management of tooth displacement injuries

Oral trauma often leads to tooth fracture; however, teeth may also become displaced, especially if the bone is less resilient, such as in young animals. The energy and direction of the impacting force greatly influence the type of injury, which may include:

- Concussion: the tooth is sensitive to percussion, but it is not mobile. In dogs and cats it may be difficult to diagnose. Treatment may be necessary in case of irreversible pulpitis, significantly increased intrapulpar pressure and ischaemic necrosis
- Subluxation: the tooth has slightly increased mobility, but it is not displaced. In dogs and cats it may be difficult to diagnose. Treatment may be necessary in case of irreversible pulpitis, as for concussion cases
- Extrusive luxation: the tooth is partially extruded out of the alveolar socket and shows increased mobility. Manual repositioning of the tooth, splinting and delayed endodontic treatment (or extraction) are necessary
- Intrusive luxation: the tooth is forced into the alveolus in an apical direction, and mobility is absent. In young children, intruded teeth may re-erupt spontaneously, but it is not known whether the same occurs in young dogs and cats. Orthodontic extrusion, splinting and delayed endodontic treatment (or extraction) may be necessary
- Lateral luxation: the tooth is displaced horizontally (Figure 9.17). The alveolar bone is typically fractured, and the mucogingival tissues are lacerated. The tooth may be 'locked' in position and shows either increased or decreased mobility. Manual repositioning of the tooth, suturing of torn soft tissues, splinting and delayed endodontic treatment (or extraction) are necessary
- Avulsion: the tooth is completely displaced from its alveolus. Manually replacing the tooth into the alveolus, suturing of torn soft tissues, splinting and delayed endodontic treatment are necessary. If the tooth is not replaced, the wound should be debrided and rinsed prior to being sutured closed.

Luxation and avulsion injuries represent dental emergencies (Gracis and Orsini, 1998). The length of time between injury and repositioning or replantation greatly influences the prognosis. In particular, prolonged drying of the tooth causes loss of vitality of the remaining periodontal ligament fibres (with additional complications such as root resorption following repositioning or replantation), and dehydration and necrosis of the pulp. The tooth should therefore be repositioned or replanted into the alveolar socket as soon as possible, ideally within 30–60 minutes of the time of injury. Meanwhile, if avulsed, the tooth should be maintained in a moist environment, using a suitable storage medium (i.e. cold low-fat milk or a commercial cell reconstitution fluid such as Hank's balanced salt solution). Antibiotic treatment should also be started immediately, and a preoperative radiographic examination needs to be performed to evaluate the injured dentoalveolar tissues as well as nearby structures.

The alveolar socket and root surface should be handled with great care. Aggressive debridement must be avoided, and blood clots or debris should be removed with gentle irrigation with lactated Ringer's solution and suction. The tooth should be held at the crown and manually repositioned (luxated tooth) or replanted (avulsed tooth). If alveolar bone fragments prevent repositioning or replantation, a blunt instrument should be used inside the alveolar socket to realign them. Loose fragments may be removed. After radiographic confirmation of its correct position, the injured tooth should be attached to adjacent teeth, ideally using a non-rigid splint. The acid-etch resin splinting technique entails the use of a composite material or acrylic resin, with or without orthopaedic wire. The splinting duration should be as short as possible, as minimizing splinting time improves the outcome of the treatment and reduces the occurrence of complications such as dentoalveolar ankylosis. Recommendations in human patients entail a 4–6 weeks splinting time for luxated teeth and 7–10 days for avulsed teeth. However, splinting time for large avulsed teeth such as canine teeth in dogs may be necessarily longer, to allow for complete periodontal healing.

In the postoperative period, systemic antibiotics (to reduce the occurrence of inflammatory resorption and pulp infection) and analgesics should be prescribed. Biting should be minimized, chew toys withdrawn and a soft diet offered. Oral home care (i.e. tooth brushing

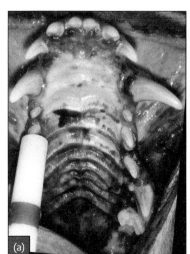 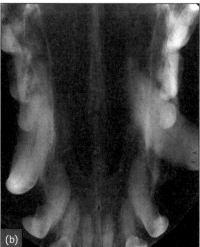 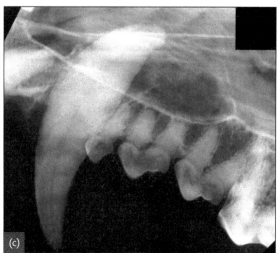

9.17 (a) Lateral luxation of the left maxillary canine tooth in a 10-year-old Beagle caused by a fight with another dog. (b) Occlusal intraoral radiographic view showing lateral displacement of the crown and nasal displacement of the root. (c) Lateral intraoral radiographic view showing distal displacement of the crown and mesial displacement of the root.
(© Dr Margherita Gracis)

and rinsing with a diluted chlorhexidine solution) should be recommended. As luxation and avulsion injuries frequently result in pulp necrosis, root canal therapy of injured teeth is necessary in most instances. It is recommended to perform it at the time of splint removal (avulsed teeth) or at least 10–14 days after repositioning (luxated teeth). In the latter case, it may be accomplished through the splint (Gracis, 2012).

Potential long-term complications following displacement and treatment include inflammatory root resorption, dentoalveolar ankylosis and root replacement resorption. Repositioned and replanted teeth should therefore be followed-up radiographically for a long period of time. Deciduous teeth should not be repositioned or replanted because of the possibility of damage to an underlying developing permanent tooth.

Management of oral bone and soft tissue trauma

Equipment for oral trauma surgery

Investing in and using the right equipment are paramount in oral trauma surgery. Operators are likely to develop a personal preference for a particular instrument or material during their careers (Reiter, 2013). The present description will deal with equipment specifically used for oral (soft tissue and bone) trauma surgery. Instruments and materials relevant to other procedures are described in other chapters of this manual.

The basic contents of a surgical pack include an instrument cassette, towel clamps, scalpel handles, retractors, thumb forceps, tissue forceps, haemostatic forceps, periosteal elevators, surgical curettes, tissue scissors, needle holders and suture scissors (Lipscomb and Reiter, 2005; Reiter, 2013). Depending on the procedure performed, other instruments and materials may be needed for the diagnosis and treatment of oral trauma (Figure 9.18).

The cassette holds a kit of select instruments for a straightforward, organized workflow.

- Backhaus or Jones towel clamps are used to attach drapes and towels to the skin. They may also be used to hold on to smaller bones or grasp flaps for manipulation during elevation and apposition prior to suturing.
- No. 3 and 5 scalpel handles are often used in oral surgery, accepting numbers 10, 11, 15 and 15C blades.
- Hand-held tissue retraction is accomplished with Seldin, Senn and Cawood-Minnesota retractors, skin hooks or stay sutures. Gelpi retractors are self-retaining versions that hold the wound open on their own.
- Thumb forceps hold and stabilize tissue during dissection and suturing. Delicate Adson 1 x 2 forceps have a fine rat-toothed grip, which causes minimal trauma to mucosal and submucosal tissue.
- Tissue forceps such as Allis forceps hold larger volumes of tissue, but are more traumatic.
- Haemostatic forceps hold delicate tissue, gently separate tissue or compress a bleeding vessel. Commonly used versions include the relatively small Halsted mosquito and the larger Kelly haemostatic forceps.
- Angled forceps are dissecting tools. However, Mixter, Rochester–Carmalt or Schnidt forceps can also be used for oesophagostomy tube placement by advancing the instrument from the oral cavity into the mid-cervical oesophagus and pushing its curved tips

- Surgical loupe (for magnification)
- Headlamp (for illumination)
- Wedge props and mouth gags (for keeping the mouth open)
- Drapes (for provision of a sterile field)
- Sterile surgical marker pen and plastic ruler (for outlining incisions)
- Dental mirror (for tissue visualization and retraction)
- Dental explorer and periodontal probe (for dental and periodontal evaluation)
- Dental elevators and extraction forceps (for removal of injured teeth and root remnants)
- Powered systems, handpieces, attachments, burs and saws (for cutting teeth and bones)
- Mallet and osteotome (for cutting bone and separating the mandibular symphysis)
- Rongeurs (for bone removal)
- No. 15 scalpel blades (for incising oral mucosa and skin)
- Cotton-tipped applicators (for absorbing blood and fluid, applying an agent or dissecting tissue)
- Swabs (for pharyngeal packing and blood/fluid absorption)
- Suture material (for vessel ligation, stay sutures and wound closure)
- Orthopaedic wire and hypodermic needles (for interdental, intraosseus and circumferential wiring)
- Resin materials (for splint fabrication)
- Wire twister and cutter (for creating twist knots and cutting wire)
- Kirschner wires and Steinmann pins (for drilling intraosseous wire holes and external skeletal fixation)
- Bone plates, screws and associated tools (for provision of rigid bone fracture stabilization)
- Bone-holding forceps (for holding on to bone or aligning bone segments)
- Wooden dowel (for manual reduction of temporomandibular joint luxation)
- Mayo bowl, bulb syringe and rinsing solutions (for lavage of wounds and cavities)
- Suction tips (for removal of blood and fluid)
- Penrose drains (for withdrawal of wound discharge)
- Culture media (for temporary storage of an avulsed tooth)
- Bone replacement materials (for bone grafting procedures)
- Topical haemostatic agents (for control of bleeding)
- Microsurgical tools (for neurovascular anastomosis during free tissue transfer)
- Feeding tubes (for postoperative nutritional support)
- Bandage tape (for custom-made muzzle fabrication)
- Elizabethan collar (for prevention of self-mutilation)
- Antimicrobial rinses and gels (for plaque control)

9.18 Instruments and materials used for the diagnosis and treatment of oral trauma in addition to the basic contents of a surgical pack.

laterally, which creates a small bulge on the skin to be incised (Terpak and Verstraete, 2012).
- Periosteal elevators commonly used in oral surgery include the Mead No. 3, Molt No. 9 or Periosteal No. EX-9M for mid-sized and larger dogs and the Glickman No. 24G or Periosteal No. EX-9 for small dogs and cats. They help in reflecting the mucoperiosteum by pressing the flat side of the instrument's working end against the bone and the convex side against the soft tissue, thus reducing the chance of tearing the elevated flap.
- Surgical curettes such as the Spratt, Volkmann or Miller are used for removal of debris and granulation tissue from a soft tissue wound, a bone surface or defect, or an alveolar socket after tooth extraction.
- Metzenbaum scissors are used for the cutting and dissecting of soft tissues. Smaller sized, curved, blunt-ended versions with serrated blades are most useful in oral surgery. They must not be used to cut suture material. Mayo scissors are used for cutting firm soft tissue and cartilage. A designated pair of Mayo scissors can be used for cutting sutures.
- Halsey (more sturdy) and DeBakey (more delicate) needle holders with serrated jaws are often used in oral surgery. They can be locked on to the needle by a ratchet mechanism to prevent needle slippage.

Initial examination and debridement

Following stabilization of the patient's condition, jaw fractures and soft tissue trauma are evaluated by inspection and palpation of the mandibular and maxillary bones, temporomandibular joints (TMJs), lips, cheeks, tongue, palate and oral and pharyngeal mucosal linings. The head is examined for asymmetry and discontinuity, exophthalmos or enophthalmos, lip avulsions and facial wounds, and the oral cavity is inspected for mucosal lacerations, haematomas and haemorrhage, fractured and displaced teeth and malocclusion (Reiter *et al.*, 2012).

Radiography and cross-sectional diagnostic imaging (computed tomography, CT) of head trauma patients should be performed under sedation or anaesthesia after stabilization of the patient. Multiple radiographic views may be necessary to assess all present injuries. Many mandibular and maxillary fractures can also be satisfactorily assessed with size 2 and 4 dental radiographic film or phosphor plates (sensor pads only come in sizes 0 and 2). Size 4 dental radiographic films or phosphor plates can also be utilized in the cat to evaluate injuries to the zygomatic arch, mandibular ramus, TMJ and tympanic bulla using extraoral radiographic techniques. CT has been shown to be superior to conventional head radiography for identification of traumatic injuries in dogs and cats (Bar-Am *et al.*, 2008) and is particularly indicated for caudal mandibular fractures, maxillary fractures and TMJ injury that cannot be assessed adequately with radiography. Patients with moderate to severe head trauma on presentation, neurological signs, failure to improve or deterioration of clinical signs, should undergo imaging studies of intracranial structures (Reiter *et al.*, 2012).

Surgical treatment is aimed at repairing hard and soft tissue injuries, establishing normal or functional occlusion, and providing acceptable cosmesis. Pharyngotomy or transmylohyoid orotracheal intubation may be performed to allow intraoperative control of occlusion without the need for extubation of the patient during surgical management of jaw fractures (Soukup and Snyder, 2015). Initially, the mouth is rinsed with 0.12% chlorhexidine digluconate, followed by wound lavage with lactated Ringer's solution (Buffa *et al.*, 1997). The injured sites are carefully debrided to remove blood clots, food particles, foreign material, small bone fragments and necrotic tissue. If teeth with fracture lines extending along the periodontal ligament space towards the root apex are retained, they should be carefully monitored for evidence of periodontal or endodontic pathology, and appropriate treatment must be initiated as soon as either is recognized (Reiter *et al.*, 2012). Severely mobile teeth, teeth with advanced periodontitis or periapical disease, and those that interfere with reduction of the bone fracture should be extracted (Schloss and Marretta, 1990). Hemisection, extraction of the crown-root segment in the fracture line, and maintenance of the non-involved crown-root segment may be an alternative to complete extraction of multi-rooted teeth (Reiter *et al.*, 2005).

Soft tissue lacerations are sutured before or after orthopaedic repair as indicated. Antibiotic therapy may be required in select cases with open bone fractures to prevent infection (Reiter *et al.*, 2012). Jaw fracture repair from a veterinary dentist's point of view utilizes the following principles:

- Use non-invasive techniques if possible
- Utilize teeth for anchorage
- Preserve sound teeth at or near the fracture site
- Concomitantly treat endodontic and periodontal lesions of teeth near or at the fracture site
- Avoid iatrogenic injury to other teeth, bone and soft tissue
- Maintain/restore proper occlusion.

Non-invasive and invasive techniques of jaw fracture repair

Muzzling

Immature, adolescent and young adult patients with little displacement of a lower jaw fracture may be fitted with a leather, nylon, plastic or adhesive tape muzzle that provides some maxillomandibular fixation with sufficient dental interlock and adequate stabilization (Reiter and Lewis, 2011; Somrak and Manfra Marretta, 2016). Such muzzles are also used as a temporary first-aid treatment for acute mandibular (particularly if bilateral) fractures while awaiting definitive treatment, for pathological mandibular fractures (to allow for adequate healing of a commissuroplasty), and as a means of additional support in active patients where the healing mandible may be subjected to excessive forces (Howard, 1981; Withrow, 1981). Caution should be exercised when concomitant upper jaw fractures or TMJ injuries are present, as placement of muzzles can lead to airway compromise and TMJ ankylosis, respectively. The adhesive tape muzzle (Figure 9.19) is applied snugly enough to maintain the dental interlock, but loosely enough (leave a gap of about 8–15 mm in cats and small dogs and 20–25 mm in medium to large dogs between the incisal edges of the maxillary and mandibular incisors) to permit the tongue to protrude and lap water and semi-liquid food (see Chapter 13). Muzzles should be changed daily to avoid development of dermatitis.

Interarch splinting

Maxillomandibular fixation for occlusal alignment and stabilization of caudal lower jaw fractures or chronic TMJ luxation can also be achieved by placement of unilateral or bilateral bis-acryl composite bridges between the maxillary and mandibular canines (or other teeth) (Figure 9.20). Pieces of cut plastic straws, into which the resin material is squeezed, may be used between the opposing canine teeth. The splints may also be reinforced with orthopaedic wire. Similar to the muzzling technique, a small gap between the maxillary and mandibular incisors must provide space for the tongue to protrude (Operative Technique 9.4). Keeping the mouth open too far, however, may lead to difficulty swallowing, improper food intake, and drooling saliva. Complications for both maxillomandibular fixation techniques include dermatitis (only for muzzling), heat prostration, dyspnoea, and – in the regurgitating or vomiting patient – aspiration pneumonia (Bennett *et al.*, 1994; Legendre, 2005). Iatrogenic tooth injury can occur at the time of splint removal, particularly when adhesive bonding and dental composite have been used for fabrication of the splints.

Alternatively, a labial reverse suture through buttons or a bignathic encircling and retaining device (BEARD) may be utilized (Kostlin *et al.*, 1996; Nicholson *et al.*, 2010; Zacher *et al.*, 2013; Goodman and Carmichael, 2016). These techniques entail the use of cerclage nylon sutures placed from the upper lip on one side, around the mandibles and back through the upper lip on the opposite side (labial reverse suture through buttons) or

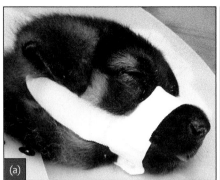
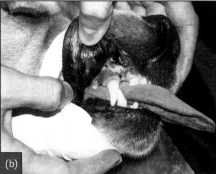
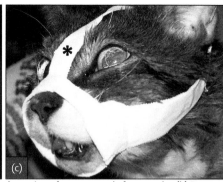

9.19 (a) Puppy with bilateral mandibular fractures treated by suturing of torn oral soft tissues and wearing of a tape muzzle for 2 weeks. (b) Dog with right caudal mandibular fracture treated with intraosseous wiring and tape muzzling; note that the muzzle is snug enough for dental interlock to be maintained, but loose enough for the tongue to protrude. (c) Cat with right mandibular fracture after gunshot injury; notice an additional third layer (∗) of the muzzle that runs over the forehead, which seems essential in cats and short-nosed dogs.
(© Dr Alexander M. Reiter)

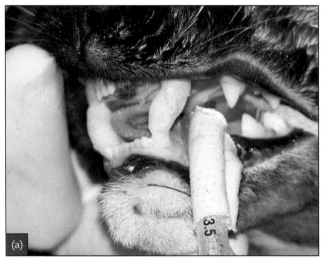

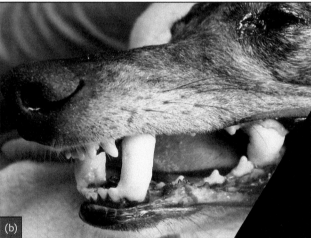

9.20 Interarch splinting performed for treatment of caudal mandibular fractures (a) between maxillary and mandibular canine teeth in a young adult cat and (b) between maxillary and mandibular canine and carnassial teeth in a young adult dog.
(© Dr Alexander M. Reiter)

subcutaneously around the mandibles and maxillae (BEARD). This type of maxillomandibular fixation allows slight TMJ mobility (depending on how much the sutures are tightened). The sutures may be easily cut and quickly removed in case of an emergency (e.g. risk of aspiration from vomiting). However, maintenance of appropriate occlusion may be less effective compared with bis-acryl composite bridges.

Circumferential wiring

Mandibular symphyseal separation or parasymphyseal fractures, common injuries in cats with high-rise or motor vehicle trauma, can be repaired with circumferential wiring (Operative Technique 9.5). The circumferential wire is removed after about 4 weeks (Reiter and Lewis, 2011). Leaving it in place for extended periods of time or overtightening carries the risk of necrosis and resorption of bone around the canine tooth roots (Figure 9.21). A twisted intraoral wire and resin splint may also be applied between the crowns of the mandibular canine teeth to give additional stabilization or as a stand-alone treatment (Legendre, 1998). A figure-of-eight wire pattern around the mandibular canine teeth may only be placed passively because twisting of the wire ends will result in linguoversion of canine and other teeth, malocclusion and TMJ pain (Reiter et al., 2012).

Interdental wiring and splinting

Alignment of mandibular as well as maxillary fracture segments can effectively be accomplished with interdental wiring techniques such as the Stout multiple-loop, crossover (Kitshoff et al., 2013) and modified Risdon (Operative Technique 9.6), which make use of the crowns of teeth for anchorage and provide additional retention surfaces for resin splints (Kern et al., 1995). Interdental wiring should never be a stand-alone treatment but always followed by stabilization with resin splinting (Muir and Gengler, 1999). Likewise, a resin splint should be reinforced by complementary wire. Although the occlusal pattern of the dog permits a splint to be placed on the buccal surface of the mandibular premolars (but not on that of the molar teeth), the splint material is applied primarily to the lingual surface of mandibular teeth and the labial/buccal surface of maxillary teeth, preferably coronal to the mucogingival junction (Legendre, 2003). Methylmethacrylate has historically been the material of choice for splint fabrication but has now been replaced by self-curing bis-acryl composite; the latter can comfortably be applied to the teeth via an applicator gun (syringe with mixing tip) (Figure 9.22).

Intraosseous wiring

Intraosseous (transosseous, interfragmentary) wiring can be used alone or in combination with interdental wiring and splinting. Open reduction and intraosseous wiring may be indicated in nasomaxillary fractures if stability cannot be achieved with less invasive techniques (Boudrieau, 2005b). Small, unattached fragments of bone are discarded, as they may become sequestra. Intraosseous

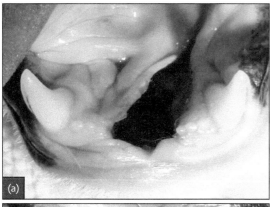

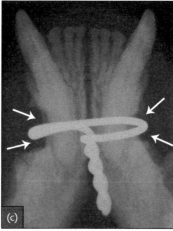

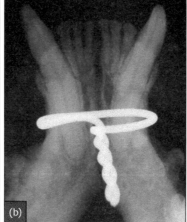

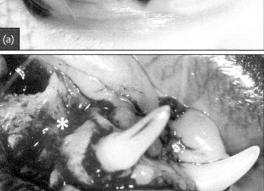

9.21 (a) An adult cat presented with separation of the mandibular symphysis. (b) Circumferential wiring was performed. (c) The patient returned 12 weeks later, showing significant loss of bone around the wire radiographically (arrowed) and (d) clinically (*) after wire removal.
(© Dr Alexander M. Reiter)

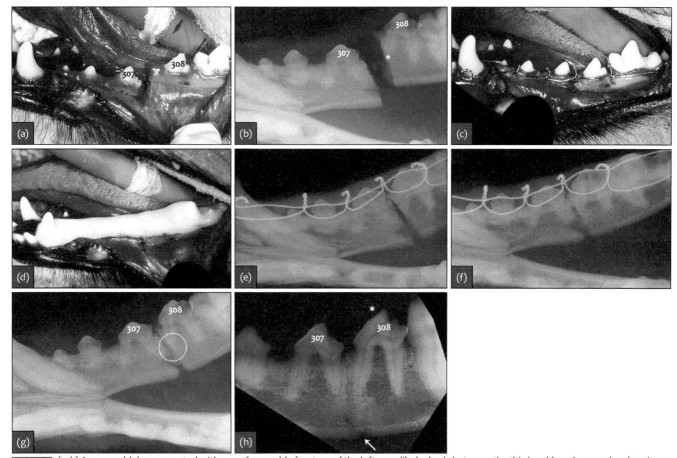

9.22 (a, b) A 2-year-old dog presented with an unfavourable fracture of the left mandibular body between the third and fourth premolars (teeth #307 and 308); note the exposed apex of the mesial root of the fourth premolar tooth (*). (c) Interdental wiring (Stout multiple loop technique) was utilized for fracture reduction, followed by (d) resin splint application. (e) A postoperative radiograph was obtained. (f) The patient returned after 4 weeks for a radiographic re-examination and – due to relocation of the client and dog – early splint removal. (g) The dotted circle outlines the area of concern, which will need to be monitored clinically and radiographically for development of periodontal and/or endodontic disease. (h) The client sent a radiograph 5 months after splint removal, showing continued healing of the previous fracture site. Note a small indentation remaining at the ventral mandibular border (arrowed) and an enamel fracture at tooth #308 (*) probably sustained at the time of splint removal.
(© Dr Alexander M. Reiter)

wiring may also be a very effective means of fracture stabilization in edentulous areas of the lower jaw or could be used when fracture segments diverge excessively at the ventral border of the mandibular body following interdental wiring and splinting.

After reflection of mucoperiosteal flaps on labial/buccal and lingual bone surfaces, holes are drilled through the mandible no closer than 3 mm to the fracture line, carefully avoiding tooth roots and the mandibular canal. A ventral approach to the mandibular body is also possible. Trocar-tipped Kirschner wires (1.6 mm (0.062 inch) or 1.1 mm (0.045 inch) K-wires) can be used for drilling intraosseous wire holes. A smooth-tipped K-wire has also been suggested for drilling a pathway through the mandibular canal, which may be less likely to damage its neurovascular bundle (Terpak and Verstraete, 2012). The drill holes should be angled towards the fracture line (e.g. from labial/buccal to lingual on the mandible), thus resulting in obtusely angled corners and enabling the wire to slide early in the tightening process (Boudrieau, 2005a). Round, surgical length carbide burs may also be used for drilling holes. Adequate cooling with lactated Ringer's solution is essential, regardless of the drilling method employed, to avoid thermal bone necrosis.

Stable fractures may sometimes be repaired with only one orthopaedic wire (18–20 G in medium to large dogs, 22 G in smaller dogs and cats) (Figure 9.23). Most commonly, however, two wires are used in a triangular or parallel configuration where two holes are made in the caudal fracture segment and two in the rostral segment (separate holes for each wire are recommended). A wire should be placed perpendicular to the fracture line, and another wire along the bisecting angle between a line perpendicular to and a line parallel to the fracture line, but other wire configurations have also been suggested. Once tightened, the wire twists are cut and bent to lie flat against the bone surface. The mucoperiosteal flaps are repositioned over the wire ends. It is also possible for an intraosseous wire to be continued as interdental wire (Figure 9.24). If the holes drilled have become larger after radiographic confirmation of fracture healing, the wires may be cut and removed. In young animals, the wires often become entirely incorporated into bone and may then not need to be removed.

External skeletal fixation

Kirschner wires or small Steinmann pins can also be used in external skeletal fixation for jaw fracture repair. This technique may be employed for maxillary and mid and caudal mandibular fractures and those associated with extensive soft tissue injury, severe comminution, and edentulous bone segments. It may also be useful in sites with missing bone fragments. At least two of the wires/pins are percutaneously placed into each bone fracture segment, carefully avoiding tooth roots and neurovascular bundles in the infraorbital or mandibular canal (Roe, 2005). The pins and screws should only engage in one mandible and not cross the intermandibular space.

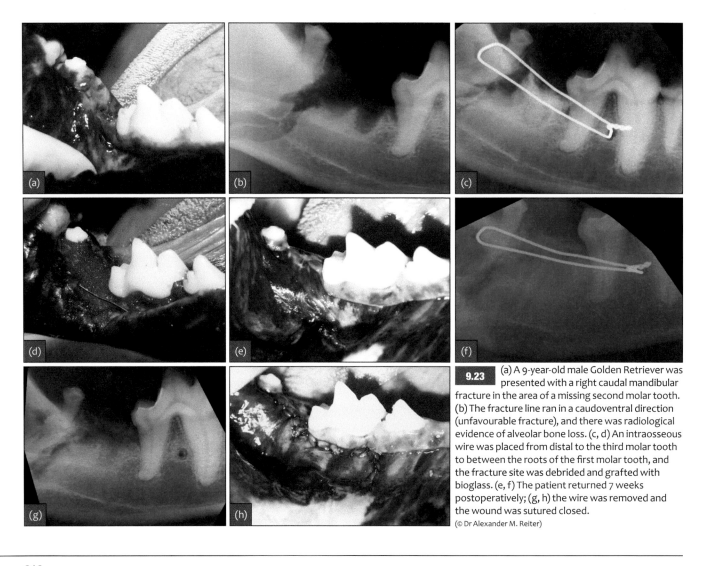

9.23 (a) A 9-year-old male Golden Retriever was presented with a right caudal mandibular fracture in the area of a missing second molar tooth. (b) The fracture line ran in a caudoventral direction (unfavourable fracture), and there was radiological evidence of alveolar bone loss. (c, d) An intraosseous wire was placed from distal to the third molar tooth to between the roots of the first molar tooth, and the fracture site was debrided and grafted with bioglass. (e, f) The patient returned 7 weeks postoperatively; (g, h) the wire was removed and the wound was sutured closed.
(© Dr Alexander M. Reiter)

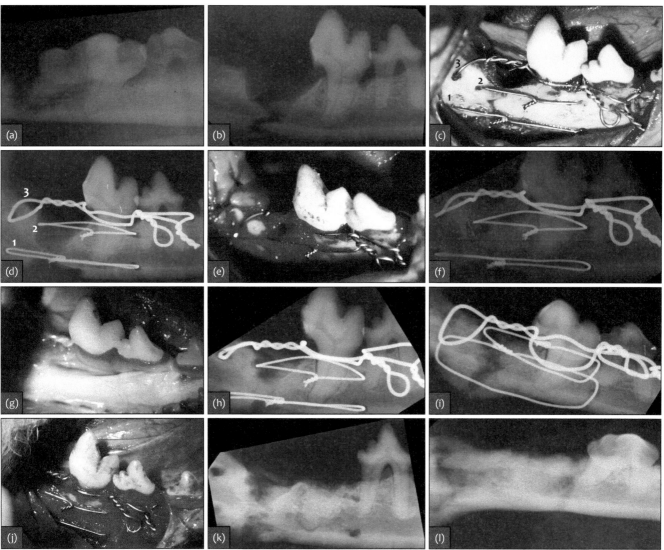

9.24 (a) A 7-year-old neutered female Bichon Frisé presented with a pathological right caudal mandibular fracture in the area of the distal root of the first molar tooth. (b) The first molar tooth was hemisected, its distal crown-root segment removed, and a temporary restoration placed in the remaining crown-root segment that was kept for anchorage of orthopaedic wire. (c, d) Two intraosseous wires (1 and 2) were placed in a near parallel fashion, and an additional wire (3) was started intraosseously in the caudal fracture segment, twisted over the extracted distal crown-root segment of the first molar tooth, looped around its remaining mesial crown-root segment, and continued rostrally as interdental wire. (e, f) The fracture site was debrided, rinsed and grafted with bioglass. (g–i) The patient returned 10 weeks postoperatively; (j, k) all wires were removed, the mesial crown-root segment of the first molar tooth was extracted, its alveolus was filled with bioglass, and the wound was sutured closed; (l) what may appear like a retained mesial root tip of the right mandibular first premolar tooth on a lateral view is actually just a bioglass filled alveolus on a more occlusal view.
(© Dr Alexander M. Reiter)

A plastic tube is placed over the exposed cut ends of the wires/pins, and while normal occlusion is maintained with the jaws closed, the tube is filled with self-curing acrylic or custom tray material (Figure 9.25). There is some risk that the external fixator will get caught on furniture, curtains or other objects, and owners must be willing to keep the pin and screw tracts clean. To remove the device, the wires/pins are cut close to the acrylic bar and then pulled from the bone. External skeletal fixation systems that include fixation pins, clamps and connecting bars are available (Terpak and Verstraete, 2012).

Bone plating

Plating provides rigid fracture stabilization and rapid return to normal function. If done correctly, fracture healing will occur with very little or no callus formation. The necessary instruments and materials are expensive, and significant

soft tissue elevation is necessary for the placement of bone plates and screws, which may further compromise the blood supply to the fractured bone segments (particularly when advanced periodontitis has already resulted in significant loss of bone) (Figure 9.26). Trauma to tooth roots and neurovascular structures may be a common complication. The development of miniplates and monocortical screws made of titanium and the possibility of angling the drill holes can reduce the occurrence of complications (Bilgili and Kurum, 2003; Reiter, 2013).

A craniomaxillofacial system may include 2.4 mm locking reconstruction plates, 2 mm locking miniplates, 2 mm, 1.5 mm, 1.3 mm and 1 mm non-locking miniplates (straight, curved, L, T, H, Y and X-shaped), meshes, various lengths and sizes of self-tapping screws and locking screws, bending screws for locking plates, drill bits, drill guides, countersink and handle, depth gauge, bending template, bending pliers, bending press, bending irons, plate cutter, bone tap,

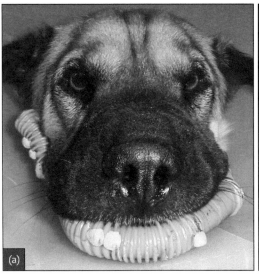
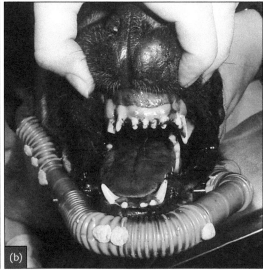

9.25 External skeletal fixation performed in a 1-year old dog. Frontal view with the mouth (a) closed and (b) slightly open. Note that the dog has a full permanent dentition which should have been used for anchorage of an interdental wiring and splinting device rather than choosing an invasive technique that has the potential of injury to the roots of the teeth and the neurovascular bundle in the mandibular canal.
(© Dr Alexander M. Reiter)

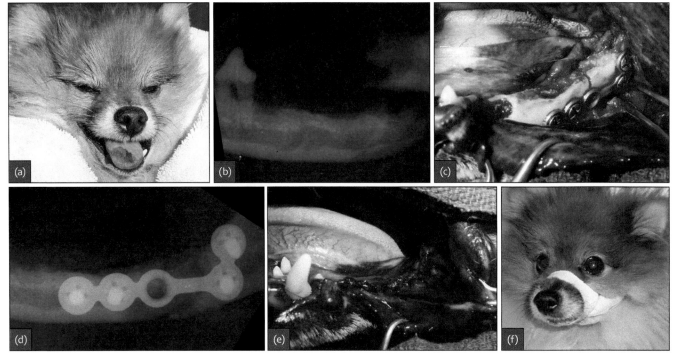

9.26 (a) An 8-year-old, neutered male Pomeranian presented with bilateral pathological mandibular fracture; note the lower jaw involuntarily hanging ventrally. (b) Intraoral radiography reveals a left mandibular body fracture. (c) Miniplate fixation was performed; only the left side is shown. (d, e) A radiograph was obtained to confirm proper fixation prior to wound closure; note that screw placement into the mandibular canal becomes challenging, if not unavoidable, with little bone height remaining. (f) The patient was fitted with a custom-made tape muzzle following bilateral miniplate fixation.
(© Dr Alexander M. Reiter)

and screwdrivers with handles (Koch, 2005; Reiter, 2013). Unless the plate can be contoured accurately to the bone, slight errors in fracture reduction may result in delayed healing and poor occlusion with the patient having difficulty in closing the mouth.

Resection of the fractured piece of jaw

Partial mandibulectomy or maxillectomy may be used in the management of jaw fractures when extensive trauma, infection or necrosis precludes proper reduction or adequate fixation. These techniques are limited to cases in which primary fracture repair is likely to fail or cases in which primary fracture repair has resulted in an inability to eat and drink. Bilateral pathological mandibular body fractures are a severe complication of advanced periodontitis in geriatric, small-breed dogs, most commonly occurring in the area of the mandibular first molars or canine teeth following minimal bony stress. Salvage procedures involve extraction of all diseased teeth. Advancing the lip commissure further rostrally (commissuroplasty) (Figure 9.27) with or without partial mandibulectomy results in a smaller oral aperture, provides support for the tongue, and permits adequate alimentation of a soft diet (Reiter and Lewis, 2011). The owner should be informed that the tongue may hang out of the mouth, and chronic drooling of saliva could result in pyoderma.

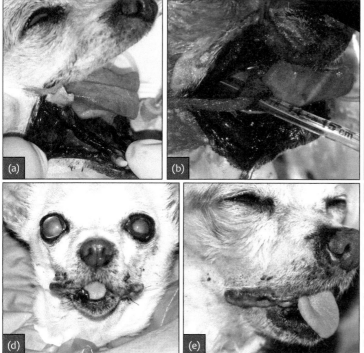

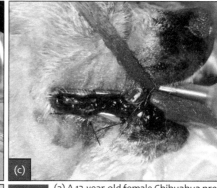

9.27 (a) A 13-year-old female Chihuahua presented with bilateral pathological mandibular fractures. (b) Following removal of teeth affected by moderate to severe periodontitis, fracture site debridement and wound closure, the upper and lower lip margins were incised, and (c) the oral mucosa and skin were closed in separate layers, thus advancing the lip commissure more rostrally. Note the tension-relieving sutures placed using fluid line cut into small segments. (d) The dog returned after 2 weeks for a re-examination. As the lip margins had been incised in the labial mucosa and not at the mucocutaneous junction (which should have been done), some oral mucosa is visible on the outside, giving the patient a 'Joker' appearance. (e) The skin sutures were removed. While the oral aperture is smaller, bilateral commissuroplasty provided sufficient support for the tongue to be kept in the mouth as much as possible. (© Dr Alexander M. Reiter)

Management of temporomandibular joint conditions

Temporomandibular joint luxation

Trauma is the usual cause of rostrodorsal luxation of the TMJ, with the mandibular condyle moving rostrally and dorsally (Klima, 2007). This results in the lower jaw shifting laterorostrally toward the contralateral side, manifesting in an acute inability of the animal to close its mouth fully due to abnormal contact between the maxillary and mandibular teeth on the opposite side. An increased width of the joint space and rostral displacement of the mandibular condyle will be noted on a dorsoventral radiographic view (Figure 9.28). Lateral oblique views are also useful in establishing a diagnosis and confirming treatment success.

Reduction of rostrodorsal TMJ luxation in cats and small dogs is achieved by placing a hexagonal pencil between the maxillary fourth premolar and mandibular first molar teeth on the affected side only and closing the lower jaw against the dowel (that functions as a fulcrum) while simultaneously rotating the pencil (clockwise when the luxation is on the left, counterclockwise when the luxation is on the right). This allows slight forward movement of the mandibular condyle to slide over the articular eminence rostrodorsal to the mandibular fossa.

The reduction is often unstable, and a tape muzzle for 2 to 3 weeks may be indicated to prevent the patient from opening the mouth wide, thus reducing the likelihood of recurring displacement. A larger wooden dowel can be used to attempt reduction of rostrodorsal TMJ luxation in mid-sized and larger dogs; however, a surgical approach should also be considered if conservative manual reduction cannot be accomplished. Chronic luxation is treated by condylectomy (Eisner, 1995).

Open-mouth jaw locking

Dysplasia of the hard and/or soft tissue structures forming the TMJ can be congenital or acquired and has primarily

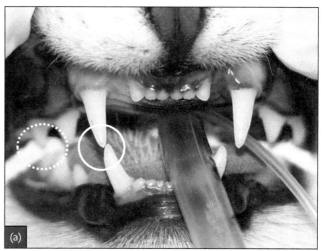

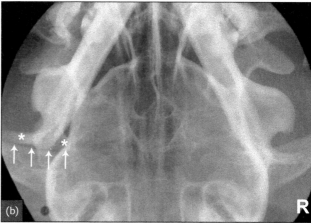

9.28 Cat presenting with luxation of the left temporomandibular joint. (a) There is incomplete closure of the mouth due to shifting of the lower jaw to the right, resulting in maxillary and mandibular canine (full circle) and cheek teeth (dotted circle) on the opposite side making abnormal contact. (b) A dorsoventral radiographic view reveals that the left mandibular condylar process (* indicate its lateral and medial poles) is displaced rostrally (arrowed). R = right. (© Dr Alexander M. Reiter)

been reported in Basset Hounds and Persian cats but may also occur in other dog and cat breeds (Reiter, 2004). In addition to traumatic events, a dysplastic TMJ may occasionally contribute to increased laxity of the joint capsule and displacement of the mandibular condyle. In open-mouth jaw locking (OMJL), the coronoid process of the mandible (opposite to the dysplastic TMJ) flares laterally and locks ventrolateral to the zygomatic arch. Yawning often precipitates a locking event. An ipsilateral protuberance on the ventrolateral aspect of the zygomatic arch may be palpable and sometimes even visible, and the mandible on the displaced side may be positioned slightly more ventral compared with that of the unaffected side. The patient's mouth will be wide open without any contact between maxillary and mandibular teeth. Clinical signs and radiography (dorsoventral views in locked position) are usually pathognomonic for OMJL (Figure 9.29). The addition of CT is of academic interest and may not be necessary for establishing a diagnosis, but it may allow for better evaluation of the dysplastic joint (Reiter, 2004; Soukup *et al.*, 2009).

Acute treatment of OMJL consists of opening the mouth further under sedation to release the coronoid process from the ventrolateral aspect of the zygomatic

arch, and then closing the mouth and placing a temporary tape muzzle. Surgical treatment involves partial coronoidectomy, partial zygomectomy, or a combination of both (Reiter, 2004). Both sides can be affected. Therefore, locking of the apparently unaffected side should be attempted under anaesthesia prior to surgery; both sides require surgery if locking can be elicited on either side. An incision is made along the zygomatic arch, temporal and masseter muscle insertions are dissected from the bone, and the coronoid process is identified. A segment of the zygomatic arch is removed with a rongeur or a piezoelectric surgical unit. The same instrument is then used to remove a portion of the coronoid process, followed by closure of the surgical site. If the surgery is done in the patient with the mouth locked open, it is helpful to release any muscle attachments from and grasp the coronoid process with a small towel clamp, so that it can be readily found after partial zygomectomy (Reiter, 2004).

Temporomandibular joint ankylosis

True or intracapsular ankylosis is the fusion of hard tissues within the TMJ capsule. Diagnostic imaging features are loss of joint space, irregular contour of the mandibular condyle, and excessive new bone formation (Figure 9.30). History includes a progressive inability to open the mouth following head trauma, usually in immature, adolescent and young adult animals (incidence in

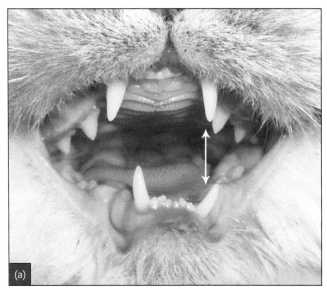

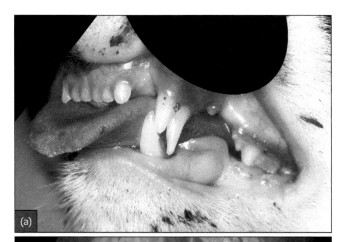

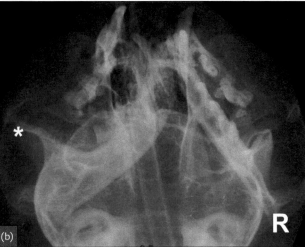

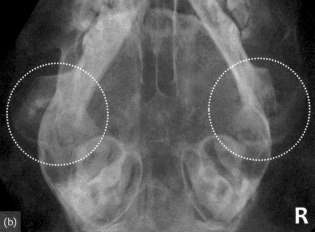

9.29 Cat presenting with open-mouth jaw locking. (a) The mouth is wide open (arrowed) with the left mandibular dental arch positioned more ventrally and no contact between maxillary and mandibular teeth. (b) A dorsoventral radiographic view reveals the left mandibular coronoid process (∗) contacting the zygomatic arch. R = right.
(© Dr Alexander M. Reiter)

9.30 (a) A kitten presented with progressive inability to open the mouth. Note the mixed dentition and mandibular distocclusion. (b) A dorsoventral radiographic view reveals bilateral temporomandibular joint ankylosis (dotted circles) with excessive new bone formation between the mandibles and the temporal bones. R = right.
(© Dr Alexander M. Reiter)

cats being greater than that in dogs). Treatment consists of condylectomy and excision of excessive new bone (which often extends extracapsularly) (Anderson *et al.*, 1996; Meomartino *et al.*, 1999; Okumura *et al.*, 1999). Transposing adjacent muscle tissue or packing fat transplants (difficult to obtain in young and lean animals) into the space between the cut bony surfaces may reduce the risk of re-ankylosis. The interposition of autologous auricular cartilage following arthroplasty is suggested for the same purpose in human patients with TMJ ankylosis (Lei, 2002; Krishnan, 2008), and may be applied in animals as well (Takaishi *et al.*, 2007).

Postoperative pain must be effectively controlled to allow physical therapy at home to be successful (repeated mouth opening several times a day). Glucocorticoids are given for several weeks after surgery in an attempt to slow the healing capacity of connective tissue such as bone. Oral prednisolone is given at 1–2 mg/kg daily divided into two doses for one week and then tapered to 0.25–0.5 mg/kg once a day over a 4-week period. Injection of repository triamcinolone into each surgical site can be used if oral prednisolone is not satisfactory (Reiter, 2012). A transdermal route is an alternative to oral administration of prednisolone.

Excessive callus formation during healing of fractures of the zygomatic arch and mandibular ramus can also lead to progressive inability to open the mouth without TMJ involvement. Such false or extracapsular ankylosis may also be a consequence of excessive new bone formation associated with middle ear disease. Surgical treatment depends on the nature and location of the ankylosis and often requires resection of the zygomatic arch, coronoid process, condylar process and excessive new bone (Reiter, 2012).

Management of oral soft tissue injuries
Lip avulsion

Lip avulsion is a degloving injury frequently associated with road traffic trauma or when the lower lip of the usually immature cat is stepped on by a person or the usually immature or smaller dog is grasped at the upper lip and muzzle (Figure 9.31) by a larger dog (Masztis, 1993). Allowing such wounds to heal by second intention would result in tissue contracture and long-term exposure of bone. The wound is debrided and rinsed, and the lip is repositioned. Securing the connective tissue side of a degloved lower lip to intermandibular tissues and the

mandibular symphysis will decrease dead space, thus reducing the risk of seroma formation (Figure 9.32). Simple interrupted sutures are made in areas with enough remaining gingiva and alveolar mucosa.

To decrease tension along the suture line on the gingival tissues, large horizontal mattress sutures can also be passed around the tooth crowns or through the mandible after drilling holes in the interradicular and/or interproximal alveolar bone with a size ¼ or ½ round surgical length carbide bur or a 1.0–1.5 mm Kirschner wire or drill bit, carefully avoiding the tooth roots. The sutures are passed full-thickness through the mandibles and lip tissues and then tied through rubber tube stents on the cutaneous side. When necessary, a Penrose drain can be placed through a stab incision at the skin ventral to the intermandibular tissues to decrease fluid accumulation in dead spaces. Lacerations of the cheek or lip are debrided and sutured for apposition of the mucosa and skin (Lewis and Reiter, 2011).

Burns

Electrical burns usually occur in young animals that chew on power cords (Lewis and Reiter, 2011). Neurogenic pulmonary oedema and smoke inhalation can be life-threatening. Burns typically affect the lips, labial and buccal mucosa, alveolar mucosa, the tongue and palate (Figure 9.33). More extensive burns also affect teeth and bones (Legendre, 1993). The patient is managed conservatively (wound lavage with lactated Ringer's solution) for the first few days, allowing necrotic tissue to become evident. Careful debridement may then be initiated. Food and water intake could be compromised if a large piece of necrotic lingual tissue sloughs off. Surgical repair of a palate defect should be delayed by about 6–8 weeks following the initial trauma (to ensure vital tissue is available for flap creation).

Thermal burns resulting from exposure to hot items are sometimes seen on the nasal planum, lips, labial mucosa, tongue and palate (Figure 9.34). Owners should be advised not to overheat food and liquids when they try to make them more palatable in patients with inappetence. Possible causes of chemical burns are corrosive chemicals (if chemicals are present, clip the hair and wash the patient's skin) or gastric reflux. The lesions are acute-onset oral ulcers covered by necrotic debris (mostly on the tongue and palate); initial therapy is lavage with lactated Ringer's solution, followed by conservative management (Reiter, 2012).

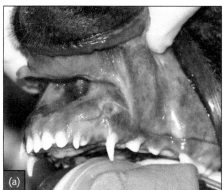 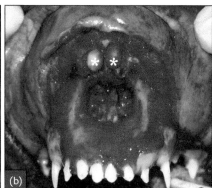 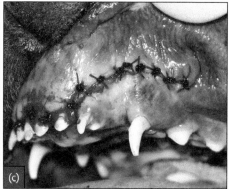

9.31 (a) A 3-month-old puppy was presented with upper lip avulsion after being grasped at its muzzle, lifted up and shaken repeatedly by another dog. (b) Cotton-tipped applicators were inserted through the nostrils to demonstrate the nasal vestibule (∗) during wound debridement. (c) The wound was rinsed and sutured closed.
(© Dr Alexander M. Reiter)

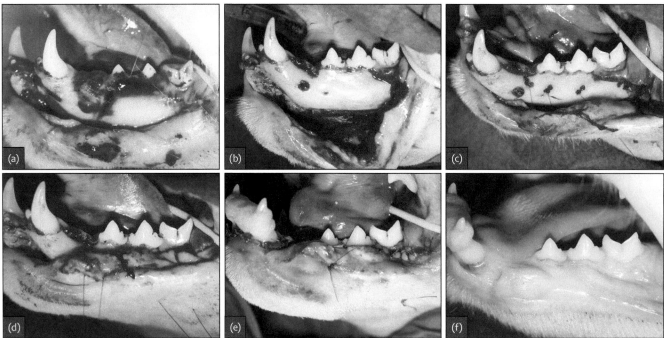

9.32 (a) An 8-month-old kitten was presented with lower lip avulsion and other maxillofacial injuries following a car accident. (b) Thorough tissue debridement was performed, and then full-thickness holes were drilled through the mandibular body. (c, d) Mattress sutures were passed through the holes and the lip tissues. Rubber tube stents should have been placed to decrease the tension on the cutanous surface. (e) The lacerated gingiva and labial/buccal mucosa were directly sutured. Some sutures were also placed around the tooth crowns. (f) At the 7-week re-examination the tissues appeared completely healed.

(© Dr Margherita Gracis)

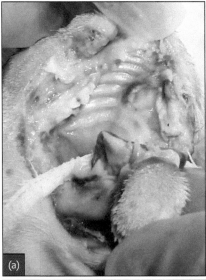

9.33 (a) A 2-month-old kitten presented with severe necrosis of the upper and lower lips, labial and buccal mucosa, alveolar mucosa, gingiva, palate and tongue 5 days after chewing on an electric power cord. (b) Following conservative treatment the patient was re-examined 5 months later. It had a significantly shorter tongue (rostral portion had sloughed off), a right lower lip defect (with previously exposed bone now fully epithelialized), and abnormally developed permanent teeth (underdeveloped right maxillary fourth premolar tooth, missing all right mandibular cheek teeth, mesioverted right maxillary canine tooth).

(© Dr Alexander M. Reiter)

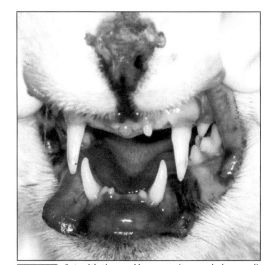

9.34 Cat with thermal burns on its nasal planum, lips and tongue as a result of being fed soft food that had been carelessly warmed in the microwave.

(© Dr Alexander M. Reiter)

Projectile injuries

In gunshot trauma, projectile injury to soft and hard tissues is by means of laceration and crushing, shock waves and cavitation. Bones are shattered and soft tissue damage can occur well beyond the visible injury due to progressive vascular compromise (Lewis and Reiter, 2011). Once airway compromise from tissue swelling and severe bleeding (Figure 9.35) is under control, the injured tissues are debrided, projectile fragments are removed, and the wound is closed. Larger wounds may be only temporarily sutured closed to allow tissue swelling to decrease and sloughing of necrotic tissue to take place. Treating the

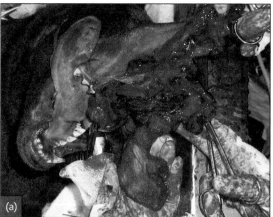
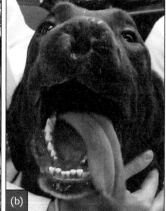
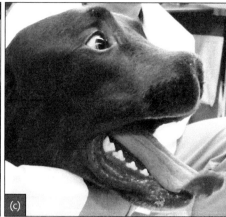

9.35 (a) A dog presented with gunshot trauma, showing severe haemorrhage from injured soft and hard tissues of the nose and upper jaw. This image shows the anaesthetized dog in the emergency room, before proper surgical preparation was implemented. (b, c) The same patient was re-examined 3 months and multiple surgeries later. Note the missing mandibular canine teeth (which had been extracted due to complicated fracture) and one large opening replacing the lost nasal planum and nostrils.
(© Dr Alexander M. Reiter)

patient conservatively for a few days allows determination of viable tissues available for definitive repair at a later time (Reiter, 2012).

Dogs and cats shot by an arrow may present with a wound of unknown origin if the arrow breaks off below the skin or if the arrow grazes the patient. Arrowheads designed for hunting often have three razor-sharp triangular projections that widen further from the tip (Lewis and Reiter, 2011). Blindly pulling the arrow from the entrance wound or advancing one that has not fully exited is not recommended due to the risk of causing further trauma. Surgical dissection to the level of the arrowhead should be performed; once it is exposed, dissection is continued to expose its barbs that can be removed at the level of the shaft to prevent further injury, prior to removing the rest of the arrow (Lewis and Reiter, 2011).

Lacerations, foreign bodies and bite wounds

Labial, buccal, lingual and palatal lacerations are debrided and sutured closed with a synthetic absorbable monofilament suture material. Severe tongue injury may occur during fights with other animals, and tongue avulsion has been reported due to entrapment in a paper shredder. Trauma to the mandibular or sublingual salivary gland ducts or salivary gland capsule and parenchyma may result in extravasation of saliva into submucosal and subcutaneous spaces, causing sublingual, pharyngeal or cervical sialoceles (Smith and Reiter, 2011).

Foreign bodies tend to penetrate the oral mucosa in the sublingual area (Figure 9.36), palatoglossal fold, soft palate, tonsil, floor of the orbit, or pharyngeal wall (Walshaw, 2011). They could also be lodged across the hard palate between maxillary cheek teeth (e.g. a wooden stick) or get caught around the tongue and saw their way into the lingual frenulum (e.g. a needle with thread). Clinical signs depend on the location of the foreign body (decreased appetite and water intake, pawing at the face, swelling in the intermandibular or neck region, intra- and/or extraoral sinus tracts, drooling of clear or blood-tinged saliva, and retching, gagging or vomiting). Because many foreign bodies are not radiopaque, ultrasonography, CT and magnetic resonance imaging (MRI) are often more helpful than radiographs in pinpointing their location (Lewis and Reiter, 2011).

Contamination of open wounds (including those from animal bites) can be minimized by clipping the hair, rinsing

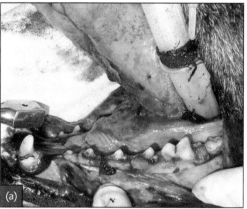
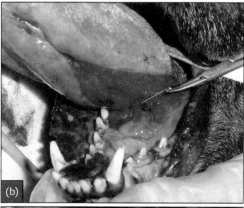
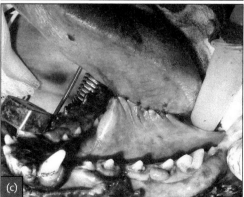

9.36 (a) A dog presented with a non-healing wound in the sublingual region. (b) The wound was explored and a linear foreign body retrieved. (c) The wound was lavaged and sutured closed.
(© Dr Alexander M. Reiter)

with 0.12% chlorhexidine digluconate and lactated Ringer's solutions, applying sterile lubricant, and covering with a sterile gauze dressing until further assessment. Good blood supply and excellent immune defences of oral tissues mean that intraoral wounds often require only debridement and lavage prior to closure. Extraoral wounds of older full-thickness lacerations are often left to heal by second intention whereas intraoral wounds are closed at the time of initial debridement (Lewis and Reiter, 2011).

The intraoral wound entrance may have healed by the time the patient presents with clinical signs. Thus, if a foreign body is present or suspected, the wound should be explored, the foreign body removed and the wound cleansed and sutured. Drainage (e.g. with a Penrose drain directed to an extraoral opening in a location as ventral as possible) should be performed if significant dead space has been created by the trauma or wound exploration. Empirical antibiotic therapy (intraoperative ampicillin at 22 mg/kg i.v. and postoperative co-amoxiclav at 12.5 mg/kg orally q12h) is instituted prior to culture and sensitivity results of infected wounds (Lewis and Reiter, 2011).

Lingual entrapment has been reported in dogs playing with hollow chew toys, which once compressed can create a vacuum effect and trap the soft tissues (Rubio *et al.*, 2010). The toy should be quickly removed with the patient under general anaesthesia. Delayed intervention or forceful removal of the foreign body can cause severe vascular injury and necrosis of the tongue.

Oral bleeding

Severe oral bleeding may be due to injury of significant blood vessels, bleeding dyscrasias (e.g. von Willebrand's disease), lingual or palatal injury, severe inflammation or soft tissue trauma, oral neoplasia, and jaw fracture. Volume replacement is accomplished with crystalloids, colloids and/or blood products (Lewis and Reiter, 2011). The airway should be protected by placing a cuffed endotracheal tube to minimize the risk of aspiration of blood and subsequent pneumonia. Diffuse bleeding from nasal mucosa (e.g. after maxillectomy or palate surgery) may respond to irrigation with a mixture (0.05–0.1 ml/kg in cats; 0.1–0.2 ml/kg in dogs) of 0.25 ml phenylephrine 1% and 50 ml lidocaine 2% (Reiter, 2012). Other means of haemostasis are by vessel ligation, digital pressure, refrigerated rinsing solutions, astringents, bone wax, cellulose meshes, gelatin powder/sheets, polysaccharide powder, collagen powder/sheets, thrombin in a gelatin matrix, fibrin sealants or cyanoacrylate tissue adhesives. Pressure bandages or temporary ligation of large supplying arteries is required in cases of uncontrolled bleeding that could lead to hypovolaemic shock.

Management of salivary gland trauma

Sialocele (salivary mucocele) is an accumulation of saliva in the subcutaneous or submucosal tissue and the resulting tissue reaction to saliva. While a cyst is lined by epithelium, a sialocele has a non-epithelial, non-secretory lining that is composed primarily of fibroblasts and capillary vessels. The aetiology is not clear, but trauma to the salivary ducts or gland capsule and parenchyma has been proposed as a causative factor. The inability, however, to induce sialoceles by experimental duct injury in laboratory dogs suggests the possibility of a developmental predisposition in some animals (Smith and Reiter, 2011).

The sublingual gland is most commonly associated with sialocele. Saliva-filled structures can form in the intermandibular area (cervical sialocele), pharyngeal wall (pharyngeal sialocele) or sublingual area (sublingual sialocele or ranula) (Figure 9.37). Clinical signs depend on lesion location. A cervical sialocele often presents as a slowly enlarging, fluid-filled, non-painful mass. If appearing on the midline, it tends to shift to the originating side when the patient is placed in exact dorsal recumbency. Aspiration of a sialocele usually reveals a stringy, clear transparent or brownish-yellow fluid. Saliva of sublingual sialoceles may be blood-tinged secondary to masticatory trauma and abnormal prehension of food (Figure 9.38). Difficulty breathing and swallowing may be seen with a pharyngeal sialocele. The clinical signs for zygomatic sialocele and neoplasia are similar (visible periorbital mass and exophthalmos). Sialoliths may occur with a chronic sialocele (Smith and Reiter, 2011).

If the sublingual or mandibular salivary gland is suspected to be the origin of a sialocele, both glands will need to be removed (intracapsular resection), as they share one capsule. The skin over the glands is incised through a lateral or ventral approach. Then the capsule is identified, cut open, and gently peeled off the glands. Caudolateral traction is placed on the glands as they are dissected.

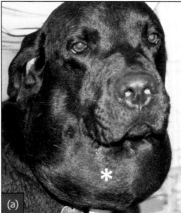
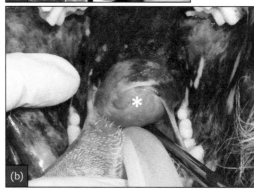
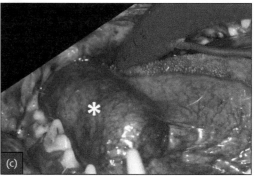

9.37 Sialoceles (*) in dogs: (a) cervical, (b) pharyngeal and (c) sublingual locations.
(© Dr Alexander M. Reiter)

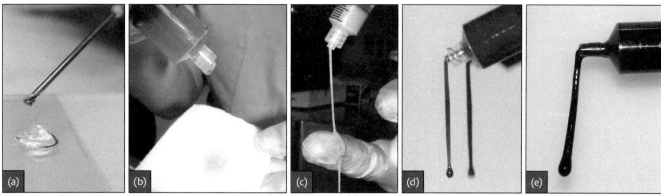

9.38 Different colour patterns of sialocele aspirates: (a) clear transparent; (b) brownish-yellow transparent; (c) brownish; (d) pink-red transparent; and (e) dark red.

(© Dr Alexander M. Reiter)

Injury to the lingual nerve traversing dorsal and rostral to the gland–duct complex must be avoided. Tunnelling of the salivary duct under the digastric muscle has been shown to facilitate removal of larger amounts of salivary tissue (Ritter *et al.*, 2006; Marsh and Adin, 2013). The ducts are ligated at the level of or beyond (when tunnelling under the digastric muscle is performed) the lingual nerve, and the glands and ducts caudal to the ligature are removed and submitted for histopathology. A Penrose drain may be placed with an exit ventral to the initial skin incision to prevent seroma formation. The drain is removed after 1 to 3 days (Figure 9.39). Marsupialization, which involves creation of a large window in the mucosa overlying a sublingual or pharyngeal sialocele to allow for intraoral drainage of saliva, is not as effective as gland resection because granulation tissue and epithelialization often results in closure of the artificial opening (Smith and Reiter, 2011).

Parotid duct migrating foreign bodies (grass seed awns) have been reported in dogs (Marques *et al.*, 2008; Goldsworthy *et al.*, 2013; Proot *et al.*, 2015). Sialadenectomy with duct excision of the affected gland is the treatment of choice. However, duct excision and ligation may also be successful and is a much simpler procedure than parotidectomy (Figure 9.40).

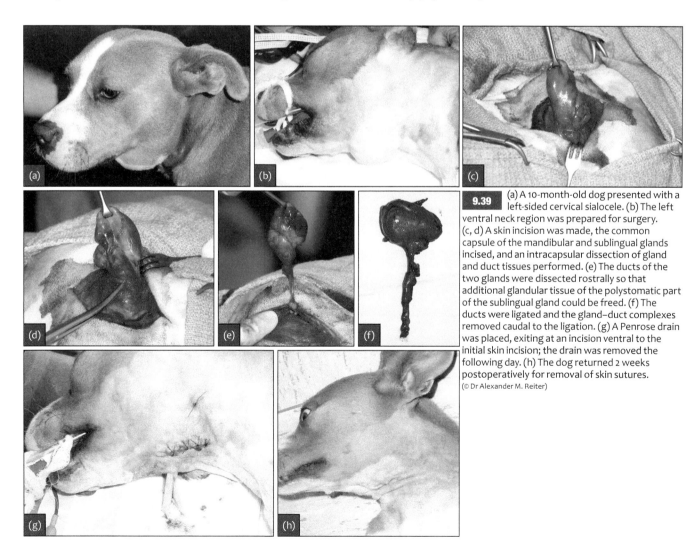

9.39 (a) A 10-month-old dog presented with a left-sided cervical sialocele. (b) The left ventral neck region was prepared for surgery. (c, d) A skin incision was made, the common capsule of the mandibular and sublingual glands incised, and an intracapsular dissection of gland and duct tissues performed. (e) The ducts of the two glands were dissected rostrally so that additional glandular tissue of the polystomatic part of the sublingual gland could be freed. (f) The ducts were ligated and the gland–duct complexes removed caudal to the ligation. (g) A Penrose drain was placed, exiting at an incision ventral to the initial skin incision; the drain was removed the following day. (h) The dog returned 2 weeks postoperatively for removal of skin sutures.

(© Dr Alexander M. Reiter)

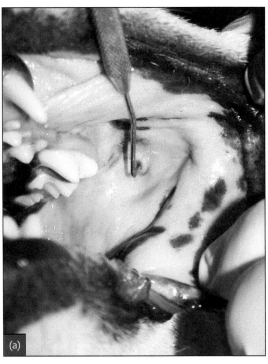

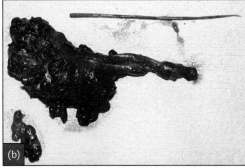

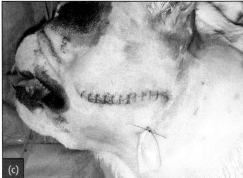

9.40 (a) Fistulous opening on the mucosa of the left cheek of a 1.5-year-old French Bulldog that presented with a persistent left facial swelling and pain on mouth opening. Head computed tomography and ultrasonography revealed a linear foreign body in a thickened tubular structure that reached the left parotid gland. (b) The parotid gland and fistulous tract (which initially seemed to be a thickened salivary duct) were surgically excised and submitted for histopathological examination. The fistulous tract was incised and a thin blade of grass was retrieved. Chronic, severe, diffuse, purulent adenitis, presence of granulation tissue and purulent cellulitis were diagnosed histologically. (c) The skin was closed routinely and a Penrose drain applied for 24 hours.
(© Dr Margherita Gracis)

Management of traumatic palate defects

In the presence of an oronasal communication, the aim of treatment is to create a partition between the oral/oropharyngeal and the nasal/nasopharyngeal compartments to eliminate the risk of rhinitis and aspiration pneumonia. However, following head trauma the management of concomitant systemic injuries should take priority; a severely compromised patient should be stabilized and monitored for at least 24–48 hours before surgery is performed. If the palate defect has developed following electric fulguration, the procedure should be postponed even longer to allow tissue necrosis to become evident and thus enable determination of tissue that will remain vital. Meanwhile, the administration of dry kibbles and/or meat is preferable over a soft, slurry diet to decrease the risk of aspiration. If the communication is large, the use of a feeding tube should be considered. If necessary, a feeding tube can be maintained during the postoperative period until surgical healing is completed. Alternatively, a soft diet should be offered for about 2 weeks postoperatively.

Preoperative thoracic radiographs should be obtained to assess any signs of aspiration pneumonia, although pulmonary involvement develops uncommonly in the case of acquired oronasal fistulas. Head and intraoral radiographs should be evaluated for concomitant skull and dental injuries, and to exclude the presence of nasal foreign bodies or bone sequestra. CT scanning is also strongly recommended, as it has been proven to be superior to conventional radiography for the evaluation of the palatal bony defects and other concomitant traumatic or congenital craniomaxillofacial abnormalities (Bar-Am et al., 2008; Nemec et al., 2015).

The choice of technique should be based on the position, shape and size of the defect, quantity and quality of neighbouring tissues (i.e. number of previous attempts at closure), presence or absence of maxillary teeth, and dental occlusion, as well as on the experience and surgical skill level of the operator. Careful planning of palatal surgical procedures is mandatory, as the availability of suitable tissues is limited. Treatment options for closure of palate defects include surgery (palatoplasty) and the use of intraosseous or interdental appliances and artificial prostheses. Surgical options include primary suturing of the defect's margins, the use of local or distant, pedicle or free, mucoperiosteal, mucogingival, mucocutaneous, cutaneous, muscle or myoperitoneal flaps (single or double-layer), and the application of distraction osteogenesis techniques. Injection and adhesion palatoplasty is an interesting potential future development in palatal surgery that has been studied in a congenital cleft palate canine model (Martinez-Alvarez et al., 2013). Bone formation along the palatal defect (and therefore reduction of the defect width) is induced by a subperiosteal injection of a bone morphogenetic protein (BMP)-2 containing hydrogel, which allows the subsequent direct suturing of the soft tissue margins.

Palatoplasty should be performed with appropriate systemic and locoregional pain management. Antibiotic prophylaxis is administered based on the patient's needs. After endotracheal intubation and placement of a pharyngeal pack, the oral cavity should be rinsed with an antiseptic solution (e.g. 0.05–0.12% chlorhexidine digluconate) and the nasal cavity thoroughly flushed with saline and then mechanically aspirated to remove any foreign bodies and debris. Abundant haemorrhage is common in palatal surgery, and appropriate haemostatic agents and techniques should be used. The use of electro- and radio-surgical units should be avoided to decrease the risk of healing complications.

Before any incision is made, the quality and quantity of available tissues should be thoroughly assessed. In recurrent palate defects, previously utilized tissues should be avoided. Exact measurements and depiction of the planned flaps using a tissue marker are strongly recommended. Tissue flaps should be significantly larger than the defect, kept moist at all times, and handled with great care using stay sutures. The suture material should be thin, synthetic, monofilament and absorbable. The most common complication of palatoplasty is wound dehiscence, frequently due to tension along the suture lines, vascular compromise and partial necrosis of the tissue flaps and making mistakes in the planning stages of palate defect surgery.

Medially positioned flaps (Von Langenbeck's technique)

Midline hard palate defects often develop following falls from a height, especially in cats. Treatment options vary based on the width of the defect and the degree of distraction of the palatal processes of the right and left maxillae. Very thin defects may be sutured closed after debridement of the wound margins and gentle approximation of the bony structures. However, if any degree of tension develops along the suture line, other techniques should be used instead (Bonner *et al.*, 2012). Bone separation may be manually reduced and a fixation device placed either intraorally or extraorally.

The Von Langenbeck's technique utilizes bipedicle mucoperiosteal palatal flaps based on the major palatine arteries, which provide excellent perfusion to the soft tissues. The unilateral technique allows placing of the suture over the palatine process of the opposite side, decreasing the chances of flap collapse and wound dehiscence (Figure 9.41). It also permits sparing of tissues that may be useful in the event of an unsuccessful outcome. If there is insufficient tension-free closure, a bilateral technique should be employed (Figure 9.42).

A full-thickness incision is made parallel to the defect and lateral to the major palatine artery, as close as possible to the dental arch (leaving 1–2 mm of gingiva/palate mucosa adjacent to the teeth) for a slightly longer extension than the defect length. The width of the flap (the distance between the defect's margin and the lateral incision) should be at least one and a half times the width of the defect (Reiter and Smith, 2005). After debridement of the defect's margins, the flap is gently elevated with a periosteal elevator, carefully working around the major palatine artery at its exit from the major palatine foramen. To reduce tension on the flap and to avoid interruption of blood flow through the vessel, the artery may be carefully undermined from the depth of the flap for a short distance. The palatal mucosa along the opposite margin is slightly elevated from the bone surface to facilitate suturing. The flap is then sutured closed in a simple interrupted pattern. The area of exposed bone lateral to the flap is left to heal by granulation and epithelialization. There is no need to place sutures along the lateral margin of the flap.

Modified split U-flap

The modified split U-flap is used to close round or irregularly shaped defects positioned in the caudal region of the hard palate. It involves the use of two mucoperiosteal rotation flaps, requiring incision and ligation of the major palatine arteries at the most rostral aspect of the flaps. To allow a tension-free rotation of the tissue flaps, the arteries should be carefully undermined from the depth of the flaps

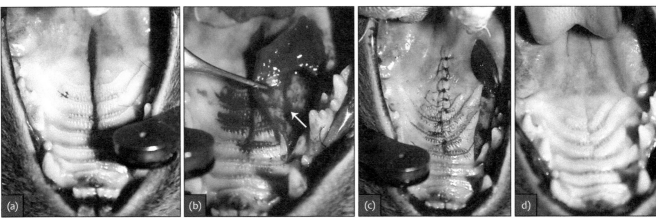

9.41 (a) A 2-year-old Domestic Shorthaired cat presented with a midline palatal fracture and tear of the hard palate mucosa following a fall from the third floor of a building. (b) A unilateral mucoperiosteal flap was elevated from the right side, carefully avoiding injury to the major palatine artery (arrowed). (c) Following marginal debridement, the flap was sutured to the opposite side of the defect. (d) A 5-week follow-up showed complete healing. Note that a spring-held mouth prop was utilized in this case, but its use should be avoided due to the reported risks of altered maxillary artery blood flow and occurrence of neurological deficits.

(© Dr Margherita Gracis)

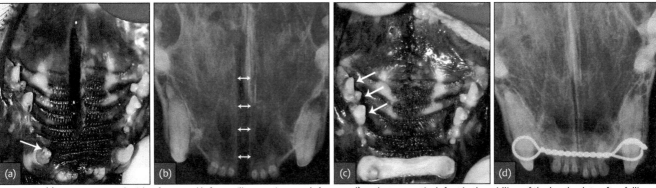

9.42 (a) A cat presented with a fractured left maxillary canine tooth (arrowed) and a traumatic defect in the midline of the hard palate after falling from a window. (b) Note the wide separation (double-ended arrows) of the left and right incisive bones and maxillae. (c) Repair was accomplished by means of approximation and suturing of medially positioned flaps after creation of bilateral releasing incisions (arrowed) into palatal mucosa along the dental arches. (d) Interquadrant splinting (twisted wire reinforced with composite resin) was performed between the maxillary canine teeth to reduce the separation.

(© Dr Alexander M. Reiter)

for a certain distance. If tension is applied on the arteries, they may be compressed against the margins of the major palatine foramina and be completely occluded, compromising the vascular supply to the flaps. The relative positions of the foramina and the palatal defect and the length of the flaps are important factors to be considered when this technique is employed. If the flaps are too short or the defect is too caudal, there is the potential risk of complete separation of the arteries from the flaps when attempting to stretch them over the defect.

The original technique entails debridement of the defect's margins followed by creation of a large U-shaped incision rostral to the defect, including most of the hard palate mucosa (Marretta *et al.*, 1991). A second incision is then made along the midline, to create two flaps of equal size that are elevated and rotated to cover the defect. In the modified technique (Reiter and Smith, 2005), the two flaps are of different lengths (Figure 9.43). The shorter flap should be sufficiently long to allow it to be rotated through

90 degrees and sutured to the lateral and caudal margins of the defect without any tension. The longer flap, which is rotated through 90 degrees and sutured to the rostral edge of the first flap, should reach the intact gingiva/palatal mucosa along the dental arch of the opposite side. If possible, a tacking suture may be placed between the rostral margin of the second flap and connective tissue intentionally left at the intermaxillary suture to obtain better apposition of the flap over the bony surface. If any tension is present along the suture lines, the flaps tend to raise and separate from the bony surface, which may lead to complications. Denuded bone rostral to the flaps is left to heal by granulation and epithelialization.

Palatal obturators

Prosthetic obturators to close oronasal communications do not provide a hermetic seal between the oral and nasal cavities. They should therefore only be employed when

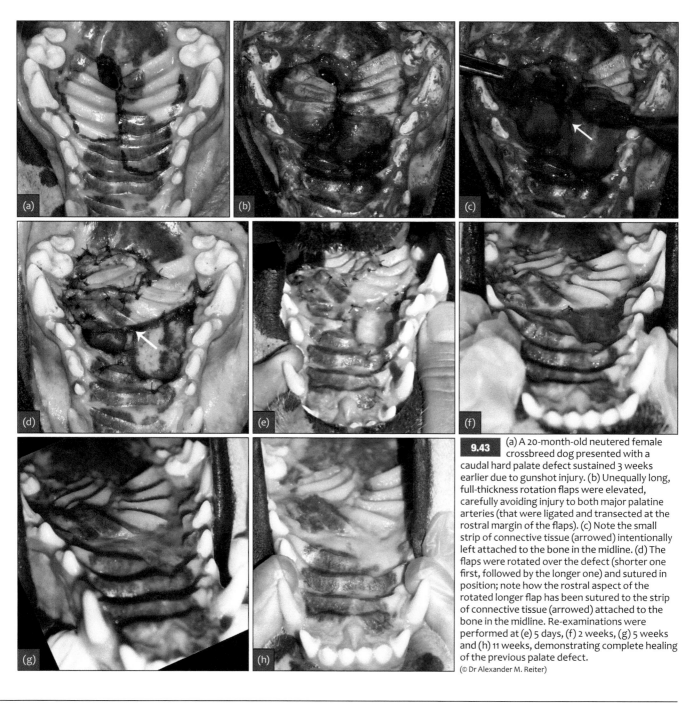

9.43 (a) A 20-month-old neutered female crossbreed dog presented with a caudal hard palate defect sustained 3 weeks earlier due to gunshot injury. (b) Unequally long, full-thickness rotation flaps were elevated, carefully avoiding injury to both major palatine arteries (that were ligated and transected at the rostral margin of the flaps). (c) Note the small strip of connective tissue (arrowed) intentionally left attached to the bone in the midline. (d) The flaps were rotated over the defect (shorter one first, followed by the longer one) and sutured in position; note how the rostral aspect of the rotated longer flap has been sutured to the strip of connective tissue (arrowed) attached to the bone in the midline. Re-examinations were performed at (e) 5 days, (f) 2 weeks, (g) 5 weeks and (h) 11 weeks, demonstrating complete healing of the previous palate defect.
(© Dr Alexander M. Reiter)

surgical repair is not feasible, has been unsuccessful or needs to be delayed. The owners should be instructed about the need for repeated follow-up visits and thorough home oral hygiene.

Prosthetic appliances may be removable or permanent, self-retaining (Figure 9.44) or requiring dental or bone attachment (Figure 9.45). Efforts to keep them in position by suturing them to soft tissues are short-lived. Inert materials that minimize tissue irritation should be used. Silicone, acrylic resins and metal alloys are most commonly utilized (Souza *et al.*, 2005). Whenever possible, it is recommended that transparent materials are used, allowing the evaluation of the nasal cavity through the appliance. It is also recommended that the owners are provided with a temporary replacement appliance in case the first prosthesis gets lost or is broken.

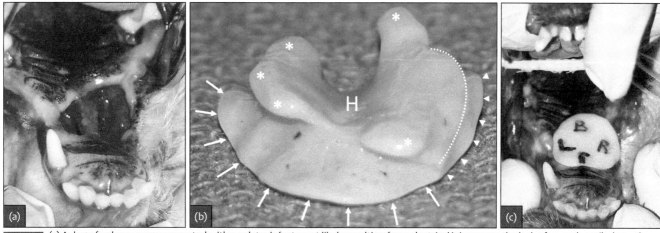

9.44 (a) A dog of unknown age presented with a palate defect most likely resulting from electrical injury; note the lack of an oral vestibule on the right side due to fusion of the upper lip with the gingiva. (b) A self-retaining permanent obturator was fabricated with bis-acryl composite; there are sufficient overhangs orally (arrowed) and nasally (*) with the exception of the side of the obturator that faces the right margin of the defect (dotted line nasally, arrowheads orally). Note that the inside of the obturator has been made hollowed out (H) to allow for free passage of nasal air and fluids. (c) The obturator has been seated in position and marked (B = back, R = right, F = front and L = left) so that a person unfamiliar with the obturator knows how to replace it in case it falls out or needs to be removed for cleansing and nasal lavage.
(© Dr Alexander M. Reiter)

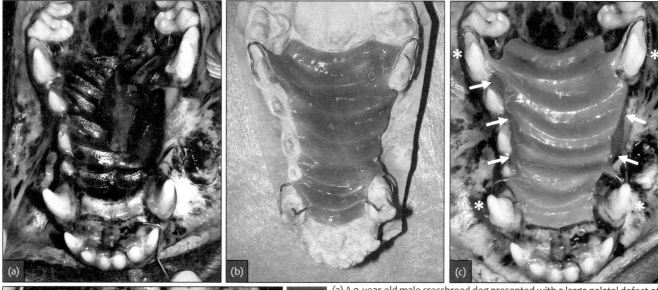

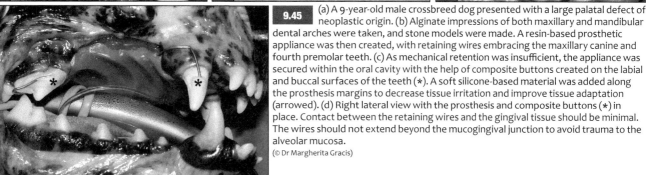

9.45 (a) A 9-year-old male crossbreed dog presented with a large palatal defect of neoplastic origin. (b) Alginate impressions of both maxillary and mandibular dental arches were taken, and stone models were made. A resin-based prosthetic appliance was then created, with retaining wires embracing the maxillary canine and fourth premolar teeth. (c) As mechanical retention was insufficient, the appliance was secured within the oral cavity with the help of composite buttons created on the labial and buccal surfaces of the teeth (*). A soft silicone-based material was added along the prosthesis margins to decrease tissue irritation and improve tissue adaptation (arrowed). (d) Right lateral view with the prosthesis and composite buttons (*) in place. Contact between the retaining wires and the gingival tissue should be minimal. The wires should not extend beyond the mucogingival junction to avoid trauma to the alveolar mucosa.
(© Dr Margherita Gracis)

Self-retaining prosthetic silicone or acrylic obturators may be fabricated directly. However, appliances created by a dental laboratory may be more precise and have a better finish. A precise impression of the defect and surrounding tissues using polyvinyl siloxane material should be submitted to the laboratory, together with alginate impressions of the upper and lower dental arches (or stone models) to evaluate the occlusion. The fit of the obturator is then evaluated on the patient under anaesthesia. If the obturator is resin-based, minor modifications may be made with appropriate burs on a dental handpiece. Self-retaining, custom-made temporary obturators can be created using polyvinyl siloxane putty (Peralta *et al.*, 2015). The impression material is mixed according to the manufacturer's instructions and placed directly into the defect, trying to obtain slight nasal overhangs providing mechanical retention. The use of this type of obturator is recommended only for short periods of time because the air and fluid flow is inhibited if the impression material has been pressed against the dorsal aspect of the nasal cavity and because the putty material will deteriorate with time.

Postoperative considerations in oral trauma patients

In patients with trauma to dental and bony tissues, occlusion should be assessed and radiographs of the surgical sites obtained after repair and prior to extubation. Patients with oral soft tissue trauma should be monitored for continued bleeding and development of oedema, seroma and haematoma. Depending on the location of trauma and treatment performed, the patient is discharged on adequate pain control, an Elizabethan collar and other restraining devices (e.g. tape muzzle), and proper feeding instructions. A feeding tube may be used for a certain period of time following severe trauma or complicated surgical procedures, particularly in severely traumatized cats that may be reluctant to resume spontaneous food and water intake. Home oral hygiene should be instituted.

Oral appliances are removed following radiographic confirmation of fracture healing, usually 3 (immature and adolescent patients) to 8 weeks postoperatively (Reiter and Lewis, 2011). Minor occlusal discrepancies after appliance removal can be corrected by crown reduction with or without endodontic treatment. If malocclusion is severe and prevents closure of the mouth, extraction of one or more teeth will be necessary to restore an acceptable functional occlusion for proper mastication. The patient should be re-evaluated in 6 and 12 months to determine appropriate healing and ensure periodontal and endodontic health of teeth near jaw fracture lines. Severe soft and hard tissue trauma in puppies and kittens can disturb normal skeletal growth and development of the teeth, resulting in maxillofacial deformities and dental abnormalities in the growing dog and cat (Reiter *et al.*, 2012).

References and further reading

Anderson MA, Orsini PG and Harvey CE (1996) Temporomandibular ankylosis: treatment by unilateral condylectomy in two dogs and two cats. *Journal of Veterinary Dentistry* 13, 23–25

Bar-Am Y, Polard RE, Kass PH *et al.* (2008) The diagnostic yield of conventional radiographs and computed tomography in dogs and cats with maxillofacial trauma. *Veterinary Surgery* 37, 294–299

Baugh D and Wallace J (2005) The role of apical instrumentation in root canal treatment: a review of the literature. *Journal of Endodontics* 31, 333–340

Bennett JW, Kapatkin AS and Marretta SM (1994) Dental composite for the fixation of mandibular fractures and luxations in 11 cats and six dogs. *Veterinary Surgery* 23, 190–194

Bilgili H and Kurum B (2003) Treatment of fractures of the mandible and maxilla by mini titanium plate fixation systems in dogs and cats. *Australian Veterinary Journal* 81, 671–673

Bonner SE, Reiter AM and Lewis JR (2012) Orofacial manifestations of high-rise syndrome: a retrospective study of 84 cats (2000–2010). *Journal of Veterinary Dentistry* 29, 10–18

Boudrieau RJ (2005a) Fractures of the mandible. In: *AO Principles of Fracture Management in the Dog and Cat, 1st edn*, ed. AL Johnson, JEF Houlton and R Vannini, pp. 99–115. Thieme, Stuttgart

Boudrieau RJ (2005b) Fractures of the maxilla. In: *AO Principles of Fracture Management in the Dog and Cat, 1st edn*, ed. AL Johnson, JEF Houlton and R Vannini, pp. 117–129. Thieme, Stuttgart

Buffa EA, Lubbe AM, Verstraete FJ *et al.* (1997) The effects of wound lavage solutions on canine fibroblasts: an *in vitro* study. *Veterinary Surgery* 26, 460–466

Clarke DE (2001) Vital pulp therapy for complicated crown fracture of permanent canine teeth in dogs: a 3-year retrospective study. *Journal of Veterinary Dentistry* 18, 117–121

Coffman CR and Visser L (2007) Crown restoration of the endodontically treated tooth: literature review. *Journal of Veterinary Dentistry* 24, 9–12

Coffman CR, Visser L and Visser CJ (2007) Tooth preparation and impression for full metal crown restoration. *Journal of Veterinary Dentistry* 24, 59–65

Colmery BH (1998) Composite restorative dentistry. *Veterinary Clinics of North America Small Animal Practice* 28, 1261–1271

de Paula-Silva FW, Wu MK, Leonardo MR *et al.* (2009) Accuracy of periapical radiography and cone-beam computed tomography scans in diagnosing apical periodontitis using histopathological findings as a gold standard. *Journal of Endodontics* 35, 1009–1012

Dominguez MS, Witherspoon DE, Gutmann JL *et al.* (2003) Histological and scanning electron microscopy assessment of various vital pulp-therapy materials. *Journal of Endodontics* 29, 324–333

Eisner ER (1990) Transcoronal approach for endodontic access to the fourth maxillary premolar in dogs. *Journal of Veterinary Dentistry* 7, 22–23

Eisner ER (1995) Bilateral mandibular condylectomy in a cat. *Journal of Veterinary Dentistry* 12, 23–26

Eisner ER (2012a) Principles of endodontic surgery. In: *Oral and Maxillofacial Surgery in Dogs and Cats, 1st edn*, ed. FJM Verstraete and MJ Lommer, pp. 217–219. Saunders Elsevier, Edinburgh

Eisner ER (2012b) Apicoectomy techniques. In: *Oral and Maxillofacial Surgery in Dogs and Cats, 1st edn*, ed. FJM Verstraete and MJ Lommer, pp. 221–232. Saunders Elsevier, Edinburgh

Fink L and Reiter AM (2015) Assessment of 68 prosthodontic crowns in 41 pet and working dogs (2000–2012). *Journal of Veterinary Dentistry* 32, 148–154

Fulton AJ, Fiani N, Arzi B *et al.* (2012) Outcome of surgical endodontic treatment in dogs: 15 cases (1995–2011). *Journal of the American Veterinary Medical Association* 241, 1633–1638

Galia Reston E and de Souza Costa CA (2009) Scanning electron microscopy evaluation of the hard tissue barrier after pulp capping with calcium hydroxide, mineral trioxide aggregate (MTA) or ProRoot MTA. *Australian Endodontic Journal* 35, 78–84

Garcia de Paula-Silva FW, Hasson B, Bezerra da Silva LA *et al.* (2009) Outcome of root canal treatment in dogs determined by periapical radiography and cone-beam computed tomography scans. *Journal of Endodontics* 35, 723–726

Girard N, Southerden P and Hennet P (2006) Root canal treatment in dogs and cats. *Journal of Veterinary Dentistry* 23, 148–160

Goldsworthy SJ, Burton C and Guilherme S (2013) Parotid duct foreign body in a dog diagnosed with CT. *Journal of the American Animal Hospital Association* 49, 250–254

Goodman AE and Carmichael DT (2016) Modified labial button technique for maintaining occlusion after caudal mandibular fracture/temporomandibular joint luxation in the cat. *Journal of Veterinary Dentistry* 33, 47–52

Gracis M (2012) Management of periodontal trauma. In: *Oral and Maxillofacial Surgery in Dogs and Cats, 1st edn*, ed. FJM Verstraete and MJ Lommer, pp. 201–215. Saunders Elsevier, Edinburgh

Gracis M and Orsini P (1998) Treatment of traumatic dental displacement in dogs: six cases of lateral luxation. *Journal of Veterinary Dentistry* 15, 65–72

Happasalo M, Shen Y, Qian W *et al.* (2010) Irrigation in endodontics. *Dental Clinics of North America* 54, 291–312

Hennet P and Girard N (2005) Surgical endodontics in dogs: a review. *Journal of Veterinary Dentistry* 22, 148–159

Howard PE (1981) Tape muzzle for mandibular fractures. *Veterinary Medicine for the Small Animal Clinician* 76, 517–519

Juriga S, Marretta SM and Weeks SM (2008) Endodontic treatment of a non-vital permanent tooth with an open root apex using mineral trioxide aggregate. *Journal of Veterinary Dentistry* 25, 189–195

Kern DA, Smith MM, Stevenson S *et al.* (1995) Evaluation of three fixation techniques for repair of mandibular fractures in dogs. *Journal of the American Veterinary Medical Association* 206, 1883–1890

Kitshoff AM, de Rooster H, Ferreira SM *et al.* (2013) The comparative biomechanics of the reinforced interdental crossover and the Stout loop composite splints for mandibular fracture repair in dogs. *Veterinary Comparative Orthopaedics and Traumatology* 26, 461–468

Klima LJ (2007) Temporomandibular joint luxation in the cat. *Journal of Veterinary Dentistry* **24**, 198–201

Koch D (2005) Screws and plates. In: *AO Principles of Fracture Management in the Dog and Cat, 1st edn*, ed. AL Johnson, JEF Houlton and R Vannini, pp. 27–50. Thieme, Stuttgart

Kostlin R, Matis U and Teske U (1996) Labial reverse through buttons – a simple technique for immobilisation of (sub)condylar fractures and luxations of the mandible in cats. *Tierarztliche Praxis* **24**, 156–163

Krishnan B (2008) Autogenous auricular cartilage graft in temporomandibular joint ankylosis – an evaluation. *Oral and Maxillofacial Surgery* **12**, 189–193

Kuntsi-Vaattovaara H, Verstraete FJM and Kass PH (2002) Results of root canal treatment in dogs: 127 cases (1995–2000). *Journal of the American Veterinary Medical Association* **220**, 775–708

Legendre L (1993) Management and long term effects of electrocution in a cat's mouth. *Journal of Veterinary Dentistry* **10**, 6–8

Legendre L (1998) Use of maxillary and mandibular splints for restoration of normal occlusion following jaw trauma in a cat: a case report. *Journal of Veterinary Dentistry* **15**, 179–181

Legendre L (2003) Intraoral acrylic splints for maxillofacial fracture repair. *Journal of Veterinary Dentistry* **20**, 70–78

Legendre L (2005) Maxillofacial fracture repairs. *Veterinary Clinics of North America Small Animal Practice* **35**, 985–1008

Lei Z (2002) Auricular cartilage graft interposition after temporomandibular joint ankylosis surgery in children. *Journal of Oral and Maxillofacial Surgery* **60**, 985–987

Lewis JR and Reiter AM (2011) Trauma-associated soft tissue injury to the head and neck. In: *Manual of Trauma Management in the Dog and Cat, 1st edn*, ed. K Drobatz, MW Beal and RS Syring, pp. 279–292. Wiley-Blackwell, Ames

Liang YH, Li G, Wesselink PR *et al.* (2011) Endodontic outcome predictors identified with periapical radiographs and cone-beam computed tomography scans. *Journal of Endodontics* **37**, 326–331

Lipscomb V and Reiter AM (2005) Surgical materials and instrumentation. In: *BSAVA Manual of Canine and Feline Head, Neck and Thoracic Surgery, 1st edn*, ed. DJ Brockman and DE Holt, pp. 16–24. BSAVA Publications, Gloucester

Luskin IR (2001) Three-quarter crown preparation. *Journal of Veterinary Dentistry* **18**, 102–105

Luotonen N, Kuntsi-Vaattovaara H, Sarkiala-Kessel E *et al.* (2014) Vital pulp therapy in dogs: 190 cases (2001–2011). *Journal of the American Veterinary Medical Association* **244**, 449–459

Lyon KF (1998) Endodontic therapy in the veterinary patient. *Veterinary Clinics of North America Small Animal Practice* **28**, 1203–1236

Marretta SM, Eurell JA and Klipperts L (1994) Development of a teaching model for surgical endodontic access sites in the dog. *Journal of Veterinary Dentistry* **11**, 89–93

Marretta SM, Golab G, Anthony JMG *et al.* (1993) Ideal coronal endodontic access points for the canine dentition. *Journal of Veterinary Dentistry* **10**, 12–15

Marretta SM, Grove TK and Grillo JF (1991) Split palatal U-flap: a new technique for repair of caudal hard palate defects. *Journal of Veterinary Dentistry* **8**, 5–8

Marsh A and Adin C (2013) Tunneling under the digastricus muscle increases salivary duct exposure and completeness of excision in mandibular and sublingual sialoadenectomy in dogs. *Veterinary Surgery* **42**, 238–242

Martinez-Alvarez C, Gonzalez-Meli B, Berenguer-Froehner B *et al.* (2013) Injection and adhesion palatoplasty: a preliminary study in a canine model. *Journal of Surgical Research* **183**, 654–662

Masztis PS (1993) Repair of labial avulsion in a cat. *Journal of Veterinary Dentistry* **10**, 14–15

Meomartino L, Fatone G, Brunetti A *et al.* (1999) Temporomandibular ankylosis in the cat: a review of seven cases. *Journal of Small Animal Practice* **40**, 7–10

Muir P and Gengler WR (1999) Interdental acrylic stabilisation of canine tooth root and mandibular fractures in a dog. *Veterinary Record* **145**, 43–45

Niemiec BA (2001) Assessment of vital pulp therapy for nine complicated crown fractures and 54 crown reductions in dogs and cats. *Journal of Veterinary Dentistry* **18**, 122–125

Niemiec BA (2005) Fundamentals of endodontics. *Veterinary Clinics of North America Small Animal Practice* **35**, 837–868

Niemiec BA and Mulligan TW (2001) Vital pulp therapy. *Journal of Veterinary Dentistry* **18**, 154–156

Okumura M, Kadosawa T and Fujinaga T (1999) Surgical correction of temporomandibular joint ankylosis in two cats. *Australian Veterinary Journal* **77**, 24–27

Peralta S, Nemec A, Fiani N and Verstraete FJ (2015) Staged double-layer closure of palatal defects in six dogs. *Veterinary Surgery* **44**, 423–431

Reiter AM (2004) Symphysiotomy, symphysiectomy and intermandibular arthrodesis in a cat with open-mouth jaw locking – case report and literature review. *Journal of Veterinary Dentistry* **21**, 147–158

Reiter AM (2012) Dental and oral diseases. In: *The Cat: Clinical Medicine and Management, 1st edn*, ed. SE Little, pp. 329–370. Saunders, St Louis

Reiter AM (2013) Equipment for oral surgery in small animals. *Veterinary Clinics of North America Small Animal Practice* **43**, 587–608

Reiter AM, Lewis JR and Harvey CE (2012) Dentistry for the surgeon. In: *Veterinary Surgery: Small Animal, 1st edn*, ed. KM Tobias and SA Johnston, pp. 1037–1053. Elsevier, St Louis

Reiter A, Lewis JR, Rawlinson JE *et al.* (2005) Hemisection and partial retention of carnassial teeth in client-owned dogs. *Journal of Veterinary Dentistry* **22**, 216–226

Reiter AM and Lewis JR (2011) Trauma-associated musculoskeletal injuries of the head. In: *Manual of Trauma Management in the Dog and Cat, 1st edn*, ed. K Drobatz, MW Beal and RS Syring, pp. 255–278. Wiley-Blackwell, Ames

Reiter AM and Smith MM (2005) The oral cavity and oropharynx. In: *BSAVA Manual of Canine and Feline Head, Neck and Thoracic Surgery, 1st edn*, ed. DJ Brockman and DE Holt, pp. 25–43. BSAVA Publications, Gloucester

Ritter MJ, von Pfeil DJF, Stanley BJ *et al.* (2006) Mandibular and sublingual sialoceles in the dog: a retrospective evaluation of 41 cases using the ventral approach for treatment. *New Zealand Veterinary Journal* **54**, 333–337

Roe SC (2005) External fixators, pins, nails, and wires. In: *AO Principles of Fracture Management in the Dog and Cat, 1st edn*, ed. AL Johnson, JEF Houlton and R Vannini, pp. 53–70. Thieme, Stuttgart

Rubio A, Van Goethem B and Verhaert L (2010) Tongue entrapment by chew toys in two dogs. *Journal of Small Animal Practice* **51**, 558–560

Schloss AJ and Marretta SM (1990) Prognostic factors affecting teeth in the line of mandibular fractures. *Journal of Veterinary Dentistry* **7**, 7–9

Shen C (2003) Dental cements. In: *Phillips' Science of Dental Materials, 11th edn*, ed. KJ Anusavice, pp. 443–494. Saunders, Philadelphia

Sigurdsson A, Trope M and Chivian N (2011) The role of endodontics after dental traumatic injuries. In: *Cohen's Pathways of the Pulp, 10th edn*, ed. KM Hargreaves, S Cohen and LH Berman, pp. 620–654. Mosby Elsevier, St Louis

Siqueira JF (2001) Aetiology of root canal treatment failure: why well-treated teeth can fail. *International Endodontic Journal* **34**, 1–10

Smith MM and Reiter AM (2011) Salivary gland disorders. In: *Clinical Veterinary Advisor, 2nd edn*, ed. E Cote, pp. 998–1001. Mosby, St Louis

Somrak AJ and Manfra Marretta S (2016) Management of temporomandibular joint luxation in a cat using a custom-made tape muzzle. *Journal of Veterinary Dentistry* **32**, 239–246

Soukup JW and Snyder CJ (2015) Transmylohyoid orotracheal intubation in surgical management of canine maxillofacial fractures: an alternative to pharyngotomy endotracheal intubation. *Veterinary Surgery* **44**, 432–436

Soukup JW, Snyder CJ and Gengler WR (2009) Computed tomography and partial coronoidectomy for open-mouth jaw locking in two cats. *Journal of Veterinary Dentistry* **26**, 226–233

Souza de HJ, Amorim FV, Corgozinho KB *et al.* (2005) Management of the traumatic oronasal fistula in the cat with a conical silastic prosthetic device. *Journal of Feline Medicine and Surgery* **7**, 129–133

Stevens RW, Strother JM and McClanahan SB (2006) Leakage and sealer penetration in smear-free dentin after a final rinse with 95% ethanol. *Journal of Endodontics* **32**, 785–788

Takaishi M, Kurita K, Matsuura H *et al.* (2007) Effect of auricular cartilage graft in the surgical treatment of temporomandibular joint ankylosis. An animal study using sheep. *Journal of Oral and Maxillofacial Surgery* **65**, 198–204

Terpak CH and Verstraete FJM (2012) Instrumentation, patient positioning and aseptic technique. In: *Oral and Maxillofacial Surgery in Dogs and Cats, 1st edn*, ed. FJM Verstraete and MJ Lommer, pp. 55–68. Saunders, Philadelphia

Visser CJ (1998) Restorative dentistry. Crown therapy. *Veterinary Clinics of North America Small Animal Practice* **28**, 1273–1284

Walshaw R (2011) Foreign body, oral. In: *Clinical Veterinary Advisor, 2nd edn*, ed. E Cote, pp. 407–409. Mosby, St Louis

Withrow SJ (1981) Taping of the mandible in treatment of mandibular fractures. *Journal of the American Animal Hospital Assocociation* **17**, 27–31

Zacher AM and Marretta SM (2013) Oral and maxillofacial surgery in dogs and cats. *Veterinary Clinics of North America Small Animal Practice* **43**, 609–649

OPERATIVE TECHNIQUE 9.1

Vital pulp therapy

Acute pulp exposure of teeth following crown fracture, crown reduction or defect preparation.

POSITIONING

Lateral, ventral or dorsal recumbency (depending on the tooth treated).

ASSISTANT

Needed.

ADDITIONAL EQUIPMENT

Rubber dam and dental clamps; round carbide bur; round diamond bur; (cross-cut) fissure bur; lactated Ringer's solution (or saline); sterile paper points; calcium hydroxide (CaOH) powder or mineral trioxide aggregate (MTA) and sterile applicator; CaOH cement; glass ionomer (or zinc oxide eugenol, ZOE); polyacrylic acid; phosphoric acid; unfilled resin; dental composite; white stone bur.

SURGICAL TECHNIQUE

Approach

Preoperative radiographs are obtained to evaluate root development, lack of complicating factors, and signs of endodontic or periodontal disease. Instruments and materials coming in direct contact with vital pulp must be sterile. The use of rubber dam and clamps (not shown below) is strongly recommended to isolate the tooth and decrease the chances of pulp infection.

Surgical manipulations

1 When indicated, and after dental scaling and polishing with pumice, perform crown reduction using a (cross-cut) fissure bur on a high-speed handpiece under cooling irrigation (remember that anything coming in contact with vital pulp needs to be sterile).

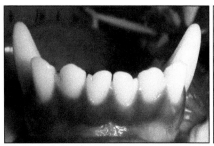 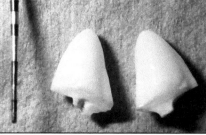

(© Dr Margherita Gracis)

2 Remove 6–8 mm of coronal pulp with a round carbide or round diamond bur to eliminate potentially inflamed and infected tissues and to provide space for the layers of materials used for direct pulp capping and restoration.

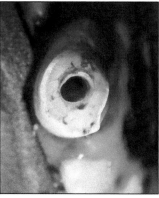

(© Dr Margherita Gracis)

→ **OPERATIVE TECHNIQUE 9.1 CONTINUED**

3 Gently apply sterile paper points to the bleeding pulp to achieve haemostasis. Leave them in place for a few minutes, and replace them until bleeding is under control.

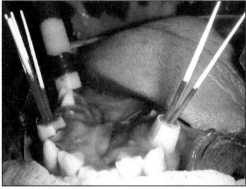 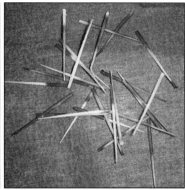

(© Dr Margherita Gracis)

4 Gently place a 1 mm layer of pulp dressing material (generally CaOH or MTA) over the pulp. Then, carefully remove any excess material and clean the dentinal walls.

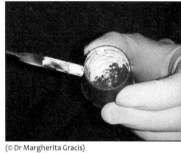 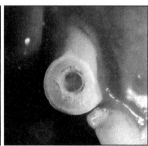

(© Dr Margherita Gracis)

5 Mix (according to the manufacturer's recommendations) and place an intermediate base layer (e.g. hard-setting CaOH cement, glass ionomer or ZOE).

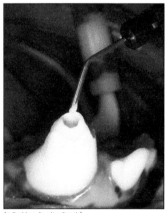 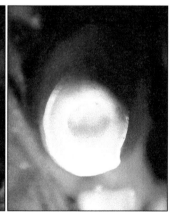

(© Dr Margherita Gracis)

6 Complete the restoration with bonded composite resins or other restorative materials.

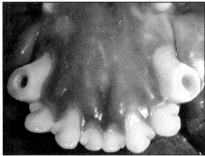 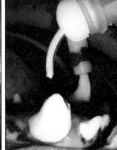 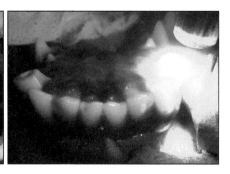

(© Dr Margherita Gracis)

→ **OPERATIVE TECHNIQUE 9.1 CONTINUED**

7 Contour and smooth the restoration, apply one or two layers of unfilled resin to seal any gaps, and then obtain a postoperative radiograph.

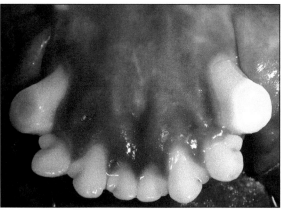

(© Dr Margherita Gracis)

PRACTICAL TIPS

- Gentle irrigation with a refrigerated solution may improve haemostasis
- Slightly moistened paper points are less likely to stick to the pulp and thus will not cause a flare-up of bleeding once removed
- In case of persistent haemorrhage, remove a few more millimetres of pulp
- It may be advisable to treat one tooth at a time (steps 1–5) to decrease the time of pulp exposure for each tooth

POSTOPERATIVE CARE

Dental radiographs should be obtained after 3–6 months and then yearly thereafter to ensure continued vitality of the pulp.

OPERATIVE TECHNIQUE 9.2

Standard root canal therapy (standardized filing technique and cold lateral condensation)

INDICATIONS

Irreversible pulpitis (with or without pulp exposure), complicated crown (and sometimes crown-root) fractures, and iatrogenic pulp exposure of a mature (with a closed apex) tooth.

POSITIONING

Lateral, ventral or dorsal recumbency (depending on tooth treated).

ASSISTANT

Needed.

ADDITIONAL EQUIPMENT

Rubber dam and clamps; round or pear-shaped carbide bur; round diamond bur; pathfinder; Gates Glidden drills; barbed broaches; hand- or motor-driven files; lubricating paste; rinsing solutions; paper points; endodontic sealer; gutta-percha (GP) points; spiral filler; spreader; heated instrument; plugger; instruments and materials for defect preparation and restoration.

SURGICAL TECHNIQUE

Approach

Preoperative radiographs are obtained to evaluate root development, lack of complicating factors, and signs of endodontic or periodontal disease. The procedure must be performed aseptically, possibly using a rubber dam. Placing a suction tip next to the access hole is recommended while rinsing the root canal, to reduce the risk of

→ **OPERATIVE TECHNIQUE 9.2 CONTINUED**

contact between the rinsing solution (in particular sodium hypochlorite) and the oral soft tissues. For the same reason, copious rinsing of the area with water from the three-way syringe should also be performed each time the rinsing solution is used.

Surgical manipulations

1 Access to the pulp chamber is accomplished by means of a small round or pear-shaped carbide bur that is initially angled perpendicularly to the tooth surface, and then directed towards the apex.

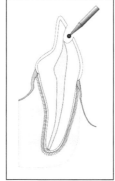

(Courtesy of D Crossley)

2 A pathfinder and lubricating paste may be used to locate the pulp cavity. The access hole is then slightly enlarged with a Gates Glidden drill to a size that allows easy insertion of the instruments.

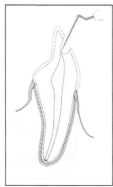

(Courtesy of D Crossley)

3 A relatively thin barbed broach is inserted to the apical portion of the root canal, rotated clockwise, and gently withdrawn to retrieve any intact pulp tissue.

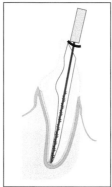

(Redrawn after D Crossley)

4 The root canal is rinsed with an appropriate solution (e.g. sodium hypochlorite) and the outside area of the tooth and surrounding soft tissues rinsed with water.

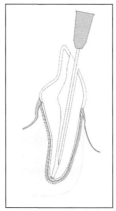

(Courtesy of D Crossley)

5 Working length is determined by inserting a relatively thin endodontic file (the first file) to the apex and placing a rubber stop to a repeatable position. A radiograph is obtained to confirm apical placement. The file is then used to start cleaning and shaping the root canal.

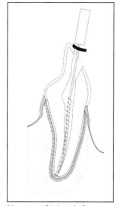

(Courtesy of D Crossley)

6 The pulp cavity is abundantly irrigated. In thin canals a lubricating agent can be applied to facilitate insertion and use of small instruments.

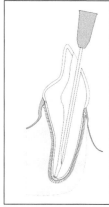

(Courtesy of D Crossley)

7 Files of progressively increasing sizes (*) are used, recapitulating frequently (using finer instruments after each file to ensure removal of all dentinal debris from the apical area of the root canal) (arrowheads).

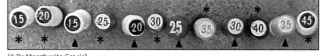

(© Dr Margherita Gracis)

8 After the use of each file, the root canal is abundantly irrigated and the outside area of the tooth and surrounding soft tissues rinsed with water.

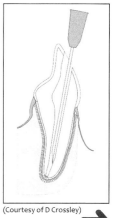

(Courtesy of D Crossley)

→ **OPERATIVE TECHNIQUE 9.2 CONTINUED**

9 A radiograph is obtained to confirm apical placement of the last file able to reach the apex (master apical file).

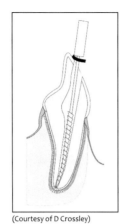
(Courtesy of D Crossley)

13 The GP master point is identified, and its apical fit is confirmed radiographically, before it is retrieved and put aside.

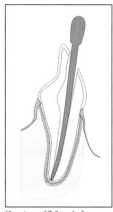
(Courtesy of D Crossley)

10 The pulp cavity is irrigated once more with sodium hypochlorite and the solution is aspirated with the same syringe. The same procedure is repeated using saline and then a 17% EDTA solution, which is left in place for about 1 minute, to remove the smear layer.

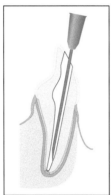
(Redrawn after D Crossley)

14 The root canal's walls are coated with an endodontic sealer, using a spiral filler.

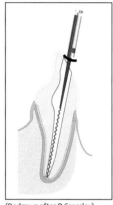
(Redrawn after D Crossley)

11 The pulp cavity is finally abundantly rinsed with saline. Sodium hypochlorite and 95% ethanol may also be used as final solutions. The outside area of the tooth and surrounding soft tissues are rinsed once more with water.

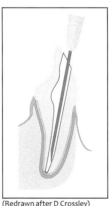
(Redrawn after D Crossley)

15 Then the GP master point is coated with a thin layer of sealer and inserted into the root canal down to the apex. A spreader is inserted next to it to condense the GP master point apically and laterally, and then removed.

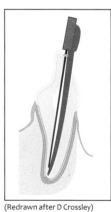
(Redrawn after D Crossley)

12 Paper points are used to dry the pulp cavity.

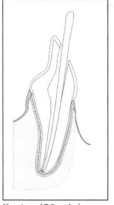
(Courtesy of D Crossley)

16 The spreader is inserted again to create room for an initially relatively large accessory GP point. The accessory GP point is inserted, and the same steps are repeated as previously described. The root canal is filled with multiple, progressively thinner, accessory GP points until it appears completely obturated.

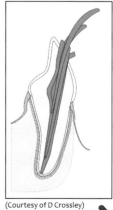
(Courtesy of D Crossley)

→ **OPERATIVE TECHNIQUE 9.2 CONTINUED**

17 The remaining GP points are cut off at the coronal access and plugged apically.

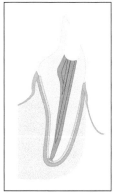

(Redrawn after D Crossley)

18 The coronal access is then restored, and radiographs are obtained to confirm appropriate obturation and restoration.

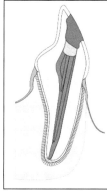

(Courtesy of D Crossley)

PRACTICAL TIPS

- One should master a standardized filing technique and cold lateral condensation before engaging in motor-driven filing techniques and warm condensation methods
- It may be avisable to cut and remove the distal end of each GP point as deeply as possible with a heated instrument prior to inserting other points, to avoid congestion of the pulp chamber with GP and to ensure a uniform obturation of the root canal (note that this is a slightly different technique compared with that shown in point 16)
- In multi-rooted teeth, the pulp chamber should not be forgotten in terms of filing, shaping, disinfecting and restoring, as furcation canals connecting the pulp chamber with the periodontal ligament have been reported

POSTOPERATIVE CARE

Dental radiographs should be obtained after 6 months and then yearly thereafter to ensure continued periapical health of the treated tooth.

OPERATIVE TECHNIQUE 9.3

Dental defect preparation and restoration

INDICATIONS

Restoration of a dental defect such as that created when accessing the pulp chamber during endodontic treatment.

POSITIONING

Lateral, ventral or dorsal recumbency (depending on the tooth treated).

ASSISTANT

Needed.

ADDITIONAL EQUIPMENT

Appropriate burs (diamond round, carbide round and cross-cut fissure) and instruments for defect preparation including materials for dentine conditioning, enamel etching and adhesive bonding; glass ionomer; dental composite; and finishing burs (such as a cone-shaped white stone).

→ **OPERATIVE TECHNIQUE 9.3 CONTINUED**

SURGICAL TECHNIQUE

Approach

The restoration is placed to avoid leakage into vital pulp tissue or the pulp cavity of an endodontically treated tooth. Preoperative radiographs are obtained to evaluate the defect to be restored and to assess the lack of complicating factors. The procedure must be performed aseptically, which includes using a dental dam (not shown below).

Surgical manipulations

1 The crown of the tooth is scaled and polished with a glycerin-free product (such as pumice powder) and then rinsed and air-dried. Residual gutta-percha (GP) and endodontic sealer are removed from the walls of the pulp chamber with an excavator or a pear-shaped bur (which should not be used for any of the successive steps to avoid GP contamination of the restorative materials). The access site should be free from GP.

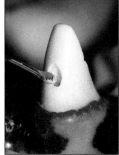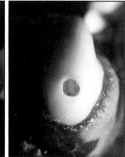

(© Dr Margherita Gracis)

2 To remove the smear layer and any residual endodontic sealer from the pulp cavity, the dentinal walls are conditioned for 15 seconds with 10% polyacrylic acid applied with a microbrush or a syringe applicator, avoiding any contact with soft tissues.

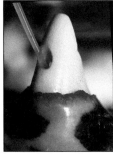

(© Dr Margherita Gracis)

5 After the intermediate layer has set, the access area is prepared again removing any residual material from the dentinal walls with an excavator (or a bur of appropriate configuration), creating a slightly retentive shape into the dentine, and using a brush to clean the enamel surface.

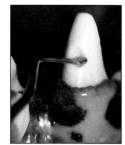

(© Dr Margherita Gracis)

3 The conditioning gel is then flushed out with a gentle stream of water and air from the three-way syringe for a minimum of 20 seconds, followed by drying of the area (but avoiding dessication).

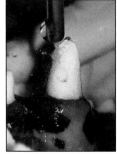

(© Dr Margherita Gracis)

6 Enamel margins should be slightly bevelled outwards to increase the bonding surface and to remove any unsupported enamel. This may be accomplished with an excavator, a chisel, or a powered instrument.

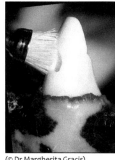

(© Dr Margherita Gracis)

4 Based on the sealer used for obturation, an intermediate layer may be necessary (such as chemically-cured or light-cured glass ionomer or CaOH paste), applied following the manufacturer's instructions. The base material should completely cover and seal the GP and cement and be more than 1 mm thick.

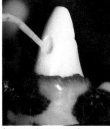

(© Dr Margherita Gracis)

7 To improve bonding of the restorative material, the dentine is conditioned again, and enamel surrounding the access site is etched. Etched enamel should have a chalky appearance, and contact with saliva or other contaminants should be avoided before the restoration is completed.

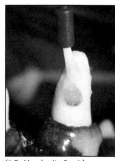

(© Dr Margherita Gracis)

→ OPERATIVE TECHNIQUE 9.3 CONTINUED

8 A dentine primer and a bonding agent (unfilled resin or adhesive) are applied to the tooth surface. Many contemporary bonding systems combine the primer and adhesive into a single bottle. The solution is applied and dried for a few seconds; application and light-curing of the primer/bonding agent must be performed strictly in accordance with the manufacturer's instructions. The previously etched surfaces should look glossy.

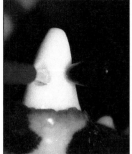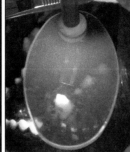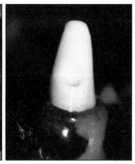

(© Dr Margherita Gracis)

9 The composite (filled resin) is usually dispensed from a syringe and applied to the prepared defect with the aid of a plastic or other composite instrument.

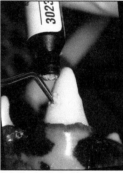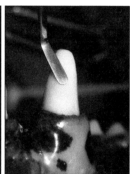

(© Dr Margherita Gracis)

10 To minimize polymerization shrinkage (a phenomenon affecting all composite materials that tend to contract towards the bulk of the material during hardening) and improve curing efficiency, sequential layers of about 2 mm thickness should be placed, shaped and light-cured, until the whole defect is filled or slightly overfilled. When curing, the light tip is kept as close as possible to the material, and the restoration should be cured from different angles.

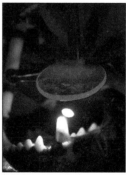

(© Dr Margherita Gracis)

11 After complete polymerization, the material in excess can be removed and the restoration contoured using 12-fluted finishing burs, diamond finishing burs, abrasive-coated disks or white stones.

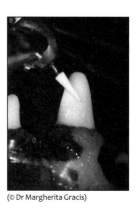

(© Dr Margherita Gracis)

→ **OPERATIVE TECHNIQUE 9.3 CONTINUED**

12 Finally, the restoration is polished with very fine polishing disks, finishing rubber burs and appropriate polishing paste. An extra layer of unfilled resin may be applied and light-cured to fill any microscopic voids and to make the restoration surface smoother.

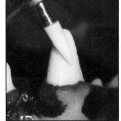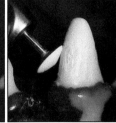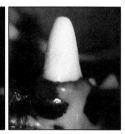

(© Dr Margherita Gracis)

PRACTICAL TIP

- Manual undermining of a defect restoration site by means of subtle dentine removal and proper defect preparation greatly increases the successful outcome of dental restoration in veterinary patients

POSTOPERATIVE CARE

None, unless other procedures have been performed.

OPERATIVE TECHNIQUE 9.4

Interarch splinting

INDICATIONS

Provision of maxillomandibular fixation for occlusal alignment and stabilization of caudal lower jaw fractures or chronic temporomandibular joint luxation.

POSITIONING

Lateral, dorsal or ventral recumbency.

ASSISTANT

Needed.

ADDITIONAL EQUIPMENT

Coarse pumice; materials for acid etching and adhesive bonding; dental composite and/or bis-acryl composite; power tools for trimming of the splints.

SURGICAL TECHNIQUE

Approach

Resin bridges are fabricated between the maxillary and mandibular canines (or other teeth) with the mouth slightly open but the jaws in proper occlusal alignment.

Surgical manipulations

1 The teeth to be involved in the splints are scaled, dried and acid-etched for 15 seconds.

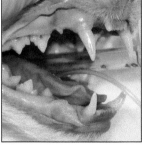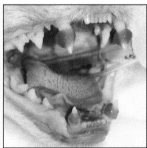

(© Dr Alexander M. Reiter)

→ **OPERATIVE TECHNIQUE 9.4 CONTINUED**

2 The acid and any oral debris are rinsed from the mouth.

3 Avoiding any contact with the etched teeth, the endotracheal tube is positioned so that it emerges from the mouth in the median plane.

4 The teeth are air-dried, and an unfilled resin is applied and light-cured.

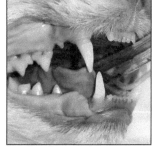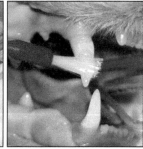

(© Dr Alexander M. Reiter)

5 The assistant stabilizes the upper and lower jaws in proper occlusal alignment with the mouth slightly opened and the tips of the canine teeth slightly overlapping (gap of about 8–15 mm in cats and small dogs and 20–25 mm in medium to large dogs between the incisal edges of the maxillary and mandibular incisors). Alternatively, a twisted wire can be applied, which helps keep the mandible in proper occlusion and increases mechanical retention of the resin.

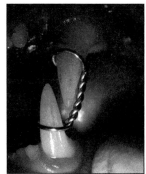

(© Dr Margherita Gracis)

6 Composite is then applied to create bridges that connect the maxillary and mandibular canine (or other) teeth on each side; dental composite (left) needs to be light-cured, while bis-acryl composite (right) hardens on its own in a few minutes.

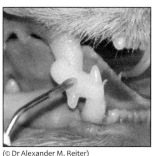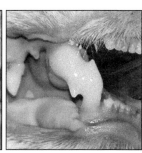

(© Dr Alexander M. Reiter)

7 The interarch splints are trimmed (followed by polishing) so that enough space is created for the tongue to freely move in and out of the mouth.

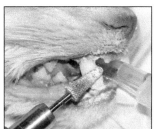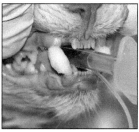

(© Dr Alexander M. Reiter)

8 The patient is extubated with the mouth hanging over the edge of the table to allow any remaining oral fluid to flow from the mouth.

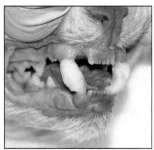

(© Dr Alexander M. Reiter)

→ **OPERATIVE TECHNIQUE 9.4 CONTINUED**

9 The splints are removed after 2–4 weeks (or after radiographic confirmation of healing) by making narrow grooves into them and breaking off small pieces.

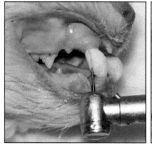 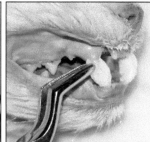

(© Dr Alexander M. Reiter)

10 The tooth surfaces are polished.

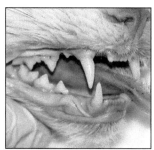

(© Dr Alexander M. Reiter)

PRACTICAL TIPS

- Pieces of plastic straws (cut to the desired length) may be placed between opposing canine teeth into which the resin material can flow
- Additional retention is achieved by treating the scaled tooth surface with coarse pumice (which creates tiny scratches for micromechanical retention) and by applying unfilled resin to the acid-etched and dried enamel surface (which improves retention, but complicates the resin's removal)
- Unfilled resins should only be applied to a small area of the surface of the crown and not to the tip, to reduce the risk of crown fracture at the time of splint removal
- Providing the pet owner with extraction forceps allows breakage of the splints in case of sudden respiratory compromise (e.g. after aspiration of food matter)

POSTOPERATIVE CARE

Elizabethan collar as needed; soft food until splint removal; no hard toys or treats.

OPERATIVE TECHNIQUE 9.5

Circumferential wiring

Primarily used for repair of mandibular symphysis separation or parasymphyseal fracture.

POSITIONING

Lateral or dorsal recumbency.

ASSISTANT

Not needed.

ADDITIONAL EQUIPMENT

No. 15 scalpel blade; 18 G hypodermic needle; 22 G (or thicker in dogs) orthopaedic wire; wire twister; wire cutter.

SURGICAL TECHNIQUE

Approach

An orthopaedic wire is brought around both mandibles immediately distal to the mandibular canine teeth, leaving the least amount of soft tissue between the wire and bone surface, and twisted below the chin. Images shown here were obtained from a cadaver specimen. In a clinical patient, the hair should be adequately clipped, the skin prepared for aseptic surgery, and the surgical site draped.

Surgical manipulations

1 The injured site is debrided and rinsed.

2 A stab incision is made in the chin at the ventral midline.

3 An 18 G needle is inserted between bone and soft tissues to exit into the mouth distal to the canine teeth.

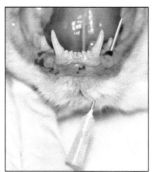

(© Dr Alexander M. Reiter)

4 A 20–22 G orthopaedic wire is passed through the needle.

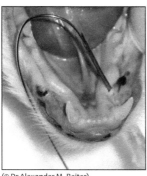

(© Dr Alexander M. Reiter)

5 The needle is removed and reinserted on the other side, and the oral wire end is passed through the needle opening.

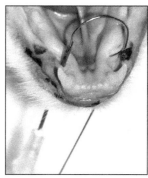

(© Dr Alexander M. Reiter)

6 The needle is again removed, the symphysis is held in proper alignment, and the wire ends are twisted below the chin until the lower jaw is stable.

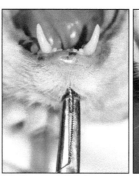
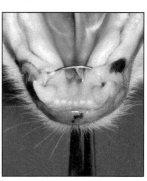

(© Dr Alexander M. Reiter)

→

→ **OPERATIVE TECHNIQUE 9.5 CONTINUED**

7 The twisted wire is trimmed (left), and the 0.5 to 1 cm portion of twisted wire is bent caudally so that the skin covers it (one nylon suture may be placed near the most caudal aspect of the incision) (right). If the twisted wire is not bent, a protective covering (made of resin) should be placed over the cut end of the twisted wire to prevent the exposed portion from catching on fabric and/or causing laceration.

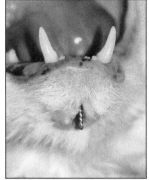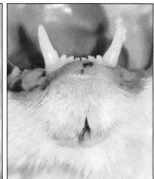

(© Dr Alexander M. Reiter)

8 A radiograph is obtained to confirm proper alignment of the separation.

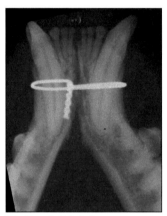

(© Dr Alexander M. Reiter)

9 The wire is removed after about 4 weeks, following radiographic confirmation of healing, by cutting it intraorally and straightening its ends, incising the skin at the chin, grasping the twisted wire and pulling it out.

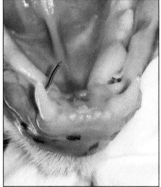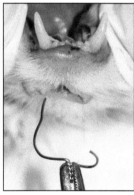

(© Dr Alexander M. Reiter)

10 The intraoral and skin wounds are rinsed and left to granulate and epithelialize.

PRACTICAL TIP

- When bending twisted wire, the wire may loosen or become fatigued, especially if the bend is created where the first twist occurs. Creating the bend further away from the junction between the loop and twisted wire may make this less likely
- Twisting the wire excessively will result in pressure necrosis of the bone, linguoversion of canine and other teeth, malocclusion and TMJ pain

POSTOPERATIVE CARE

Soft food for 2 weeks; no hard toys or treats.

Interdental wiring and splinting

INDICATIONS

Upper and lower jaw fractures with sufficient numbers of teeth available for anchorage of wire and resin.

POSITIONING

Lateral, ventral or dorsal recumbency.

ASSISTANT

May be needed.

ADDITIONAL EQUIPMENT

Hypodermic needle; orthopaedic wire; coarse pumice; materials for acid etching and adhesive bonding; dental composite; bis-acryl composite; pencil; power tools for trimming and shaping of the splint.

SURGICAL TECHNIQUE

Approach

A wire-reinforced interdental splint is fabricated on teeth within a dental arch.

Surgical manipulations

1   Scale and polish the teeth to be involved in the splint.

2   Use orthopaedic wire (22–26 G in dogs and 24–28 G in cats) and place it intragingivally below the dental bulge, where possible (via a hypodermic needle that is inserted through gingiva between teeth).

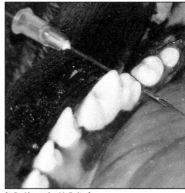

(© Dr Alexander M. Reiter)

3   Interdental wiring:

  a. Stout multiple-loop technique (imagine a fracture between the right mandibular third and fourth premolar teeth):
      –   Start caudally and, as you proceed rostrally, include two or more teeth in each fracture segment
      –   Make wire loops lingually (or labially/buccally, but be aware of occlusion) for lower jaw fractures and labially/buccally for upper jaw fractures
      –   Insert an appropriately sized hypodermic needle through the gingiva in between teeth, and then guide a fitting wire through the needle opening
      –   Leave the 'working' wire (the one used to make loops) longer than the 'static' wire (the one threaded through the loops once they have been created)
      –   Hand twist the wire ends in edentulous areas (if present), and then continue the loop technique
      –   Once sufficient teeth have been included in the wiring procedure, twist the rostral wire ends and interdental loops in a pull-and-twist fashion (slight ventral pull for the lower jaw and dorsal pull for the upper jaw)
      –   Trim the twisted rostral wire end until a 5–7 mm knot remains which is bent towards the tooth without interfering with occlusion
      –   Curve the twisted loops interdentally without interfering with occlusion.

→ **OPERATIVE TECHNIQUE 9.6 CONTINUED**

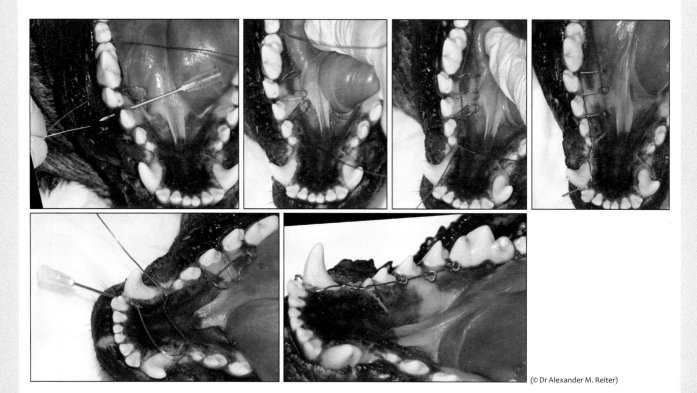

(© Dr Alexander M. Reiter)

b. Modified Risdon technique (imagine several fractures between the stable right maxillary fourth premolar tooth and left maxillary canine tooth):
    –   Start caudally and secure a wire around a tooth with sufficient periodontal attachment (intragingivally distally and – if possible – also mesially)
    –   Hand twist the two equally long wire ends along the dental arch (lingually for the lower jaw and labially/buccally for the upper jaw) and anchor them to a tooth rostral to the bone fracture(s); one can also cross towards the other side or have twisted wires meet rostrally from either side
    –   Use a strong synthetic absorbable monofilament suture material and secure the twisted wire to gingiva at several locations in between the two anchor teeth, which effectively aligns displaced fracture segments.

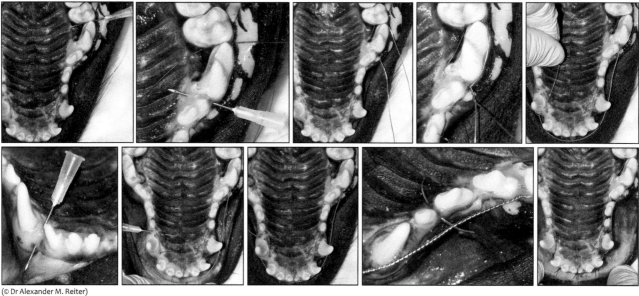

→ **OPERATIVE TECHNIQUE 9.6 CONTINUED**

4 Acid-etch the surfaces of the teeth that will be covered with bis-acryl composite.

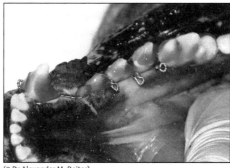
(© Dr Alexander M. Reiter)

5 Rinse acid and any oral debris from the mouth, and air-dry the teeth (ensuring that their crowns are not re-contaminated with blood, saliva or other fluids).

6 Apply bis-acryl composite primarily to the lingual surface of mandibular teeth and the labial/buccal surface of maxillary teeth (leave the tips of the crowns uncovered to ease splint removal upon healing).

When possible, the composite resin should be applied at a distance from the gingiva. If not possible, it should not extend beyond the mucogingival junction.

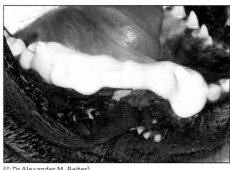
(© Dr Alexander M. Reiter)

7 Once the material has set, trim and shape the splint with an acrylic bur on a low-speed handpiece and/or with crown-preparation diamond burs on a high-speed handpiece, under water cooling.

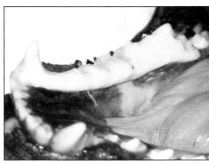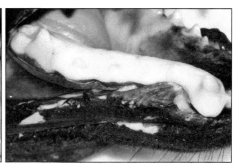
(© Dr Alexander M. Reiter)

8 Check the occlusion; occlusal contact points can be marked with a pencil prior to further splint trimming and shaping.

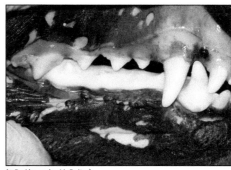
(© Dr Alexander M. Reiter)

9 Polish the splint once adequate mouth closure is confirmed.

10 Rinse debris from the mouth and remove the pharyngeal packing.

11 Obtain a postoperative radiograph.

12 Extubate and recover the patient.

→ **OPERATIVE TECHNIQUE 9.6 CONTINUED**

13 Institute home oral hygiene (oral application of chlorhexidine gel and daily tooth and splint brushing).

14 Remove the splint after 4–8 weeks (or after radiographic confirmation of healing) by interdental sectioning with a bur and detaching the material in segments, using an extraction or band remover forceps and a dental elevator; then clean and polish the teeth.

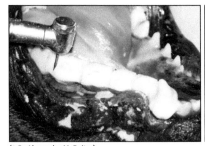 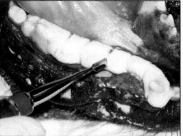 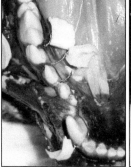 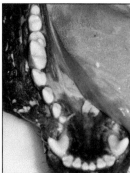

(© Dr Alexander M. Reiter)

PRACTICAL TIPS

- Pharyngotomy or transmylohyoid orotracheal intubation may be used to allow intraoperative control of occlusion without the need for extubation of the patient during the procedure
- Wire slippage from the teeth can be prevented by:
  - Placing the wire intragingivally between the teeth and below the dental bulge
  - Placing drops of dental composite at the gingival third of the mesial and distal crown surfaces of the teeth to create overhangs that allow the wire to remain in position (particularly useful in cats)
- Additional retention is achieved by:
  - Treating the scaled tooth surface with coarse pumice (which creates tiny scratches for micromechanical retention)
  - Applying unfilled resin to the acid etched and dried enamel surface (which improves micromechanical retention) at select areas with or without also applying dental composite
  - Leaving the twisted interdental loop ends intact, thus allowing resin material to flow into them
- Coloured resin aids in visualization during splint application and removal
- Before complete removal, it is recommended to section the splint at the level of the bone fracture lines, and gently test the mandibular/maxillary segment mobility
- If stabilization is satisfactory, then the entire splint is removed. Otherwise, the splint is repaired by simply adding new bis-acryl composite resin at the sectioned sites and maintained in place for a longer time. Any fracture of the resin happening during the healing period may be repaired in similar fashion

POSTOPERATIVE CARE

Elizabethan collar as needed; soft food until splint removal, with no hard toys or treats; gingival inflammation from splint and wire trauma usually subsides within a few days after splint removal.

Chapter 10

Management of dental, oral and maxillofacial developmental disorders

Loic Legendre and Alexander M. Reiter

Occlusion and malocclusion

The relationship between the teeth of the upper and lower dental arches is called 'occlusion'. With the ever expanding number of dog and cat breeds, there is also increasing variation in the shapes and sizes of heads and jaws. Establishing what is normal occlusion is somewhat problematic because what is considered to be normal for a Shih Tzu might be abnormal for a Borzoi. In the same way, a Persian and an Oriental Shorthair cat have different relationships between the upper and lower jaw, although cats show less variation than dogs. Three types of head conformation are recognized: long (dolichocephalic), medium (mesocephalic or mesaticephalic) and short (brachycephalic). When describing a 'normal' occlusion (or orthocclusion), we are referring to a mesocephalic head. The Nomenclature Committee of the American Veterinary Dental College (AVDC) has reviewed malocclusion and its various forms in order to clarify and standardize the diverse conditions encompassed under this term (AVDC, 2015).

Normal occlusion (orthocclusion)

A closed mouth inspection is necessary to fully evaluate dental occlusion. In mesocephalic and dolichocephalic dogs, the maxillary incisor teeth are positioned labial to the corresponding mandibular incisor teeth (Figure 10.1; see Chapter 2). The incisal tips of the mandibular incisor teeth contact the cingula of the maxillary incisor teeth. The mandibular canine tooth is inclined labially and bisects the interproximal (interdental) space between the opposing maxillary third incisor and canine teeth. The maxillary premolar teeth do not contact the mandibular premolar teeth. The crown cusps of the mandibular premolar teeth are positioned slightly lingual to the arch formed by the maxillary premolar teeth. The cusps of the mandibular premolar teeth bisect the interproximal (interdental) spaces mesial to the corresponding maxillary premolar teeth. The mesial cusp of the maxillary fourth premolar tooth is positioned buccal to the space between the mandibular fourth premolar and first molar teeth.

Normal occlusion in cats is similar (Figure 10.2). The maxillary incisor teeth are labial to the mandibular incisor teeth, with the incisal tips of the mandibular teeth contacting the cingula of the maxillary teeth or occluding just palatal to them. The mandibular canine tooth fits in the diastema between the maxillary third incisor and canine

teeth, equidistant between the two and touching neither. The incisor bite and canine interdigitation form the dental interlock. Each mandibular premolar tooth is positioned mesial to the corresponding maxillary premolar tooth. The maxillary second premolar tooth points into a space between the mandibular canine and third premolar teeth. The subsequent teeth interdigitate, with the mandibular premolar teeth and first molar teeth being situated lingual to the maxillary teeth. The buccal surface of the mandibular first molar tooth occludes with the palatal surface of the maxillary fourth premolar tooth. The maxillary first molar tooth is located distopalatal to the maxillary fourth premolar tooth and does not occlude with any other tooth (Milella, 2015).

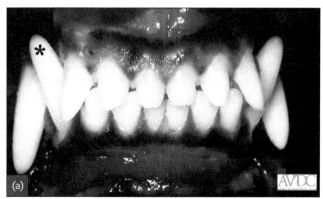

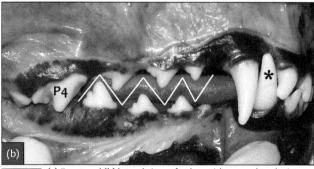

10.1 (a) Front and (b) lateral view of a dog with normal occlusion. Note the position of the mandibular canine tooth (∗) and the interdigitation of the cusps of the maxillary and mandibular premolar teeth (white zig-zag pattern). The maxillary fourth premolar tooth (P4) conceals the mandibular first molar tooth when the mouth is closed.
(a, © AVDC® used with permission; b, © Dr Margherita Gracis)

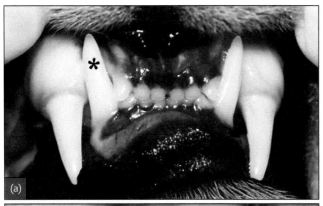

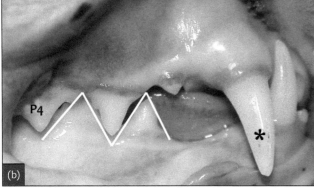

10.2 (a) Front and (b) lateral view of a cat with normal occlusion. (a) Note the position of the mandibular canine tooth (∗). (b) Note the position of the maxillary canine tooth (∗) and the interdigitation of the cusps of the maxillary and mandibular premolar teeth (white zig-zag pattern). The maxillary fourth premolar tooth (P4) conceals the mandibular first molar tooth when the mouth is closed.
(© Dr Alexander M. Reiter)

Malocclusion

Causes

Malocclusion is a misalignment of the teeth and/or jaws. It can be atraumatic, cause discomfort or result in severe pathology. The cause may be genetic, developmental or accidental (Lobprise *et al*., 1999; Gracis *et al*., 2000; Sarkiala-Kessel, 2001). It can involve the teeth (size, shape and position) and/or the jaws (size, shape and relation to each other). Head shape, jaw length, tooth size and position are inherited and characteristic of each breed.

Classification

Dental malocclusion (neutrocclusion or class 1 malocclusion): Dental malocclusion refers to malposition of one or more teeth regardless of the presence or absence of a normal rostrocaudal relationship of the upper and lower dental arches; the terminology used to describe malocclusion is defined in Figure 10.3.

Symmetrical skeletal malocclusion: Mandibular distocclusion (class 2 malocclusion) refers to an abnormal rostrocaudal relationship between the dental arches in which the lower dental arch occludes caudal to its normal position relative to the upper dental arch (Figure 10.4).
   Mandibular mesiocclusion (class 3 malocclusion) refers to an abnormal rostrocaudal relationship between the dental arches in which the lower dental arch occludes rostral to its normal position relative to the upper dental arch (Figure 10.5).

Term	Description
Distoversion	Describes a tooth that is in its anatomically correct position in the dental arch but which is abnormally angled in a distal direction
Mesioversion	Describes a tooth that is in its anatomically correct position in the dental arch but which is abnormally angled in a mesial direction
Linguoversion or palatoversion	Describes a tooth that is in its anatomically correct position in the dental arch but which is abnormally angled in a lingual or palatal direction
Labioversion	Describes an incisor or canine tooth that is in its anatomically correct position in the dental arch but which is abnormally angled in a labial direction
Buccoversion	Describes a premolar or molar tooth that is in its anatomically correct position in the dental arch but which is abnormally angled in a buccal direction
Rotation	Describes a tooth that is in its anatomically correct position in the dental arch but which is abnormally turned along its longitudinal axis due to lack of rotation of the developing tooth germ
Supraocclusion	Describes a tooth that is in its anatomically correct position in the dental arch but which extends beyond the occlusal plane
Infraocclusion	Describes a tooth that is in its anatomically correct position in the dental arch but which failed to reach the occlusal plane
Displacement	Describes a tooth that is abnormally positioned in the dental arch due to bodily movement
Crossbite	Describes a dental malocclusion in which one or more mandibular teeth have a more labial or buccal position than the antagonist maxillary tooth and can be classified as rostral or caudal
Rostral crossbite	One or more of the mandibular incisor teeth is situated labial to the opposing maxillary incisor teeth when the mouth is closed
Caudal crossbite	One or more of the mandibular cheek teeth is situated buccal to the opposing maxillary cheek teeth when the mouth is closed

10.3 Dental malocclusion terminology.
(Adapted from AVDC (http://www.avdc.org))

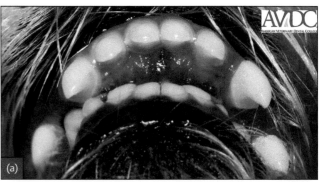

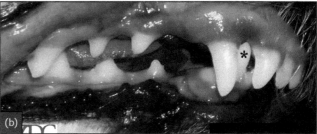

10.4 (a) Front and (b) lateral view of a dog with a class 2 malocclusion. Note that the lower jaw is too short with the mandibular canine tooth (∗) and the incisor teeth impinging on the hard palate mucosa.
(© AVDC® used with permission)

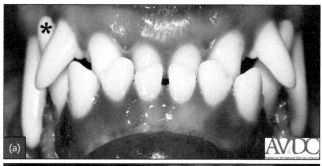

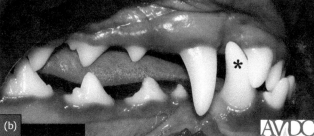

10.5 (a) Front and (b) lateral view of a dog with class 3 malocclusion. Note the upper jaw is too short with the mandibular canine tooth (*) hitting the distal aspect of the maxillary third incisor tooth upon closure of the mouth. Several maxillary incisor teeth bite into the gingiva lingual to the mandibular incisor teeth. (© AVDC® used with permission)

Asymmetrical skeletal malocclusion (class 4 malocclusion): Maxillomandibular asymmetry describes skeletal malocclusions that can occur in a rostrocaudal, side-to-side or dorsoventral direction.

Maxillomandibular asymmetry in a rostrocaudal direction occurs when mandibular mesioclusion or distocclusion is present on one side of the head while the contralateral side retains normal dental alignment (Figure 10.6). It is sometimes referred to as a wry bite. It is fairly rare and can be associated with side-to-side asymmetry.

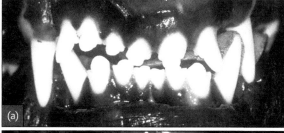

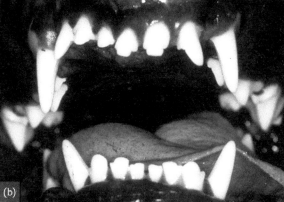

10.6 Maxillomandibular asymmetry in a rostrocaudal direction in a dog. Front views with the mouth (a) nearly closed and (b) moderately open. Note that the right upper jaw appears shorter compared with the left, and that there is no longer midline alignment between the upper and lower jaws. (© Dr Alexander M. Reiter)

Maxillomandibular asymmetry in a side-to-side direction occurs when there is loss of the midline alignment of the upper and lower jaws. Causes can be genetic but are primarily traumatic, such as when a puppy gets bitten in the face and the affected quadrant slows or stops growing, resulting in a deviation of the jaw to the side of the trauma (Figure 10.7). The deviation can be severe, and the patient may present with multiple teeth in traumatic malocclusion.

Maxillomandibular asymmetry in a dorsoventral direction results in an open bite, which is defined as an abnormal vertical space between the upper and lower dental arches when the mouth is closed (Figure 10.8). In some cases, interference with the growth of the lower jaw causes one or both mandibles to bow ventrally, creating a unilateral or bilateral open bite. In others, the cause for the jaw deviation is not found.

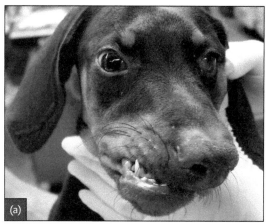

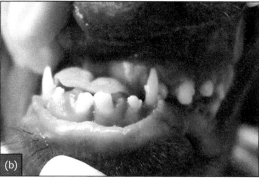

10.7 Maxillomandibular asymmetry in a side-to-side direction in a dog with mixed dentition. Front views with (a) the mouth closed and (b) the lips retracted. Note the loss of the midline alignment of the upper and lower jaws due to severe deviation. (© Dr Alexander M. Reiter)

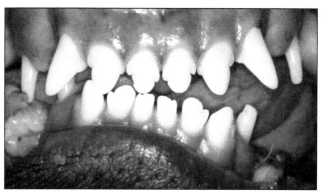

10.8 Maxillomandibular asymmetry in a dorsoventral direction resulting in an open bite in a 7-month-old dog. Note that all four deciduous canine teeth are still present, and there appears delayed eruption of the permanent canine teeth. (© Dr Alexander M. Reiter)

Equipment, instruments and materials used in orthodontics

A specific set of instruments and materials is needed for orthodontic treatment (Ross, 1986a; Wiggs and Lobprise, 1997) (Figure 10.9).

Impression trays

Trays made of hard plastic or metal can be purchased, or they can be fabricated using thermoplastic beads. They should follow the shape of the upper and lower dental arches, but must be several millimetres wider than the actual arch and deep enough to accommodate the height of the crowns of the teeth. Considering the varied sizes of our veterinary patients, an assortment of different trays should be available. They are filled with alginate or other impression materials to obtain full-mouth impressions.

Rubber mixing bowls and mixing spatulas

Bowls and mixing spatulas are used to mix alginate impression materials to obtain full-mouth impressions and dental stone to create dental models.

Impression material

Polyvinyl siloxane putty and light body impression compound are indicated for obtaining detailed impressions of the teeth or portion of the dental arch involved in orthodontic movement. Alginate impression compound is normally used for full dental arch impressions.

Bite registration material

Baseplate wax or polyvinyl siloxane compound may be used for bite registration (see Operative Technique 10.1). Baseplate wax is produced as a sheet that is hard at room temperature. It is softened under warm water, folded to create a double-layered sheet, and placed between the maxillary and mandibular incisor and canine teeth. The mouth is closed, which allows the maxillary and mandibular incisor and canine teeth to indent the wax in the process. Cold water is sprayed on to the wax to harden it before removing it from the mouth. The indents marked into the wax help the dental laboratory technician to align the stone models obtained from the upper and lower jaws. The same result can be obtained using polyvinyl siloxane which, however, is more expensive.

Dental stone

Type III and IV dental stone (the latter is preferred due to its hardness) are used for pouring models in veterinary dentistry. Both are stronger than type I (plaster of Paris) and type II (dental plaster) stone and therefore have less chance of breaking when being removed from the impression trays. They have specific mixing ratios (water to powder) that have to be followed when preparing them.

Dental vibrator

This equipment provides a mixing platform that vibrates at three speeds. The vibration helps with the mixing of powder and water in alginate and dental stone and the elimination of air bubbles trapped in the mixture.

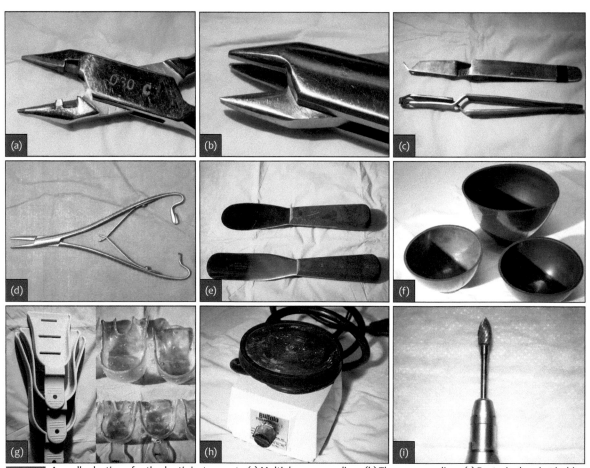

| 10.9 | A small selection of orthodontic instruments. (a) Multiple purpose pliers. (b) Three-prong pliers. (c) Posterior bracket holders. (d) Mathieu needle holder. (e) Mixing spatulas. (f) Rubber mixing bowls. (g) Two versions of impression trays. (h) Dental vibrator. (i) Acrylic contouring bur mounted on a straight cone on a low-speed handpiece. |

Plaster cutters and water-cooled power trimmer

Plaster cutters are large cutting pliers designed to lop off superfluous chunks of dental stone. To obtain a professional looking stone model, all sides not containing teeth are reduced using a power trimmer, which is a large water-cooled sanding disk against which the base and sides of the models are flattened.

Orthodontic wire

Orthodontic wire has memory (i.e. it returns to its straight shape after being bent). This allows it to be distinguished from orthopaedic wire, which retains its shape once bent. Orthodontic wire of sizes 22–32 G is most commonly used.

Orthodontic pliers

Pliers are used to bend wires, create spring loops, activate appliances and adjust orthodontic wires. Among the most commonly utilized instruments are the three-prong, the bird beak, the Howe, and the tweed loop-forming pliers. A Mathieu driver comes in very handy to twist wires evenly, preventing kinks that weaken the wires.

Wire cutters

Wire cutters, also called universal scissors, possess serrated edges and a notch to catch the wire and prevent it from slipping while being cut. They work better with smaller gauge wires.

Brackets, buttons and bands

Brackets can be rectangular and flat. Their base may be bent slightly to fit canine and premolar teeth where they are most commonly used. They may be used for anchorage of orthodontic wires and elastics. Buttons are round and ideal for anchorage of ligature orthopaedic wires and elastics. A band is a thin plate of stainless-steel metal that wraps around a tooth. It may have attachments welded to it (e.g. brackets) or be used to anchor an appliance to the teeth. Brackets, buttons and bands are cemented to the teeth.

Hypodermic needles

Hypodermic needles, 25 mm (1 inch) in length, size 18 or 21 G, may be used to build the telescopic part of an inclined plane.

Bracket holders and tweezers

Bracket holders are designed to hold brackets and buttons, and tweezers are for placing them on the surface of teeth.

Bracket-removing pliers

These pliers are specifically designed with one side Teflon-covered and one shorter side with a straight bevel. The Teflon-covered side is placed on the cusp tip of the tooth while the straight bevel is placed on the gingival aspect of the bracket or button. Closing the pliers dislodges the bracket or button without damaging the tooth.

Elastic chains, tubes and threads

Elastic chains (short link, medium link, long link), tubes (hollow) and threads (solid) are attached to anchor devices on teeth and extended between them, to effect movement of the target tooth. Dynamometers are available to measure the tension applied to these elastic devices.

Orthodontic bonding cements

Resin-based cements are used to bond orthodontic appliances, including brackets, buttons and bands, to teeth.

Orthodontic and acrylic composites

Orthodontic composites are commonly used to attach brackets, buttons and bands to teeth or to fabricate self-made buttons. Self-curing, non-exothermic bis-acryl composites are used to build inclined planes, bite blocks and crown extensions.

Trimming and finishing burs

Acrylic contouring burs mounted on to a straight cone that is attached to a low-speed dental handpiece are used to shape orthodontic appliances such as an inclined plane.

Treatment of malocclusion affecting the deciduous dentition
Adverse dental interlock

The presence of malocclusion in immature animals often creates an 'adverse dental interlock', which results in trauma and interferes with proper growth of the jaws. Occasionally, there is no trauma, but interference only. Treatment is simple and consists of removing the teeth creating the interlock. Extraction should be performed as early as possible to allow the maximum time for spontaneous correction of the abnormal occlusion prior to eruption of the permanent teeth (Figure 10.10). Removing a dental interlock in a deciduous dentition is called 'interceptive orthodontics' (Hale, 2005). Unfortunately, it does not guarantee that occlusion will be normal in the adult patient; extraction of teeth interfering with normal jaw growth only allows the patient to express its full genetic potential. The final occlusion will depend on the hereditary baggage of the patient. Occlusion is then re-evaluated when the permanent teeth have erupted.

Persistent deciduous teeth

Persistent deciduous teeth should also be extracted, as they may contribute to the displacement of the permanent successor. Any tooth displacement can result in trauma (Figure 10.11). The persistent deciduous tooth also causes crowding, which could exacerbate periodontal disease (Legendre, 1994c; Fulton et al., 2014).

Extracting deciduous teeth requires finesse, pre- and postoperative dental radiographs, appropriate instruments, and good technique (see Chapter 12). Trying to rush these extractions is a grave mistake. With the help of fine and curved luxators, deciduous canine teeth can be gently luxated without causing damage to the developing permanent dentition. An open extraction technique is recommended if the tooth fractures or cannot be removed in a closed fashion. It should be remembered to keep the instrument away from that surface of the deciduous tooth facing its permanent successor (Hobson, 2005).

Cutting off the crowns of deciduous teeth must not be contemplated; it is the root of the deciduous tooth that may cause deviation of the permanent tooth. Furthermore,

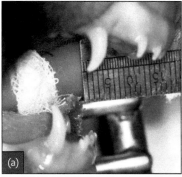

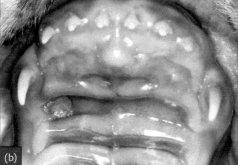

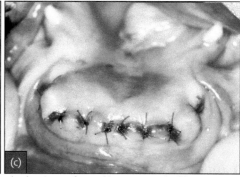

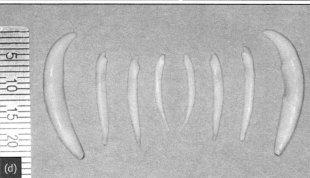

10.10 Interceptive orthodontics performed in a 2.5-month-old puppy. (a) Note the discrepancy in length between the upper and lower jaws. (b) Impressions left in the hard palate mucosa by the deciduous mandibular canine and incisor teeth. (c) Sutured extraction sites. (d) Note the crown-root relationships of extracted deciduous teeth.
(© Dr Alexander M. Reiter)

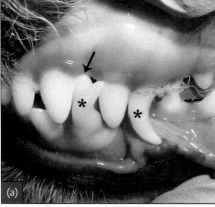

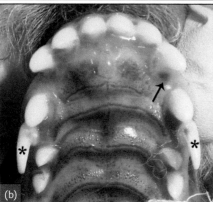

10.11 (a) Lateral view of the closed mouth and (b) occlusal view of the rostral upper jaw in a 7-month-old dog. Note the presence of persistent deciduous canine teeth (*), accompanied by a displaced permanent left mandibular canine tooth leaving an impression in the gingiva immediately distal to the third incisor tooth (arrowed).

removal of the crown opens the pulp cavity of the tooth and thus leads to formation of endodontic and periapical disease that can ultimately cause damage to the permanent tooth. Finally, it may be considered to be negligence and places the operator in an ethically and legally precarious position.

Treatment of specific malocclusions affecting the permanent dentition

Treatment depends on the condition, each of which may have more than one possible treatment option. Before initiating any of the following treatments, the veterinary dentist should discuss ethical considerations of such treatment, and orthognathic surgery to correct skeletal malocclusion should be carefully considered (see Chapter 1) (Emily, 1992; Buchet and Boudrieau, 1999; Carvalho et al., 2014). For the sake of argument, we shall assume that all the treatments described below are to be applied to neutered patients, whether pure-bred or not, to eliminate the chance of transmitting poor genes to the next generation.

In most cases full-mouth impressions should be obtained and stone models created. Stone models permit the evaluation of occlusion of a patient in its absence, may be used as a preoperative database and are sometimes utilized to build an appliance (Operative Technique 10.1). Scaling and polishing the teeth included in any appliance with pumice powder is necessary to allow proper bonding of dental composites or acrylic resins.

There are various options for treatment of maloccluding teeth, including extraction, crown reduction and vital pulp therapy, passive and active orthodontic movement, and surgical orthodontics (Ross, 1986b; Goldstein, 1990; Amimoto et al., 1993; Wiggs and Lobprise, 1997; Surgeon, 2005).

The timing and removal of orthodontic appliances (e.g. inclined planes, active orthodontic devices, crown extensions) must be carefully planned, as early removal may allow teeth to move back to their original position and careless removal may lead to injury of teeth and soft tissues. Retainers (devices that keep teeth, once having reached their perfect position, in that position without exerting an active force) should be placed until the 'memory' of the periodontal ligament has faded (which can take several months). Leaving the tips of the cusps of teeth visible at the time of appliance instalment will reduce the risk that one accidentally injures a tooth when removing a bis-acryl composite appliance.

Linguoversion of mandibular canine teeth

Breeds with narrow lower jaws such as poodles seem to be over-represented. The lingual displacement of the permanent mandibular canine teeth is often associated with persistence of the deciduous canine teeth (Bannon and Baker, 2008). Linguoversion may be the only abnormality (Figure 10.12) or it may be part of a class 2 malocclusion where the mandibular canine teeth become 'trapped' palatal or distal to the maxillary canine teeth. The aetiology affects the ethics of treatment, but not the treatment itself. The linguoverted mandibular canine teeth may impact the mucosa in the interproximal space between the maxillary third incisor and canine teeth or the palate, creating a soft tissue defect or, in the worst case scenario, an oronasal fistula.

Treatment: The treatment includes extraction, crown reduction with endodontic therapy, or corrective orthodontic movement of the affected tooth. Extraction is rarely recommended, as it is traumatic and can lead to complications such as mandibular fracture, alveolar osteitis, osteomyelitis, haemorrhage, lingual ptosis and loss of defensive capacity (Bannon and Baker, 2008). Crown reduction with vital pulp therapy is a viable option that has the advantage of sparing the gingival third of the crown and supporting root and being performed in one anaesthetic session (Figure 10.13) (Legendre, 1994a). This technique preserves function and vitality of the tooth, which continues to provide support for the tongue. A major disadvantage includes the risk of introduction of pulpal infection and inflammation; thus, some veterinary dentists prefer standard root canal therapy over vital pulp therapy in mature patients with closed root apices (Greenfield, 2011). Radiographic follow-ups are necessary to monitor the success of this procedure.

Corrective orthodontics may involve one of several techniques, such as rubber ball therapy, W-wire, expansion screw, composite resin inclined plane, composite resin telescopic inclined plane, and cast metal telescopic inclined plane (Oakes and Beard, 1992; Pavlica and Cestnik, 1995; Wiggs and Lobprise, 1997; Verhaert, 1999). The rubber ball, being a removable appliance, is the simplest. Unfortunately, it is reserved for cases presenting with a neutrocclusion or some severe class 2 malocclusion (with the mandibular canine teeth occluding distal to their maxillary counterparts). The patient needs to carry the ball for a certain amount of time during the day for the treatment to be effective. Both an expansion screw and W-wire

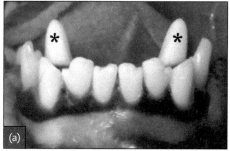

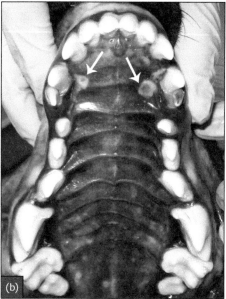

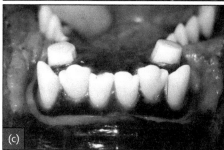

10.13 (a) Linguoversion of mandibular canine teeth (∗) in a dog with class 2 malocclusion. (b) Impressions are left in the hard palate mucosa (arrowed) by the displaced mandibular canine teeth. Note the presence of four persistent deciduous canine teeth. (c) The deciduous canine teeth were extracted and the crowns of the permanent canine teeth were reduced to the level of the mandibular incisor teeth, followed by vital pulp therapy.
(© Dr Alexander M. Reiter)

need to be activated regularly and can only move teeth in one direction (labial) (Wiggs and Lobprise, 1997; van de Wetering, 2007).

An inclined plane, on the other hand, can tip teeth in two directions, labial and mesial or, in rare cases, labial and distal (Figure 10.14) (Hale, 1996; Ulbricht and Marretta, 2005; Blazejewski, 2013; Furman and Niemiec, 2013; Kim *et al.*, 2015). It does not require activation, and the telescopic variation expands as the young patient's palate continues to grow (Legendre, 1994b, 2010). The appliance can be fabricated by a laboratory (indirect inclined plane) or built inside the mouth by the operator (direct inclined plane; see Operative Technique 10.2). If the canine tooth is only slightly displaced palatally, crown lengthening by means of a composite resin extension (Figure 10.15) can be performed or a natural inclined plane (Figure 10.16) may be created (Blazejewski, 2013; Smith, 2013).

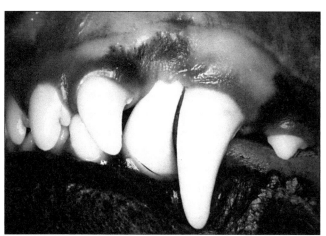

10.12 Linguoversion of the left mandibular canine tooth in a dog, causing a soft tissue lesion mesial to the left maxillary canine tooth.

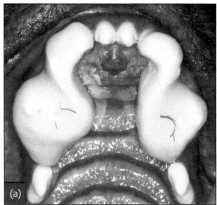

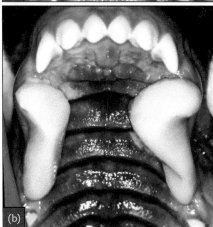

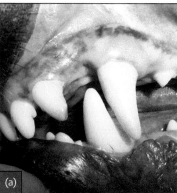

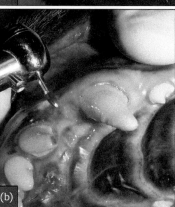

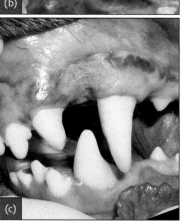

10.14 Two different designs of direct inclined planes: (a) one design moves the mandibular canine teeth mesiolabially and (b) the other design moves the mandibular canine teeth distolabially.
(© Dr Alexander M. Reiter)

10.16 (a) The lingually displaced left mandibular tooth has left an impression in the gingiva between the left maxillary third incisor and canine teeth. (b) A natural inclined plane is created with a 12-fluted bur (bullet- or egg-shaped) on a water-cooled high-speed handpiece to create space for and allow the lingually displaced left mandibular canine tooth to move labially. (c) The cut gingiva is coated with a layer of tissue protectant (such as tincture of myrrh and benzoin).
(© Dr Alexander M. Reiter)

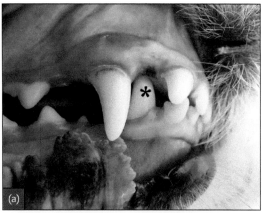

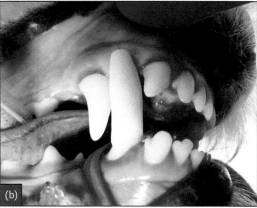

10.15 (a) Linguoversion of the right mandibular canine tooth (∗) in a dog. (b) Composite resin extension has been bonded to the displaced tooth in order to tip it labially upon occluding into the space between the ipsilateral maxillary third incisor and canine tooth. The appliance should be built bilaterally to avoid mandibular deviation and allow for proper tooth tipping.
(© Dr Sigbjorn Storli)

Mesioversion of the maxillary canine tooth

This is primarily encountered in small- and toy-breed dogs and seen in Persian and Siamese cats (Figure 10.17). The most commonly affected dog breed is the Shetland Sheepdog, with a few other breeds such as the Italian Greyhound and Miniature Schnauzer occasionally also exhibiting this trait (Wiggs and Lobprise, 1997; Legendre and Stepaniuk, 2008). Mesioversion may be idiopathic or associated with the persistence of a deciduous maxillary canine tooth. The tooth displacement closes the interdental space between the maxillary third incisor and canine teeth, and prevents the mandibular canine tooth from moving labially. In some cases the mesioversion is extreme and the affected maxillary canine tooth erupts horizontally just distal to the third incisor tooth. These cases are referred to as 'lance canine' and are believed to be hereditary. As the maxillary canine tooth occupies the space where the mandibular canine tooth occludes, the latter is displaced either lingually into palatal gingiva or hard palate mucosa or, more commonly, labially into the upper lip. It may even end up on the outside of the upper lip, causing ulceration of the lip skin (Verhaert, 2007).

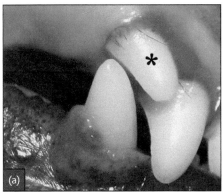

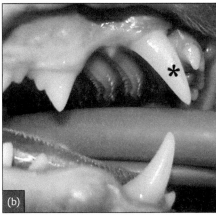

10.17 (a) Dog with a 'lance canine', an extreme form of mesioversion, of the right maxillary canine tooth (∗). (b) Mesioversion of the right maxillary canine tooth (∗) in a cat.

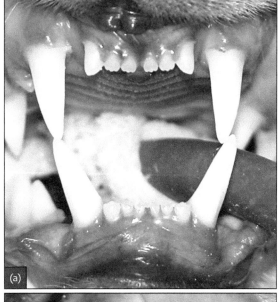

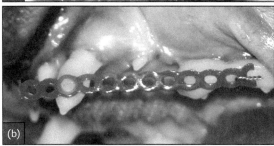

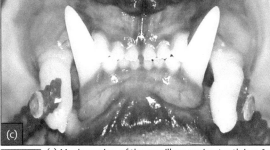

Treatment: Extraction of the affected tooth is a treatment option; however, this may lead to entrapment of the upper lip by the mandibular canine tooth. If the maxillary canine tooth is not in the direct path of the mandibular canine tooth, crown reduction with vital pulp therapy of the mandibular tooth can be performed. Active orthodontic movement usually has a superior outcome (Figure 10.18), thus often remaining the treatment of choice (Wiggs and Lobprise, 1997; Gengler, 2004) (Operative Technique 10.3).

Crossbite and level bite

Crossbite describes a malocclusion in which one or more mandibular teeth are situated more labial or buccal than the opposing maxillary teeth. It may be secondary to palatoversion of the maxillary teeth or labioversion/buccoversion of the mandibular teeth. It can be classified as rostral or caudal.

In rostral crossbite one or more mandibular incisor teeth are labial to the opposing maxillary incisor teeth when the mouth is closed (Figure 10.19). It may be associated with class 3 malocclusion and is considered normal or acceptable in most brachycephalic breeds. If the upper jaw is short or the lower jaw too long, the mandibular incisor teeth occlude labial to the maxillary incisor teeth. Less frequently, it is diagnosed in a patient with neutrocclusion (class 1 malocclusion). The crossbite may cause traumatic contact between the teeth and/or with the opposite soft tissues. The maxillary incisor teeth may also contact the mandibular incisor teeth or the opposing oral mucosa upon closing of the mouth. The mandibular canine teeth may also contact the maxillary second or third incisor teeth. Repeated trauma may result in tooth attrition, crown fracture, tooth mobility, tooth displacement or exacerbation of periodontal disease.

10.18 (a) Mesioversion of the maxillary canine teeth in a 6-month-old Siamese cat. (b) Active orthodontic movement is performed. Note the elastic chain spanning from a transparent plastic button on the left maxillary canine tooth to a wire hook attached to an anchorage unit built on the maxillary third and fourth premolar teeth. (c) Front view 1 week after the start of treatment.
(© Dr Alexander M. Reiter)

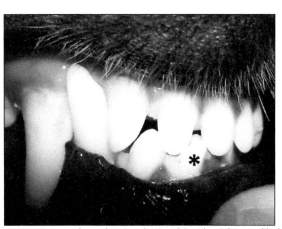

10.19 Rostral crossbite in a dog involving the right mandibular second incisor tooth (∗).
(© Dr Alexander M. Reiter)

In caudal crossbite one or more mandibular cheek teeth are buccal to the opposing maxillary cheek teeth when the mouth is closed (Figure 10.20). This type of malocclusion is more frequently seen in Collies and other dolichocephalic breeds. Treatment is necessary only in case of traumatic contact between the teeth and injury of opposite soft tissues, generally entailing extraction of involved teeth.

A level bite is a condition where maxillary and mandibular incisor teeth occlude edge to edge. As with rostral crossbite, it is often associated with a class 3 malocclusion and may also result in attrition, fracture, mobility and displacement of teeth (Figure 10.21).

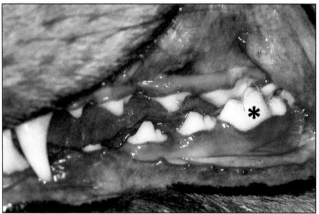

10.20 Caudal crossbite in a dog with the left mandibular first molar tooth (∗) occluding buccal to the left maxillary fourth premolar tooth.
(© Dr Alexander M. Reiter)

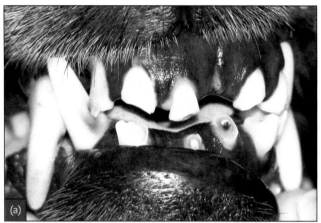

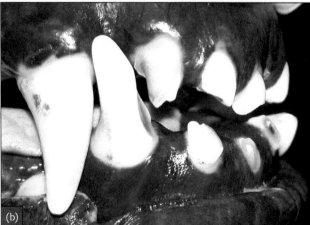

10.21 (a) Front and (b) side views of severely worn teeth resulting in pulp exposure in a dog with 'level bite' malocclusion.
(© Dr Alexander M. Reiter)

Treatment: Correction of rostral crossbite and some cases of level bite consists in re-establishing a 'scissor bite'. If this is not possible, treatment may involve crown reduction with vital pulp therapy or serial extraction to eliminate traumatic contact. Orthodontic correction should be attempted only in cases where the crossbite is not associated with a class 3 malocclusion. Class 3 malocclusion is usually considered to have a genetic cause and should not be masked in a breeding population. There are several ways to correct a rostral crossbite, but no matter which technique is used three goals remain important: moving the maxillary incisor teeth labially; moving the mandibular incisor teeth lingually; and keeping the mouth slightly open during treatment to allow movement to take place. The mouth is kept open with the help of bite blocks or bite shelves (i.e. appliances that impede complete closure of the oral cavity during orthodontic treatment). The teeth can be moved using universal screws, memory wires, labial and lingual arch bars, inclined planes, or even surgical intervention (Legendre, 1991; Peak *et al.*, 1999).

Developmental abnormalities of teeth

Abnormalities in the differentiation of the dental lamina and the tooth germs are responsible for several anomalies, which may be inherited, acquired or idiopathic.

Structural abnormalities of teeth

Genetic and/or developmental enamel formation and maturation abnormalities, such as enamel hypoplasia and enamel hypomineralization, may affect the teeth of dogs and cats (Mannerfelt and Lindgren, 2009). Genetic factors tend to affect the whole amelogenetic process; thus, defects are widespread in the teeth (amelogenesis imperfecta). Developmental factors act for a finite amount of time during amelogenesis, resulting in defects only in the enamel being formed during that finite time. One usually sees banded enamel defects at the same level on teeth forming at the same time. Examples of exogenous factors for structural abnormalities of teeth are hypocalcaemia, excessive fluoride ingestion, local infection, localized trauma, nutritional deficiencies, and most commonly epitheliotropic virus infections (Bittegeko *et al.*, 1995). The presentation can vary in severity from mild forms with only a few small pitting deficiencies, in otherwise normal crowns, to extensive defects that reduce the crowns to knobs and shorten the roots.

Enamel hypoplasia and hypomineralization

Enamel hypoplasia refers to inadequate deposition of enamel matrix; it affects one or several teeth and may be focal or multifocal. The crowns of affected teeth can have areas of normal enamel next to areas of hypoplastic or missing enamel (Figure 10.22). It may be associated with enamel hypomineralization, which refers to inadequate mineralization of enamel matrix, often affecting several or all teeth (Boy *et al.*, 2016). The crowns of such teeth are covered by soft or flaky enamel that may be worn rapidly (Figure 10.23).

In both conditions the patient ends up with rough-surfaced, discoloured teeth. Plaque and calculus accumulate more rapidly and result in a more acute form of

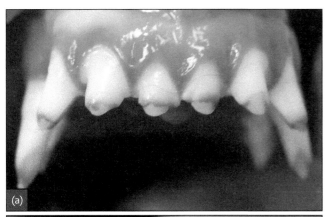

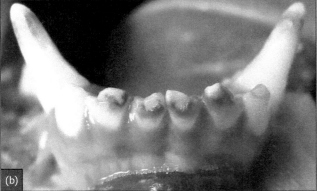

10.22 Enamel hypoplasia of (a) maxillary and (b) mandibular teeth in a dog. The banded enamel defects affecting multiple teeth indicate that some systemic disturbance occurred for a finite amount of time during amelogenesis.

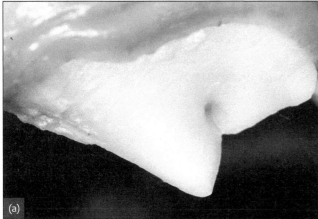

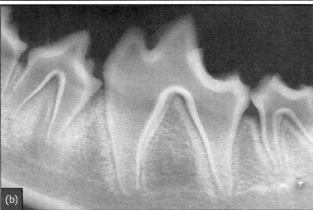

10.23 Enamel hypomineralization in a dog. (a) Note the scratches made in the crown surface of the left maxillary fourth premolar tooth upon scaling. (b) Note the lack of a dense enamel layer on the radiograph showing the left mandibular cheek teeth.
(© Dr Alexander M. Reiter)

periodontal disease. Treatment consists of first obtaining radiographs of the full dentition to determine if some teeth are already non-vital. Such teeth, when still immature, need to be extracted. The crown surface of vital teeth affected by enamel hypoplasia and hypomineralization can be sealed with an unfilled resin to prevent toxins percolating through exposed dentinal tubules, which is an inciting cause of pulpitis, pulp necrosis and periapical disease. In addition, sealing decreases dentine hypersensitivity resulting from exposure of dentinal tubules. Radiographs should be repeated 6 months later. If the teeth have matured normally, they will show thicker dentinal walls and a decreased size of the pulp cavity. Strategically important teeth can be restored with composite resin to improve cosmetic results and to smooth the crown surface. They can also undergo prosthodontic treatment to increase function and prevent fracture. Frequent professional dental cleaning will be necessary. Scaling should be performed with great care, to avoid removal of softened dental tissues. Sonic and ultrasonic scalers should be used at low power, and manual instruments used with a light touch. Meticulous home care is recommended to prevent plaque and calculus accumulation and reduce the need for professional treatment.

Dentinogenesis imperfecta

Dentinogenesis imperfecta is a hereditary disorder resulting in defective dentine in both the primary and secondary dentitions. It results in discoloured and easily worn teeth that are prone to fracture (Figure 10.24). It has been seen in families of Standard Poodles and Akitas and in a few

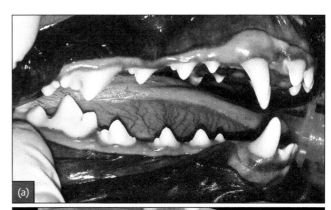

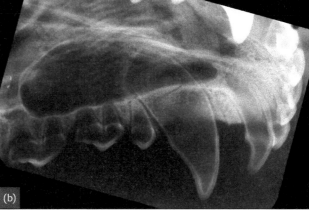

10.24 (a) Clinical and (b) radiographic appearance of some of the teeth of a 6-month-old crossbreed dog affected by dentinogenesis imperfecta. All teeth showed similar radiographic features, with a thinner than normal layer of dentine. Histologically, the presence of cementum on an extracted tooth was inconsistent, and the presence of dentine was unremarkable with a poor or absent tubular architecture.
(© Dr Margherita Gracis)

other breeds. The complications of dentinogenesis imperfecta are difficult to manage, and fractured teeth should be treated by extraction.

Regional odontodysplasia

Regional odontodysplasia is a very rare dental anomaly involving both deciduous and permanent teeth, so far only described in one young cat (Hoffman, 2008). In humans, it usually affects teeth in only one jaw quadrant. Salient signs include soft discoloured teeth, gingivitis, swelling or abscess. Enamel and dentine are hypomineralized and hypoplastic, giving the affected teeth a ghostly appearance on radiographs. The aetiology is unknown, and recommendations are to extract all affected and unerupted teeth.

Odontoblastic dysplasia

Odontoblastic dysplasia, also known as dentine dysplasia type III, is another rare condition with only one report in the veterinary literature (Smithson *et al.*, 2010). The name comes from the human literature where cases are linked to an autosomal dominant trait. It is difficult to speculate about an exact cause of the disease. Upon presentation, both developmental sets of teeth are normal in length and appearance. On radiographs there is partial obliteration of the pulp chamber, and the density of contrast is poor. The root canals are so irregular that any needed endodontic treatment carries a poor prognosis.

Size abnormalities of teeth

Macrodontia refers to teeth larger than normal. Microdontia refers to teeth smaller than normal. Both conditions are rarely reported. They are of limited clinical importance except perhaps when macrodont teeth result in crowding, correction of which requires extraction.

Numerical abnormalities of teeth

Anodontia refers to the failure of all teeth to develop. This is often hereditary and very rare in both dogs and cats (Vieira *et al.*, 2009).

Hypodontia refers to the developmental absence of a few teeth, and oligodontia refers to the developmental absence of numerous teeth (Figure 10.25). The cause can be genetic, traumatic or the result of medications or intrauterine disturbances. It may be associated with ectodermal dysplasia (Lewis *et al.*, 2010). Premolars are the most commonly missing teeth. The mandibular third molar teeth are often missing in small-breed dogs. On the other hand, canine and carnassial teeth are rarely missing. Presentation is simple; there is a bare part of the dental arch where a tooth should be present. The alveolar margin height in edentulous areas may be lower than in areas where teeth are present. Confirmation requires dental radiography. Treatment is not required.

Hyperdontia refers to the presence of an extra (supernumerary) tooth (Figure 10.26). Incisor and premolar teeth are most commonly involved, but it can happen with any type of teeth. The operator should verify that the supernumerary tooth has a normal crown and root and that there is adequate space for avoidance of traumatic malocclusion. If crown and root are normal and there is adequate space for the supernumerary tooth, then no treatment is necessary. The presence of an abnormal crown may require restoration or extraction. An abnormal root may require endodontic treatment or extraction. Traumatic malocclusion would require orthodontic movement or extraction.

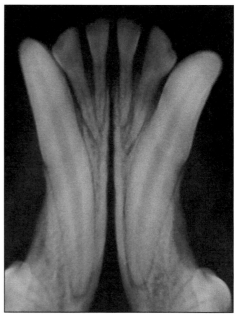

10.25 Developmentally missing mandibular third incisor and first premolar teeth in a dog.
(© Dr Alexander M. Reiter)

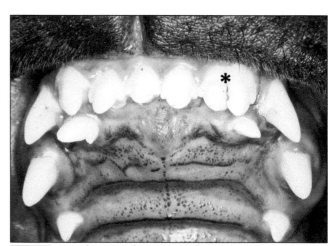

10.26 Hyperdontia in a dog. There are five right maxillary incisor and four left maxillary incisor teeth; the left maxillary second incisor tooth (∗) shows gemination.

Shape abnormalities of teeth
Gemination, fusion and concrescence

Gemination (twinning) refers to a single tooth bud's attempt to divide partially (invagination of the crown) or completely (presence of an identical supernumerary tooth) (Verstraete, 1985) (Figure 10.27). The operator needs to verify that there is adequate space to accommodate the larger crown or supernumerary tooth and confirm normal crown and root radiographically. If crown and root are normal, no further treatment is necessary. Otherwise, treatment will be similar to that described above for hyperdontia.

Fusion (synodontia) is caused by the combination of adjacent tooth germs, resulting in union of the developing teeth. This may be partial or complete, depending on the stage of odontogenesis and the proximity of the developing teeth (Menzies *et al.*, 2012). There may be a single tooth of normal or abnormal size, a bifid crown or two recognizable teeth (Figure 10.28). The teeth are joined at the dentine or enamel level. The operator needs to follow the same steps as when encountering geminated teeth.

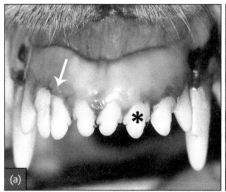

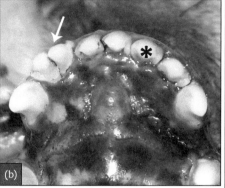

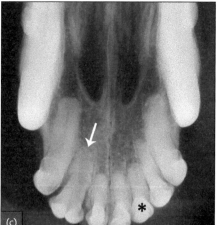

10.27 (a) Front view, (b) ventral view and (c) dental radiograph of a dog showing gemination of the right maxillary second incisor tooth (arrowed) and a supernumerary left maxillary first (or second) incisor tooth (*).
(© Dr Alexander M. Reiter)

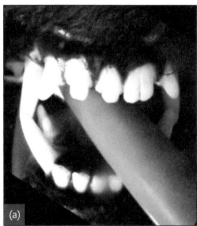

10.28 (a) Front view and (b) dental radiograph showing fusion of the left maxillary first and second incisor teeth in a dog.
(© Dr Alexander M. Reiter)

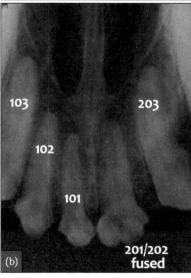

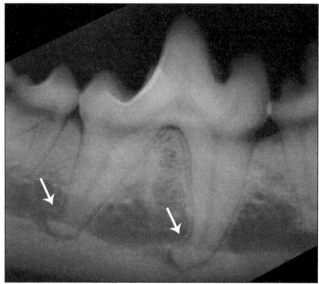

10.29 Radiograph of a right mandibular first molar tooth in a dog, showing dilacerated root ends (arrowed).
(© Dr Alexander M. Reiter)

Roots are more often bent than crowns, especially in toy breeds where the roots of the mandibular first molar teeth bounce off the ventral mandibular cortices. A dilacerated crown may be cosmetically disturbing, and its roughness may exacerbate plaque and calculus accumulation. Cosmetic restoration with composite resin may be all that is needed for treatment. Dilacerated roots become problematic during tooth extraction or endodontic therapy.

Dens invaginatus

Dens invaginatus (dens in dente) results from an infolding of the outer surface of a tooth into the interior. This can occur in either the crown (involving the pulp chamber) or the root (involving the root canal). Coronal invagination results from an infolding of the enamel organ into the dental papilla, while radicular invagination is due to an infolding of the Hertwig's epithelial root sheath. In contrast to the coronal type (lined with enamel), the radicular type is lined with cementum. Enamel overlying the coronal invagination is often thin, of poor quality or missing, and the defect may be separated from the pulp cavity by a relatively thin layer of hard tissue. Thus, there is a greater risk of development of caries and endodontic disease (Figure 10.30). Affected teeth can sometimes be detected in time by an astute

Concrescence refers to fusion of the roots of two or more teeth at the cementum level. True concrescence is present when the fusion occurs during tooth development. If the condition occurs later, it is called acquired concrescence. The diagnostic and treatment protocols are the same as above.

Dilaceration

Dilaceration refers to a disturbance in tooth development, causing the crown or root to be abruptly bent or crooked (Figure 10.29). Causes are local trauma or lack of space.

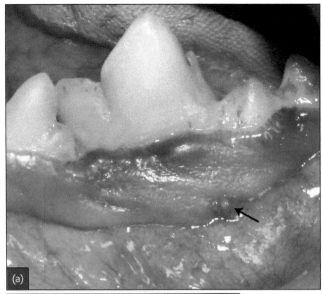

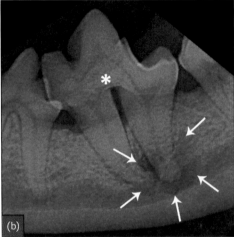

10.30 Dens invaginatus of a left mandibular first molar tooth in a dog. (a) There is a sinus tract (arrowed) at the mucogingival junction. (b) There is evidence of coronal invagination (*) and periapical disease (arrowed) on the dental radiograph of this tooth.
(© Dr Alexander M. Reiter)

clinician, but they usually present with periapical disease secondary to infection invading the invagination (Duncan, 2010). Treatment of the tooth is by means of endodontic therapy followed by restoration of the defect, if possible, or extraction (Stein *et al*., 2005; Coffman *et al*., 2009).

Enamel pearls

An enamel pearl (enamel drop, enamel nodule or enameloma) is a small, spherical growth on the root of a tooth. It is probably formed by the Hertwig's epithelial root sheath and made mostly of enamel with a small dentine core and sometimes a covering of cementum. They can cause periodontal irritation and may require surgical removal.

Supernumerary roots

Extra (supernumerary) roots can be seen on any multi-rooted tooth, but the maxillary third premolar followed by the mandibular fourth premolar teeth are most commonly involved in dogs, whereas in the cat it is the maxillary third premolar followed closely by the maxillary second premolar teeth (Verstraete and Terpak, 1997). The condition does not cause a problem, until exodontic or endodontic therapy is

attempted. Thus, it is imperative to obtain dental radiographs before starting any dental or oral surgical procedure.

Ectodermal dysplasia

Ectodermal dysplasia is a genetic (autosomal dominant) disorder seen in dogs, mice, cattle and humans. Affected individuals are born with absent or abnormal ectodermal structures such as skin, lacrimal glands and teeth. Hypodontia and oligodontia are the most common dental findings in dogs. Both deciduous and permanent teeth may be conical and have a reduced number of cusps (Figure 10.31). The roots may be decreased in number and size, fused or dilacerated. Possible other dental anomalies are persistent deciduous teeth, mesioversion of maxillary canine teeth and caudal crossbite (Lewis *et al*., 2010). 'Peg tooth' is a morphological term, referring to a small, conical, single-rooted tooth often seen in patients suffering from ectodermal dysplasia, such as Chinese Crested Dogs.

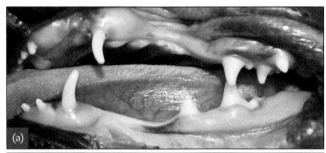

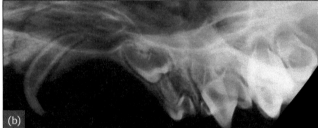

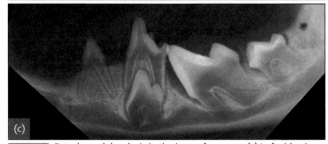

10.31 Ectodermal dysplasia in the jaws of a puppy. (a) Left side view. (b) Dental radiograph of the left upper jaw. (c) Dental radiograph of the left lower jaw. Note the presence of oligodontia, reduced number of cusps, and conical shape of the cusps of both the deciduous and permanent teeth.
(© Dr Alexander M. Reiter)

Eruption and exfoliation abnormalities of teeth

An unerupted tooth is defined as one that has not yet perforated the oral mucosa. An embedded tooth is an unerupted tooth whose eruption is compromised by lack of eruptive force. Previous trauma to the area could account for the presence of unerupted teeth (Figure 10.32). Embedded teeth without a history of trauma seem to be

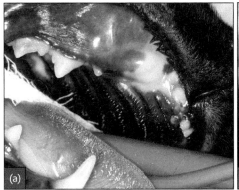
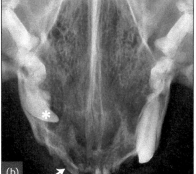
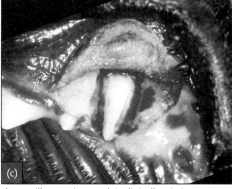
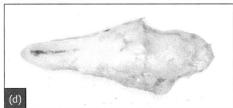

10.32 Embedded tooth in a cat. (a) The right maxillary canine tooth is clinically missing. (b) Dental radiography shows the tooth (∗) to be present with an abnormally shaped root. Note also the displaced right maxillary third incisor tooth (arrowed), consistent with a previous history of trauma. (c) A small flap was raised, and (d) the malformed canine and incisor teeth were extracted.

(© Dr Alexander M. Reiter)

rare both in dogs and cats (Carle and Shope, 2014). An impacted tooth is an unerupted or partially erupted tooth whose eruption is prevented by contact with a physical barrier (Figure 10.33). This condition is most commonly seen in toy and brachycephalic dog breeds where crowding of teeth may cause impaction (Domnick, 2014).

Eruption is sometimes delayed for weeks and occasionally for months. Familial delayed eruption occurs in Tibetan and Wheaten Terriers and probably also in other dog breeds (Harvey and Emily, 1992). A radiographic examination is required to ascertain that an unerupted tooth is not congenitally missing and to identify its exact position.

Treatment

If the patient is young and the crown of the unerupted tooth is pointing in the correct direction, treatment may consist of operculectomy. A circular incision is made over the crown of the affected tooth, and the overlying gingiva is removed. The surgical site should be rechecked in 1–2 weeks to ensure that the gingiva has healed properly and to evaluate the degree of eruption (Stapleton and Clarke, 1999). Forced eruption of an impacted maxillary canine tooth in a cat by means of surgical exposure and orthodontic extrusion has also been described (Surgeon, 2000).

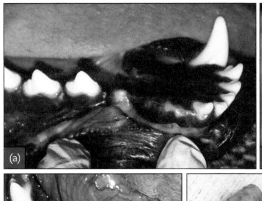
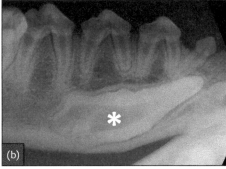

10.33 Impacted tooth in a dog. (a) The right mandibular canine tooth is clinically missing. (b) Dental radiography shows the tooth (∗) to be present. (c) A lingual approach was undertaken and (d) the malformed tooth (together with the second incisor and first, second and third premolar teeth) was extracted. (e) The wound was then sutured closed.

(© Dr Alexander M. Reiter)

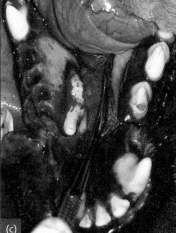
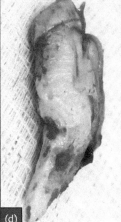
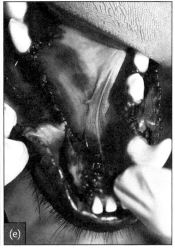

Dentigerous cyst

With deeply impacted or abnormally positioned unerupted teeth, extraction is necessary to prevent dentigerous cyst formation (Verstraete *et al.*, 2011; Edstrom *et al.*, 2013; Babbit *et al.*, 2016). The cells responsible for cyst formation originate from epithelial cell rests of Malassez. The crown of the unerupted tooth is initially enclosed by tissue that attaches at the cementoenamel junction. With continued fluid deposition into the space between this tissue and the crown, a cyst develops (Figure 10.34) that at some point may encompass the entire tooth and affect the adjacent teeth and jaw bone (Gioso and Carvalho, 2003; D'Astous, 2011; MacGee *et al.*, 2012). Several radiographs, obtained at different angles, help determine the exact position of the unerupted tooth and decide how to access it without trauma to adjacent structures. Cysts are smaller and easier to deal with in the younger patient. It is therefore recommended that all the teeth are counted at around 6 months of age when patients are presented for vaccinations or neutering and any edentulous areas (areas of apparently missing teeth) are radiographed. Treatment of a dentigerous cyst consists of extraction of the unerupted tooth with an open technique, drainage of cyst fluid, and removal of the entire cystic lining. If the defect is large and the risk of pathological jaw fracture is increased due to the loss of bone, a bone graft may be placed. The cystic lining should be submitted for histopathological examination, as malignant transformation of dentigerous cysts has been reported.

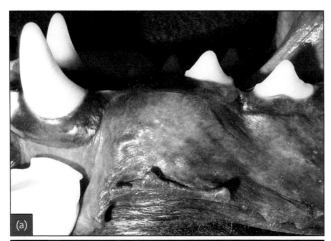
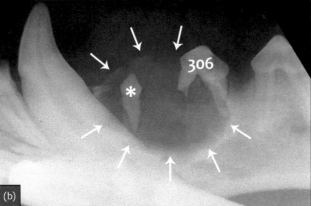

10.34 Dentigerous cyst in a dog. (a) Lateral view of the left rostral mandible. Note the swelling in the area of a missing first premolar tooth and the distally displaced second premolar tooth. (b) Dental radiography shows an unerupted left mandibular first premolar tooth (*) to be surrounded by a cyst-like lesion (arrowed), causing pressure resorption of the roots of the caudally displaced second premolar tooth (306).
(© Dr Alexander M. Reiter)

Congenital lip and palate defects

Development of the head begins during the fourth week of gestation. While in many species the medial nasal and maxillary prominences fuse to form the primary palate (upper lip and the most rostral hard palate), it has been suggested that the medial nasal prominences do not really contribute to upper lip formation in dogs and cats (Senders *et al.*, 1986). The secondary palate is formed from bilateral palatal shelves that grow out from the maxillary processes and join with each other and the developing nasal septum (Reiter and Holt, 2012).

Congenital lip and palate defects can be inherited. Clefts may also develop if an intrauterine insult (trauma, stress, glucocorticoids, antimitotic drugs, nutritional, hormonal, viral and toxic factors) occurs at a very specific time in fetal development (25th to 28th day in dogs). The growth of the palatine portions of facial bones in broad-headed fetuses may not always successfully keep up with the growth of the head, and thus brachycephalic breeds tend to be at higher risk of developing defects of the primary and secondary palates (Reiter and Holt, 2012).

Cleft lip

Defects of the primary palate are obvious at birth as an abnormal fissure in the upper lip and/or a cleft of the most rostral hard palate (Figure 10.35). They are fairly rare congenital defects that are considered to be secondary to intrauterine stress or trauma. Cleft lips can be unilateral or bilateral and may be associated with a cleft palate

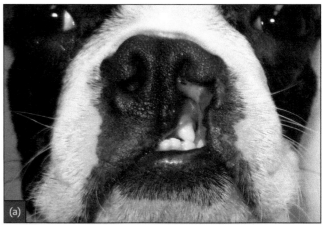
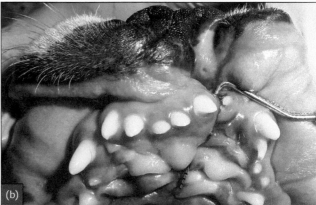

10.35 Defect of the primary palate, manifesting as a left-sided cleft lip and a cleft of the most rostral hard palate in an 8-month-old Boston Terrier. (a) Front view and (b) with the upper lips retracted.
(© Dr Alexander M. Reiter)

(Peralta *et al.*, 2017). Some may also be associated with a bifid nose (Arzi and Verstraete, 2011). The incisive bone fails to fuse properly with the maxilla, resulting in a defect of the upper lip and most rostral portion of the hard palate, normally between the third incisor and canine teeth. Supernumerary incisor teeth (some of them located on the maxillary side of the palatal defect) are common in affected individuals. Except for being externally visible, cleft lips rarely result in clinical signs beyond mild rhinitis and dryness of the exposed oral mucosa, and repair may be performed for purely aesthetic reasons (Reiter and Holt, 2012). Those that extend into the hard palate require surgical treatment to separate the oral cavity from the nasal cavity.

Cleft lip repair

Closure of defects of the lip and most rostral hard palate is challenging and complex (Howard *et al.*, 1976; Kirby *et al.*, 1988). The floor of the nasal vestibule and most rostral hard palate are reconstructed by creating flaps of both oral and nasal soft tissue or flaps that are harvested from oral soft tissue only. Closed extraction of selected teeth (incisors and canines) prior to lip and palate surgery will facilitate future flap management. Repair is achieved with advancement, rotation, transposition or overlapping flaps, followed by reconstructive cutaneous surgery to provide symmetry (Reiter, 2010; 2015).

Cleft palate

Clefts of the secondary palate (cleft hard and/or soft palate) are more common and more serious, although they may not be visible externally. They are almost always along the midline (Peralta *et al.*, 2017). As fusion of the palatine shelves during intrauterine life starts rostrally and continues in a caudal direction, defects of the hard palate are usually associated with a midline soft palate abnormality (Figure 10.36). Soft palate defects without hard palate defects may occur in the midline or may be laterally located (caused by lack of fusion between the soft palate and the pharyngeal walls). Rarely, the soft palate may be hypoplastic (markedly reduced in length).

Clinical signs and history associated with congenital secondary palate defects include difficulty nursing, nasal discharge, sneezing, rhinitis, coughing, gagging, laryngotracheitis, aspiration pneumonia, poor weight gain and general unthriftiness (Reiter, 2010, 2015). Middle ear disease and other craniofacial abnormalities have been reported with congenital defects of the secondary palate (Gregory, 2000; White *et al.*, 2009; Woodbridge *et al.*, 2012; Nemec *et al.*, 2015).

Preoperative management

Management of patients with defects of the secondary palate usually requires nursing care in the form of tube feeding to avoid aspiration pneumonia. Surgery prior to 2 months of age is challenging due to the presence of delicate and friable soft tissues and an increased anaesthetic risk in very young animals. Postponing surgery until after 5 months of age may result in a relatively wider cleft, as the animal grows, and in compounded management problems, which are not desirable. Thus, congenital palate defects in cats and dogs are best repaired at 3–4 months of age (Reiter and Holt, 2012). Several complex surgical procedures exist to resolve these conditions (Marretta, 2012).

Cleft palate repair

Though the (unilateral or bilateral) medially positioned flap technique (Beckman, 2011) can be used for repair of narrow midline clefts of the hard palate (Figure 10.37), the overlapping flap technique (Howard *et al.*, 1974) is preferred for wider midline clefts of the hard palate for the following reasons (Figure 10.38):

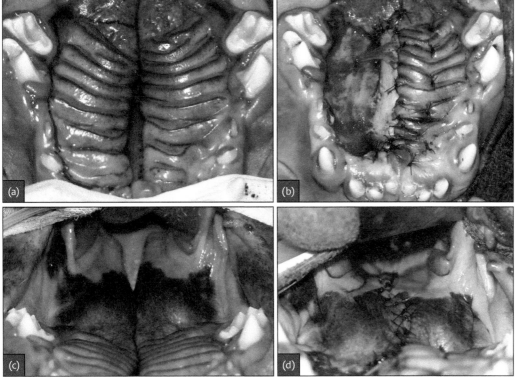

10.36 Complete defect of the secondary palate, manifesting as a midline cleft of the hard and soft palate in a 5-month-old Bulldog. (a) View towards the hard palate cleft. (b) The defect is repaired with an overlapping flap technique. (c) View towards the soft palate cleft. (d) The defect is repaired with a medially positioned flap technique.
(© Dr Alexander M. Reiter)

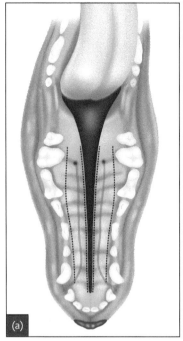

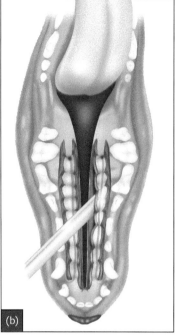

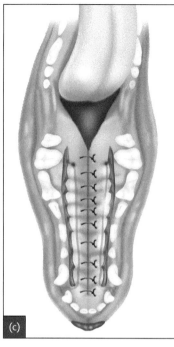

10.37 For narrow congenital hard palate clefts, the medially positioned flap technique may be utilized. (a) Incisions are made at the medial edges of the hard palate defect. Releasing incisions 1–2 mm away from the teeth are often necessary for accommodation of flaps. (b) The periosteum is undermined without injuring the major palatine arteries. (c) The flaps are slid together and sutured over the defect.
(Reproduced from the *BSAVA Manual of Canine and Feline Head, Neck and Thoracic Surgery*)

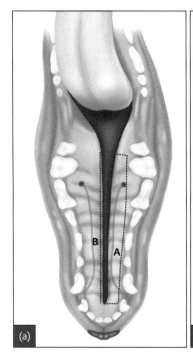

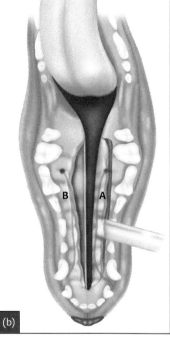

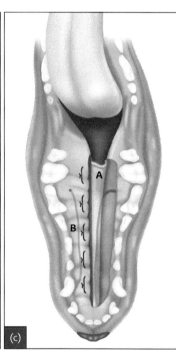

10.38 For wider congenital hard palate clefts, the overlapping flap technique is utilized. (a) Incisions are made in the mucoperiosteum of the hard palate. (b) Flap A is elevated and flap B is undermined. (c) Flap A is turned on itself and sutured under flap B so that the connective tissue surfaces are in contact. Care should be taken to not injure the major palatine arteries during elevation of flap A and undermining flap B.
(Reproduced from the *BSAVA Manual of Canine and Feline Head, Neck and Thoracic Surgery*)

- Less tension on the suture line
- Suture line not located directly over the defect
- Large area of opposing connective tissue, resulting in a stronger scar.

Incisions are made in the mucoperiosteum to the bone along the dental arch about 1–2 mm away from the teeth and to the rostral and caudal margins of the hard palate defect on one side, forming an overlapped flap, and at the medial margin of the defect on the other side, forming an envelope flap (Reiter and Smith, 2005). Each flap is undermined with a periosteal elevator, carefully avoiding injury to the major palatine artery as it exits the major palatine foramen at the palatine shelf of the maxilla about 0.5–1 cm palatal to the maxillary fourth premolar tooth (more rostral in the cat than the dog). Careful dissection of the major palatine artery at the connective tissue side of the overlapped flap will release it from surrounding tissue to accommodate the rotation of this flap (Reiter and Holt, 2012). A pocket is created at the medial margin of the envelope flap to create space for the overlapped flap. The overlapped flap is inverted at its base, turned and secured under the envelope flap with horizontal mattress sutures so that large connective tissue surfaces are in contact. Granulation and epithelialization of exposed bone generally are completed in 3 to 4 weeks (Reiter and Smith, 2005). Free tissue transfer (grafting) of cortico-cancellous tibial bone for a congenital hard palate cleft in a dog has also been described (Ishikawa *et al.*, 1994). Another option would be a double-layer technique following extraction of cheek teeth, using both hard palate mucosa and labial/buccal mucosa to close congenital defects of the secondary palate in dogs (Peralta *et al.*, 2015).

The medially positioned flap technique is typically employed for repair of midline clefts of the soft palate (Reiter and Holt, 2012). Incisions are made along the medial margins of the defect to the level of the middle or caudal aspect of the palatine tonsils (see Figures 10.36 and 10.39). The palatal tissues are separated with blunt-ended scissors to form a dorsal and ventral flap on each side. The two dorsal and the two ventral flaps are sutured separately in a simple interrupted pattern to the midpoint or caudal end of the palatine tonsils (Reiter and Smith, 2005). A bilateral overlapping flap technique for a midline soft palate cleft has also been described (Griffiths and Sullivan, 2001).

Repair of a unilateral cleft of the soft palate is best performed after removal of the ipsilateral palatine tonsil (Reiter and Smith, 2005). The tonsillectomy incision can be extended rostrally to the most rostral location of the soft palate defect and continued along the medial edge of the soft palate defect (Figure 10.40). The pharyngeal and palatal tissues are separated, and two dorsal and two ventral flaps are sutured separately in a simple interrupted pattern to the midpoint or caudal end of the contralateral palatine tonsil (Warzee et al., 2001).

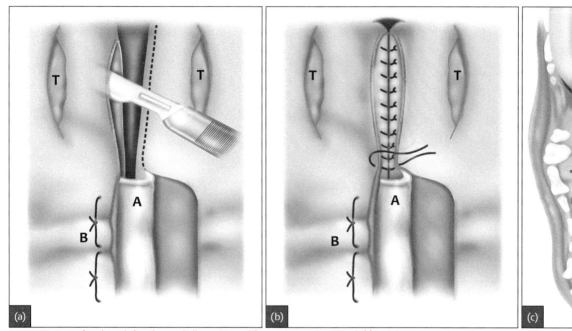
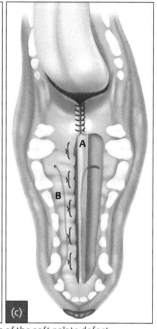

10.39 For soft palate clefts, the medially positioned flap technique is utilized. (a) Incisions are made at the margins of the soft palate defect. (b) Dorsal and ventral flaps are sutured separately. (c) Both hard (overlapping flap technique) and soft palate defects closed. T = palatine tonsil.
(Reproduced from the BSAVA Manual of Canine and Feline Head, Neck and Thoracic Surgery)

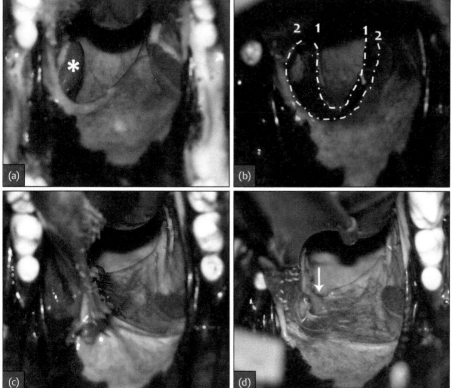

10.40 Repair of unilateral clefts of the soft palate. (a) First remove the ipsilateral palatine tonsil (∗) and then (b) extend the tonsillectomy incision rostrally to the most rostral location of the soft palate defect and continue along the medial edge of the soft palate defect. The pharyngeal and palatal tissues are separated, and two dorsal (1) and two ventral (2) flaps are created. (c) These flaps are sutured separately in a simple interrupted pattern to the level of the midpoint or caudal end of the contralateral tonsil. (d) The 2-month re-examination shows slight dehiscence at the caudal margin of the sutured site. However, the caudal edge of the soft palate (arrowed) still correctly lines up with the caudal end of the contralateral tonsil.
(© Dr Alexander M. Reiter)

Treatment of congenital hypoplasia of the soft palate is challenging, but may be conducted in similar fashion after bilateral tonsillectomy and extension and continuation of incisions into the rudimentary, uvula-like soft palate tissue. Dorsal and ventral flaps are created and sutured separately in a simple interrupted pattern to the midpoint or caudal end of the tonsillectomy sites (Sylvestre and Sharma, 1997; Reiter and Holt, 2012). Bilateral buccal mucosa flaps have also been employed for repair of soft palate hypoplasia in dogs (Sager and Nefen, 1998). The use of bilateral pharyngeal advancement flaps and one overlapping hard palate flap was described for repair of soft palate hypoplasia in a cat (Headrick and McAnulty, 2004).

Other developmental abnormalities of hard and soft tissues of the head

Temporomandibular joint dysplasia and open-mouth jaw locking

Dysplasia of the temporomandibular joint (TMJ) refers to a condition where one or both mandibular condyles, mandibular fossae and/or the surrounding soft tissue structures (capsule, lateral TMJ ligament) are malformed (Dickie *et al.*, 2002; Lerer *et al.*, 2014) (Figure 10.41). Upon full opening of the mouth (e.g. yawning, vocalizing, trying to catch a large ball) and just prior to closing the mouth, the mandibular condyle may luxate to a degree that the coronoid process gets locked ventrolateral to the zygomatic arch. The condition has been reported in the Basset Hound, Dachshund, Irish Setter, American Cocker Spaniel, Cavalier King Charles Spaniel, Pekingese, Boxer, Dobermann, Golden Retriever, Labrador Retriever, Bernese Mountain Dog, and primarily the Persian cat (Robins and Grandage, 1977; Lantz and Cantwell, 1986; Reiter, 2004; Soukup *et al.*, 2009). TMJ dysplasia is not always present, though, and other causative and or predisposing factors (e.g. mandibular symphyseal laxity) may play a role in the development of open-mouth jaw locking (OMJL). The patient presents in a state of acute agitation with its mouth wide open, drooling

and with the mandible slightly rotated ventrally, towards the locked side (Figure 10.42). Immediate relief is provided by sedating the patient, replacing the lower jaw (by manually unlocking the coronoid process from the zygomatic arch), and placing a tape muzzle. Anti-inflammatory drugs and soft food should be prescribed. After 2 weeks the muzzle may be removed. In recurrent cases, treatment consists of surgical correction (partial zygomectomy, partial coronoidectomy, or a combination of both) (Figure 10.43).

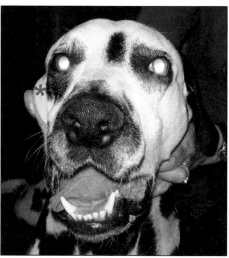

10.42 Dalmatian dog with open-mouth jaw locking. The mouth is locked open with no contact between the upper and lower teeth, the lower jaw is rotated ventrolaterally towards the right side, and the tip of the coronoid process (*) of the displaced right mandible is locked ventrolateral to the zygomatic arch.
(© Dr Margherita Gracis)

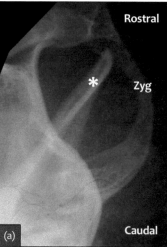

10.43 Dorsoventral radiographic views of a dog with open-mouth jaw locking. (a) Before partial zygomectomy. (b) Following surgery. Note the position of the coronoid process (*), the zygomatic arch (Zyg) and the area where the surgery was performed (arrowed).

10.41 Temporomandibular joint dysplasia in a dog shown on a lateral oblique radiographic view. Note the lack of congruence of the mandibular condyle (MC), the flattened mandibular fossa (MF), and the short retroarticular process (RP). B = tympanic bulla.

Craniomandibular osteopathy

Craniomandibular osteopathy (CMO) is a disease usually bilaterally involving the body of the mandible, TMJ and tympanic bulla. There may be a genetic component considering that breeds such as West Highland White, Scottish and Cairn Terriers seem to be primarily affected (Padgett and Mostosky, 1986); however, other dog breeds can also have CMO (Taylor *et al.*, 1995; Franch *et al.*, 1998; Huchkowsky, 2002). The mandibles are thickened due to woven bone proliferation (Figure 10.44). In severe cases, the condition extends to the TMJ and tympanic bulla (Shorenstein *et al.*, 2014). Occasionally, a thickening of the calvarium, the tentorium cerebelli and the extremities may also be observed (Pettit *et al.*, 2012). Patients present with discomfort, inability to fully open the mouth and reluctance to eat. Hyperthermia may be present, and neurological signs may occasionally be seen (Ratterree *et al.*, 2011).

Treatment consists of anti-inflammatory drugs (non-steroidal anti-inflammatory drugs (NSAIDs) or glucocorticoids), analgesic drugs and nutritional support.Anti-inflammatory doses of glucocorticoids are the authors' preferred choice of treatment due to their catabolic effects on connective tissue such as bone. If there is extensive bone proliferation between the angular process of the mandible, TMJ and tympanic bulla, the patient may not be able to open its mouth as a result of a mechanical lock, resulting in problems with food intake. Surgery may then be necessary to remove excess bone to regain function. The worst cases occasionally warrant euthanasia.

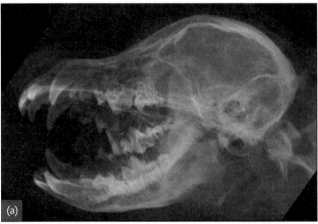

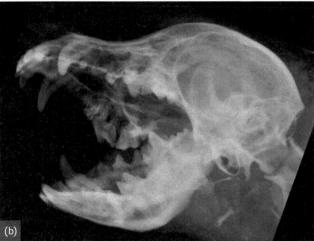

10.44 (a) Craniomandibular osteopathy in a dog, manifesting as thickened mandibles and calvarial bones. (b) The patient 1 year later, showing resolution of clinical signs but continued thickening of the ventral mandibular borders.

Calvarial hyperostosis

Calvarial hyperostosis is a disease seen particularly in young Bullmastiffs (Pastor *et al.*, 2000; McConnell *et al.*, 2006; Thompson *et al.*, 2011; Mathes *et al.*, 2012) and is similar to human infantile cortical hyperostosis. It is characterized by progressive bony proliferation and thickening of the cortical bone of the calvarium (see Chapter 4). It manifests as a smooth thickening of various calvarial bones, making it different from the irregular thickening seen in craniomandibular osteopathy. Clinical signs include painful swelling of the skull, exophthalmos, fever and lymph node swelling (McConnell *et al.*, 2006). In most cases it is self-limiting (Pastor *et al.*, 2000).

Periostitis ossificans

The few cases reported in the veterinary literature show that this is a condition that affects puppies with a mixed dentition. It usually presents with a unilateral swelling on the buccal surface of the caudal mandible. Parallel radiographs reveal the presence of a double-cortex appearance at the ventral aspect of the mandible. This double-cortex formation can sometimes also be appreciated on the lingual and buccal surfaces of the affected mandible on occlusal views (Figure 10.45). An incisional biopsy is recommended to eliminate differential diagnoses (such as cysts, craniomandibular osteopathy, trauma or neoplasia). The aetiology seems to be an inflamed or infected dental follicle related to a developing unerupted tooth and/or is secondary to pericoronitis. Treatment occasionally requires an anti-inflammatory regimen, but the condition may also resolve on its own (Blazejewski *et al.*, 2010).

Fibrous osteodystrophy

Fibrous osteodystrophy can be a congenital condition associated with primary hyperparathyroidism and nutritional or renal secondary hyperparathyroidism (Norrdin, 1975; Kyle *et al.*, 1985; Sarkiala *et al.*, 1994; Carmichael *et al.*, 1995). There is generalized osteopenia, but it is more marked in the bones of the jaws. The bone demineralization results in partial or total loss of the lamina dura. This in turn causes tooth mobility, drifting and malocclusion. The patient presents with facial swelling and a history of poor growth. Examination reveals thickened rubbery jaws and ulcerated oral mucosa. Palpation shows mobile teeth. Radiographs are striking; they display marked decrease of bone density, loss of normal trabecular bone structure and loss of lamina dura. Unlike bone, however, the teeth do not appear to be demineralized and rarely undergo resorption, though exceptions do exist (Figure 10.46). Treatment is rarely successful and prognosis is very poor, except in the case of nutritional secondary hyperparathyroidism, which may be treated by feeding an appropriately formulated diet and oral calcium supplementation, if necessary.

Brachycephalic obstructive airway syndrome

The term brachycephalic obstructive airway syndrome refers to the combination of anatomical variations commonly seen in chondrodystrophic breeds (e.g. Pugs, English Bulldogs, French Bulldogs), including stenotic nares, shortened nose, presence of rhinopharyngeal turbinates, relative macroglossia and relatively elongated soft palate. Some of these dogs may also have malformed, aberrant, obstructive

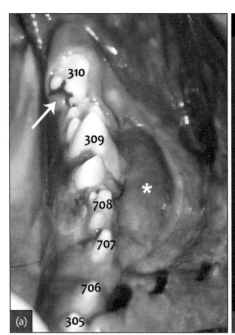

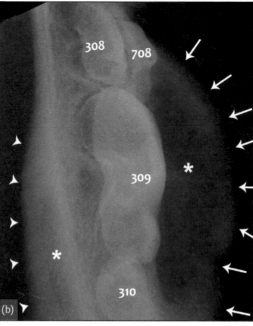

10.45 A 4.5-month-old male Labrador Retriever with periostitis ossificans. (a) Note the fluid-filled swelling (∗) in the area of the left mandibular deciduous fourth premolar (708) and permanent first molar (309) teeth and the clinical signs of pericoronitis (arrowed) at the incompletely erupted left mandibular second molar (310) tooth. (b) The occlusal radiograph of the left mandibular body shows the double-cortex formation lingually and buccally (arrowed) with a space between the two cortices (∗).
(From Blazejewski *et al.* (2010), *Journal of Veterinary Dentistry*, with permission; © Dr Alexander M. Reiter)

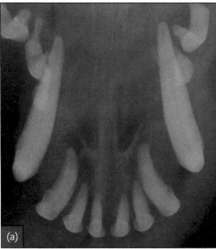

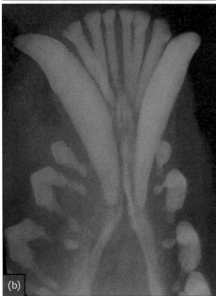

10.46 Dental radiographs of the (a) rostral upper jaw and (b) rostral lower jaw in a 10-year-old dog with renal secondary hyperparathyroidism and fibrous osteodystrophy clinically manifesting as 'rubber jaw'.
(© Dr Alexander M. Reiter)

nasal conchae and a narrow trachea (Oechtering *et al.*, 2016a). Increased resistance to air flow through the upper respiratory tract and continuous inspiratory effort may lead to secondary manifestations, such as an abnormally thickened and hyperplastic soft palate, everted and enlarged palatine tonsils, collapse or paralysis of the laryngeal cartilages, everted laryngeal saccules and bronchial collapse, all of which exacerbate respiratory effort (Crosse *et al.*, 2015).

The patient may show stertor or stridor, gagging, coughing, exercise or stress intolerance and, in more severe cases, cyanosis and collapse (Fasanella *et al.*, 2010). A high prevalence of gastrointestinal tract problems (i.e. oesophageal, gastric and, less commonly, duodenal anomalies) has been described in brachycephalic dogs with respiratory problems, suggesting a possible influence of upper respiratory tract disease on gastro-oesophageal disease and *vice versa* (Poncet *et al.*, 2006).

Treatment

Oxygen supplementation and medical management may be necessary in preparation for surgery of cases showing acute severe respiratory distress. Corrective surgical procedures include partial resection of the nares, shortening/thinning of the soft palate, laryngeal saccu-lectomy, and tonsillectomy (Davidson *et al.*, 2001; Riecks *et al.*, 2007; Dunié-Mérigot *et al.*, 2010; Cantatore *et al.*, 2012). Laser-assisted turbinectomy of obstructive nasal conchae using a diode laser has also been shown to improve endonasal airway patency in brachycephalic dogs with intranasal obstruction (Oechtering *et al.*, 2016b). Arytenoid lateralization may be necessary in dogs showing laryngeal paralysis.

Correction of stenotic nares (naroplasty) helps improve breathing. The nostrils are opened by taking a pie wedge out of the alar folds and suturing the cut edges to each other (Figure 10.47). Several other techniques have been described (Ellison, 2004; Huck *et al.*, 2008; Trostel and Frankel, 2010).

Partial resection of the soft palate (staphylectomy) may be performed using a scalpel blade, scissors, diathermy or CO_2 laser (Brdecka *et al.*, 2008). Use of a laser offers multiple advantages, making the surgery simpler and

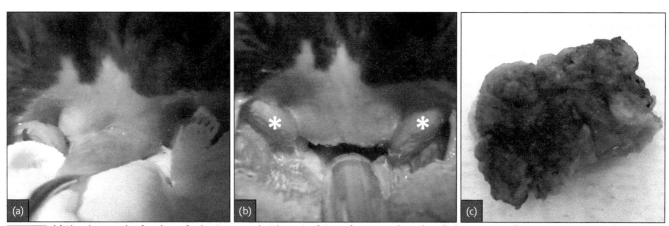

10.47 (a) Severely stenotic nares in a young French Bulldog. (b, c) Bilateral naroplasty has been performed.

faster, controlling bleeding and reducing swelling. The surgical technique involves grasping the caudal point of the soft palate with tissue forceps and pulling it rostroventrally. Excess soft palate tissue is resected from the caudal edge of one tonsil to the caudal edge of the other (Figure 10.48). However, simply trimming an elongated soft palate may not address any associated hyperplasia. A portion of the oropharyngeal mucosa and underlying soft tissue of the soft palate can be excised, and the caudal edge of the soft palate is then folded rostrally on to itself. This folded flap palatoplasty technique will both shorten and thin an elongated and hyperplastic soft palate to also relieve nasopharyngeal obstruction (Findji and Dupre, 2009).

If the laryngeal saccules are everted, they may be removed at the same time as the soft palate resection, or they may be left in and allowed to return to a more normal position. The saccules are gently held with forceps and resected flush with the lateral walls of the larynx.

The prognosis is good for young animals if treated before secondary manifestations occur. Surgically treated animals will generally breathe much more easily and with significantly reduced respiratory distress (Torrez and Hunt, 2006). Their activity level will also markedly improve. Older animals may have a less favourable prognosis, especially if the process of laryngeal collapse or paralysis has already started. If laryngeal collapse is advanced, the prognosis is poor unless additional procedures are performed to address this serious problem.

Tight lower lip

Tight lower lip is a genetic condition seen mostly in Shar-Pei dogs (McCoy, 1997; Holmstrom, 2012), but the authors have recently seen a few cases in Mastiff dogs. The patients present with the lower lip rolled over the mandibular incisor teeth in such a way that, when the mouth is closed, the lower lip is caught between the maxillary and mandibular incisor teeth. In severe cases, the lower lip even rolls over the mandibular canine teeth. Not only is the lip traumatized, but it can interfere with the normal growth of the lower jaw, resulting in class 2 malocclusion. The goal of treatment is to increase the oral vestibule by means of a vestibuloplasty.

The patient is placed in ventral recumbency with its head elevated and its lower jaw hanging open. The alveolar mucosa of the lower lip is incised at or near the mucogingival junction, from one lateral lip frenulum to the other. The submucosal tissues and muscular attachments are dissected free. The labial mucosa attached to the freed lip is tacked to the deeper tissues to prevent it from reattaching to the gingiva or alveolar mucosa (McCoy, 1997). At the re-examination visit the lip should be in the correct anatomical position (Figure 10.49).

To keep the cut edges from reattaching to each other and to preserve a deeper oral vestibule, the operator can also place a buccal mucosal graft in between the incision margins. This complicates the surgery markedly. One easier option is to use a Penrose drain as a stent to separate the edges and force the tissue to epithelialize

10.48 (a) The elongated soft palate of a dog is grasped with a pair of tissue forceps and gently pulled rostroventrally. Wet gauzes are used to protect the other soft tissues and the endotracheal tube while using the CO_2 laser scalpel. (b) The soft palate is resected from the caudal edge of one tonsil to the caudal edge of the other (*). Use of the laser scalpel eliminates the need to suture the incised margin. (c) The piece resected with the laser shows a non-bleeding cutting edge.

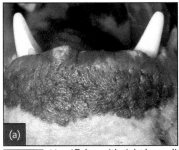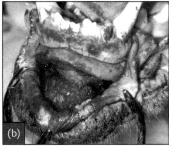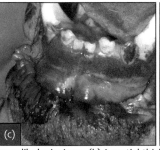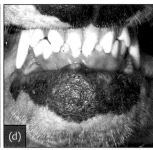

10.49 Mastiff dog with tight lower lip. (a) The lower lip rolls caudally over the mandibular incisors. (b) A partial-thickness incision is made into alveolar mucosa near the mucogingival junction. The lip is dissected free and allowed to hang down. (c) The edges of the labial mucosa of the freed lip are sutured down to the periosteum to prevent them from re-attaching to the alveolar mucosa. The defect is left to granulate in by second intention. This creates a new band of epithelialized tissue that releases the tension on the lip. When the surgery is complete, the lower lip should rest in a lower position than before, and the incisor teeth should be visible. (d) At the 3-week recheck visit, the lower lip is still below the incisor teeth.

over the defect. The Penrose drain is measured, cut, sutured around the circumference of the defect, and tacked in the middle to the depth of the new oral vestibule. Epithelialization takes 2–3 weeks to occur. The drain must therefore be sutured with slowly absorbable or non-absorbable sutures.

Tongue anomalies

Ankyloglossia, also known as 'tongue-tie', is a congenital oral anomaly that decreases the mobility of the tongue and is caused by a short lingual frenulum (Temizsoylu and Avki, 2003; Karahan and Kul, 2009). The lingual frenulum extends up to the tip or near the tip of the tongue. The tip of the tongue is often notched. It seems to be diagnosed most often in Kangal Shepherd Dogs, but its genetic aetiology is still under investigation. Treatment consists of lingual frenuloplasty for partial ankyloglossia or lingual frenulotomy for complete ankyloglossia (Alkan *et al.*, 2013). The prognosis is good.

Macroglossia (Figure 10.50) has been reported in Giant Schnauzer puppies with congenital hypothyroid dwarfism and in adult German Shepherd Dogs with acromegaly (Greco *et al.*, 1991; Fracassi *et al.*, 2014). Dogs with severe macroglossia may benefit from partial resection of the tongue.

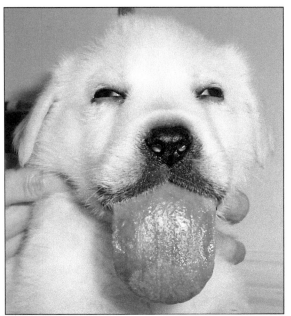

10.50 Puppy with macroglossia. Note the erosions at the rostral aspect of the dorsum of the tongue.
(© Dr Alexander M. Reiter)

Microglossia, also known as 'bird tongue', is a rare genetic disorder manifesting as a small abnormally shaped tongue that prevents normal nursing. Upward and inward curling of the fimbriated margins of the tongue gives it a narrow and pointed appearance. Despite intensive nursing care, affected puppies may not survive (Wiggs *et al.*, 1994).

References and further reading

Alkan F, Koc Y, Tepeli C *et al.* (2013) Management of complete and partial ankyloglossia in Kangal Shepherd Dogs. *Research Opinions in Animal and Veterinary Sciences* **3**, 462–465

American Veterinary Dental College (2015) *Classification of Dental Occlusion in Dogs.* Available at: https://www.avdc.org/Nomenclature/Nomen-Occlusion.html

Amimoto A, Iwamoto S, Taura Y *et al.* (1993) Effects of surgical orthodontic treatment for malalignment due to the prolonged retention of deciduous canines in young dogs. *Journal of Veterinary Medical Science* **55**, 73–79

Arzi B and Verstraete FJ (2011) Repair of a bifid nose combined with a cleft of the primary palate in a 1-year-old dog. *Veterinary Surgery* **40**, 865–869

Babbit SG, Krakowski Volker M and Luskin IR (2016) Incidence of radiographic cystic lesions associated with unerupted teeth in dogs. *Journal of Veterinary Dentistry* **33**, 226–233

Bannon K and Baker L (2008) Cast metal bilateral telescoping incline plane for malocclusion in a dog. *Journal of Veterinary Dentistry* **25**, 250–258

Beckman B (2011) Repair of secondary cleft palate in the dog. *Journal of Veterinary Dentistry* **28**, 58–62

Bittegeko SB, Arnbjerg J, Nkya R *et al.* (1995) Multiple dental developmental abnormalities following canine distemper infection. *Journal of the American Animal Hospital Association* **31**, 42–45

Blazejewski SW (2013) Thermoplastic inclined plane aligner for correction of bilateral mandibular canine tooth distoclusion in a cat. *Journal of Veterinary Dentistry* **30**, 236–247

Blazejewski SW, Lewis JR, Gracis M *et al.* (2010) Mandibular periostitis ossificans in immature large breed dogs: five cases (1999–2006). *Journal of Veterinary Dentistry* **27**, 148–159

Boy S, Crossley D and Steenkamp G (2016) Developmental structural tooth defects in dogs – Experience from veterinary dental referral practice and review of the literature. *Frontiers in Veterinary Science* **3**. doi: 10.3389/fvets.2016.00009

Brdecka DJ, Rawlings CA, Perry AC *et al.* (2008) Use of an electrothermal, feedback-controlled, bipolar sealing device for resection of the elongated soft palate in dogs with obstructive upper airway disease. *Journal of the American Veterinary Medical Association* **233**, 1265–1269

Buchet M and Boudrieau RJ (1999) Correction of malocclusion secondary to maxillary impaction fractures using a mandibular symphyseal realignment in eight cats. *Journal of the American Animal Hospital Association* **35**, 68–76

Cantatore M, Gobbetti M, Romussi S *et al.* (2012) Medium term endoscopic assessment of the surgical outcome following laryngeal saccule resection in brachycephalic dogs. *Veterinary Record* **170**, 518–523

Carle D and Shope B (2014) Soft tissue tooth impaction in a dog. *Journal of Veterinary Dentistry* **31**, 96–105

Carmichael DT, Williams CA and Aller SM (1995) Renal dysplasia with secondary hyperparathyroidism and loose teeth in a young dog. *Journal of Veterinary Dentistry* **12**, 143–146

Carvalho VG, Gioso MA, Carvalho PE *et al.* (2014) Intra-oral mandibular sagittal osteotomy technique to correct mandibular distoclusion and mesio-occlusion. Study in canine cadavers. *Veterinary and Comparative Orthopaedics and Traumatology* **27**, 27–35

Coffman CR, Visser CJ and Visser L (2009) Endodontic treatment of dens invaginatus in a dog. *Journal of Veterinary Dentistry* **26**, 220–225

Crosse KR, Bray JP, Orbell GM et al. (2015) Histological evaluation of the soft palate in dogs affected by brachycephalic obstructive airway syndrome. New Zealand Veterinary Journal 15, 1–20

D'Astous J (2011) An overview of dentigerous cysts in dogs and cats. Canadian Veterinary Journal 52, 905–907

Davidson EB, Davis MS, Campbell GA et al. (2001) Evaluation of carbon dioxide laser and conventional incisional techniques for resection of soft palates in brachycephalic dogs. Journal of the American Veterinary Medical Association 219, 776–781

Dickie AM, Schwarz T and Sullivan M (2002) Temporomandibular joint morphology in Cavalier King Charles Spaniels. Veterinary Radiology and Ultrasound 43, 260–266

Domnick ED (2014) Diagnostic imaging in veterinary dental practice. Impaction of the right mandibular canine tooth. Journal of the American Veterinary Medical Association 245, 281–283

Duncan HL (2010) Diagnostic imaging in veterinary dental practice. Dens invaginatus leading to arrested maturation of the right and left mandibular first molar teeth. Journal of the American Veterinary Medical Association 237, 1251–1253

Dunié-Mérigot A, Bouvy B and Poncet C (2010) Comparative use of CO_2 laser, diode laser and monopolar electrocautery for resection of the soft palate in dogs with brachycephalic airway obstructive syndrome. Veterinary Record 167, 700–704

Edstrom EJ, Smith MM and Taney K (2013) Extraction of the impacted mandibular canine tooth in the dog. Journal of Veterinary Dentistry 30, 56–61

Ellison GW (2004) Alapexy: an alternative technique for repair of stenotic nares in dogs. Journal of the American Animal Hospital Association 40, 484–489

Emily P (1992) Feline malocclusion. Veterinary Clinics of North America: Small Animal Practice 22, 1453–1460

Fasanella FJ, Shivley JM, Wardlaw JL et al. (2010) Brachycephalic airway obstructive syndrome in dogs: 90 cases (1991–2008) Journal of the American Veterinary Medical Association 237, 1048–1051

Findje L and Dupre G (2009) Folded flap palatoplasty for treatment of elongated soft palate in 55 dogs. European Journal of Companion Animal Practice 19, 125–132

Fracassi F, Zagnoli L, Rosenberg D et al. (2014) Spontaneous acromegaly: a retrospective case control study in German Shepherd Dogs. Veterinary Journal 202, 69–75

Franch J, Cesari JR and Font J (1998) Craniomandibular osteopathy in two Pyrenean Mountain Dogs. Veterinary Record 142, 455–459

Fulton AJ, Fiani N and Verstraete FJ (2014) Canine pediatric dentistry. Veterinary Clinics of North America: Small Animal Practice 44, 303–324

Furman R and Niemiec B (2013) Variation in acrylic inclined plane application. Journal of Veterinary Dentistry 30, 161–166

Gengler WR (2004) Masel chain appliance for orthodontic treatment. Journal of Veterinary Dentistry 21, 258–261

Gioso MA and Carvalho VG (2003) Maxillary dentigerous cyst in a cat. Journal of Veterinary Dentistry 20, 28–30

Goldstein GS (1990) The diagnosis and treatment of orthodontic problems. Problems in Veterinary Medicine 2, 195–219

Gracis M, Keith D and Vite CH (2000) Dental and craniofacial findings in eight Miniature Schnauzer dogs affected by myotonia congenita: preliminary results. Journal of Veterinary Dentistry 17, 119–127

Greco DS, Feldman EC, Peterson ME et al. (1991) Congenital hypothyroid dwarfism in a family of Giant Schnauzers. Journal of Veterinary Internal Medicine 5, 57–65

Greenfield B (2011) Crown reduction and root canal therapy for malocclusion in a dog. Journal of Veterinary Dentistry 28, 102–109

Gregory SP (2000) Middle ear disease associated with congenital palatine defects in seven dogs and one cat. Journal of Small Animal Practice 41, 398–401

Griffiths LG and Sullivan M (2001) Bilateral overlapping mucosal single-pedicle flaps for correction of soft palate defects. Journal of the American Animal Hospital Association 37, 183–186

Hale FA (1996) Orthodontic correction of lingually displaced canine teeth in a young dog using light-cured acrylic resin. Journal of Veterinary Dentistry 13, 69–73

Hale FA (2005) Juvenile veterinary dentistry. Veterinary Clinics of North America: Small Animal Practice 35, 789–817

Harvey CE and Emily P (1992) Occlusion, occlusive abnormalities and orthodontic treatment. In: Small Animal Dentistry, 1st edn, pp. 266–296. Mosby, St Louis

Headrick JF and McAnulty JF (2004) Reconstruction of a bilateral hypoplastic soft palate in a cat. Journal of the American Animal Hospital Association 40, 86–90

Hobson P (2005) Extraction of retained primary canine teeth in the dog. Journal of Veterinary Dentistry 22, 132–137

Hoffman S (2008) Abnormal tooth eruption in a cat. Journal of Veterinary Dentistry 25, 118–122

Holmstrom SE (2012) Inferior labial frenoplasty and tight lip syndrome. In: Oral and Maxillofacial Surgery in Dogs and Cats, ed. FMJ Verstraete and MJ Lommer, pp. 515–518. Saunders Elsevier, Philadelphia

Howard DR, Davis DG, Merkley DF et al. (1974) Mucoperiosteal flap technique for cleft palate repair in dogs. Journal of the American Veterinary Medical Association 165, 352–354

Howard DR, Merkley DF, Lammerding JJ et al. (1976) Primary cleft palate (harelip) and closure repair in puppies. Journal of the American Animal Hospital Association 12, 636–640

Huchkowsky SL (2002) Craniomandibular osteopathy in a Bullmastiff. Canadian Veterinary Journal 43, 883–885

Huck JL, Stanley BJ and Hauptman JG (2008) Technique and outcome of nares amputation (Trader's technique) in immature Shih Tzus. Journal of the American Animal Hospital Association 44, 82–85

Ishikawa Y, Goris RC and Nagaoka K (1994) Use of a cortico-cancellous bone graft in the repair of a cleft palate in a dog. Veterinary Surgery 23, 201–205

Karahan S and Kul BC (2009) Ankyloglossia in dogs: a morphological and immunohistochemical study. Anatomia, Histologia and Embryologia 38, 118–121

Kim CG, Lee SY and Park HM (2015) Staged orthodontic movement of mesiolinguoversion of the mandibular canine tooth in a dog. Journal of the American Animal Hospital Association 51, 49–55

Kirby BM, Bjorling DE and Mixter RC (1988) Surgical repair of a cleft lip in a dog. Journal of the American Animal Hospital Association 24, 683–687

Kyle MG, Davis GB and Thompson KG (1985) Renal osteodystrophy with facial hyperostosis and 'rubber jaw' in an adult dog. New Zealand Veterinary Journal 33, 118–120

Lantz GC and Cantwell HD (1986) Intermittent open-mouth lower jaw locking in five dogs. Journal of the American Veterinary Medical Association 188, 1403–1405

Legendre LF (1991) Anterior crossbite correction in a dog using a lingual bar, a labial bow, lingual buttons and elastic threads. Journal of Veterinary Dentistry 8, 21–25

Legendre LF (1994a) Bilateral vital pulpotomies as a treatment of a class 2 malocclusion. Canadian Veterinary Journal 35, 583–585

Legendre LF (1994b) Treatment of a malocclusion in a dog using both exodontic and orthodontic procedures. Canadian Veterinary Journal 35, 454–456

Legendre LF (1994c) Dentistry on deciduous teeth: what, when and how. Canadian Veterinary Journal 35, 793–794

Legendre LF (2010) Building a telescopic inclined plane intraorally. Journal of Veterinary Dentistry 27, 62–65

Legendre LF and Stepaniuk K (2008) Correction of maxillary canine tooth mesioversion in dogs. Journal of Veterinary Dentistry 25, 216–221

Lerer A, Chalmers HJ, Moens NM et al. (2014) Imaging diagnosis – temporomandibular joint dysplasia in a Basset Hound. Veterinary Radiology and Ultrasound 55, 547–551

Lewis JR, Reiter AM, Mauldin EA et al. (2010) Dental abnormalities associated with X-linked hypohidrotic ectodermal dysplasia in dogs. Orthodontics and Craniofacial Research 13, 40–47

Lobprise HB, Wiggs RB and Peak RM (1999) Dental diseases of puppies and kittens. Veterinary Clinics of North America: Small Animal Practice 29, 871–893

MacGee S, Pinson DM and Shaiken L (2012) Bilateral dentigerous cysts in a dog. Journal of Veterinary Dentistry 29, 242–249

Mannerfelt T and Lindgren I (2009) Enamel defects in Standard Poodle dogs in Sweden. Journal of Veterinary Dentistry 26, 213–215

Marretta SM (2012) Cleft palate repair techniques. In: Oral and Maxillofacial Surgery in Dogs and Cats, ed. FJM Verstraete and MJ Lommer, pp. 351–362. Saunders Elsevier, Philadelphia

Mathes RL, Holmes SP, Coleman KD et al. (2012) Calvarial hyperostosis presenting as unilateral exophthalmos in a female English Springer Spaniel. Veterinary Ophthalmology 15, 263–270

McConnell JF, Hayes A, Platt SR et al. (2006) Calvarial hyperostosis syndrome in two Bullmastiffs. Veterinary Radiology and Ultrasound 47, 72–77

McCoy DE (1997) Surgical management of the tight lip syndrome in the Shar-Pei dog. Journal of Veterinary Dentistry 14, 95–96

Menzies RA, Reiter AM and Lewis JR (2012) Developmental tooth anomaly in a cat. Journal of Veterinary Dentistry 29, 112–113

Milella L (2015) Occlusion and malocclusion in the cat: what's normal, what's not and when's the best time to intervene? Journal of Feline Medicine and Surgery 17, 5–20

Nemec A, Daniaux L, Johnson E et al. (2015) Craniomaxillofacial abnormalities in dogs with congenital palatal defects: computed tomographic findings. Veterinary Surgery 44, 417–422

Norrdin RW (1975) Fibrous osteodystrophy with facial hyperostosis in a dog with renal cortical hypoplasia. The Cornell Veterinarian 65, 173–186

Oakes AB and Beard GB (1992) Lingually displaced mandibular canine teeth: orthodontic treatment alternatives in the dog. Journal of Veterinary Dentistry 9, 20–25

Oechtering GU, Pohl S, Schlueter C et al. (2016a) A novel approach to brachycephalic syndrome. 1. Evaluation of anatomical intranasal airway obstruction. Veterinary Surgery 45, 165–172

Oechtering GU, Pohl S, Schlueter C et al. (2016b) A novel approach to brachycephalic syndrome. 2. Laser-assisted turbinectomy (LATE). Veterinary Surgery 45, 173–181

Padgett GA and Mostosky UV (1986) The mode of inheritance of craniomandibular osteopathy in West Highland White Terrier dogs. American Journal of Medical Genetics 25, 9–13

Pastor KF, Boulay JP, Schelling SH et al. (2000) Idiopathic hyperostosis of the calvaria in five young Bullmastiffs. Journal of the American Animal Hospital Association 36, 439–445

Pavlica Z and Cestnik V (1995) Management of lingually displaced mandibular canine teeth in five Bull Terrier dogs. *Journal of Veterinary Dentistry* **12**, 127–129

Peak RM, Lobprise HB and Wiggs RB (1999) Fabrication of a labial maxillary arch bar from orthodontic wire, acrylic and orthodontic buttons. *Journal of Veterinary Dentistry* **16**, 30–34

Peralta S, Fiani N, Kan-Rohrer KH *et al.* (2017) Morphological evaluation of clefts of the lip, palate, or both in dogs. *American Journal of Veterinary Research* **78**, 926–933

Peralta S, Nemec A, Fiani N *et al.* (2015) Staged double-layer closure of palatal defects in 6 dogs. *Veterinary Surgery* **44**, 423–431

Pettit R, Fox R, Comerford EJ *et al.* (2012) Bilateral angular carpal deformity in a dog with craniomandibular osteopathy. *Veterinary Comparative Orthopaedics and Traumatology* **25**, 149–154

Poncet CM, Dupre GP, Freiche VG *et al.* (2006) Long term results of upper respiratory syndrome surgery and gastrointestinal tract medical treatment in 51 brachycephalic dogs. *Journal of Small Animal Practice* **47**, 137–142

Ratterree WO, Glassman MM, Driskell EA *et al.* (2011) Craniomandibular osteopathy with a unique neurological manifestation in a young Akita. *Journal of the American Animal Hospital Association* **47**, e7–12

Reiter AM (2004) Symphysiotomy, symphysiectomy and intermandibular arthrodesis in a cat with open-mouth jaw locking – case report and literature review. *Journal of Veterinary Dentistry* **21**, 147–158

Reiter AM (2010) Palate defect. In: *Mechanisms of Disease in Small Animal Surgery, 3rd edn*, ed. MJ Bojrab and E Monnet, pp. 118–124. Teton NewMedia, Jackson

Reiter AM (2015) Cleft palate and acquired palate defects. In: *Clinical Veterinary Advisor, 3rd edn*, ed. E Cote, pp. 188–201. Mosby, St Louis

Reiter AM and Holt D (2012) Palate surgery. In: *Veterinary Surgery: Small Animal, 1st edn*, ed. KM Tobias and SA Johnston, pp. 1707–1717. Elsevier, St Louis

Reiter AM and Smith MM (2005) The oral cavity and oropharynx. In: *BSAVA Manual of Canine and Feline Head, Neck and Thoracic Surgery, 1st edn*, ed. DJ Brockman and DE Holt, pp. 25–43. BSAVA Publications, Gloucester

Riecks TW, Birchard SJ and Stephens JA (2007) Surgical correction of brachycephalic syndrome in dogs: 62 cases (1991–2004). *Journal of the American Veterinary Medical Association* **230**, 1324–1328

Robins G and Grandage J (1977) Temporomandibular joint dysplasia and open-mouth jaw locking in the dog. *Journal of the American Veterinary Medical Association* **171**, 1072–1076

Ross DL (1986a) Orthodontics for the dog. Bite evaluation, basic concepts, and equipment. *Veterinary Clinics of North America: Small Animal Practice* **16**, 955–966

Ross DL (1986b) Orthodontics for the dog. Treatment methods. *Veterinary Clinics of North America: Small Animal Practice* **16**, 939–954

Sager M and Nefen S (1998) Use of buccal mucosal flaps for the correction of congenital soft palate defects in three dogs. *Veterinary Surgery* **27**, 358–363

Sarkiala EM, Dambach D and Harvey CE (1994) Jaw lesions resulting from renal hyperparathyroidism in a young dog – a case report. *Journal of Veterinary Dentistry* **11**, 121–124

Sarkiala-Kessel E (2001) Malocclusion in a cat. *Journal of Veterinary Dentistry* **18**, 76–77

Senders CW, Eisele P, Freeman LE *et al.* (1986) Observations about the normal and abnormal embryogenesis of the canine lip and palate. *Journal of Craniofacial Genetics and Developmental Biology* **2**, 241–248

Shorenstein B, Schwartz P and Kross PH (2014) What is your diagnosis? Craniomandibular osteopathy. *Journal of the American Veterinary Medical Association* **245**, 491–492

Smith MM (2013) Gingivectomy, gingivoplasty and osteoplasty for mandibular canine tooth malocclusion. *Journal of Veterinary Dentistry* **30**, 184–197

Smithson CW, Smith MM and Gamble DA (2010) Multifocal odontoblastic dysplasia in a dog. *Journal of Veterinary Dentistry* **27**, 242–247

Soukup JW, Snyder CJ and Gengler WR (2009) Computed tomography and partial coronoidectomy for open-mouth jaw locking in two cats. *Journal of Veterinary Dentistry* **26**, 226–233

Stapleton BL and Clarke LL (1999) Mandibular canine tooth impaction in a young dog – treatment and subsequent eruption: a case report. *Journal of Veterinary Dentistry* **16**, 105–108

Stein KE, Marretta SM and Eurell JA (2005) Dens invaginatus of the mandibular first molars in a dog. *Journal of Veterinary Dentistry* **22**, 21–25

Surgeon TW (2000) Surgical exposure and orthodontic extrusion of an impacted canine tooth in a cat: a case report. *Journal of Veterinary Dentistry* **17**, 81–85

Surgeon TW (2005) Fundamentals of small animal orthodontics. *Veterinary Clinics of North America: Small Animal Practice* **35**, 869–889

Sylvestre AM and Sharma A (1997) Management of a congenitally shortened soft palate in a dog. *Journal of the American Veterinary Medical Association* **211**, 875–877

Taylor SM, Remedios A and Myers S (1995) Craniomandibular osteopathy in a Shetland Sheepdog. *Canadian Veterinary Journal* **36**, 437–439

Temizsoylu MD and Avki S (2003) Complete ventral ankyloglossia in three related dogs. *Journal of the American Veterinary Medical Association* **223**, 1443–1445

Thompson DJ, Rogers W, Owen MC *et al.* (2011) Idiopathic canine juvenile cranial hyperostosis in a Pit Bull Terrier. *New Zealand Veterinary Journal* **59**, 201–205

Torrez CV and Hunt GB (2006) Results of surgical correction of abnormalities associated with brachycephalic airway obstruction syndrome in dogs in Australia. *Journal of Small Animal Practice* **47**, 150–154

Trostel CT and Frankel DJ (2010) Punch resection alaplasty technique in dogs and cats with stenotic nares: 14 cases. *Journal of the American Animal Hospital Association* **46**, 5–11

Ulbricht RD and Marretta SM (2005) Orthodontic treatment using a direct acrylic inclined plane. *Journal of Veterinary Dentistry* **22**, 60–65

van de Wetering A (2007) Orthodontic correction of a base narrow mandibular canine tooth in a dog. *Journal of Veterinary Dentistry* **24**, 22–28

Verhaert L (1999) A removable orthodontic device for the treatment of lingually displaced mandibular canine teeth in young dogs. *Journal of Veterinary Dentistry* **16**, 69–75

Verhaert L (2007) Developmental oral and dental conditions. In: *BSAVA Manual of Canine and Feline Dentistry, 3rd edn*, ed. C Tutt, J Deeprose and DA Crossley, pp. 77–95. BSAVA Publications, Gloucester

Verstraete FJM (1985) Anomalous development of the upper third premolar in a dog and a cat. *Journal of the South African Veterinary Association* **56**, 131–134

Verstraete FJM, Bliss PZ, Hass PH *et al.* (2011) Clinical signs and histological findings in dogs with odontogenic cysts: 41 cases (1995–2010). *Journal of the American Animal Hospital Association* **239**, 1470–1476

Verstraete FJM and Terpak CH (1997) Anatomical variations in the dentition of the domestic cat. *Journal of Veterinary Dentistry* **14**, 137–140

Vieira AL, Ocarino Nde M, Boeloni JN *et al.* (2009) Congenital oligodontia of the deciduous teeth and anodontia of the permanent teeth in a cat. *Journal of Feline Medicine and Surgery* **11**, 156–158

Warzee CC, Bellah JR and Richards D (2001) Congenital unilateral cleft of the soft palate in six dogs. *Journal of Small Animal Practice* **42**, 338–340

White RN, Hawkins HL, Alemi VP *et al.* (2009) Soft palate hypoplasia and concurrent middle ear pathology in six dogs. *Journal of Small Animal Practice* **50**, 364–372

Wiggs RR and Lobprise HB (1997) Basics of orthodontics. In: *Veterinary Dentistry Principles and Practice, 1st edn*, pp. 435–481. Lippincott-Raven, Philadelphia

Wiggs RB, Lobprise HB and de Lahunta A (1994) Microglossia in three littermate puppies. *Journal of Veterinary Dentistry* **11**, 129–133

Woodbridge NT, Baines EA and Baines SJ (2012) Otitis media in five cats associated with soft palate abnormalities. *Veterinary Record* **171**, 124–125

Useful websites

Nomenclature information of the American Veterinary Dental College (AVDC): www.avdc.org

OPERATIVE TECHNIQUE 10.1

Obtaining a full-mouth impression, bite registration and creating stone models

INDICATIONS

Full-mouth impression and bite registration are necessary to create stone models. The models can be used as a preoperative database or to build an appliance.

POSITIONING

Dorsal and ventral recumbency.

ASSISTANT

Needed.

ADDITIONAL EQUIPMENT

Impression trays; alginate; water; flexible plastic bowl; spatula; boxing wax; rope wax; bandage tape; slightly damped paper towels; baseplate wax or polyvinyl siloxane; dental stone type III or IV; dental laboratory knife; power trimmer, plaster cutter or laboratory bur.

TECHNIQUES

Full-mouth impression

1 Scale, polish, rinse and dry the teeth.

2 Select the appropriately sized tray (there should be at least 5 mm of space between the teeth and the edge of the tray, which must have holes, otherwise a tray adhesive will need to be used).

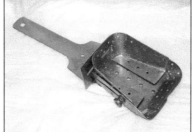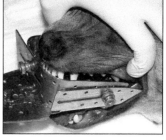

(© Dr Alexander M. Reiter)

3 Pre-measure the amount of alginate impression material and water to be used; follow the manufacturer's instructions (polyvinyl siloxane could also be used, but alginate is less expensive and gives adequate results).

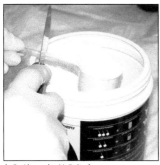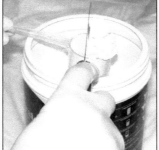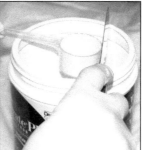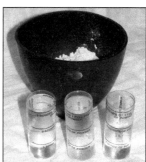

(© Dr Alexander M. Reiter)

→ **OPERATIVE TECHNIQUE 10.1 CONTINUED**

4 Pour the cold water on to the powder in the flexible plastic bowl and start mixing vigorously with a spatula, working the mix against the walls of the bowl to minimize air bubble formation. As soon as the mix is homogenous, transfer it to the tray.

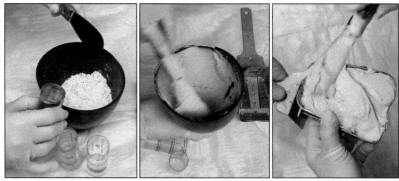

(© Dr Alexander M. Reiter)

5 Seat the tray on the teeth of the upper or lower jaw, making sure that the lips and tongue are not in the way when taking the impression.

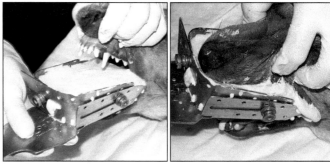

(© Dr Alexander M. Reiter)

6 Wait until the alginate is set. Then carefully pull the tray off of the teeth. Inspect the impression for voids, and if necessary take a new impression. Clean any debris from the impression, trim any redundant material, wrap it in a slightly damped paper towel (to prevent dehydration), and set aside.

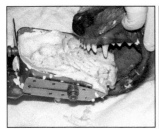 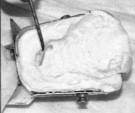 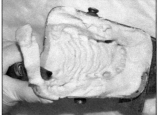 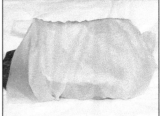

(© Dr Alexander M. Reiter)

7 Repeat the process for the opposite jaw.

Bite registration

1 Soften a sheet of baseplate wax under warm water (a roll of polyvinyl siloxane wide and long enough to include incisor and canine teeth can be used instead).

2 Fold it to create a double-layered sheet, extubate the patient (or detach the endotracheal (ET) tube from the anaesthesia machine, deflate its cuff, and carefully insert the tube further down the trachea) and roll the tongue to the back of the mouth just enough to allow complete closure of the mouth, but carefully preventing obstruction of the larynx.

→ **OPERATIVE TECHNIQUE 10.1 CONTINUED**

3 Place the sheet (or roll) in between the incisor and canine teeth and close the mouth tightly enough to imprint the sheet (or polyvinyl siloxane roll).

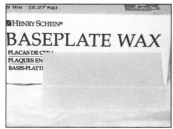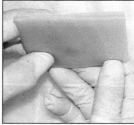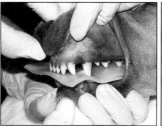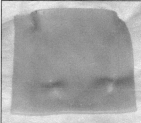

(© Dr Alexander M. Reiter)

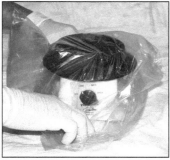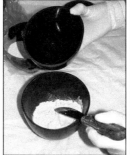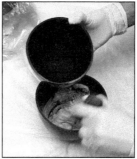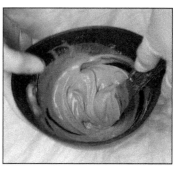

(© Dr Alexander M. Reiter)

4 Open the mouth, remove the sheet (or roll), retrieve the tongue, re-intubate (or reposition the endotracheal tube), inflate the ET tube cuff, and reattach the tube to the anaesthesia machine. The imprinted sheet or roll will allow the dental laboratory technician to properly align the stone models produced of the upper and lower jaws.

Stone model fabrication

1 If using alginate impression material, models have to be poured within 30 minutes of taking the impressions. If using polyvinyl siloxane, models may be poured within 14 days without seeing any significant shrinkage. Use a dental stone type III (moderate strength) or type III (high strength) gypsum material. Types I and II are not strong enough.

2 Cover the dental vibrator with a plastic bag to protect it from being soiled. Add water to dental stone powder in a flexible plastic bowl (follow the manufacturer's instructions) and mix it with a spatula.

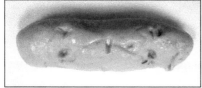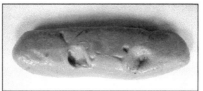

(© Dr Alexander M. Reiter)

3 Place the bowl on the dental vibrator to eliminate air bubbles introduced into the mix during the mixing process.

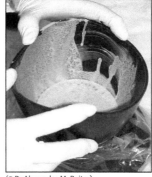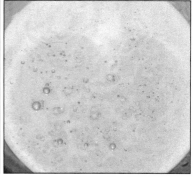

(© Dr Alexander M. Reiter)

→ **OPERATIVE TECHNIQUE 10.1 CONTINUED**

4 Wet the impression such that the dental indents are slightly filled with water.

5 Place the impression on the vibrator on an incline. With the help of a small spatula, add a small amount of stone at the caudal end of the impression and let it run down into the dental indents, displacing the water in the process (without water, the stone is more likely to trap air, creating bubble defects in the model).

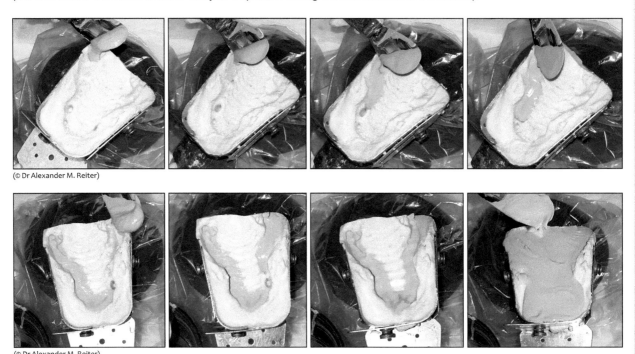

(© Dr Alexander M. Reiter)

(© Dr Alexander M. Reiter)

6 When all the dental indents are coated with stone, pour the surplus water out.

7 Place boxing wax secured with bandage tape around the tray and impression. Build up the base of the model with additional dental stone. Leave undisturbed until dry.

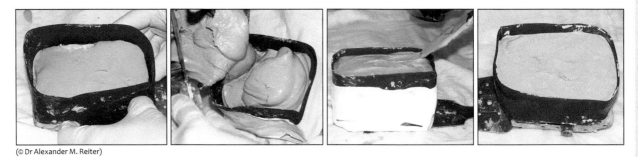

(© Dr Alexander M. Reiter)

8 From 4 to 6 hours later, remove the trays from the impression materials. Incise the impression material by making numerous cross-cuts. Remove the sections gently, one at a time to prevent damage to the model.

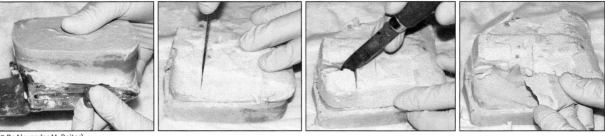

(© Dr Alexander M. Reiter)

→

→ **OPERATIVE TECHNIQUE 10.1 CONTINUED**

9 Inspect the model for voids. Trim the model with the help of a water-cooled power trimmer, plaster cutter or laboratory bur.

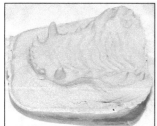 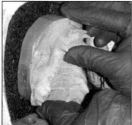 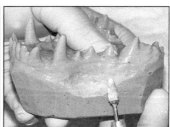 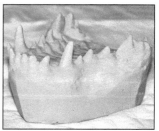

(© Dr Alexander M. Reiter)

OPERATIVE TECHNIQUE 10.2

Fabrication of a direct inclined plane

INDICATIONS

This appliance is utilized to correct linguoversion of mandibular canine teeth in patients with class 1 malocclusion. Due to ethical considerations, orthodontic treatment is not recommended in patients suffering from a class 2 malocclusion of genetic origin, unless they are neutered.

POSITIONING

Dorsal recumbency.

ASSISTANT

Needed.

ADDITIONAL EQUIPMENT

Ligature wire; wire cutter; hypodermic needles; 37% phosphoric acid etching gel; dental brush; unfilled resin; light-curing gun; light-cured dental composite; self-curing bis-acryl composite; shaping composite instruments; trimming burs.

TECHNIQUE

1 The canine and other selected teeth (e.g. incisors and rostral premolars), depending on the size of the inclined plane and direction of tooth movement, are cleaned, etched, rinsed and dried.

a. Drops of dental composite may be placed and an orthopaedic wire (24 G) secured between the canine and third incisor teeth to reinforce the appliance.

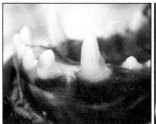 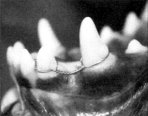 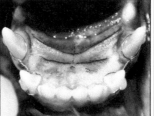 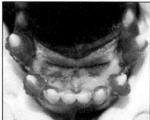

(© Dr Alexander M. Reiter)

→ **OPERATIVE TECHNIQUE 10.2 CONTINUED**

b. A telescopic bar, constructed from two differently sized hypodermic needles, may be placed between the canine teeth to allow for continued growth of the upper jaw.

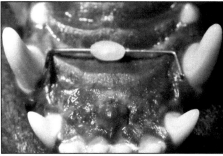
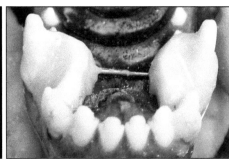

(© Dr Alexander M. Reiter)

2 A self-curing composite resin is used to create inclined planes extending from where the tips of the mandibular canine teeth contact the hard palate mucosa, two-thirds of the way up the crowns of the maxillary canine teeth, to where they should normally be. The inclined planes incorporate several incisor teeth and/or rostral premolar teeth for added stability. The deposition of composite resin can be controlled by using utility wax to delineate the areas to be built up.

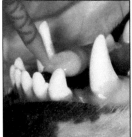
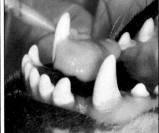
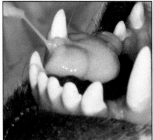
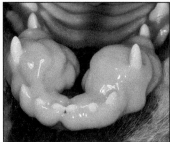

(© Dr Alexander M. Reiter)

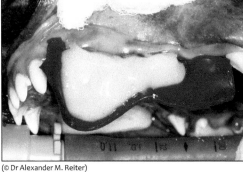
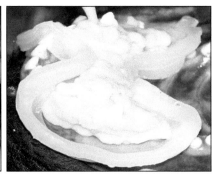

(© Dr Alexander M. Reiter)

3 The appliance is trimmed, shaped and smoothed. The inclined surfaces need to be as smooth as possible and should follow a minimum of a 45-degree angle with the surface of the palate.

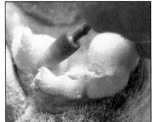
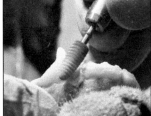
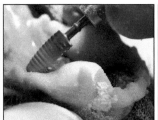
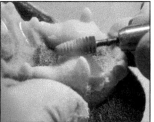

(© Dr Alexander M. Reiter)

→ **OPERATIVE TECHNIQUE 10.2 CONTINUED**

4 The final inclined plane should cover the least amount of gingiva and hard palate mucosa and not extend into alveolar mucosa.

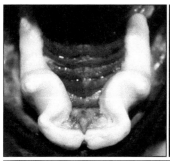
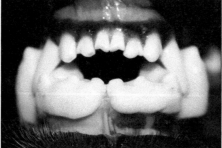
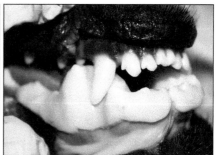

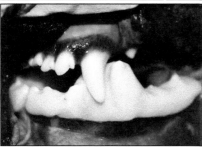

(© Dr Alexander M. Reiter)

OPERATIVE TECHNIQUE 10.3

Active orthodontic appliance with brackets, buttons or ligature wires and elastic chain

INDICATIONS

One of the most common indications for the use of active orthodontic appliances with brackets, buttons or hooks, wires and elastic chains is the treatment of a mesioverted maxillary canine tooth. The goal is to pull the displaced canine tooth distally.

POSITIONING

Lateral recumbency.

ASSISTANT

Needed.

ADDITIONAL EQUIPMENT

Metal brackets or buttons; plastic buttons; ligature wire; wire cutter; 37% phosphoric acid etching gel; dental brush; unfilled resin; light-curing gun; light-cured dental composite; self-curing bis-acryl composite; shaping composite instruments; trimming burs; elastic chain (continuous filament pattern); rope wax to cover areas that could cause discomfort upon contact.

TECHNIQUE

1 The displaced maxillary canine tooth and the anchor teeth are scaled and polished with pumice, then rinsed, etched, rinsed again and dried.

→ OPERATIVE TECHNIQUE 10.3 CONTINUED

2   Various designs of anchorage are possible for the movement of the canine tooth, including a 'snowman', custom-made composite button, wire-reinforced resin hook, metal button or plastic button.

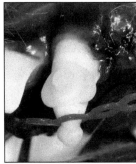
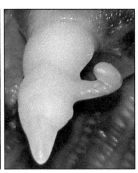
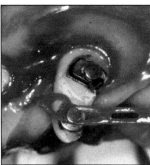
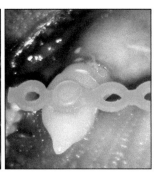

(© Dr Alexander M. Reiter)

3   An anchorage unit is created by connecting the maxillary fourth premolar to the first molar teeth (dog) or the maxillary third premolar to the fourth premolar teeth (cat). This is achieved using metal brackets, metal or plastic buttons, and/or custom-made composite buttons that are connected with each other by a twisted ligature wire (the twisted wire end may then also be used as a hook that is covered with some resin).

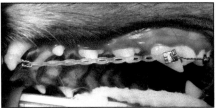
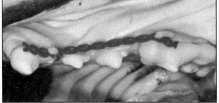
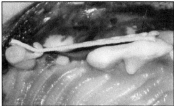

(© Dr Alexander M. Reiter)

4   The resting length of the chain between the anchorage unit and the anchorage device on the canine tooth is measured in holes. The chain should not be reduced to less than 75% of its resting length when stretched between the anchorage unit and the anchorage device on the canine tooth (e.g. if the resting length is 10 holes, then the chain should not be stretched to fewer than eight holes).

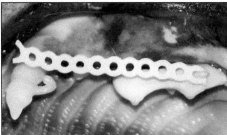
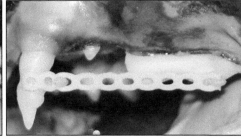

(© Dr Alexander M. Reiter)

5   The chain is changed every 10–14 days. In most cases, the movement is completed in 6–10 weeks. It may be wise to leave a 'neutral' chain as a retainer in place for several more weeks or months to avoid movement of the treated tooth to its original position.

6   Occasionally, the mandibular canine tooth gets tipped labially while the maxillary canine tooth moves distally. If the mandibular canine tooth does not relapse into its original position, a second appliance is constructed to tip the tooth distolingually.

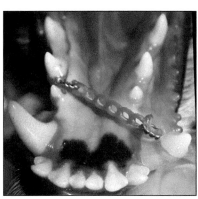

(© Dr Alexander M. Reiter)

Chapter 11

Management of oral and maxillofacial neoplasia

Giorgio Romanelli and John R. Lewis

The term *tumour* refers to a swollen or distended area. The term has evolved to be interpreted specifically as benign or malignant neoplastic disease. Benign and malignant oral and maxillofacial tumours are common in dogs, whereas oral and maxillofacial neoplasia in cats tends to be malignant. Benign tumours may be locally invasive but do not metastasize to distant sites. Oral tumours account for 6% of all canine tumours and up to 12% of feline tumours (Stebbins *et al.*, 1989; Liptak and Withrow, 2010). In dogs, the oral cavity is the fourth most common site of neoplasia. There is not a definitive breed predilection, but many purebred dogs, including Cocker Spaniels, German Shepherd Dogs, retrievers and poodles may have a higher risk of developing oral and maxillofacial cancer. A list of important oral and maxillofacial tumours in dogs and cats is seen in Figure 11.1.

Benign
• Acanthomatous ameloblastoma
• Adenoma
• Amyloid-producing odontogenic tumour
• Benign peripheral nerve sheath tumour
• Canine papilloma
• Cementoma
• Feline inductive odontogenic tumour
• Giant cell granuloma
• Granular cell tumour
• Lipoma
• Melanocytoma
• Osteoma
• Papillary squamous cell carcinoma
• Peripheral odontogenic fibroma
• Plasma cell tumour

Malignant
• Adenocarcinoma
• Anaplastic neoplasm
• Fibrosarcoma
• Haemangiosarcoma
• Lymphosarcoma
• Malignant melanoma
• Malignant peripheral nerve sheath tumour
• Mast cell tumour
• Multilobular tumour of bone
• Osteosarcoma
• Rhabdomyosarcoma
• Squamous cell carcinoma
• Undifferentiated neoplasm

11.1 Important oral and maxillofacial tumour types in dogs and cats.

Malignant oral and maxillofacial tumours

The most common malignant oral and maxillofacial tumour in the dog is malignant melanoma (MM), followed by squamous cell carcinoma (SCC) and fibrosarcoma (FSA). In the cat, SCC is the most common malignant oral and maxillofacial tumour (60–70% of cases), followed by FSA.

Malignant melanoma

Malignant melanoma (MM) is the most common oral and maxillofacial tumour in dogs, but it is rare in the mouths of cats. Breeds with pigmented oral mucosa may be predisposed to MM. It presents as a single, friable, often ulcerated and/or necrotic mass, usually located on the gingiva, tongue and alveolar, labial or buccal mucosa (Figure 11.2). Large pigmented tumours are likely to be MM. However, up to 40% of MM may be amelanotic (Figure 11.3). Histologically, MM may show a lack of differentiation and be diagnosed as undifferentiated malignant tumour or anaplastic sarcoma. An immunohistochemical stain, Melan-A, can be used to differentiate between MM and other tumours, although Melan-A is less sensitive as neoplasms become more undifferentiated. PNL2 stain seems slightly more sensitive than Melan-A (Ramos-Vara *et al.*, 2000; Ramos-Vara and Miller, 2011). Malignant melanomas are often highly invasive and usually require radical resection

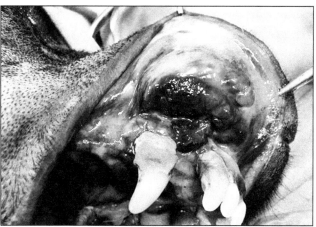

11.2 Malignant melanoma of the right upper lip in a 13-year-old entire male Miniature Schnauzer.
(© Giorgio Romanelli)

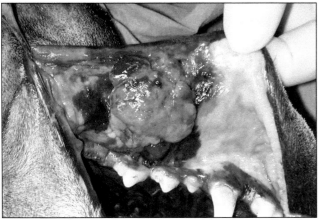

11.3 Amelanotic malignant melanoma of the right upper lip and cheek in a 9-year-old neutered female crossbreed dog.
(© Giorgio Romanelli)

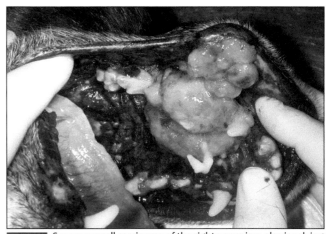

11.5 Squamous cell carcinoma of the right upper jaw, also involving the hard palate and lip, in an 11-year-old entire male crossbreed dog.
(© Giorgio Romanelli)

(1.5–2 cm margins in all directions, including skin) to prevent local recurrence (Tuohy *et al.*, 2014). A benign variant of oral melanoma, sometimes referred to as oral melanocytoma, has been described. Melanocytomas tend to be very well circumscribed, less than 1 cm in diameter at the time of diagnosis and respond well to marginal or wide excision rather than radical mandibulectomy or maxillectomy (Esplin, 2008). Oral MM has a variable metastatic rate, depending on site, size and biological behaviour of the individual tumour. The authors have seen a great degree of variation in the aggressiveness of MM and survival times of affected patients.

Squamous cell carcinoma

Squamous cell carcinoma (SCC) is the most common oral and maxillofacial tumour in cats and the second most common malignant tumour of the mouth in dogs. It usually has the appearance of a pink or red ulcerated mass that may bleed very easily (Figures 11.4, 11.5 and 11.6). SCC may be evident as ulceration of the soft tissues of the upper or lower jaw, with no evidence of an overt mass. Occasionally, cats or dogs with SCC will present with the clinical finding of a loose tooth or teeth, which may be mistaken for periodontal disease. Risk factors in cats may include use of flea collars and eating canned tuna and canned cat food. Exposure to environmental tobacco smoke increased the risk for having SCC by a factor of two but was not found to be statistically significant (Bertone *et al.*, 2003). Tumour biopsy samples from cats exposed to environmental tobacco smoke were 4.5 times more likely to overexpress p53 than were tumours from unexposed

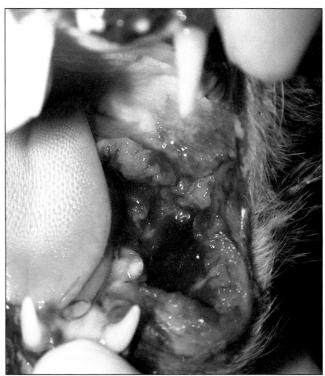

11.6 Squamous cell carcinoma of the left mandible in a 7-year-old neutered male Domestic Shorthaired cat.
(© Giorgio Romanelli)

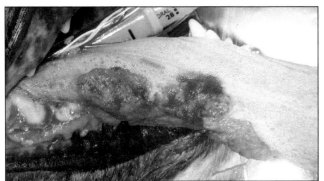

11.4 Squamous cell carcinoma of the right lateral aspect of the tongue in a 10-year-old entire male Labrador Retriever.
(© Giorgio Romanelli)

cats (Snyder *et al.*, 2004). SCC rapidly infiltrates bone, especially in the cat. In dogs, the metastatic rate is considered to be low for rostral tumours and high for lingual and tonsillar tumours (Figure 11.7). Wide excision (10 mm margin or more) may be sufficient to prevent recurrence of small SCCs; however, depending on location and radiographic evidence of invasion, radical resection may be a better approach. Lingual SCC, if small at the time of diagnosis, may be cured by radical glossectomy, but micrometastasis to regional lymph nodes may become apparent after surgery. Though glossectomy may cause significant functional issues in both canine and feline patients, dogs appear to adapt better than cats to radical resection of lingual tissue. A multi-centre study of 44 dogs with tonsillar SCC showed a median survival time of 179 days. Clinical signs of anorexia and lethargy were significantly associated with a poor prognosis (Mas *et al.*, 2011). In cats with

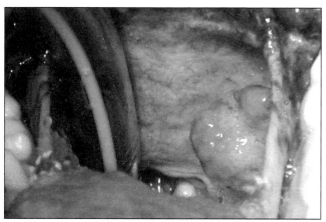

11.7 Squamous cell carcinoma of the left palatine tonsil in an 8-year-old entire male crossbreed dog.
(© Giorgio Romanelli)

SCC, the prevalence of metastasis has historically been considered to be low, but recent studies suggest a metastatic rate of approximately 30% to the mandibular lymph nodes (Gendler *et al.*, 2010; Soltero-Rivera *et al.*, 2014).

A less aggressive variant, termed papillary SCC, is seen most commonly in young dogs. The authors have seen papillary SCC in puppies as young as 5 months of age. However, papillary SCC can be seen in dogs of any age (Nemec *et al.*, 2014). The typical appearance is a verrucous pink mass arising from the gingiva of the rostral maxilla or mandible. Papillary SCC has not been documented to metastasize, and thus aggressive local treatment (partial maxillectomy or mandibulectomy) is often curative (Soukup *et al.*, 2013; Nemec *et al.*, 2014).

Fibrosarcoma

Fibrosarcoma (FSA) is the second most common malignant oral and maxillofacial tumour in cats and the third most common in dogs. It tends to occur in large-breed dogs with a possible breed predilection for retrievers. FSA often presents as a raised, broad-based, maxillary mass, growing on the palate or lateral muzzle (Figure 11.8). In some cases, FSA can appear benign histologically and

may be misdiagnosed as a fibroma or a low-grade FSA even with large biopsy samples because it may not show typical histopathological criteria of malignancy (Ciekot *et al.*, 1994). Sending tissue samples to pathologists with an interest in, and experience with, the varying manifestations of oral and maxillofacial neoplasia will increase the odds of an accurate diagnosis. Treatment of histologically low-grade, biologically high-grade FSA (so-called 'high-low FSA') must be very aggressive. FSA is very infiltrative, and even with advanced diagnostics, it is challenging to discern the full extent of the tumour in dogs and cats. Therefore, radical surgery, and possibly postsurgical radiation therapy, is often required for a chance of a cure (Frazier *et al.*, 2012; Gardner *et al.*, 2015). In one study, prevalence of pulmonary metastasis in dogs with high-low FSA was 12% (3/25 dogs), and regional lymph node metastasis was 20% (5/25 dogs) (Ciekot *et al.*, 1994).

Malignant peripheral nerve sheath tumour

Malignant peripheral nerve sheath tumour (MPNST) is an uncommon neoplasm of the oral cavity, but when it occurs it manifests as a diffuse, poorly delineated mass involving a large portion of the mandible or maxilla. The authors have seen MPNST arising in the area rostral to the infra-orbital foramen, and as a fleshy mass arising from the inferior alveolar neurovascular bundle, seen on dental radiographs as concentric bone loss in the mandibular canal. MPNST may be most challenging to treat and prevent local recurrence due to tracking of the tumour along nerve sheaths, though benign versions may exist. When malignant, radical excision (2 cm or greater margins) may be necessary to obtain a possible cure.

Osteosarcoma

Osteosarcoma (OSA) of the oral cavity tends to manifest as fleshy, red, friable soft tissue masses with bone lysis rather than hard tissue proliferation (Figure 11.9). Mandibular OSA appears to have a better prognosis than

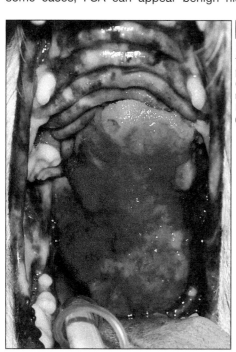

11.8
Fibrosarcoma of the hard and soft palate in a 6-year-old entire male Golden Retriever dog.
(© Giorgio Romanelli)

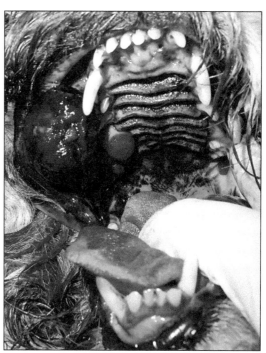

11.9 Osteosarcoma of the right maxilla in a 5-year-old neutered female Lhasa Apso dog.
(© John R. Lewis)

appendicular OSA (Farcas *et al.*, 2014). In a recent study of canine mandibular OSA, median survival time was 525 days, and 58% of dogs developed metastatic disease (Coyle *et al.*, 2015).

Multilobular tumour of bone

Multilobular tumour of bone (osteochondrosarcoma, chondroma rodens) is a hard, well-circumscribed, non-ulcerated mass, occurring most commonly on the caudal mandible, hard palate, zygomatic arch, base of the skull and cranium. Radiographic appearance is a characteristic combination of mineralized and non-mineralized tissue, usually well circumscribed, such that it has been referred to as a 'popcorn ball' appearance. One study of 39 dogs showed a metastatic rate of 56%, and 47% of treated dogs had local recurrence. However, median survival times were quite good at 797 days (Dernell *et al.*, 1998).

Mast cell tumour

Mast cell tumour (MCT) occurs rarely in the oral cavity, though MCT may arise from the gingiva, the skin lateral to the nasal plane, lips and tongue (Wright and Chretin, 2006; Elliott *et al.*, 2013). MCT should be considered as a differential diagnosis with any waxing and waning oral or perioral mass. A retrospective study of 44 cases of canine oral and perioral mast cell tumours showed 59% of dogs had metastasis at the time of presentation. Overall median survival time was 52 months, which dropped to 14 months for dogs with the presence of lymph node metastasis. Median survival time in dogs without lymph node metastasis was not reached during the study period (Hillman *et al.*, 2010).

Others

Less common malignant tumours include adenocarcinoma, haemangiosarcoma, lymphosarcoma, rhabdomyosarcoma, and anaplastic and undifferentiated neoplasms. The adenocarcinoma is of epithelial origin, deriving from glandular tissue of either the oral cavity, nasal cavity or salivary gland duct tissue (major or accessory). The haemangiosarcoma is a tumour of vascular endothelial origin characterized by extensive metastasis and has been reported in the gingiva, tongue and hard palate. The lymphosarcoma, also known as lymphoma, is a tumour defined by a proliferation of lymphocytes within solid organs, such as the lymph nodes and tonsils, or the skin, nasal cavity, and mouth. The rhabdomyosarcoma originates from skeletal muscle (such as in the tongue) or embryonic mesenchymal cells. An anaplastic neoplasm is a tumour whose cells are generally undifferentiated and pleomorphic (displaying variability in size, shape and pattern of cells and/or their nuclei). An undifferentiated neoplasm is a tumour whose cells are generally immature and lack distinctive features of a particular tissue type.

Benign oral and maxillofacial tumours

'Epulis' is a non-specific clinical descriptive term referring to a proliferative growth on the gingiva (which could essentially be benign or malignant); therefore, the use of this term is discouraged.

Peripheral odontogenic fibromas (fibromatous epulis and ossifying epulis) are common in dogs, but rare in cats, and present as firm gingival masses adjacent to a tooth that are usually covered by normal mucosa. Since these tumours arise from epithelial clusters within gingival connective tissue or periodontal ligament, the tooth or teeth from which the tumour arose often require extraction to prevent recurrence. However, since these masses are slow growing and do not metastasize, marginal resection is often a good place to start to confirm the diagnosis and, in some cases, prevent recurrence. Though cats are rarely affected, when they are, peripheral odontogenic fibromas may arise from multiple teeth in the same patient (Colgin *et al.*, 2001; Knaake and Verhaert, 2010).

Acanthomatous ameloblastoma (acanthomatous epulis) (Figure 11.10), seen commonly in the rostral mandible of dogs, has never been documented to metastasize and carries a good prognosis with surgical resection when 1 cm margins of clinically and radiographically normal tissue are removed beyond the tumour (Fiani *et al.*, 2011; Goldschmidt *et al.*, 2017). Other potentially effective treatments include radiation therapy and intralesional bleomycin chemotherapy (Thrall, 1984; Yoshida *et al.*, 1998).

Osteomas are benign, well circumscribed bony masses that may occur in dogs or cats. They have been reported on the hard palate, zygomatic arch and caudal mandible (Soltero-Rivera *et al.*, 2015). Biopsy results may show a histopathological diagnosis of normal woven bone rather than obvious characteristics of neoplasia. Of four cats treated in one study, surgical treatment of mandibulectomy, maxillectomy or debulking resulted in greater than 1-year survival in all cats (Fiani *et al.*, 2011).

Oral plasmacytoma may arise at various locations (Wright *et al.*, 2008; Smithson *et al.*, 2012), but perhaps the most common location is the dorsal surface of the tongue, where it manifests as a well circumscribed red mass, often less than 1 cm in diameter. Surgical margins of less than 1 cm have been curative in cases seen by the authors.

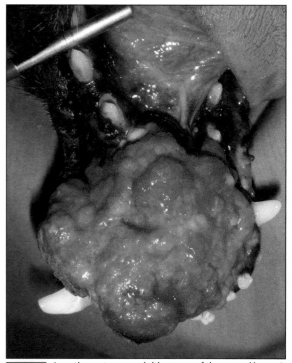

11.10 Acanthomatous ameloblastoma of the rostral lower jaw in an 18-year-old entire male crossbreed dog.
(© Dr Margherita Gracis)

Amyloid-producing odontogenic tumours can be very locally invasive with significant bone destruction. However, they have not been documented to metastasize in dogs and cats. Curative-intent surgery may require 1 cm clinical and radiographic margins. If the tumour is in a location that is not amenable to surgery, or if pet owners would rather treat with radiation therapy, good responses have been seen (Moore *et al.*, 2000).

Feline inductive odontogenic tumour (FIOT) has also been previously referred to as inductive fibroameloblastoma (Gardner and Dubielzig, 1995). This tumour occurs most commonly in young cats, with a possible predilection for the rostral maxilla. Although this tumour does not appear to metastasize, FIOT grows by expansion and can infiltrate underlying bone to cause considerable local destruction (Beatty *et al.*, 2000). The term 'inductive' refers to a reciprocal interaction between developmental cells, which results in formation of tooth-like tissue.

Another example of an inductive mass is the odontoma. Odontomas, however, are considered hamartomas, rather than a true neoplasia. Hamartomas are composed of tissue elements normally found at the site, showing a normal rate of tissue growth, but these tissues develop as a disorganized mass to resemble neoplasia. Odontomas occur as either complex or compound varieties, depending on whether mineralized tooth-like structures form within the mass. Compound odontomas contain tooth-like structures, whereas complex odontomas contain an amorphous mineralized pattern rather than tooth-like structures (Walker *et al.*, 2009).

Giant cell granuloma, formerly known as giant cell epulis, is rare in dogs and extremely rare in cats. These masses arise from the gingiva and often present as red, fleshy, friable, readily bleeding masses. They have been known to recur after conservative resection, and therefore wide surgical excision may be preferred over intralesional or marginal resection, especially when dealing with recurrent masses. Positive staining with TRAP (tartrate-resistant acid phosphatase) is consistent with osteoclastic origin (Desoutter *et al.*, 2012).

Papilloma is an exophytic, pedunculated, cauliflower-like tumour of epithelium. Canine papillomatosis is thought to be due to infection with canine papillomavirus in typically young dogs; severe papillomatosis may be recognized in older dogs that are immunocompromised (see Chapter 8 for further information).

Less common benign tumours include adenoma, cementoma, granular cell tumour, and lipoma. The adenoma is an epithelial tumour in which the cells form recognizable glandular structures or in which the cells are derived from glandular epithelium. The cementoma is an odontogenic tumour of mesenchymal origin, consisting of cementum-like tissue deposited by cells resembling cementoblasts. The granular cell tumour, also called myoblastoma, is a neoplasm of the skin or mucosa with uncertain histogenesis, most commonly occurring on the tongue. The lipoma is a mesenchymal tumour originating from lipocytes.

History and clinical signs

Dogs and cats are often presented after an oral or maxillofacial mass is identified by the owner or during routine examination by the veterinary professional. Some patients have a history of mobile teeth. Animals that have neoplasia in the caudal maxilla or palatine tonsils are usually diagnosed later in the course of the disease. Clinical signs include halitosis, haemorrhage (spontaneous or after feeding, drinking, chewing or playing with objects), drooling, maxillofacial deformity, difficulty or pain upon opening the mouth, and weight loss. Some patients are diagnosed during a professional dental cleaning procedure or are presented for an enlarged mandibular or retropharyngeal lymph node. In advanced maxillary tumours, there may be invasion of the nasal cavity and/or retrobulbar space with subsequent sneezing, nasal discharge/haemorrhage, exophthalmos, orbital deformity and decreased ocular retropulsion.

Work-up

Before examining the face and mouth, a thorough physical examination is performed. A complete blood count, serum biochemistry and urine examination should be completed. Anaemia may be seen due to continuous blood loss or chronic disease. Hypercalcaemia can be seen in some animals with MM, SCC, other carcinomas or keratinizing and acanthomatous ameloblastomas (Reiter, 2002; Dhaliwal and Tang, 2005).

Staging

The term 'staging' describes the classification of neoplasms according to the extent of the tumour. The TNM staging system described by the World Health Organization is an international standard for the extent of tumour involvement according to three basic elements: primary tumour (T), regional lymph nodes (N), and metastasis (M). Subscripts are used to denote size and degree of involvement; for example, 0 indicates undetectable, and 1, 2, 3 and 4 refer to a progressive increase in tumour size or changes in the lymph nodes. Substages a and b are used to indicate absence or presence of bony invasion of the tumour or metastatic disease within the lymph nodes. The TNM staging for oral and maxillofacial tumours, tumours of the lips and tumours of the oropharynx are described in Figures 11.11, 11.12 and 11.13, respectively.

Clinical examination of the face and mouth

Dogs and cats with an oral or maxillofacial tumour must be thoroughly evaluated, and there is often a benefit to performing an examination under general anaesthesia. The tumour is palpated, and three-dimensional measurements are taken. A probe can be used to inspect the insertion of the tumour on the mandible or the maxilla and to assess its connection to the deeper tissues. The teeth are assessed for mobility, and the bone is assessed for soft areas or pathological fractures.

- MM is usually ulcerated and friable, readily bleeding and often pigmented; however, pigmentation may not be present in amelanotic melanomas.
- FSA is firm, broad-based, and often maxillary in origin, sometimes with secondary ulceration.
- SCC is pink–red, friable, verrucous, ulcerative and bleeding.
- Peripheral odontogenic fibromas tend to be firm to hard masses covered by normal mucosa and with a broad-based or pedunculated attachment to the gingiva.
- Acanthomatous ameloblastoma is often pink, proliferative and verrucous (see Figure 11.10).

Tumour (T)	
Tis	Tumour *in situ*
To	No evidence of tumour
T1	Tumour <2 cm diameter at greatest dimension: a. Without evidence of bone invasion b. With evidence of bone invasion
T2	Tumour 2–4 cm diameter at greatest dimension: a. Without evidence of bone invasion b. With evidence of bone invasion
T3	Tumour >4 cm diameter at greatest dimension: a. Without evidence of bone invasion b. With evidence of bone invasion
Regional lymph nodes (N)	
No	No regional lymph node metastasis
N1	Movable ipsilateral lymph nodes a. Nodes not considered to contain growth b. Nodes considered to contain growth
N2	Movable contralateral lymph nodes a. Nodes not considered to contain growth b. Nodes considered to contain growth
N3	Fixed lymph nodes
Distant metastasis (M)	
Mo	No distant metastasis
M1	Distant metastasis

Stage grouping			
Stage	*T*	*N*	*M*
I	T1	No, N1a or N2a	Mo
II	T2	No, N1a or N2a	Mo
III[a]	T3	No, N1a or N2a	Mo
	Any T	N1b	Mo
IV	Any T	N2b or N3	Mo
		Any N	M1

11.11 Clinical staging (TNM) of oral and maxillofacial tumours. [a] Any bone involvement.
(Data from Owen, 1980)

Tumour (T)	
Tis	Tumour *in situ*
To	No evidence of tumour
T1	Tumour <2 cm diameter at greatest dimension, superficial or exophytic
T2	Tumour <2 cm diameter at greatest dimension, with minimal invasion in depth
T3	Tumour ≥2 cm diameter at greatest dimension, or with deep invasion irrespective of size
T4	Tumour invading bone
Regional lymph nodes (N)	
No	No regional lymph node metastasis
N1	Movable ipsilateral lymph nodes: a. No evidence of lymph node metastasis b. Evidence of lymph node metastasis
N2	Movable contralateral or bilateral lymph nodes: a. No evidence of lymph node metastasis b. Evidence of lymph node metastasis
N3	Fixed lymph nodes
Distant metastasis (M)	
Mo	No distant metastasis
M1	Distant metastasis

11.12 Clinical staging (TNM) of tumours of the lips.
(Data from Owen, 1980)

Tumour (T)	
Tis	Tumour *in situ*
To	No evidence of tumour
T1	Tumour superficial or exophytic: a. Without systemic signs b. With systemic signs
T2	Tumour with invasion of palatine tonsil only: a. Without systemic signs b. With systemic signs
T3	Tumour with invasion of surrounding tissues: a. Without systemic signs b. With systemic signs
Regional lymph nodes (N)	
No	No regional lymph node metastasis
N1	Movable ipsilateral lymph nodes: a. No evidence of lymph node metastasis b. Evidence of lymph node metastasis
N2	Movable contralateral or bilateral lymph nodes: a. No evidence of lymph node metastasis b. Evidence of lymph node metastasis
N3	Fixed lymph nodes
Distant metastasis (M)	
Mo	No distant metastasis
M1	Distant metastasis

11.13 Clinical staging (TNM) of tumours of the oropharynx.
(Data from Owen, 1980)

Diagnostic imaging of the tumour

Intraoral radiography is essential in evaluating bony involvement and treatment planning (Figure 11.14). The radiographic appearance of malignant oral and maxillofacial tumours is variable. However, there is often a mixed appearance of bone lysis and periosteal proliferation. Since radiographic evidence of demineralization may sometimes not be evident until 40% or more bone loss has occurred, radical surgery may still be necessary in the absence of significant bony changes if the tumour type warrants aggressive treatment. When performing radiographs of the head, the most important views for the oral cavity are the intraoral, open-mouth, lateral, dorsoventral and lateral oblique. Intraoral dental radiographs are performed with a size 4 phosphor plate or conventional dental radiographic film.

Since the full extent of caudal mandibular and maxillary tumours may be difficult to assess with dental or head radiography, other modalities are helpful for maxillary, caudal mandibular and pharyngeal masses. Computed tomography (CT) is a diagnostic procedure that utilizes computer-processed X-rays to produce tomographic images or 'slices' of specific areas of the body. CT allows for simultaneous evaluation of bone and soft tissue with a high spatial resolution, high contrast and excellent anatomical detail. Moreover, CT-guided biopsy of deep structures is helpful to obtain a diagnosis. CT is particularly useful in imaging tumours invading the nasal cavity and the retrobulbar space (Figure 11.15). Head and neck CT may show enlargement of the medial retropharyngeal lymph nodes, which may not be evident on clinical examination. CT provides a more sensitive evaluation than thoracic radiography for the detection of small nodule pulmonary metastasis and is also very useful for the assessment of metastatic disease affecting the abdominal organs (Nemanic *et al.*, 2006). Three-dimensional reconstructions can be very helpful for surgical planning.

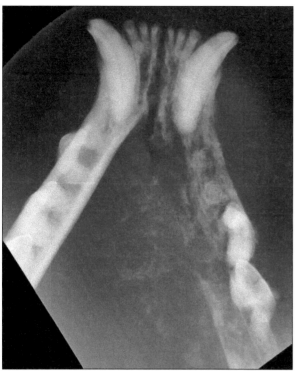

11.14 Intraoral radiograph of a 13-year-old female neutered Domestic Shorthaired cat with a left mandibular squamous cell carcinoma. Note the extensive lysis with minimal bone production. (© Margherita Gracis)

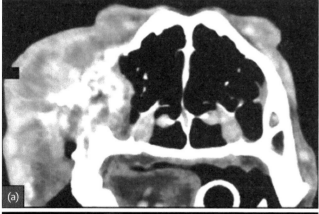

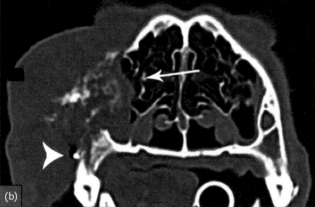

11.15 Computed tomography images obtained via (a) a soft tissue and (b) a bone window of an 8-year-old entire male German Shepherd Dog with a right maxillary osteosarcoma. Note the involvement of the maxilla (arrowhead) and the nasal turbinates (arrowed).

Magnetic resonance imaging (MRI) utilizes a large encircling magnet to create a magnetic field that affects electrons in tissues of the body. MRI allows a high contrast between different tissues with a high spatial resolution, providing very detailed pictures. Evaluation of soft tissue masses with MRI may be very helpful in planning surgical margins. However, since evaluation of bony structures is often important with oral and maxillofacial tumours, CT is usually the advanced diagnostic test of choice in imaging the mouth, face and other structures of the head.

Biopsy

Biopsy is the most important step in the diagnosis and staging of oral and maxillofacial tumours and can be accomplished using cytological or histological methods (Arzi and Verstraete, 2012). Cytopathology and histopathology are complementary, and any inconclusive cytological result must always be confirmed by means of a histological examination (Bonfanti *et al.*, 2015).

Cytology: Cytological samples can be obtained using a fine-needle aspiration (FNA) or a non-aspiration fine-needle (NAFN) technique. When using the FNA technique, the needle, connected to a 5 to 10 ml syringe, is inserted into the lesion, and negative pressure is applied on the syringe to maintain vacuum and aspirate cells into the needle and hub. At the end of the procedure the vacuum is slowly released, the needle extracted from the tumour and detached from the syringe, the syringe is filled with air, the needle reattached, and its content expelled on to a glass slide. When using the NAFN technique, only the needle is held between the thumb, index and middle finger, and it is rapidly and repeatedly inserted into the tumour, at the same time rotating the needle on its axis and redirecting it into the lesion. The needle contents are then sprayed on to a slide after attaching it to an air-filled syringe. To prepare the slide, a second slide is placed on the first and the two are gently pressed and pulled apart in parallel, aiming to obtain a monolayer of intact cells. One should avoid using needles larger than 22 G to obtain a sheet of single cells without excessive haemodilution of the sampled tissue. The FNA technique usually results in samples that are more cellular. It is therefore indicated in very firm and compact lesions that exfoliate poorly. In samples obtained with the NAFN technique, the cells are less traumatized. This technique may be preferred to sample lymph nodes, mucosal, cutaneous and subcutaneous lesions as well as thoracic and abdominal organs in staging oncological patients. More accurate results can be obtained by avoiding aspiration of areas that are necrotic or ulcerated. Similarly, touch preparations or scrapings are often unrewarding due to the heavily contaminated or inflamed ulcerated surface of an oral tumour. Cytological samples should always be obtained by inserting the needle through oral tissue, and not through the cutaneous surface of the lip or cheek, to avoid contamination of unaffected tissues and difficulties during curative-intent surgery.

Histology: A tissue biopsy and histological examination is essential in the diagnostic process of every tumour. It may be a simple but mandatory task, with a few simple rules to follow:

* The best method to acquire a representative sample is a large incisional biopsy using a blade or a large punch (and not a diathermy instrument that can distort the margins of the specimen, making histopathological diagnosis challenging). Areas of necrosis and severe

ulceration should be avoided. Other methods of biopsy (small punch, needle core) may provide only very small samples, and their interpretation can be difficult. If these instruments are used, multiple samples may be necessary to obtain a diagnosis. Grasping instruments (e.g. uterine biopsy forceps, rongeurs) are sometimes helpful to retrieve multiple biopsies from deeper areas of an oral or maxillofacial tumour, including bone and soft tissue structures

- Oral and maxillofacial tumours should be biopsied through the oral cavity and not from the cutaneous surface or the lip to avoid cutaneous contamination and difficulties during curative-intent surgery. Subcutaneous masses of the muzzle may be biopsied through the skin if a representative sample cannot be obtained intraorally; however, care should be taken during incisional biopsy to avoid spreading tumour cells into new sites, making it more difficult to achieve clean margins during future curative-intent surgery
- Small lesions, especially if not involving bone, can be treated with an excisional biopsy, bearing in mind that, if margins are incomplete, a larger revision surgery will be required to obtain complete excision
- Debulking of oral tumours is largely unrewarding, unless the mass is pedunculated and an area of large ulceration can be traded for an area of smaller ulceration by removing the tumour at its narrow base. Sometimes, very large lesions have a narrow base and can be removed with clean margins
- Lesions that can impair swallowing or breathing (e.g. tonsillar and palatal masses) may require prompt excision, prior to obtaining a histopathological diagnosis. A final plan is then made once histopathology is available.

Clinical examination of the regional lymph nodes

Regional lymph nodes (parotid, mandibular and medial retropharyngeal) are palpated to assess consistency, size and mobility. Lymph node enlargement may be the first visible sign associated with the oral mass, especially in the case of tonsillar SCC; however, lymph nodes affected by metastasis are not always enlarged (Williams and Packer, 2003). Medial retropharyngeal lymph node enlargement can be difficult to discern because this lymph node is deeply seated in the neck, caudomedial to the mandibular salivary gland, resulting in lateral displacement of the salivary gland that must not be confused with the node itself. From the mandibular lymph nodes, lymph may flow to the ipsilateral medial retropharyngeal lymph node, or along anastomotic connections to the contralateral medial retropharyngeal node (Belz and Heath, 1995). During the staging process, regional lymph nodes should also be aspirated when possible, since palpation is known to be neither sensitive nor specific in detecting regional lymph node metastasis (Williams and Packer, 2003). While fine-needle aspiration of the mandibular lymph nodes is easily accomplished in most dogs and cats, aspirating the parotid node is difficult or impossible if it is not enlarged. Medial retropharyngeal lymph nodes may be aspirated under sedation or anaesthesia by CT or ultrasound guidance (Figure 11.16).

Thoracic and abdominal radiography, computed tomography and ultrasonography

Thoracic radiographs are a common first step in staging tumours since they can often be obtained in the conscious patient. Taking three views (left and right lateral

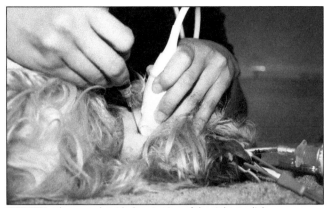

11.16 Ultrasound-guided aspiration of the right medial retropharyngeal lymph node in an 8-year-old neutered female Yorkshire Terrier dog with right mandibular malignant melanoma.
(© John R. Lewis)

and one ventrodorsal or dorsoventral) increases the chances of detection of true metastases compared with two views. Pulmonary metastasis may be seen as a solitary nodule, multiple nodules (Figure 11.17), or a diffuse 'snowstorm' pattern throughout the lung field. Very small lesions, less than 5 mm in diameter, may not be visible on thoracic radiographs and, therefore, 'normal' thoracic radiographs do not completely rule out the possibility of pulmonary metastasis.

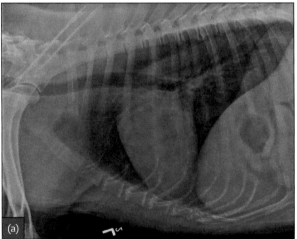

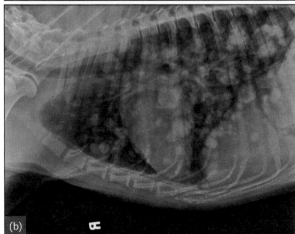

11.17 A 7-year-old neutered female German Shepherd Dog presented with a left mandibular myxosarcoma. (a) Preoperative thoracic radiograph appears to be within normal limits. (b) The patient was presented 3 months after the mandibulectomy due to a decreased appetite. The thoracic radiograph reveals multiple metastatic lesions.
(© John R. Lewis)

CT produces data that can be manipulated through a process known as 'windowing' to demonstrate various bodily structures based on their ability to block the X-ray beam, and has several advantages over traditional radiography. CT avoids the superimposition of structures that lie outside the area of interest. Because of the inherent high-contrast resolution of CT, differences can be distinguished between tissues that differ in physical density by less than 1%. Data from a single CT imaging procedure consisting of either multiple contiguous or one helical scan can be viewed as images in the axial, dorsal or sagittal planes, depending on the diagnostic task. This is referred to as multi-planar reformatted imaging. CT shows high sensitivity and is currently the technique of choice for imaging the thorax (Alexander *et al.*, 2012). The pulmonary parenchyma can be investigated even in the presence of pleural effusion, and metastatic nodules less than 2 mm in diameter may be clearly seen. CT, moreover, allows image-guided biopsy of surgically less accessible areas. The multi-slice CT scanner refers to a special system equipped with a multiple-row detector array to simultaneously collect data at different slice locations. With these newer multi-slice machines it is possible to obtain a total body scan in a few seconds.

Ultrasonography has many benefits and some limitations in staging oncological patients. It is a non-invasive technique, well tolerated and usually does not require the use of sedation or general anaesthesia. It is, moreover, widely available, inexpensive, and allows 'real-time' biopsies for cytological or histological examination to be carried out. Limitations include low specificity, dependence on operator skill and low value for evaluation of most lung lesions where an air interface exists. Ultrasonography has its maximal application in imaging and sampling abdominal lesions, for example hepatic nodules suspected to be metastatic.

Equipment, instruments and materials for surgery

Oral and maxillofacial tumour surgery requires certain instruments and materials in addition to a standard surgical pack:

- An electrosurgery unit (diathermy machine) is helpful, and it must be of adequate power for coagulation and cutting. The mucosal cutaneous incisions must not be made with the monopolar handpiece because it will cause thermal damage to the tissues and result in impaired healing. Incisions made with a cold scalpel undergo faster re-epithelialization. Using electrosurgery near bone can cause bone necrosis. Dehiscence rates of maxillectomy sites were found to be very high when electrosurgery was used (Salisbury *et al.*, 1985)
- Radiosurgery uses radio waves in place of an electric current and is associated with less iatrogenic damage than traditional electrosurgery
- Periosteal elevators of different shapes and sizes to elevate the mucosa from the bone should be available
- Retractors of different sizes and shapes to reflect soft tissue structures should be available
- An osteotome and a mallet may be used to split the mandibular symphysis. These instruments lack the finesse necessary for fine osteotomy and should be used with caution
- Oscillating and sagittal saws are very helpful in oral and maxillofacial tumour surgery, and an ample choice of blades of different length, width and thickness should be available to cut the bone with extreme precision

- A high-speed dental handpiece or electric drill designed for oral and maxillofacial surgery is helpful to cut the bone in very small patients or to perform a variety of maxillectomies and mandibulectomies. Burs for the high-speed dental handpiece include FG type 701, surgical length 702, diamond crown preparation burs, Lindemann burs, and a variety of round carbide and round diamond burs
- A piezoelectric surgical device (piezotome) may also be used to perform precise bone cuts during maxillectomies and mandibulectomies. Key features of piezosurgery include the selective cutting of only mineralized structures without damaging soft tissues (e.g. vessels, nerves or mucosa), which remain undamaged even in the case of accidental contact. It also ensures precise cutting action and at the same time maintains a blood-free site because of the physical phenomenon of cavitation (Vercellotti, 2004)
- Rongeurs of different sizes should be available to smooth rough edges of cut bone. This can also be accomplished using a large round diamond bur on a high-speed dental handpiece
- Sterile saline or lactated Ringer's and a bulb syringe should be available to cool the bone during osteotomy and to wash debris from the wound
- Surgical suction with a fine Frazier tip is helpful to aspirate blood and fluids
- CO_2 and diode lasers may be helpful in certain surgeries to diminish bleeding, such as during tonsillectomy, glossectomy, and removal of palatal masses.

The authors do not recommend using a Gigli saw in oral and maxillofacial surgery.

Client education

Communication is extremely important prior to embarking upon an involved oral or maxillofacial surgical procedure. These involved procedures are not ones that should be entered into lightly due to potential intraoperative and postoperative complications, changes in function, and changes in aesthetic appearance. Effective communication is a two-way street. Input and historical information from the client allows the veterinary surgeon (veterinarian) to make appropriate treatment recommendations, which allow the client to make choices that are right for the pet and family. It is common for the initial consultation to require an hour or more of discussion. What is the biological behaviour of the tumour? What intraoperative complications may occur? What can the client expect in terms of aesthetics, long-term function and quality of life of the pet? What care will be necessary in the immediate postoperative period? Which patients are suboptimal candidates for surgery? What can we expect for life expectancy after the procedure? What is the patient's life expectancy if surgery is not performed?

Perioperative considerations
Biological nature of the tumour

The histopathological appearance of some oral and maxillofacial tumours does not allow for a straightforward diagnosis (e.g. high-low FSA). Without a definitive diagnosis via incisional biopsy, the clinician cannot provide much information about the biological behaviour of the tumour.

Intraoperative complications

Haemorrhage is one of the most common intraoperative complications of oncological oral and maxillofacial surgery due to the ample blood supply of the head. Prior to maxillectomy and mandibulectomy procedures, a patient should be blood-typed. Dogs that have had previous transfusions and cats should receive a cross-match to check for compatibility of available units of packed red cells. Serial packed cell volume/total protein measurements may be done intraoperatively, with the caveat that decreased values may not be immediately apparent after significant blood loss. Other possible intraoperative problems include hypotension due to blood loss or inhalant anaesthesia. If haemorrhage subsides intraoperatively, this may be due to adequate haemostasis, but it may also be due to hypotension, resulting in a false sense of security until the patient becomes normotensive.

Postoperative complications

Dehiscence may occur in 7–33% of maxillectomy cases. Obtaining a tension-free closure and judicious use of cautery appear to be key to minimizing the likelihood of dehiscence. Inadvertent or intended transection of major salivary ducts may result in abnormal accumulation of saliva in the form of a sublingual, pharyngeal or cervical sialocele. Trauma from occlusion may occur to the surgical site if a large tooth in the opposing jaw is impinging upon it. This should be taken into consideration at the time of surgery, with consideration given to crown reduction and vital pulp therapy or extraction as necessary to ensure comfort and appropriate healing. In cases of segmental or total mandibulectomy, mandibular drift of the other mandible will occur towards the side of the surgery and may result in palatal trauma from a remaining mandibular canine tooth. The use of orthodontic buttons and a power chain has been suggested for preventing mandibular drift after mandibulectomy in dogs (Bar-Am and Verstraete, 2010).

Immediate postoperative period

Aggressive surgery warrants multimodal pain therapy, including long-acting nerve blocks, opioids and anti-inflammatory medications. Patients undergoing radical surgery invariably benefit from placement of a fentanyl transdermal patch with injectable opioid supplementation until the patch achieves adequate blood levels. If fentanyl patches are placed preoperatively, care must be taken not to place heating pads directly on the patch to avoid excessive and rapid transdermal drug absorption.

The postoperative period after major oral and maxillofacial resections requires a learning curve for the patient, in particular for the most basic functions such as eating and drinking. Hydration may be maintained with intravenous fluids. Water is offered once the animal has recovered from anaesthesia. Soft food is offered 6–12 hours after surgery and maintained for about 2 weeks. In contrast to cats, dogs that undergo very involved oral and maxillofacial surgeries rarely require placement of a temporary feeding tube if the patient's appetite was good prior to the procedure. Most dogs will eat and drink autonomously within 24 hours after the procedure. Cats require more time to rebound from mandibulectomy or maxillectomy, and due to concerns of hepatic lipidosis an oesophagostomy tube is often placed at the time of radical oral or maxillofacial surgery. This tube may be removed within a few weeks, or once the patient eats and drinks on its own. No hard toys or treats are allowed during this period. An Elizabethan collar may be necessary for 1–2 weeks postoperatively, especially if the resection required skin removal. Custom-made tape muzzles or nylon muzzles may be utilized if they will help to minimize the risk of dehiscence, such as when a commissuroplasty has been performed.

Postoperative antibiotic treatment is not generally required after oral and maxillofacial surgeries in the otherwise healthy patient. Intraoperative antibiotics may be given intravenously (e.g. ampicillin, cefazolin). Broad-spectrum antibiotics (e.g. co-amoxiclav), clindamycin, cefalexin, spiramycin/metronidazole) are given perioperatively in debilitated and immunosuppressed patients and those suffering from organ disease, endocrine disorders, cardiovascular disease, severely contaminated wounds and systemic infections.

Aesthetics and long-term function

Approximately 12% of cats undergoing mandibulectomy may never regain the ability to eat or drink again after surgery, in particular if more than 50% of the mandible is removed (Northrup et al., 2006). Dogs virtually always find a way to become self-sufficient; one exception might be near-total or total glossectomy where, although many dogs adapt, a patient may occasionally require a permanent feeding tube due to difficulty swallowing. Aesthetically, any maxillofacial deformation caused by surgery is less obvious once the hair has grown back. Maxillectomy patients may have a dished-in appearance or enophthalmos if a partial orbitectomy was necessary. Mandibulectomy patients may have mandibular drift, tongue protrusion, drooling and subsequent moist dermatitis. Maintenance or reconstruction of the oral vestibule during wound closure will help to minimize drooling. The quality of life provided by maxillectomy and mandibulectomy procedures is very good in the vast majority of patients.

Decision-making

Unlike in human medicine, the ability to assess histopathological margins of the excised tumour intraoperatively via frozen sections is not usually possible in most veterinary oral and maxillofacial surgery facilities. Therefore, the clinician must use all available information to decide how aggressive one must be to obtain a cure, while maintaining as much function as possible. Each case is different. However, obtaining a definitive diagnosis by means of biopsy is helpful to provide information regarding how much unaffected tissue around the tumour needs to be removed. Removing a tumour with clean margins should be envisioned in three dimensions, which often requires removal of skin in addition to mucosa, teeth and bone. To the authors' knowledge, no studies have been done to assess optimal margins for different tumour types; the authors generally attempt to achieve at least 1 cm margins with acanthomatous ameloblastoma and squamous cell carcinoma. Margins obtained around a malignant melanoma may be variable (usually in the 1–2 cm range) depending on the level of suspicion for an aggressive versus a non-aggressive variant. Sarcomas such as fibrosarcoma and malignant peripheral nerve sheath tumours require the greatest margin of normal tissue to prevent recurrence; the authors often aim to achieve at least 2 cm margins around these tumours.

Expected outcomes

It may not be in the patient's best interest to perform major oral or maxillofacial surgery if there is no chance for a good long-term prognosis, i.e. years rather than months of functional, pain-free living. Therefore, the authors typically recommend aggressive mandibulectomy or maxillectomy procedures only in those patients whose staging shows no metastasis (or where metastatic disease is likely to be well controlled) and whose primary tumour is of a size and location that lends itself to being completely excised with clean margins.

Invasive tumours should not be treated by conservative surgery. Debulking of oral masses is generally unrewarding and may actually cause more morbidity than doing nothing, due to lack of normal healing of tumour tissue. One exception where debulking may be helpful is with pedunculated tumours; debulking these may provide the opportunity to exchange a large area of ulceration, bleeding and secondary infection with a smaller lesion.

Re-examinations are scheduled at 2 weeks (removal of skin sutures) and at 2, 6 and 12 months postoperatively. Collaboration with an oncologist is helpful after results of histological examination of surgical margins are known, to discuss the need for further treatment (surgery, radiation therapy, immunotherapy and/or chemotherapy). Palpation of non-resected regional lymph nodes should be performed frequently (with aspiration and cytological examination or resection and histological examination of enlarged nodes), and thoracic radiographs are repeated at 2, 6 and 12 months to monitor for distant metastasis.

Definitive surgical treatment

Knowledge of tumour type allows for a greater understanding of what kind of resection is necessary. The extent of tumour resection can be categorized as:

- Intralesional/intracapsular: incisional biopsy or a debulking procedure
- Marginal: removal of a tumour within its suspected reactive zone (e.g. removal of a pedunculated peripheral odontogenic fibroma at the level of its most coronal attachment to the gingival margin)
- Wide: removal of the neoplasm including the pseudocapsule, reactive zone, and a small margin (millimetres) of normal tissue (e.g. rim excision of a small acanthomatous ameloblastoma at the dorsal aspect of the mandible)
- Radical: removal of the tumour, pseudocapsule, reactive zone, and a large margin (centimetres) of normal tissue (e.g. from partial to total mandibulectomy/maxillectomy for malignant tumours).

Maxillectomy

Resection techniques depend on size and location of the mass. Partial resection of the rostral upper jaw on one or both sides (rostral maxillectomy or incisivectomy) may be curative for small masses located around the maxillary incisor or canine teeth (Operative Technique 11.1). Resection of a central or caudal portion of the maxilla (central or caudal maxillectomy) is necessary for masses arising in the premolar and molar teeth regions. Resection of the entire dental arch on one side, including the palate to or beyond the midline (right or left total maxillectomy) may be

necessary for large and invasive tumours. For caudally located tumours that extend on to the side of the face, the bones forming the ventral and lateral limits of the orbit (caudal maxilla and zygomatic arch) can be resected via a partial orbitectomy. A combined dorsolateral and intraoral approach has been described for surgery of the caudal maxilla (Lascelles *et al.*, 2003). However, this approach may not be feasible if obtaining clean margins requires removal of skin. When large amounts of skin need to be removed, reconstruction efforts may be necessary in the form of a rotational skin flap or other reconstructive flap. In cats, the relatively small size of the head and limited oral mucosa make radical maxillectomy more challenging in terms of closure and obtaining margins while maintaining function.

Tumour excision

The extent of the margin of apparently normal tissue removed around the tumour will depend on tumour type, but the removal of skin, labial and buccal mucosa, alveolar mucosa, gingiva, palatal mucosa and bone should generally be at least 1 cm away from the gross and radiographic evidence of the tumour. Uninvolved teeth on either side of the desired area of excision may be extracted so that the resected area can be 'tapered' at each end. The mucosa of the upper jaw and palate is incised with a scalpel blade to the bone and reflected with a periosteal elevator to expose the underlying bone. Haemorrhage at palatal incisions is often profuse but can usually be controlled by digital pressure until the resected tissue is lifted out. The use of electrosurgery along the incised mucosal edges is to be avoided due to the high likelihood of postoperative dehiscence (Salisbury *et al.*, 1985).

Once the soft tissues are sufficiently reflected to prevent trauma during osteotomy, the incisive, maxillary and palatine bones are cut along the incision line with a dental bur (surgical 702 or Lindemann bur) on a sterile high-speed dental handpiece, using irrigation with sterile saline or lactated Ringer's solution to minimize thermal damage of tissues. Alternatively, a sagittal/oscillating bone saw or piezotome unit with varying blades may be used. A piezotome unit is very helpful, as it avoids damage to soft tissue structures. The decision of which of these bone-cutting instruments to use depends on the size of the piece of tissue being removed, the adjacent structures, and the degree of finesse needed to avoid collateral damage in a particular area. More than one of these devices may be helpful at different stages of the same procedure. Haemorrhage may be so profuse that continued 'blind' cutting of bone (especially the palatine process of the maxilla) with high-speed equipment might be necessary to allow quick removal and access to deeper bleeding vessels. A large periosteal elevator (such as a Seldin elevator) or large winged dental elevator (size 8) is inserted into bone cutting lines and gently rotated to break any remaining bony attachments while keeping neurovascular bundles still attached for easy ligation and transection. If the line of excision includes the infraorbital canal, its neurovascular bundle is identified and ligated once the resected piece is lifted out. Remaining attachments are separated, and the section is removed *en bloc*. A radiograph is obtained of the wound to ensure complete removal of root remnants as well as the excised piece to provide a sense of whether the resected tissue may be sufficient to obtain adequate bony margins.

Haemorrhage is controlled, and the remaining tissues are examined. If nasal conchae were partially severed or traumatized during the resection, they are cut with curved

Mayo scissors to leave a clean edge. Haemorrhage that cannot be controlled by ligation or pressure may respond to surface application of a mixture (0.05–0.1 ml/kg in cats; 0.1–0.2 ml/kg in dogs) of 0.25 ml phenylephrine 1% and 50 ml lidocaine 2% (Reiter, 2012). Other materials aiding in haemostasis include absorbable gelatin sponges, thrombin in a gelatin matrix, and microporous polysaccharide beads. Unilateral carotid artery ligation should be considered if haemorrhage continues and cannot be controlled.

Wound closure

The defect between the nasal and oral cavities is covered with a flap of labial or buccal mucosa and submucosal connective tissue that is gently undermined until sufficient tissue is available to cover the defect without tension. A two- or three-layer closure is preferred. When possible, a series of small holes is drilled into the bone with a small round carbide bur. These holes allow for tacking of the first layer, the submucosal connective tissue, to the bone adjacent to the defect. The next layer involves apposing connective tissue of the labial/buccal flap to connective tissue of the palatal soft tissue, often in a horizontal mattress pattern, to relieve tension on the epithelial edges. Finally, the mucosa is apposed with absorbable suture in a simple interrupted pattern, spaced 3–4 mm apart. Blood-tinged nasal discharge will be present for several days after surgery, as the nasal tissues heal. Ipsilateral mandibular teeth that could irritate or create tension on the flap may be surgically reduced under sterile conditions with concurrent vital pulp therapy, or they may be extracted. Aesthetically, maxillectomy in most circumstances causes minor maxillofacial abnormality (e.g. visible concavity on the side of the face). If the resection includes the entire incisive bone and one or both canine teeth, the ventral support for the nasal cartilages and nasal plane is lost, and the nose will tip ventrally.

Mandibulectomy

Limits for resection are very wide, including rim excision (marginal mandibulectomy of the dorsal aspect of the mandibular body) (Operative Technique 11.2), unilateral or bilateral rostral mandibulectomy (Operative Technique 11.3), partial mandibular body resection (segmental mandibulectomy), resection of one entire mandible (total mandibulectomy), or resection of one entire mandible and a portion of the contralateral mandible. For more caudally located lesions, the mandibular ramus or a portion of it (e.g. the coronoid process) can be resected by an approach through the zygomatic arch and the masseter muscle. Resection of bilateral rostral mandibular sections to the level of the first or second premolar teeth in dogs and just caudal to the canine teeth in cats, provides good function and very good aesthetic results. Bilateral resections caudal to this level result in progressively greater issues with retention of the tongue and ability to eat and groom. The ability to adapt to such surgeries appears to be species-related, with dogs adapting more readily than cats. Resection of the full length of the mandibular symphysis causes the two remaining mandibular sections to 'float', which is functionally and aesthetically acceptable. New reconstruction and regenerating techniques using internal fixation and a compression resistant matrix infused with recombinant human bone morphogenetic proteins (rhBMP-2) have been described in dogs undergoing segmental and bilateral rostral mandibulectomies (Boudrieau et al., 2004; Lewis et al., 2008; Arzi et al., 2014, 2015).

Tumour excision

The extent and location of the mucosal incisions and possible extraction of additional teeth on either side of the desired area of excision are determined in a similar fashion as for maxillectomies. The labial, buccal, alveolar and sublingual mucosa and the gingiva are incised to the bone with a No. 15 scalpel blade, and the soft tissues are reflected with a periosteal elevator to expose the underlying bone. Haemorrhage can usually be controlled by digital pressure, and identifiable vessels are ligated. The use of electrosurgery along the incised mucosal edges is to be avoided.

The bone is channelled along the resection lines with a dental bur, sagittal/oscillating bone saw or piezotome unit, deep enough to reach near to the mandibular canal (mandibulectomies rostral to the mesial root of the mandibular second premolar tooth will leave the mandibular canal and middle mental foramen unharmed). When cutting through the mandibular body with a bur, the osteotomy is made circumferentially and deep enough to weaken the bone, but not into the mandibular canal. If unilateral resection is performed, the mandibular symphysis can be separated with a scalpel blade in cats or an osteotome and mallet in dogs. The scored piece is separated by inserting and rotating a Seldin elevator or winged dental elevator in the bone groove created by the osteotomy until the remaining bony attachments break. The pieces are separated to allow visualization of the inferior alveolar neurovascular bundle as it crosses to the isolated segment; then the bundle is ligated and transected. A radiograph is obtained of the wound to ensure complete removal of root remnants as well as the excised piece to provide a sense of whether the resected tissue may be sufficient to obtain adequate bony margins. Rough edges of bone are burred smooth, and the connective tissue is sutured to decrease dead space (holes in the bone can be created here for tacking of soft tissue), followed by suturing the labial/buccal and sublingual mucosal edges across the remaining mandible. Skin may need to be removed to improve closure of bilateral rostral mandibulectomies or to ensure margins in all directions. Adjacent skin can be undermined, advanced and rotated into the area as needed to close the wound.

Right or left total mandibulectomy (previously mistakenly termed hemimandibulectomy, even though there are no hemimandibles in dogs and cats) gives a greater likelihood of complete resection of vascular and perineural invasion within bone. The skin overlying the ventrolateral aspect of the mandible is often removed to ensure margins in every dimension. Intermandibular musculature (mylohyoideus and geniohyoideus muscles) is transected as needed. The mandibular symphysis is separated with a scalpel blade or osteotome and mallet. Incisions are made well away from the tumour in the gingiva, alveolar, sublingual, labial and buccal mucosa (or skin lateral to the vestibular (i.e. labial/buccal) mucosa). The attachments of the tongue (genioglossus and hyoglossus muscles) are separated, leaving the mandibular and sublingual gland ducts intact if they can be identified and are beyond the proposed margins of removal. These salivary ducts can be transected and ligated if necessary to obtain adequate margins. The attachment of the digastricus muscle at the ventral margin of the mandible is incised. The mandible can then be swung laterally, which facilitates dissection of the masseter, medial and lateral pterygoid and temporal muscles from their attachments, exposing the mandibular ramus. The inferior alveolar neurovascular bundle enters the mandibular canal through the mandibular foramen located on the medial surface of the caudal aspect of the mandible and is hidden beneath the rostral attachments of the medial pterygoid muscle, which must be dissected carefully to avoid transecting the bundle accidentally; the bundle is then ligated and transected. The temporomandibular joint capsule and lateral ligament are exposed, and the capsule is incised. The remaining medial and lateral pterygoid muscle attachments on the angular and condylar processes and the temporal muscle attachments on the rostral and dorsal edges of the coronoid process are dissected free and cut with scissors, and the mandible is lifted out.

Wound closure

The incision is closed with absorbable sutures, apposing connective tissue, incised oral mucosal edges and the skin. If skin overlying the mandible was removed, the incised edge of skin is attached to the incised edge of the upper lip.

When a large amount of mandible is removed from one side, the tongue will deviate to this side, resulting in drooling and chronic dermatitis. This can be partially corrected by rostral advancement of the lip commissure on one or both sides to create support for the tongue. Commissuroplasty is performed by incising the mucocutaneous junction of the upper and lower lips rostrally to the level of the maxillary second premolar tooth. The mucosa at the incised edges of the upper and lower lips is sutured, followed by suturing of the skin. Because the rostral portion of the commissuroplasty may dehisce if the patient is allowed to excessively open its mouth during the immediate postoperative period, a loose custom-made tape or nylon muzzle should be kept in place for 2–4 weeks after surgery. Tension-relieving suture techniques may also be helpful. After total mandibulectomy, the remaining mandible will drift towards the midline, which may result in palatal trauma from the mandibular canine tooth when the mouth is closed. To prevent this, the tooth is extracted (better before mandibulectomy is performed, to reduce the risk of fracturing the remaining rostral mandibular bone during exodontics) or its crown surgically reduced under sterile conditions with concurrent vital pulp therapy or standard root canal therapy. Elastic training may also be utilized to reduce mandibular drift and traumatic malocclusion (Bar-Am and Verstraete, 2010).

Glossectomy

Lingual tumours may be resected with good results if the resection can be confined to the rostral or middle portions of the tongue. Partial surgical resection is likely to result in significant haemorrhage. Clamping the tongue caudal to the excision site with non-crushing Doyen intestinal forceps aids in control of bleeding, but to avoid excessive trauma to remaining tissue, it should be considered that only the tips of the forceps are non-crushing. Ideally, tongue tissue is removed as a wedge so that muscle and mucosa can be apposed with absorbable sutures. Malignant lesions located deep in the root of the tongue or causing the tongue to be immovable are not amenable to resection. Similar to mandibulectomies, cats are likely to adapt more poorly to glossectomy procedures than dogs. A recent retrospective study in dogs showed a 28% recurrence rate in dogs undergoing glossectomy. Procedures ranged from marginal to near-total glossectomy (Culp *et al.*, 2013).

Radical lip and cheek resection

Surgical principles for resection of malignant tumours of the lip and cheek include maintenance of a functional lip commissure so that the mouth can open adequately, separate closure of the incisions in the mucosa and the skin when the resection is full-thickness, avoidance of the parotid and zygomatic salivary ducts when possible or ligation or transposition of ducts when avoidance is not possible, and cosmetic closure of any resulting maxillofacial defect by advancing or rotating tissue from the lower lip and the side of the face, head or neck (Pope, 2006). Facial nerve damage may occur when surgery of the cheek is necessary, due to the location of the dorsal and ventral buccal branches of this nerve.

Regional lymph node resection

Right and left mandibular and medial retropharyngeal lymph nodes may be removed concomitantly through a single ventral midline incision (Green and Boston, 2015). Mandibular, parotid and retropharyngeal lymph nodes can also be unilaterally removed using a single-incision approach without any described negative side effects (Smith, 1995). The parotid node is usually positioned under the rostral border of the parotid gland, on the caudal aspect of the zygomatic arch. A second node may be present and, rarely, a third. The mandibular lymph centre consists of a group of two to five nodes located caudoventral to the angular process of the mandible and rostral to the mandibular salivary gland. The medial retropharyngeal node is the largest node of the head and neck area and lies deep between the muscles of the neck, caudomedial to the mandibular salivary gland.

Lymphadenectomy is not proven to increase survival time or cure rates with oral and maxillofacial tumours in dogs and cats. Therefore, removal of lymph nodes should be considered a tool for complete staging. Lymph node resection is particularly useful in the evaluation of the parotid and medial retropharyngeal nodes, which are considered difficult to sample cytologically without ultrasound or CT guidance. Assessment of all regional lymph nodes in dogs and cats with oral or maxillofacial neoplasms will detect more metastatic disease than assessing the mandibular lymph nodes only (Herring *et al.*, 2002).

Non-surgical treatment modalities

Radiation therapy

Radiation therapy can be categorized as either palliative or full-course treatment. Palliative radiation generally involves fewer treatments with higher doses per treatment, whereas full-course treatment consists of a series of more frequent treatments with a smaller fraction of radiation per treatment. High-dose fractions are more likely to result in long-term radiation side effects, thus palliative radiation should be reserved for patients who are likely to succumb to the tumour before long-term radiation side effects occur. Aggressive oral and maxillofacial tumours are usually not cured by radiation therapy alone, but radiation does play an important role in controlling microscopic disease, and in some cases (such as with odontogenic tumours) radiation can provide a high rate of clinical success as standalone therapy.

Over 90% of acanthomatous ameloblastomas responded to radiation therapy in one study (Thrall, 1984). Median survival time for patients with acanthomatous ameloblastoma treated with orthovoltage radiation therapy was 37 months, with recurrence seen in 3 of 39 dogs (Thrall, 1984). Malignant tumour formation at the site of radiation therapy was seen in 18% of the patients in this study, but a more recent study suggests that the chance of malignant tumour formation following megavoltage radiation therapy is much less common (3.5%) (McEntee, 2004). Use of radiation therapy to shrink oral tumours prior to surgery is controversial due to the concern of lack of postoperative healing and late complications. Whenever possible, the authors prefer to perform surgery in the non-irradiated patient, followed by radiation therapy to treat microscopic disease if necessary. Radiation of oral malignant melanomas resulted in median survival times for dogs with stage I, II, III and IV lesions of 758, 278, 163 and 80 days, respectively, with a significant difference in survival times between stage I and other stages in one study (Kawabe et al., 2015). In another report, a combination of surgery and radiation therapy in dogs with oral fibrosarcomas resulted in a median survival time of 505 days and progression-free survival of 301 days (Gardner et al., 2015).

Immunotherapy

Immunotherapy represents a promising approach, allowing the body's immune system to fight its own cancer (Bergman, 2014). An example of immunotherapy is the human tyrosinase vaccine commercially available for dogs with malignant melanoma. By targeting tyrosinase, an enzyme essential to melanin synthesis, this plasmid DNA vaccine provides an immunotherapy specific to melanocytes. One study evaluated survival times of dogs with stage II and III oral malignant melanomas that were surgically excised for local tumour control. Results showed survival time until death attributable to malignant melanoma was significantly improved for dogs that received the human tyrosinase vaccine, compared with that of historical controls (Grosenbaugh et al., 2011). A more recent study evaluated the efficacy of a human chondroitin sulfate proteoglycan-4 (CSPG4) DNA-based vaccine administered by electroporation in dogs with stage II–III disease after surgical resection of CSPG4-positive oral malignant melanomas, resulting in significantly longer overall and disease-free survival times in vaccinated compared with non-vaccinated dogs (Riccardo et al., 2014).

Chemotherapy

The role of chemotherapy is limited in the treatment of oral and maxillofacial tumours. Systemic medical therapy is often pursued for oral manifestations of cutaneous T-cell lymphoma (mycosis fungoides). Intralesional bleomycin therapy has been described in two reports for treatment of acanthomatous ameloblastoma with good results in limited numbers of patients (Yoshida et al., 1998; Kelly et al., 2010). Bone exposure at the site of the tumour was noted in four of seven dogs in one of the studies (Kelly et al., 2010). An example of success with chemotherapy is seen in the treatment of canine tonsillar SCC, where piroxicam and carboplatin resulted in complete regression of the tumour and prevention of the need for further surgery in four of seven dogs in one study (de Vos et al., 2005). Electrochemogene therapy shows promise as a possible future therapy (Reed et al., 2010).

Multimodal therapeutic approach

Oral and maxillofacial tumours can also be treated combining surgery, radiotherapy, chemotherapy and new therapies using tyrosine kinase inhibitors and anti-angiogenic drugs. This is especially true for tumours considered resistant to radiation therapy alone or considered not amenable to surgical resection, such as fibrosarcoma or feline SCC. A study of oral malignant melanoma in dogs, however, found no significant improvement in survival time with systemic adjuvant therapy (e.g. radiation therapy, various chemotherapeutic regimens, or immunotherapy) (Boston et al., 2014).

A recent study evaluated the survival of six cats with oral SCC in different locations following multimodal therapy (medical treatment with piroxicam, thalidomide and bleomycin plus radiation therapy and surgery); three patients with sublingual SCC were alive and in complete remission after 759, 458 and 362 days, when data analysis ceased (Marconato et al., 2013). Radiosensitization may improve response to radiation therapy, but gemcitabine is not recommended in cats due to haematological toxicity.

Following successful surgery of the oral or maxillofacial tumour, 'adjuvant' therapy is given to prevent local recurrence or the development of metastasis. Adjuvant therapy may include chemotherapy, radiation therapy, targeted therapy or biological therapy. In contrast, 'neoadjuvant' therapy serves to shrink a tumour before its definitive treatment (usually surgery). Examples of neoadjuvant therapy include chemotherapy and radiation therapy.

References and further reading

Alexander K, Joly H, Blond L et al. (2012) A comparison of computed tomography, computed radiography and film-screen radiography for the detection of canine pulmonary nodules. Veterinary Radiology and Ultrasound 53, 258–265

Arzi B, Cissell DD, Pollard RE et al. (2015) Regenerative approach to bilateral rostral mandibular reconstruction in a case series of dogs. Frontiers in Veterinary Science, Veterinary Dentistry and Oromaxillofacial Surgery 2, 1–7

Arzi B and Verstraete FJM (2012) Clinical staging and biopsy of maxillofacial tumors. In: Oral and Maxillofacial Surgery in Dogs and Cats, ed. FJM Verstraete and MJ Lommer, pp. 373–486. Saunders Elsevier, Edinburgh

Arzi B, Verstraete FJM, Huey DJ et al. (2014) Regenerating mandibular bone using rhBMP-2: Part 1 – Immediate reconstruction of segmental mandibulectomies. Veterinary Surgery 44, 403–409

Bar-Am Y and Verstraete FJM (2010) Elastic training for the prevention of mandibular drift following mandibulectomy in dogs: 18 cases (2005–2008). Veterinary Surgery 39, 574–580

Beatty JA, Charles JA, Malik R et al. (2000) Feline inductive odontogenic tumour in a Burmese cat. Australian Veterinary Journal 78, 452–455

Belz GT and Heath TJ (1995) Lymph pathways of the medial retropharyngeal lymph node in dogs. Journal of Anatomy 186, 517–526

Bergman PJ (2014) Immunotherapy in veterinary oncology. Veterinary Clinics of North America: Small Animal Practice 44, 925–939

Bertone ER, Snyder LA and Moore AS (2003) Environmental and lifestyle risk factors for oral squamous cell carcinoma in domestic cats. Journal of Veterinary Internal Medicine 17, 557–562

Bonfanti U, Bertazzolo W, Gracis M et al. (2015) Diagnostic value of cytological analysis of tumours and tumour-like lesions of the oral cavity in dogs and cats: a prospective study on 114 cases. Veterinary Journal 205, 322–327

Boston SE, Lu X, Culp WT et al. (2014) Efficacy of systemic adjuvant therapies administered to dogs after excision of oral malignant melanomas: 151 cases (2001–2012). Journal of the American Veterinary Medical Association 245, 401–407

Boudrieau RJ, Mitchell SL and Seeherman H (2004) Mandibular reconstruction of a partial hemimandibulectomy in a dog with severe malocclusion. Veterinary Surgery 33, 119–130

Ciekot PA, Powers BE, Withrow SJ et al. (1994) Histologically low-grade, yet biologically high-grade, fibrosarcomas of the mandible and maxilla in dogs: 25 cases (1982–1991). Journal of the American Veterinary Medical Association 204, 610–615

Colgin MA, Schulman FY and Dubielzig RR (2001) Multiple epulides in 13 cats. Veterinary Pathology 38, 227–229

Coyle VJ, Rassnick KM, Borst LB et al. (2015) Biological behaviour of canine mandibular osteosarcoma. A retrospective study of 50 cases (1999–2007). Veterinary and Comparative Oncology 13, 89–97

Culp WT, Ehrhart N, Withrow SJ et al. (2013) Results of surgical excision and evaluation of factors associated with survival time in dogs with lingual neoplasia: 97 cases (1995–2008). Journal of the American Veterinary Medical Association 242, 1392–1397

de Vos JP, Burm AG, Focker AP et al. (2005) Piroxicam and carboplatin as a combination treatment of canine oral non-tonsillar squamous cell carcinoma: a pilot study and literature review of a canine model of human head and neck squamous cell carcinoma. Veterinary Comparative Oncology 3, 16–24

Dernell WS, Straw RC, Cooper MF et al. (1998) Multilobular osteochondrosarcoma in 39 dogs: 1979–1993. Journal of the American Animal Hospital Association 34, 11–18

Desoutter AV, Goldschmidt MH and Sánchez MD (2012) Clinical and histologic features of 26 canine peripheral giant cell granulomas (formerly giant cell epulis). Veterinary Pathology 49, 1018–1023

Dhaliwal RS and Tang KN (2005) Parathyroid hormone-related peptide and hypercalcaemia in a dog with functional keratinizing ameloblastoma. Veterinary Comparative Oncology 3, 98–100

Elliott JW, Cripps P, Blackwood L et al. (2013) Canine oral mucosal mast cell tumours. Veterinary and Comparative Oncology 14, 101–111

Esplin DG (2008) Survival of dogs following surgical excision of histologically well-differentiated melanocytic neoplasms of the mucous membranes of the lips and oral cavity. Veterinary Pathology 45, 889–896

Farcas N, Arzi B and Verstraete FJ (2014) Oral and maxillofacial osteosarcoma in dogs: a review. Veterinary and Comparative Oncology 12, 169–180

Fiani N, Arzi B, Johnson EG et al. (2011) Osteoma of the oral and maxillofacial regions in cats: seven cases (1999–2009). Journal of the American Veterinary Medical Association 238, 1470–1475

Fiani N, Verstraete FJ, Kass PH et al. (2011) Clinicopathologic characterization of odontogenic tumors and focal fibrous hyperplasia in dogs: 152 cases (1995–2005). Journal of the American Veterinary Medical Association 238, 495–500

Frazier SA, Johns SM, Ortega J et al. (2012) Outcome in dogs with surgically resected oral fibrosarcoma (1997–2008). Veterinary and Comparative Oncology 10, 33–43

Gardner DG and Dubielzig RR (1995) Feline inductive odontogenic tumor (inductive fibroameloblastoma) – a tumor unique to cats. Journal of Oral Pathology and Medicine 24, 185–190

Gardner H, Fidel J, Haldorson G et al. (2015) Canine oral fibrosarcomas: a retrospective analysis of 65 cases (1998–2010). Veterinary and Comparative Oncology 13, 40–47

Gendler A, Lewis JR, Reetz JA et al. (2010) Computed tomographic features of oral squamous cell carcinoma in cats: 18 cases (2002–2008). Journal of the American Veterinary Medical Association 236, 319–325

Goldschmidt SL, Bell CM, Hetzel S et al. (2017) Clinical characterization of canine acanthomatous ameloblastoma (CAA) in 263 dogs and the influence of postsurgical histopathological margin on local recurrence. Journal of Veterinary Dentistry 34, 241–247

Green K and Boston SE (2015) Bilateral removal of mandibular and medial retropharyngeal lymph nodes through a single ventral midline incision for staging of head and neck cancers in dogs: a description of surgical technique. Veterinary and Comparative Oncology doi: 10.1111/vco.12154

Grosenbaugh DA, Leard AT, Bergman PJ et al. (2011) Safety and efficacy of a xenogeneic DNA vaccine encoding for human tyrosinase as adjunctive treatment for oral malignant melanoma in dogs following surgical excision of the primary tumor. American Journal of Veterinary Research 72, 1631–1638

Herring ES, Smith MM and Robertson JL (2002) Lymph node staging of oral and maxillofacial neoplasms in 31 dogs and cats. Journal of Veterinary Dentistry 19, 122–126

Hillman LA, Garrett LD, de Lorimier LP et al. (2010) Biological behavior of oral and perioral mast cell tumors in dogs: 44 cases (1996–2006). Journal of the American Veterinary Medical Association 237, 936–942

Kawabe M, Mori T, Ito Y et al. (2015) Outcomes of dogs undergoing radiotherapy for treatment of oral malignant melanoma: 111 cases (2006–2012). Journal of the American Veterinary Medical Association 247, 1146–1153

Kelly JM, Belding BA and Schaefer AK (2010) Acanthomatous ameloblastoma in dogs treated with intralesional bleomycin. Veterinary and Comparative Oncology 8, 81–86

Knaake FAC and Verhaert L (2010) Histopathology and treatment of nine cats with multiple epulides. Vlaams Diergeneeskundig Tijdschrift 79, 48–53

Lascelles BD, Thomson MJ, Dernell WS et al. (2003) Combined dorsolateral and intraoral approach for the resection of tumors of the maxilla in the dog. Journal of the American Animal Hospital Association 39, 294–305

Lewis JR, Boudrieau RJ, Reiter AM et al. (2008) Mandibular reconstruction after gunshot trauma in a dog using recombinant human bone morphogenetic protein-2. Journal of the American Veterinary Medical Association 233, 1598–1604

Liptak JM and Withrow SJ (2010) Oral tumors. In: Small Animal Clinical Oncology, 4th edn, ed. SJ Withrow and DM Vail, pp. 455–475. Saunders Elsevier, Edinburgh

Marconato L, Buchholz J, Keller M et al. (2013) Multimodal therapeutic approach and interdisciplinary challenge for the treatment of unresectable head and neck squamous cell carcinoma in six cats: a pilot study. Veterinary and Comparative Oncology 11, 101–112

Mas A, Blackwood L, Cripps P et al. (2011) Canine tonsillar squamous cell carcinoma – a multi-centre retrospective review of 44 clinical cases. Journal of Small Animal Practice 52, 359–364

McEntee MC, Page RL, Théon A et al. (2004) Malignant tumor formation in dogs previously irradiated for acanthomatous epulis. Veterinary Radiology and Ultrasound 45, 357–361

Moore AS, Wood CA, Engler SJ et al. (2000) Radiation therapy for long-term control of odontogenic tumours and epulis in three cats. Journal of Feline Medicine and Surgery 2, 57–60

Nemanic S, London CA and Wisner ER (2006) Comparison of thoracic radiographs and single breath-hold helical CT for detection of pulmonary nodules in dogs with metastatic neoplasia. Journal of Veterinary Internal Medicine 20, 508–515

Nemec A, Murphy BG, Jordan RC et al. (2014) Oral papillary squamous cell carcinoma in twelve dogs. Journal of Comparative Pathology 150, 155–161

Northrup NC, Selting KA, Rassnick KM et al. (2006) Outcomes of cats with oral tumors treated with mandibulectomy: 42 cases. Journal of the American Animal Hospital Association 42, 350–360

Owen LN (1980) TNM Classification of Tumors in Domestic Animals, 1st edn. World Health Organisation, Geneva

Pope ER (2006) Head and facial wounds in dogs and cats. Veterinary Clinics of North America: Small Animal Practice 36, 793–817

Ramos-Vara JA, Beissenherz ME, Miller MA et al. (2000) Retrospective study of 338 canine oral melanomas with clinical, histologic, and immunohistochemical review of 129 cases. Veterinary Pathology 37, 597–608

Ramos-Vara JA and Miller MA (2011) Immunohistochemical identification of canine melanocytic neoplasms with antibodies to melanocytic antigen PNL2 and tyrosinase: comparison with Melan A. Veterinary Pathology 48, 443–450

Reed SD, Fulmer A, Buckholz J et al. (2010) Bleomycin/interleukin-12 electrochemogene therapy for treating naturally occurring spontaneous neoplasms in dogs. Cancer Gene Therapy 17, 457–464

Reiter AM (2002) Hypercalcaemia in dogs with acanthomatous epulides – case report and retrospective study on 59 cases (1986–2002). Proceedings of the 16th Annual Veterinary Dental Forum, Savannah, GA, USA. pp. 107–110

Reiter AM (2012) Dental and oral diseases. In: The Cat: Clinical Medicine and Management, 1st edn, ed. SE Little, pp. 329–370. Saunders, St Louis

Riccardo F, Iussich S, Maniscalco L et al. (2014) CSPG4-specific immunity and survival prolongation in dogs with oral malignant melanoma immunized with human CSPG4 DNA. Clinical Cancer Research 20, 3756–3762

Salisbury SK, Thacker HL, Pantzer EE et al. (1985) Partial maxillectomy in the dog. Comparison of suture material and closure techniques. Veterinary Surgery 14, 265–276

Smith MM (1995) Surgical approach for lymph node staging of oral and maxillofacial neoplasms in dogs. Journal of the American Animal Hospital Association 31, 514–518

Smithson CW, Smith MM, Tappe J et al. (2012) Multicentric oral plasmacytoma in three dogs. Journal of Veterinary Dentistry 29, 96–110

Snyder LA, Bertone ER, Jakowski RM et al. (2004) p53 expression and environmental tobacco smoke exposure in feline oral squamous cell carcinoma. Veterinary Pathology 41, 209–214

Soltero-Rivera MM, Engiles JB, Reiter AM et al. (2015) Benign and malignant proliferative fibro-osseous and osseous lesions of the oral cavity of dogs. Veterinary Pathology 52, 894–902

Soltero-Rivera MM, Krick EL, Reiter AM et al. (2014) Prevalence of regional and distant metastasis in cats with advanced oral squamous cell carcinoma: 49 cases (2005–2011). Journal of Feline Medicine and Surgery 16, 164–169

Soukup JW, Snyder CJ, Simmons BT et al. (2013) Clinical, histologic and computed tomographic features of oral papillary squamous cell carcinoma in dogs: nine cases (2008–2011). Journal of Veterinary Dentistry 30, 18–24

Stebbins KE, Morse CC and Goldschmidt MH (1989) Feline oral neoplasia: a ten-year survey. Veterinary Pathology 26, 121–128

Thrall DE (1984) Orthovoltage radiotherapy of acanthomatous epulides in 39 dogs. Journal of the American Veterinary Medical Association 184, 826–829

Tuohy JL, Selmic LE, Worley DR et al. (2014) Outcome following curative-intent surgery for oral melanomas in dogs: 70 cases (1998–2011). Journal of the American Veterinary Medical Association 245, 1266–1273

Vercellotti T (2004) Technological characteristics and clinical indications of piezoelectric bone surgery. Minerva Stomatologica 53, 207–214

Walker KS, Lewis JR, Durham AC et al. (2009) Diagnostic imaging in veterinary dental practice. Odontoma and impacted premolar. Journal of the American Veterinary Medical Association 235, 1279–1281

Williams LA and Packer RA (2003) Association between lymph node size and metastasis in dogs with oral malignant melanoma: 100 cases (1987–2001). Journal of the American Veterinary Medical Association 222, 1234–1236

Wright ZM and Chretin JD (2006) Diagnosis and treatment of a feline oral mast cell tumor. Journal of Feline Medicine and Surgery 8, 285–289

Wright ZM, Rogers KS and Mansell J (2008) Survival data for canine oral extramedullary plasmacytomas: a retrospective analysis (1996–2006). Journal of the American Animal Hospital Association 44, 75–81

Yoshida K, Watarai Y, Sakai Y et al. (1998) The effect of intralesional bleomycin on canine acanthomatous epulis. Journal of the American Animal Hospital Association 34, 457–461

OPERATIVE TECHNIQUE 11.1

Unilateral rostral maxillectomy

INDICATIONS

Unilateral rostral maxillectomy may be chosen as a curative-intent surgery for small, lateralized masses where diagnostic imaging and histotype suggest a unilateral approach to be sufficient.

POSITIONING

Lateral or dorsal recumbency.

ASSISTANT

Necessary.

ADDITIONAL EQUIPMENT

High-speed dental drill; cross-cut fissure surgical length bur; small round carbide bur; periosteal elevators of various sizes; No. 15 scalpel blades; winged dental elevators; Seldin elevator; large round diamond bur; cooling solutions.

SURGICAL TECHNIQUE

Approach

Gingiva, alveolar, labial and palatal mucosa, bone, teeth ± nasal conchae are removed *en bloc* from the rostral upper jaw with an intraoral approach to allow for removal of the tumour with clean margins. Images shown in this operative technique were obtained from a cadaver specimen. In a clinical patient, the hair should be adequately clipped, the skin prepared for aseptic surgery, and the surgical site draped.

Surgical manipulations

1   Margins are pre-measured, and a sterile marking pen is used to guide the line of cut. The arch of cut is semicircular on the labial and palatal aspects of the gingival mass.

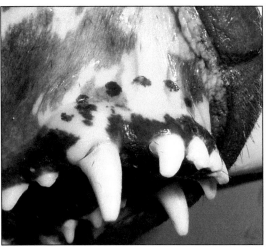
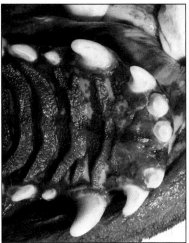

(© John R. Lewis)

→ **OPERATIVE TECHNIQUE 11.1 CONTINUED**

2 A No. 15 scalpel blade is used to incise through gingiva, alveolar and labial mucosa, and submucosa of the rostrolateral upper jaw to expose the bone. Edges of the incised soft tissues may be lifted with a periosteal elevator, and the soft tissues retracted with 1–2 sutures or an appropriate instrument prior to performing osteotomy.

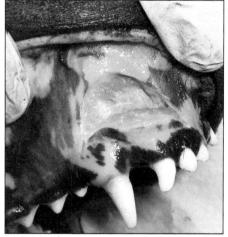

(© John R. Lewis)

3 A cross-cut fissure surgical length bur is used to perform osteotomy on the labial surface, full-thickness through the root of the canine tooth and a less deep score line elsewhere. Sterile saline or lactated Ringer's solution is used to cool the bur. There is potential risk of tumour invasion along the periodontal ligament space. Thus, the entire tooth is ideally removed in one piece together with a malignant tumour. However, it may be decided on a case-by-case basis whether the piece resected should contain entire teeth or one can cut through teeth at sufficient distance from the tumour margins.

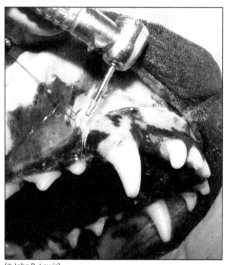

(© John R. Lewis)

4 The palatal mucosa is incised with a No. 15 blade and is lifted and retracted to expose the bone. Significant bleeding will occur from the diffuse venous plexus of the palatal soft tissues. Digital pressure over the major palatine artery caudal to the incision will decrease blood loss. Significantly bleeding vessels may be ligated. Avoid use of electrosurgery, radiosurgery or laser on cut edges of mucosa.

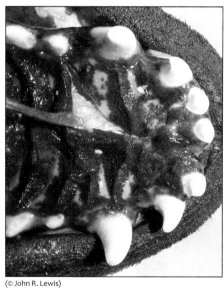

(© John R. Lewis)

→ **OPERATIVE TECHNIQUE 11.1 CONTINUED**

5   A cross-cut fissure surgical length bur is used to cut full-thickness through the incisive bone and maxilla and their palatine processes. Sterile saline or lactated Ringer's solution is used to cool the bur.

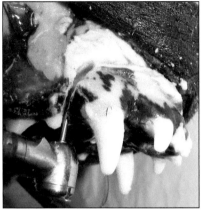

(© John R. Lewis)

6   A winged dental elevator or Seldin elevator is placed in the score line and the piece is lifted *en bloc* from the surgery site by breaking any remaining bony attachments. If the piece is still too attached to remove, the score lines are made deeper until it can be gently removed. Any vessels attached to the dislodged piece are ligated with absorbable monofilament suture material and transected.

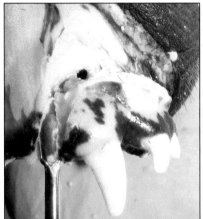

(© John R. Lewis)

7   Dental radiographs are taken of the excised piece and the wound to assess bony margins and visualize retained roots or crown-root segments that may require extraction. The bony edges are made smooth with a large round diamond bur prior to wound closure.

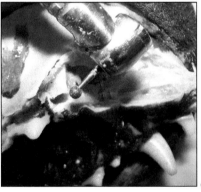

(© John R. Lewis)

8   The mucosa and submucosal tissues of the rostral upper lip are undermined dorsally with a combination of blunt and sharp dissection towards the mucocutaneous junction to allow for a tension-free closure. One or two releasing incisions may be necessary to allow for a tension-free mucoperiosteal flap.

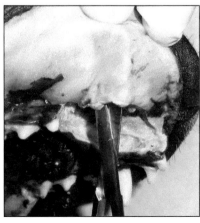

(© John R. Lewis)

→ **OPERATIVE TECHNIQUE 11.1 CONTINUED**

9 Holes may be drilled in the bone adjacent to the wound (being careful not to damage remaining teeth) with a small round carbide bur to allow for 2 metric (3/0 USP) absorbable tacking suture placement, thus minimizing dead space and tension on the mucosal suture line.

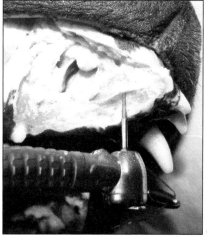
(© John R. Lewis)

The submucosal tissues are closed with 2 metric (3/0 USP) or 1.5 metric (4/0 USP) absorbable monofilament suture material in a simple interrupted or horizontal mattress pattern. The mucosa is closed with 1.5 metric (4/0 USP) absorbable monofilament suture material in a simple interrupted pattern.

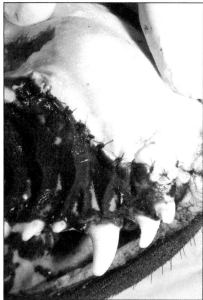
(© John R. Lewis)

PRACTICAL TIP

- Having blood products available is important for major oral and maxillofacial surgical procedures, particularly maxillectomies

POSTOPERATIVE CARE

Use of an Elizabethan collar and soft food for 2 weeks, with no access to hard toys or treats. Expect some serosanguineous oral and nasal discharge for a few days postoperatively.

OPERATIVE TECHNIQUE 11.2

Mandibular rim excision (dorsal marginal mandibulectomy)

Mandibular rim excision, also known as dorsal marginal mandibulectomy, is a procedure reserved for small, dorsally located tumours of the lower jaw that require 1 cm or less of normal tissue margins for a surgical cure. The size of the patient plays a role in determining if this technique will result in a functional mandible or one that will be prone to future jaw fracture due to minimal remaining bone. In small patients, a segmental mandibulectomy may be advisable rather than a mandibular rim excision.

POSITIONING

Lateral recumbency.

ASSISTANT

Optional.

ADDITIONAL EQUIPMENT

High-speed dental drill; cross-cut fissure surgical length bur; small round carbide bur; periosteal elevators of varied sizes; No. 15 scalpel blades; winged dental elevators; Seldin elevator; large round diamond bur; cooling solutions.

SURGICAL TECHNIQUE

Approach

Gingiva, alveolar and buccal mucosa, submucosal tissue, teeth and bone are removed from the dorsal aspect of the mandible with an intraoral semilunar incision to allow for removal of the tumour with clean margins. Most images shown in this operative technique were obtained from a cadaver specimen; some are from a clinical patient. In a clinical patient, the hair should be adequately clipped, the skin prepared for aseptic surgery, and the surgical site draped.

Surgical manipulations

1   Margins of 1 cm are measured, and a sterile marking pen is used to guide the line of cut. The arch of cut is semilunar and gradual rather than rectangular or steep. A No. 15 scalpel blade is used to incise gingiva, alveolar and buccal mucosa, and submucosa of the mandibular body to expose the underlying bone, both on the buccal and the lingual sides.

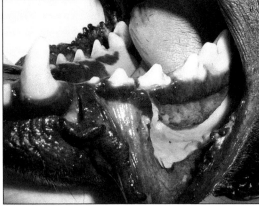
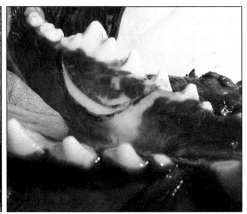

(© John R. Lewis)

→ **OPERATIVE TECHNIQUE 11.2 CONTINUED**

2 Edges of the incised mucosa may be lifted slightly with a periosteal elevator, and sutures can be placed to retract the soft tissue dorsally prior to performing the osteotomy.

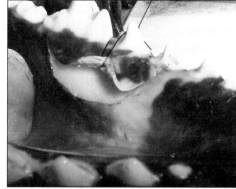
(© John R. Lewis)

3 A cross-cut fissure surgical length bur is used to perform osteotomies on the lingual and buccal portion of the mandible, beginning with full-thickness cuts on the rostrodorsal and caudodorsal surfaces of the mandible. Sterile saline or lactated Ringer's solution is used to cool the bur.

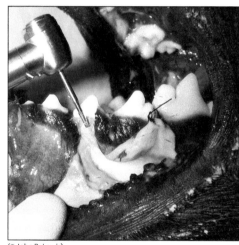
(© John R. Lewis)

4 As the bur follows the arch ventrally, a partial-thickness score line is created to match up with the full-thickness bone cuts rostrally and caudally. Care should be taken to avoid damage to the adjacent soft tissues and the inferior alveolar neurovascular bundle in the mandibular canal.

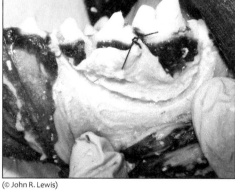
(© John R. Lewis)

5 A winged dental elevator or Seldin elevator is placed in the score line, and the piece is carefully lifted (broken away) *en bloc* from the remaining intact mandible. If the piece is still too attached to remove, the score lines are made deeper until the piece can be gently detached from the mandible while avoiding an iatrogenic mandibular body fracture.

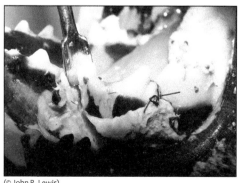
(© John R. Lewis)

→

→ **OPERATIVE TECHNIQUE 11.2 CONTINUED**

6 Dental radiographs are taken of the excised piece and the wound to assess bony margins and visualize retained roots or crown-root segments that may require removal. The teeth included in the ostectomy are ideally removed in one piece together with a malignant tumour.

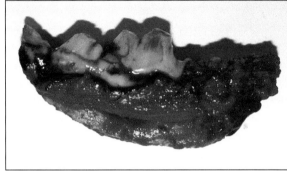
(© John R. Lewis)

7 The bony edges are made smooth with a large round diamond bur prior to wound closure.

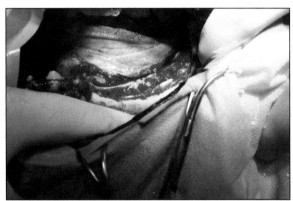
(© John R. Lewis)

The gingiva, alveolar and buccal mucosa and submucosal tissues are undermined to allow for a tension-free closure. The submucosal tissues are closed with 2 metric (3/0 USP) or 1.5 metric (4/0 USP) absorbable monofilament suture material in a simple interrupted or horizontal mattress pattern. The mucosa is closed with 1.5 metric (4/0 USP) absorbable monofilament suture material in a simple interrupted pattern.

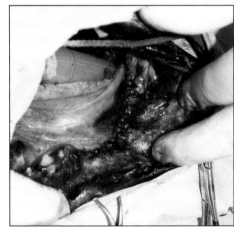
(© John R. Lewis)

PRACTICAL TIPS

- The bur will damage teeth adjacent to the line of osteotomy unless care is taken to avoid the roots and crowns
- Due to the close spacing of the teeth, cuts are best made through the crown of a tooth rather than attempting to cut between the crowns of teeth
- Residual pieces of crown and root structure are removed prior to closure

POSTOPERATIVE CARE

Soft food for 2 weeks. Expect some serosanguineous oral discharge for a few days postoperatively. If only the ventral mandibular cortex remains in place, prohibit large hard toys indefinitely to avoid fracture of the remaining portion of the mandibular body.

OPERATIVE TECHNIQUE 11.3

Bilateral rostral mandibulectomy

INDICATIONS

Bilateral rostral mandibulectomy is indicated for rostral masses of the lower jaw in which a surgical cure would be achieved by removal *en bloc* of a portion of the rostral mandibles containing incisors, canines and, if necessary, rostral premolar teeth and surrounding bone and soft tissue.

POSITIONING

Dorsal recumbency.

ASSISTANT

Necessary.

ADDITIONAL EQUIPMENT

High-speed dental drill; cross-cut fissure surgical length bur; small round carbide bur; periosteal elevators of various sizes; No. 15 scalpel blades; winged dental elevators; large round diamond bur; cooling solutions.

SURGICAL TECHNIQUE

Approach

Skin, bone, teeth and mucosa are removed *en bloc* to allow for removal of the tumour with clean margins. The rostral lip is reconstructed to minimize postoperative drooling and moist dermatitis. Images shown in this operative technique were obtained from a cadaver specimen. In a clinical patient, the hair should be adequately clipped, the skin prepared for aseptic surgery and the surgical site draped.

Surgical manipulations

1   A V-shaped wedge of skin of the rostral lower jaw is included with the piece of jaw to be resected to allow for reconstruction of the oral vestibule after removal of the rostral aspects of the mandibles.

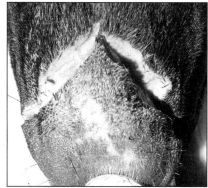

(© John R. Lewis)

2   Mucosa of the lateral aspect of the lower lip and alveolar mucosa and gingiva of the rostral lower jaw are incised. Branches of mental vessels are ligated as necessary. The sublingual mucosa is also incised, possibly rostral to the salivary gland duct openings, as dictated by the margins of the tumour.

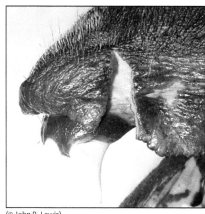

(© John R. Lewis)

→ **OPERATIVE TECHNIQUE 11.3 CONTINUED**

3 A periosteal elevator is used to remove soft tissue along the desired line of osteotomy.

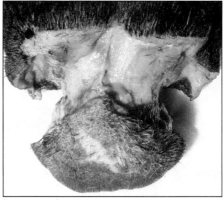

(© John R. Lewis)

4 A cross-cut fissure surgical length bur is used to cut through the rostral aspects of the mandibles. Sterile saline or lactated Ringer's solution is used to cool the bur. If the line of cut is rostral to the mesial root of the second premolar teeth, a full-thickness cut can be made through the bones and canine tooth roots. Caudal to the mesial root of the mandibular second premolar tooth, the mandible is scored to nearly the level of the mandibular canal, and the remaining bony attachments are fractured to allow for safe ligation of the inferior alveolar neurovascular bundle. There is a potential risk of tumour invasion along the periodonteal space. Thus, the entire tooth is ideally removed in one piece together with a malignant tumour. However, it may be decided on a case-by-case basis whether the piece resected should contain entire teeth or one can cut through teeth at sufficient distance from the tumour margins.

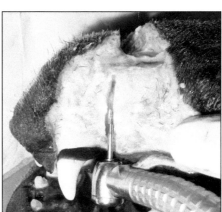

(© John R. Lewis)

5 Roots of any transected teeth are removed. Dental radiographs are taken of the excised piece and the remaining mandibles, to ensure that root remnants are not retained.

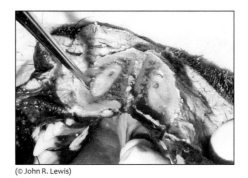

(© John R. Lewis)

6 A small round carbide bur may be used to create tacking holes in the bone for tension-relieving sutures to minimize dehiscence. Rough edges of bone are made smooth with a large round diamond bur, and the area is lavaged and prepared for closure.

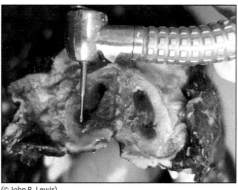

(© John R. Lewis)

→ **OPERATIVE TECHNIQUE 11.3 CONTINUED**

7   A 3 metric (2/0 USP) or 2 metric (3/0 USP) absorbable monofilament suture material is passed through the drilled holes and tacked to the subcutaneous tissue of the lip and chin. The submucosal and subcutaneous tissues are closed with 2 metric (3/0 USP) or 1.5 metric (4/0 USP) absorbable sutures in a simple interrupted or horizontal mattress pattern.

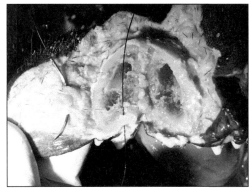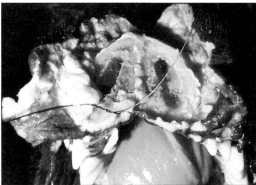

(© John R. Lewis)

8   The mucosa of the lip and sublingual area are apposed with 1.5 metric (4/0 USP) or 1 metric (5/0 USP) absorbable sutures in a simple interrupted pattern.

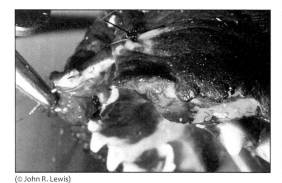

(© John R. Lewis)

9   The skin is closed with 2 metric (3/0 USP) nylon sutures in a cruciate or simple interrupted pattern.

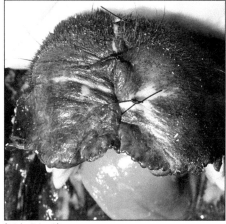

(© John R. Lewis)

PRACTICAL TIP

- Removal of a wedge of skin, though perhaps not necessary to obtain clean margins on a dorsally located rostral mandibular tumour, will allow for a more anatomically accurate reconstruction of the lower lip, by bringing the edges of the labial mucosa together at the midline, which will also maintain an oral vestibule

POSTOPERATIVE CARE

Elizabethan collar and soft food for 2 weeks, with no access to hard toys or treats. Expect some serosanguineous oral discharge for a few days postoperatively. Transient, mild central lingual ptosis and drooling of saliva may develop.

Chapter 12

Closed and open tooth extraction

Alexander M. Reiter

Extraction of teeth (exodontics) is one of the most frequently performed procedures in small animal practice (Harvey and Emily, 1993; Clark et al., 2002). It should not be treated lightly, as 'extraction' is final. The client must consent to the number of teeth to be removed prior to performing the procedure, and the veterinary surgeon (veterinarian) must be familiar with the tissues that hold the teeth in the jaws (Lommer, 2012a). Utilizing good instrumentation and applying proper techniques can help to provide a stress-free and controlled procedure for the operator with minimal trauma to the patient, faster recovery and healing, and more dependable long-term results (Kertesz, 1993; Scheels and Howard, 1993). The entire tooth must be removed to avoid local or systemic infection. If a root remains in the jaw, it must be recorded in the patient's medical record. Tension is probably the most common reason for flap dehiscence (Reiter and Soltero-Rivera, 2014).

Indications

If any disease process is too advanced for the teeth to be saved, extraction is necessary. Financial and other considerations may also lead the client to request extraction (Harvey and Emily, 1993). Indications for extraction are listed below.

- Periodontal disease: teeth affected by periodontal disease are usually extracted if periodontal health cannot be restored, or if the client is unwilling to commit to a combination of oral home hygiene and periodic professional oral care.
- Tooth resorption: about one-third of domestic cats (Reiter and Mendoza, 2002) suffer from idiopathic resorption of multiple permanent teeth. Extraction of affected teeth is the currently recommended treatment of choice.
- Tooth fracture with pulp exposure: a tooth fractured beyond repair, or beyond the owner's financial means to preserve it, must be extracted.
- Endodontic or periapical disease: teeth with pulpitis, pulp necrosis or periapical disease for which endodontic treatment is inappropriate, or is declined by the owner, must be extracted (Reiter et al., 2012).
- Caries: maxillary and mandibular first and second molar teeth in dogs are most commonly affected. These teeth must be extracted if restoration or endodontic treatment is not feasible.

- Persistent deciduous teeth: two homologous teeth should never be in the mouth at the same time and at the same location (i.e. permanent tooth has erupted and corresponding deciduous tooth has not yet exfoliated). Deciduous canine teeth may represent an exception to the rule, as they are normally present for several days or weeks after eruption of the permanent counterparts. However, they can interfere with the normal eruption pathway of their permanent successors by competing for the same space in the mouth, which may result in malocclusion and crowding, predisposing to periodontal disease (Legendre, 1994; Hobson, 2005).
- Malocclusion: maloccluding teeth should be extracted if they interfere with masticatory function, cause trauma to other tissues or lead to periodontal disease. Extraction is also indicated when orthodontic treatment, occlusal equilibration or other corrective techniques are not feasible or are declined by the client.
- Supernumerary teeth: extra teeth can cause crowding and may interfere with normal occlusion and periodontal health.
- Non-functional malformed teeth: malformed teeth may interfere with normal occlusion and periodontal health. Restoration is often not feasible because of the extent or type of malformation or for economic reasons.
- Unerupted or partially erupted teeth: if no cause can be identified for a tooth to remain unerupted, it is termed an embedded tooth. An unerupted or partially erupted tooth is considered to be impacted if the path of eruption is blocked or impaired. Unerupted teeth in adult animals must be removed using open extraction principles to prevent infection, pressure necrosis and the potential formation of a dentigerous cyst and/or neoplasia (MacGee et al., 2012).
- Fractured and retained roots: these must always be extracted, with the possible exception of ones that are affected by advanced replacement resorption. Extraction is particularly indicated if retained roots communicate with the oral cavity or are associated with periodontal, endodontic or periapical disease (Moore and Niemiec, 2014). Roots may also be identified radiographically following radical jaw resections.
- Teeth in areas of osteomyelitis and osteonecrosis: antimicrobial therapy is supported by extraction of involved teeth and aggressive debridement of infected tissues (Boutoille and Hennet, 2011).

- Teeth in a jaw fracture line: the general opinion that teeth in fracture lines must always be extracted, regardless of health, should be rejected, as they may be used as anchor points during jaw fracture repair, favour bone healing and provide stability to the fracture site. Teeth affected by mild periodontal disease should be treated at the time of fracture fixation. However, those with moderate to severe periodontitis should be extracted. A multi-rooted tooth may be sectioned and the loose crown-root segment removed, while the solid crown-root segment surrounded by reasonably healthy periodontium may be retained. Endodontic treatment must be performed on the remaining tooth segment(s) (Reiter et al., 2005).
- Traumatically displaced teeth: luxated teeth should be extracted if they cannot be repositioned and treated endodontically. Nasally intruded teeth must be extracted to prevent chronic secondary rhinitis and intermittent epistaxis.
- Client preference: extraction is performed when the client desires less expensive but definitive treatment. Alternative treatments for strategic teeth (i.e. canines and carnassials) should be recommended if the periodontium is sound.

The most common indications for tooth extraction in dogs are probably periodontal disease and tooth fracture, and in cats tooth resorption and stomatitis.

Contraindications

Tooth extraction may be contraindicated or less optimal over tooth-saving procedures (Holmstrom et al., 1998) in:

- Patients with high anaesthetic risk due to health concerns
- Patients undergoing radiation therapy involving the jaws that would inhibit healing; if one has to extract a tooth in the area of previous radiation therapy, it is recommended to perform the procedure soon after the acute side effects have worn off (e.g. after 6–8 weeks) rather than waiting months or years, as the potential for wound healing will become progressively worse and not better (Reiter and Soltero-Rivera, 2014)
- Patients with uncontrolled bleeding disorders
- Patients on medications that may cause prolonged bleeding times or prevent healing
- Patients with oral neoplasia; extraction of teeth involved with or surrounded by malignant neoplasia may predispose to the development of regional and distant metastasis.

Preparation

Client communication

The available treatment options should always be discussed with the client. The client's approval must be obtained for the extent of treatment, the cost anticipated by the clinician and a plan of action in the event that an unexpected problem requiring further treatment is discovered during the extraction procedure (Holmstrom et al., 1998). This is essential to avoid the potential for future litigation. Thus, obtaining signed consent from the client, including the number of teeth to be removed, is important prior to performing any tooth extraction.

Patient preparation

Reasonable health, determined by physical examination and laboratory tests where indicated, is required when an animal is to undergo general anaesthesia.

- An endotracheal tube with inflated cuff and an oropharyngeal pack will prevent blood, calculus and other debris from entering the trachea or oesophagus.
- The jaws should be securely propped open without unnecessary strain on the temporomandibular joints. The use of spring-loaded mouth gags is to be avoided, particularly in cats (Reiter, 2014).
- A towel beneath the patient's head will cushion it from pressure during the procedure.
- Ophthalmic lubricating ointment will protect eyes from drying, and a cloth covering the face will prevent soiling of the skin and fur.
- The anaesthetized animal should be placed in a comfortable position that allows easy access to the side of the mouth being operated on.
- A surgical drape should be fixed with delicate towel clamps to the lip margins to delimit the surgical field and reduce the risk of contamination of surgical sites by hair and other debris.

Oral tissues have an abundant blood supply, and their epithelial surface is constantly bathed by saliva, a fluid rich in antimicrobial properties. Healing of incisional wounds in oral mucosa is therefore more rapid than in skin, with superior phagocytic activity and earlier epithelialization. Infections after oral surgery procedures are rare despite preoperative preparation of the oral mucosa being more difficult than skin, and despite the inability to isolate the affected area postoperatively (Reiter, 2007).

Extractions should ideally be performed in a clean mouth. Scaling and polishing the teeth followed by preoperative rinsing with dilute chlorhexidine gluconate (0.12%) may aid in reducing bacteraemia and bacterial aerosols. Care should be taken in preventing calculus and other debris from contaminating the alveolar sockets and interfering with normal wound healing. Perioperative broad-spectrum antibiotics are given in selected cases, such as:

- Debilitated and immunocompromised patients
- Patients suffering from organ disease, endocrine disorders, cardiovascular disease or severe local or systemic infection
- Patients with permanent implants and transplants.

Dental radiographs should be obtained prior to tooth extraction to evaluate alveolar bone health and variations in root anatomy, and to determine the presence of dento-alveolar ankylosis or replacement resorption of roots that could potentially complicate the extraction procedure. Perioperative pain control is achieved by the use of systemic analgesic drugs and by the administration of nerve blocks using long-lasting local anaesthetics (see Chapter 6).

Role of veterinary nurses and technicians

Laws vary with regard to extraction of teeth performed by registered veterinary nurses or technicians. The law in most countries forbids them from performing surgery. However, closed extractions are often referred to as 'non-surgical', thus presenting a potential conflict for the veterinary nurse or technician (Holmstrom, 2000).

The American Veterinary Dental College (AVDC) developed a position statement regarding veterinary dental health care providers (adopted 5 April, 1998): 'Only veterinarians shall determine which teeth are to be extracted and perform extraction procedures…' In the United Kingdom at present Schedule 3 does not allow veterinary nurses to perform open (surgical) extractions, but they may extract loose teeth under the direct supervision of the veterinary surgeon who has made the diagnosis requiring this treatment option (Reiter, 2007).

However, every tooth extraction should be considered a surgical procedure. Rather than distinguishing between simple (or non-surgical) extraction and complex (or surgical) extraction, one should consider using the terms closed extraction (without a flap) and open extraction (with a flap).

Operator considerations

Practice on a cadaver and familiarity with dental anatomy are mandatory prior to performing new techniques on a patient (Figure 12.1). Safety measures during extraction procedures include the wearing of safety glasses, masks (or face shields) and gloves. Adequate lighting, magnification, suction, use of an air/water syringe, and relative position of the clinician and patient are all factors affecting visibility.

During maxillary tooth extractions, the patient's head is cradled with the palm of the free hand over the bridge of the upper jaw. During mandibular tooth extractions, the lower jaw can be cradled in the palm of the free hand, or the individual side can be grasped between the thumb and forefinger. These positions help to prevent iatrogenic trauma and jaw fracture by neutralizing pressure applied to the bone during extraction. Luxators and elevators are

grasped with the butt of the handle seated in the palm and the index finger extended along the blade of the instrument to act as a stop should the instrument slip. Used in this way, iatrogenic damage is prevented (Harvey and Emily, 1993).

Mechanics of tooth extraction

Teeth are anchored to the alveolar bone of the incisive bones, maxillae and mandibles by soft tissue components of the periodontium, the gingiva and periodontal ligament. During the extraction process, these tissues must be severed (junctional epithelium and gingival connective tissue) or stretched and torn (periodontal ligament fibres) to allow delivery of the tooth being extracted. Gentle tissue handling is important to minimize trauma and to allow rapid healing of both soft and hard tissues (Reiter, 2007).

The roots of carnivores' incisor teeth are often curved and flattened oval in cross-section, providing anti-rotational retention. The canine tooth of the dog has a curved root with an oval cross-section. Its maximum bulbosity (circumference) is not at the cementoenamel junction or the alveolar margin, but at some distance apical to them. Through this feature, alveolar bone locks the root into the jaw. Divergence of premolar and molar tooth roots is another important retention aid. The distal aspect of the mesial root of the mandibular first molar tooth in the dog has a prominent indentation that corresponds with a bony extension of its alveolus, thus increasing contact area between tooth and bone and providing additional anti-rotational retention (Figure 12.2). Cheek teeth in cats often have bulbous apices due to hypercementosis, which

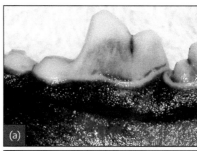
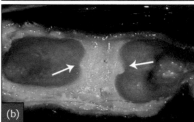
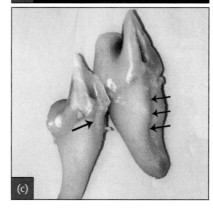

12.2 (a) Right mandibular first molar tooth in a dog. (b) Note the bony extensions (arrowed) within the empty alveoli. (c) These bony extensions correspond to indentations (arrowed) along the distal surface of the mesial root and to some extent the mesial surface of the distal root.

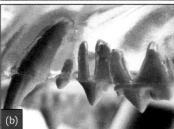
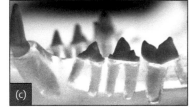

12.1 (a) Labial and buccal alveolar bone has been removed in this dog skull to visualize the roots of the left maxillary and mandibular teeth. Transparent plastic models are also available to review root anatomy, as shown here for (b) the maxillary and (c) the mandibular teeth in the cat.

increases retention. Cheek teeth in small dogs may have apically curved roots reaching into the ventral mandibular cortex. All of these clinical scenarios can make extraction of the teeth a challenging process (Kertesz, 1993). In the dog the incisor, canine, first premolar and mandibular third molar teeth are single-rooted; in the cat, the incisor, canine and commonly the maxillary second premolar teeth are single-rooted. The cat's maxillary first molar teeth may be treated as single-rooted teeth, even though they often have more than one root, as these roots are usually fused together.

Three basic types of lever (Figure 12.3) are involved in tooth extraction (Holmstrom *et al.*, 1998):

- A first-class lever, with a fulcrum between the resistance and the force
- A wedge lever
- A wheel and axle lever.

Equipment

Air-powered systems are equipped with irrigating mechanisms to cool the burs used in high- and low-speed dental handpieces. High-speed handpieces accept a number of different friction-grip (FG) burs, including round (to remove alveolar bone), cross-cut fissure (to section multi-rooted teeth) and round diamond burs (to smooth alveolar bone) (Figure 12.4). Burs in low-speed handpieces are used for cutting bone only (Reiter and Soltero-Rivera, 2014).

Extraction is considered to be a surgical procedure, and since the instruments will enter tissue they must be sterile. Instruments are cleaned, autoclaved and stored in closed cassettes, which are then placed on a sterile field and opened ready for use (Reiter, 2013). The basic contents of a tooth extraction pack are listed in Figure 12.5 and shown in Figure 12.6.

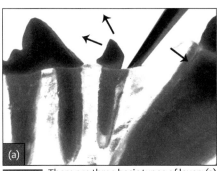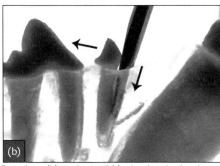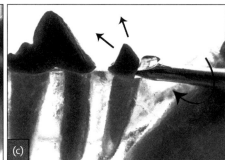

12.3 There are three basic types of lever: (a) first-class, (b) wedge and (c) wheel and axle. The arrows indicate the direction of force applied against the tooth as well as the direction the tooth is moved in.

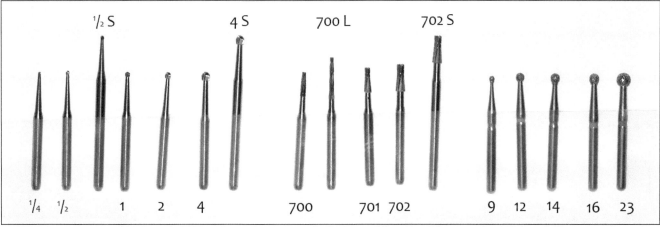

12.4 An assortment of friction-grip (FG) burs for use in a water-cooled high-speed dental handpiece: round carbide burs (left), cross-cut fissure burs (middle) and round medium-coarse diamond burs (right). L = long (i.e. the working end is longer than normal); S = surgical (i.e. the shank is longer than normal).
(© Dr Alexander M. Reiter)

- Dental radiographic equipment
- High-speed dental equipment with water irrigation
- Non-surgical and surgical-length dental friction-grip (FG) burs: cross-cut fissure (700, 701, 702), round (¼, ½, 1, 2, 4) and round diamond (9, 14, 23)
- No. 3 or 5 scalpel handle with 11, 15 or 15C blades
- Sharp and narrow-tipped (2–6 mm) periosteal elevators (such as Mead No. 3 or Periosteal EX-9M for medium-sized and larger dogs, Glickman No. 24G or Periosteal EX-9 for small dogs and cats)
- Adson 1 x 2 thumb forceps (smaller version)
- Dental elevators (1, 2, 3, 4, 6)
- Dental luxators

- Small and large extraction forceps
- Root tip elevators
- Root tip forceps
- Small spoon curettes
- Irrigation solutions (dilute chlorhexidine, lactated Ringer's solution)
- Gauze sponges
- Small Metzenbaum scissors
- Needle holders
- Synthetic, absorbable monofilament suture material, 1 and 1.5 metric (5/0 and 4/0 USP), with swaged on, taper-point, round, non-cutting needle
- Suture scissors (or designated pair of Mayo scissors)

12.5 Basic contents of a tooth extraction pack.

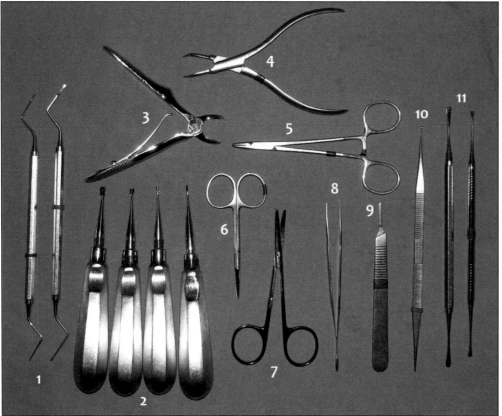

12.6 Tooth extraction kit for the cat (larger versions of the instruments may be used in the dog). 1 = root tip elevators; 2 = winged luxating elevators; 3 = extraction forceps; 4 = root tip forceps; 5 = needle holder; 6 = suture scissors; 7 = curved Metzenbaum scissors; 8 = Adson 1 x 2 thumb forceps; 9 = scalpel handle; 10 = surgical curette; 11 = periosteal elevators.
(© Dr Alexander M. Reiter)

Oral flaps should be grasped on their connective tissue side rather than at their margins so that the latter will not get traumatized prior to suturing; thumb forceps providing a fine rat-toothed grip are ideal for that purpose (Figure 12.7). Periosteal elevators are used to raise oral flaps, engaging the flat or concave side of the instrument against the bone and its convex side against the soft tissue, thus reducing the chance of tearing or puncturing the elevated soft tissue (Reiter and Soltero-Rivera, 2014).

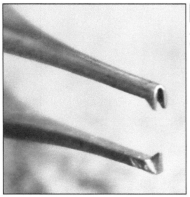

12.7 Close-up of the tips of a pair of Adson 1 x 2 thumb forceps.
(© Dr Alexander M. Reiter)

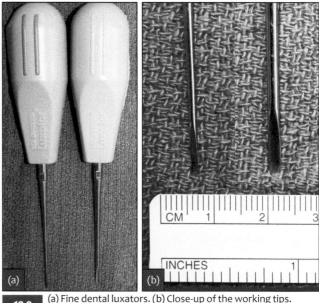

(a) (b)

12.8 (a) Fine dental luxators. (b) Close-up of the working tips.
(© Dr Alexander M. Reiter)

Instruments for luxating, elevating and extracting teeth

Dental luxators have sharp and often flat-tipped blades designed to penetrate into the narrow periodontal ligament space and cut periodontal ligament fibres between the tooth and alveolar bone (Figure 12.8). Luxators are made of softer steel than elevators and should not be used with a leverage technique for large teeth or root fragments, as they can easily bend or break (Reiter, 2013).

The size of dental elevators should closely approximate the size of the tooth or crown-root segment being elevated. Most are made of hard steel. The relative thickness of some elevator tips often makes them less suitable for wedging between the tooth and alveolar bone (unless space has been created by a luxator) (Figure 12.9). 'Luxating elevators' are now available with thin, sharp tips (Reiter, 2013).

Similar to elevators, the instruments are grasped with the butt of the handle seated in the palm, and the index finger is extended along the blade to act as a stop in case the instrument slips (Reiter and Soltero-Rivera, 2014). The blade of the instrument is gently worked into the space

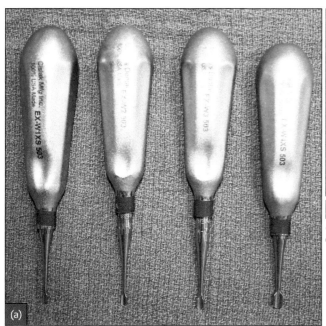

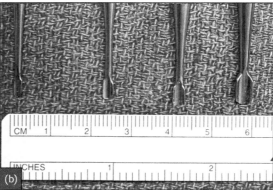

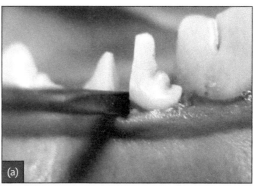

12.9 (a) Winged dental elevators (from left to right: sizes 1–4) whose curved blades should fit the circumference of a tooth. (b) Close-up of the working tips.
(© Dr Alexander M. Reiter)

between the tooth or crown-root segment and the alveolar bone. A well controlled rotational motion around the shank's long axis between the root and a fulcrum point (vertical rotation) (Figure 12.10) is performed to create a slow, gentle and steady pressure on the tooth or crown-root segment. This pressure is held for at least 10 seconds to break down the periodontal ligament fibres. The elevator can also be placed perpendicular to the tooth or crown-root segment to lever it out of the alveolus through the line of least resistance, with a fulcrum point preferably on alveolar bone (horizontal rotation) and not on adjacent teeth (unless the tooth used as a fulcrum is to be extracted as well) (Figure 12.11) (Reiter, 2007).

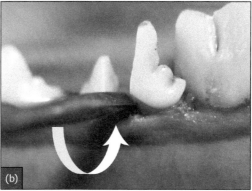

12.11 Horizontal rotation with (a) the elevator being inserted perpendicular to and in between two crown-root segments and then (b) rotated along its long axis.

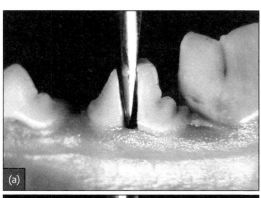

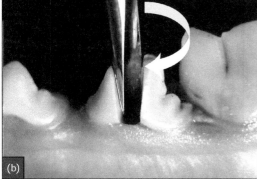

12.10 Vertical rotation with (a) the elevator being inserted parallel to and in between two crown-root segments and then (b) rotated along its long axis.

Extraction forceps should have a narrow beak, fit the tooth as closely as possible and be applied as far apically on the tooth as possible to reduce the chances of root fracture. They should only be applied when the tooth is very loose. Forceps can easily apply excessive or improper forces resulting in tooth fracture (Harvey and Emily, 1993). Extraction forceps may have beaks that fully close or not (Figure 12.12). They should still fit the circumference of the teeth, crown-root segments or roots to be extracted, and be used gently to minimize the risk of tooth fracture. Small root tip elevators (Figure 12.13) and forceps (Figure 12.14) are available for elevation and removal of root remnants (Reiter and Soltero-Rivera, 2014).

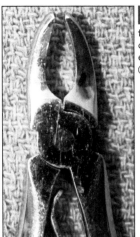

12.12 Extraction forceps with beaks that do not fully close but still fit the circumference of the teeth, crown-root segments or roots to be extracted.
(© Dr Alexander M. Reiter)

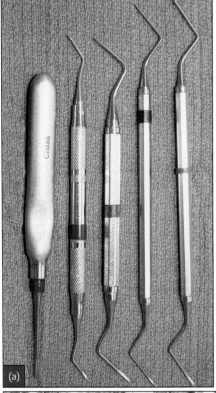

12.13 (a) Small root tip elevators ('teasers') for removal of root remnants. (b) Close-up of the working tips.
(© Dr Alexander M. Reiter)

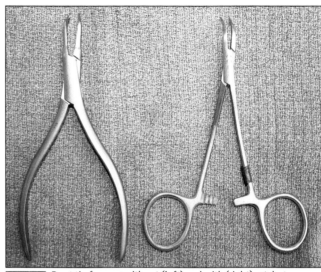

12.14 Root tip forceps without (left) and with (right) ratchet mechanism for removal of root remnants.
(© Dr Alexander M. Reiter)

Instruments and materials for extraction site management

Surgical curettes remove debris and granulation tissue from an alveolar socket after tooth extraction or the connective tissue side of a flap prior to closure. Curved, blunt-ended Metzenbaum scissors with serrated blades are used for dissecting the connective tissue side of oral flaps and fine cutting of their edges prior to wound closure (Reiter and Soltero-Rivera, 2014). Specific suture scissors or a designated pair of Mayo scissors should be reserved for cutting sutures (Lipscomb and Reiter, 2005).

Autogenous bone (cancellous bone and cortical bone chips) as well as allograft-based (demineralized bone of the same species) and ceramic-based (calcium phosphate, calcium sulphate and bioglass) bone graft substitutes are most commonly used in veterinary dentistry (Reiter and Soltero-Rivera, 2014), although their routine use in extraction sites may not be needed (Araújo and Lindhe, 2005; Blanco *et al.*, 2011; Da Silva *et al.*, 2012, 2013; Discepoli *et al.*, 2013).

Size 7.5 x 7.5 cm (3 x 3 inches) gauze swabs allow digital control of haemorrhage during tooth extraction procedures. Lavage with refrigerated lactated Ringer's solution may also provide good haemostasis. Excessive bleeding from tooth extraction sites near tubular structures such as the mandibular and infraorbital canals can effectively be controlled by packing the alveolar sockets with a small amount of bone wax (a sterile beeswax-based compound) (Reiter, 2013; Reiter and Soltero-Rivera, 2014). However, the use of bone wax should be weighed against possible complications (i.e. infection, embolization, chronic foreign body reaction and delayed healing) (Anderson, 2012).

Instruments and materials for extraction site closure

Halsey or DeBakey needle holders with serrated jaws are used to lock on to curved needles by a ratchet mechanism. An absorbable suture material is preferred for wound closure in the oral cavity so that sedation or anaesthesia for suture removal can be avoided (Lipscomb and Reiter, 2005; Reiter, 2007, 2013).

- Chromic catgut persists for 4–7 days and elicits the greatest inflammatory tissue reaction of all suture materials. Its use is not recommended. Therefore, a longer-lasting, synthetic and absorbable material is preferred in dogs and cats to avoid early wound breakdown.
- Polyglactin 910 and polyglycolic acid are good for procedures in which healing is relatively rapid, but they may elicit an inflammatory tissue reaction due to their multifilament nature.
- Synthetic monofilament sutures induce the least foreign body reaction in oral tissues:
  - The use of polydioxanone for closure of tooth extraction sites is discouraged due to its prolonged persistence (6–8 weeks)
  - Poliglecaprone 25 (1.5 metric (4/0 USP) for dogs or 1 metric (5/0 USP) for cats and small dogs) with a swaged-on ½-circle taper-point, round, non-cutting needle is the preferred suture material for most oral surgeries (Figure 12.15). This avoids the need for suture removal, minimizes the inflammatory oral tissue reaction around sutures, and reduces trauma to already inflamed or friable tissues. It persists for about 3–5 weeks
  - Small swaged-on ⅜-circle reverse-cutting needles may cause minimal tissue drag, but they can readily tear through delicate or inflamed oral mucosal tissues.

Simple interrupted square or surgeon's knots should be followed by three more throws to ensure knot security (Reiter, 2013). Some veterinary dentists prefer a continuous suture pattern, thus increasing the speed of closure of large flaps, reducing anaesthesia time, and minimizing an inflammatory tissue reaction by having fewer knots exposed to the oral cavity.

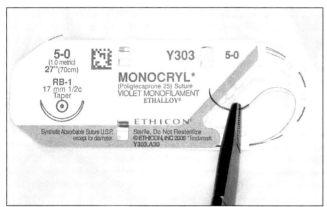

12.15 1 metric (5/0 USP) synthetic, absorbable monofilament material with a swaged-on, taper-point, round, non-cutting needle.
(© Dr Alexander M. Reiter)

Techniques for tooth extraction

The principles of tooth extraction (Figure 12.16) are to reduce or eliminate the retentive factors that hold a tooth in the jaw. Forceps should not be applied to teeth until such a level of mobility has been obtained that the instrument can be used solely for the delivery of the tooth or crown-root segments (Kertesz, 1993; Niemiec, 2008). It is best to slowly stretch, sever and tear the periodontal ligament fibres using luxators and elevators. Little benefit is achieved by working forcefully against the mechanical

- Obtain preoperative dental radiographs
- Cut the gingival attachment first
- Section multi-rooted teeth into single-rooted crown-root segments
- Perform open extraction where indicated
- Do not create incision lines over a future void
- Minimize thermal damage by using water irrigation
- Place vertical incisions only at the line angles of the teeth or in sufficiently wide interdental spaces
- Avoid excessive alveolectomy
- Stretch and tear the periodontal ligament fibres
- Keep the index finger close to the instrument tip
- Use your free hand to support the jaw
- Do not use force; use slow steady pressure
- Do not leave root fragments behind
- Smooth any rough alveolar bone edges
- Provide fresh soft tissue margins
- Cover any exposed bone with soft tissue
- Avoid trauma to the flap
- Do not suture flaps under tension
- Use appropriate suture material for wound closure
- Possibly obtain postoperative radiographs

12.16 Principles of tooth extraction.

factors that retain the teeth. A rotational motion should be used and the tooth eased out of the socket rather than forced. The entire root must be removed. The key to effective tooth extraction is patience. Extractions can be performed using the closed technique, i.e. without raising a mucoperiosteal flap, or using the open technique, i.e. raising a mucoperiosteal flap to expose alveolar bone (Gorrel and Robinson, 1995; DeBowes, 2005; Gengler, 2013).

Closed extraction

Closed extraction is primarily performed for maxillary and mandibular incisor teeth in dogs and cats, maxillary and mandibular first premolar teeth in the dog, maxillary second premolar and first molar teeth in the cat, and mobile teeth presenting with significant attachment loss (Lommer and Verstraete, 2012). Employing a closed extraction technique for other teeth risks their fracture, which then warrants an open extraction technique to remove root remnants.

Single-rooted teeth

Figure 12.17 shows closed extraction of a right maxillary first incisor tooth.

1. Insert a No. 15 scalpel blade into the gingival sulcus or periodontal pocket, direct it at 45 degrees to the long axis of the tooth to the depth of the alveolar margin, and incise the gingival attachment around the tooth.
2. Insert a luxator/elevator whose curved blade fits the circumference of the tooth between the gingival margin and the crown or exposed root at an angle of 10–20 degrees to the long axis of the tooth.
3. Gently force the luxator/elevator apically into the periodontal ligament space between the tooth and alveolar bone, using it as a wedge lever.
4. Once there is enough space created between the tooth and alveolar bone, the procedure may continue with elevators only. Apply pressure while slowly rotating the elevator through a small arc. At the end of each rotation, hold the instrument firmly against the tissues for at least 10 seconds; this will stretch and tear the periodontal ligament fibres. Place a slow, gentle, steady pressure on the tooth rather than using quick rocking motions, to

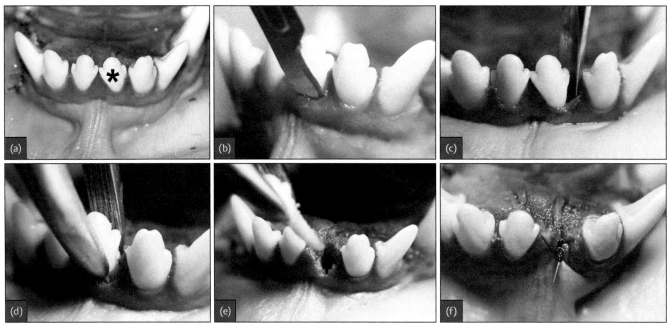

12.17 (a) Closed extraction of the right maxillary first incisor tooth (*) in a dog. (b) The gingival attachment is incised. (c) The tooth is elevated, (d) grasped with extraction forceps and (e) removed. (f) The wound is sutured closed.
(© Dr Alexander M. Reiter)

fatigue and tear the periodontal ligament fibres. Haemorrhage into the widened periodontal ligament space assists in tearing fibres through hydraulic pressure. Performing a 'wiggling' motion has the potential to crush the adjacent alveolar bone or fracture the tooth (Reiter and Soltero-Rivera, 2014).

5. As the periodontal ligament space widens, it is often helpful to change from smaller to larger instruments. Work not only in areas where progress appears to be made but return to more resistant sites. Move the elevator around the whole circumference of the tooth and gradually advance apically until the tooth begins to loosen. At this time the elevator may be used as a first-class or wheel and axle lever to elevate the tooth out of the socket.

6. When the tooth is sufficiently loose (i.e. it can move freely within its alveolar socket), extraction forceps may be placed as far apically on the tooth as possible, and the tooth rotated slightly around its long axis with a steady pull and removed from its socket. Extraction forceps are to be used with extreme care because, if incorrectly applied or used with excessive force, their use will result in crown and/or root fracture.

7. Examine the extracted tooth (primarily its apex), ensuring that the entire root has been extracted. Most roots have a smooth tip. Obtain a radiograph if there is any suspicion that a root fragment is retained in the alveolus.

8. If necessary, debride the alveolus with a spoon curette to remove granulation tissue, debris, pus and bony fragments.

9. Use a large diamond-coated round bur with water irrigation to reduce, shape and smooth the alveolar margin (alveoloplasty).

10. Gently lavage the extraction site, preferably with a polyionic solution (e.g. Ringer's lactate). Air or air/water spray must not be blown into an extraction site, as it may result in emphysema or air embolism.

11. Leave a blood clot (an essential part of socket healing) in the alveolus. If there is no bleeding into the socket, the socket should be curetted to initiate bleeding and formation of a clot.

12. Digitally compress the extraction area with a gloved finger or a damp gauze pack, and suture the gingiva using a simple interrupted tension-free pattern. Suturing may not be necessary when extracting very small teeth and if minimal damage has occurred to periodontal tissues. Suturing is required when packing the alveolus with bone grafting materials.

Two- and three-rooted teeth

A radiograph should be taken prior to extraction to determine whether a mobile multi-rooted tooth can be extracted using the closed technique. If it can, the tooth is removed as one unit by severing its gingival attachment and loosening the roots with dental luxators and elevators. An elevator can sometimes be placed into an open furcation perpendicular to the long axis of the tooth to gain good purchase, and coronally directed pressure is applied to remove the tooth, provided that the roots are not divergent or hooked (Reiter, 2007). If extraction forceps are used, each root must be completely loosened before extraction, and minimal twisting is used to remove the tooth. In selected cases where one root of the tooth is severely affected by periodontitis but the periodontium of the other root is still relatively healthy, hemisection and endodontic treatment of the remaining crown-root segment may be performed following extraction of the diseased crown-root segment (Reiter *et al.*, 2005).

Firmly attached multi-rooted teeth must be sectioned prior to extraction to avoid root fracture. This provides multiple single-rooted segments, whose extraction is no more difficult than that of multiple single-rooted teeth. Sectioning of multi-rooted teeth provides two or more single-rooted crown-root segments that are extracted as if they were single-rooted teeth (Reiter, 2007; Lommer *et al.*, 2012). Gentle reflection of the gingiva with a periosteal elevator will reveal the exact location of the furcation, decreasing the risk of damage to the gingiva during tooth sectioning. Sectioning is accomplished with a fissure bur, starting from the furcation through the crown. Two-rooted teeth are separated into two single-rooted crown-root segments. The three-rooted maxillary fourth premolar tooth of dogs and cats and the maxillary first and second molar teeth of dogs are separated into three single-rooted crown-root segments. In addition to vertical advancement of a dental elevator into the periodontal ligament space, the instrument can also be inserted horizontally in between the sectioned crown-root segments to lever them out of their alveoli (Reiter, 2007; Reiter and Soltero-Rivera, 2014).

Figure 12.18 shows closed extraction of the maxillary third and fourth premolar and first molar teeth in the dog.

1. Incise the gingival attachment around the tooth.
2. Reflect the gingiva to locate the furcation area(s).
3. Section the tooth into single-rooted crown-root segments using a cross-cut fissure bur in a high-speed handpiece with water irrigation. Sectioning is performed starting from the furcation through the crown.
    *   Two-rooted teeth: separate the tooth into one mesial and one distal single-rooted crown-root segment.
    *   Three-rooted teeth: separate the tooth first into one two-rooted and one single-rooted crown-root segment. Then separate the two-rooted crown-root segment into two single-rooted crown-root segments. For the maxillary fourth premolar tooth in dogs and cats, there is no particular sequence of sectioning. For the maxillary first and second molar teeth in dogs, the single-rooted palatal crown-root segment will first need to be separated from the two-rooted buccal portion of the tooth. Then the mesiobuccal crown-root segment can be separated from the distobuccal crown-root segment.
4. Luxate and elevate each segment as in a closed single-rooted tooth extraction. The elevator can also be placed perpendicular to the long axis of the tooth between its segments. The elevator is rotated slightly.

Hold the pressure for at least 10 seconds to loosen the crown-root segment. This action elevates one segment (wheel and axle lever) while the other (used as a fulcrum) is slightly intruded and moved mesially/distally.

5. Loosen all segments progressively, and extract them as if they were single-rooted teeth.
6. Once all segments are extracted, proceed as described for a closed extraction of a single-rooted tooth. An envelope flap may be created labially or buccally with a periosteal elevator to allow for tension-free closure.

Open extraction

The open extraction technique is employed when a tooth resists appropriate elevation due to its size and root anatomy/pathology, when multiple teeth in the same jaw quadrant need to be extracted, or if the operator is unable to retrieve a fractured or retained root. It is futile, time-consuming and damaging to the surrounding tissues to continue a closed extraction process blindly to retrieve root fragments. Raising mucoperiosteal flaps will improve visibility of and expedite access to any tooth or root that requires extraction (Reiter, 2007). When multiple teeth are affected in one jaw quadrant, the creation of large flaps is often less time-consuming than making small flaps over individual teeth.

1. Incise the gingival attachment around the tooth and extend horizontal gingival incisions to the midpoint between adjacent teeth if interdental spaces are wide.
2. Raise a mucoperiosteal flap.
    *   Make one or two releasing incisions in the alveolar mucosa down to the bone and connect them with the rostral and/or caudal end of gingival incisions. Keep in mind that suture lines should not lie over a void and that the ideal location for a releasing incision is in the interproximal space between two teeth (where bone support is present) or at the line

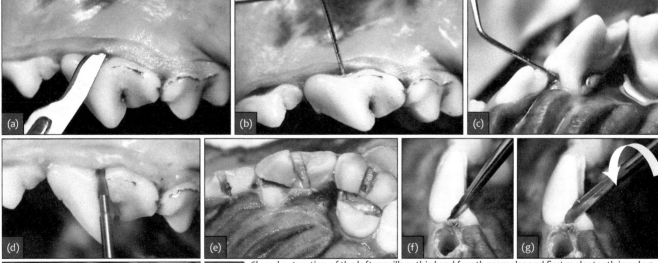

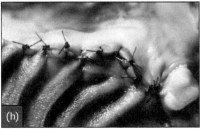

12.18 Closed extraction of the left maxillary third and fourth premolar and first molar teeth in a dog. (a) The gingival attachment is incised at 360 degrees around the teeth. The furcations between the roots are identified with a periodontal probe. Location of the fourth premolar tooth's furcations between the (b) mesiobuccal and distal roots and (c) mesiobuccal and mesiopalatal roots. (d) Sectioning between the fourth premolar tooth's mesiobuccal and distal crown-root segments is shown. (e) An occlusal view reveals completed sectioning of the three teeth. (f) A dental elevator is placed into the space created after sectioning the mesiobuccal from the mesiopalatal crown-root segments of the fourth premolar tooth and (g) is rotated along its long axis to stretch the periodontal ligament fibres. (h) The extraction sites are sutured closed, following the elevation of all crown-root segments, wound debridement and creation of a buccal envelope flap.
(© Dr Alexander M. Reiter)

angle of a tooth (point of contact between two sides of the tooth, i.e. distolabial/-buccal, distopalatal/-lingual, mesiopalatal/-lingual, and mesiolabial/-buccal). Releasing incisions should never be placed at the furcation area of a multi-rooted tooth. Releasing incisions must extend beyond the mucogingival junction and slightly diverge apically, permitting adequate blood supply to the flap. Flaps without releasing incisions (i.e. envelope flaps) can also be used, as long as there will be sufficient access to the surgical site and adequate tension release prior to wound closure.

- Near the infraorbital and middle mental foramina, split-thickness flaps may be made to avoid injury to neurovascular structures.
- Use a sharp periosteal elevator to free the attached gingiva and alveolar mucosa from the underlying bone. Care should be taken to keep the periosteal elevator close to the bone when raising a full-thickness flap and to avoid perforating the flap at the mucogingival junction.
- Utilize stay sutures or grasp the flap on its connective tissue side with thumb forceps to minimize iatrogenic trauma. The flap should be elevated beyond the end of the bony prominences (alveolar juga) covering the roots.
- Elevate the lingual or palatal gingiva as an envelope flap to expose the alveolar margin.

3. If the tooth is multi-rooted, section it appropriately. Retraction of the flap with a retraction tool or thumb forceps will protect it from iatrogenic damage during tooth sectioning.
4. Use a round bur with water irrigation to reduce the level of alveolar bone overlying the roots labially or buccally by as much as one-third to two-thirds of the length of the root(s). Continuous water irrigation is required for:

- Cooling the alveolar bone to prevent overheating and bone necrosis
- Cooling the bur to prevent overheating and loss of cutting efficiency
- Washing away bone chips that would clog the bur and maintaining good visibility to the surgical site. Septal bone does not have to be removed, except when approaching the mesiopalatal root of the maxillary fourth premolar tooth.

5. Luxate, elevate and extract the tooth or crown-root segments. If little space exists between two teeth, a fissure bur can be used to remove the dental bulge at the mesial or distal surface of the tooth to be extracted to facilitate placement of the elevator during the leverage process (care must be taken to avoid damage to the tooth that will be retained) (Figure 12.19). A small notch may be made with a bur at the neck of a crown-root segment for better instrument purchase (Figure 12.20). If progress is not achieved, remove more labial or buccal alveolar bone rather than use excessive force. Narrow slots can be created at mesial and distal aspects of each root to allow for better elevator purchase (consider the proximity of the roots of adjacent teeth to avoid damaging them).
6. Proceed with debridement, alveoloplasty and lavage of the extraction site as described for closed tooth extractions.
7. Replace the mucoperiosteal flap.

- Avoid tension on the closed flap. To increase its vertical dimension and elasticity, the flap is raised and held with thumb forceps. A scalpel blade or sharp tissue scissors is used on the exposed underside to incise the periosteum across the entire base of the flap. The tissue will advance as the inelastic periosteum is cut. The back of a scalpel blade could also be used to 'strum' and weaken the

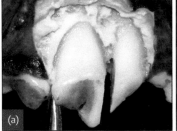
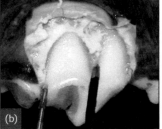
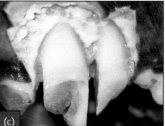
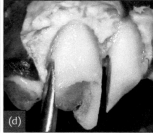

12.19 Open extraction of the right maxillary fourth premolar tooth in a dog. (a) There is usually not enough space for a dental elevator to be inserted between the maxillary fourth premolar and first molar teeth in the dog. (b, c) A cross-cut fissure bur is used to remove the dental bulge at the distal surface of the crown of the fourth premolar tooth. (d) This facilitates placement of the elevator during elevation of its distal crown-root segment.

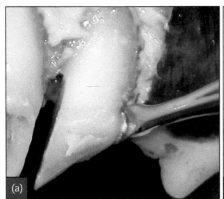
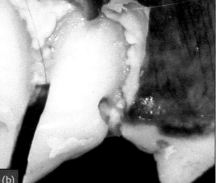
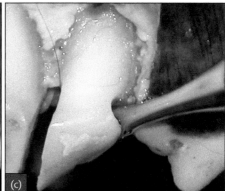

12.20 Open extraction of the right maxillary fourth premolar tooth in a dog. (a) A dental elevator is placed perpendicular to the long axis of the tooth between the mesiobuccal crown-root segment of the fourth premolar tooth and the distal aspect of the crown of the third premolar tooth. (b) A notch has been created with a bur at the neck of the mesiobuccal crown-root segment of the fourth premolar tooth. (c) This notch allows for additional elevator purchase.

periosteal layer, followed by blunt dissection with scissors. An alternative is to make a small stab incision in the periosteum through which the blade tips of closed scissors are inserted and opened to undermine the periosteal layer. Releasing incisions may also be extended and further mucosa freed until tension-free closure can be accomplished.

- Smooth any sharp spicules and reduce projections of alveolar bone prior to positioning the flap over a freshly formed blood clot. The alveolar margin may be further reduced to facilitate apposition of the flap without tension, prior to suturing.
- If required, freshen up and shape the gingival margin of the flap with fine scissors. The connective tissue side of the flap is also debrided, ensuring removal of infected and inflamed granulation tissue.
- Rinse the wound and appose the flap to the palatal/ lingual gingiva by means of simple interrupted sutures (some prefer a continuous suture pattern for large flaps). The corners of the flap are sutured first, and additional sutures are placed 2–3 mm apart and 2–3 mm from the flap edges.
- Suture the releasing incision(s), ensuring that suture lines do not lie over a void.

Extraction of specific teeth

Deciduous teeth

If the clinician identifies a permanent tooth erupting, and the corresponding deciduous tooth has not yet exfoliated, it may be wise to wait a week or two before hastily extracting the deciduous tooth (Reiter, 2007). Compared with their permanent successors, the roots of deciduous teeth are longer and thinner and may be partly resorbed. They are therefore more likely to fracture during extraction. A preoperative radiograph should be obtained to determine the proximity of the deciduous tooth root to the permanent tooth and to evaluate to what extent the root of the deciduous tooth has undergone resorption. Deciduous teeth are removed with closed or open extraction techniques, taking great care not to damage underlying tooth buds or the erupting permanent teeth. The keys to success are gentle technique (no force) and patience (Hobson, 2005).

Persistent deciduous canine teeth are common candidates for extraction. The maxillary deciduous canine tooth is always distal to the permanent canine tooth, whereas the mandibular deciduous canine tooth is labial to the permanent canine tooth (Kertesz, 1993). The extraction technique is much the same as for single-rooted permanent teeth. The deciduous tooth is loosened using fine luxators and elevators between the root and bone. Luxation/elevation may also be accomplished with a 22 G needle as a wedge lever.

Despite extra care being taken by the clinician, the client should always be informed about potential complications associated with extraction of deciduous teeth near (developing) permanent teeth. Depending on the developmental stage of permanent successors, iatrogenic trauma may result in discoloration, enamel hypomineralization and hypoplasia, and crown/root dilacerations (bending) of the permanent tooth. Most deciduous tooth extractions are carried out after the permanent successor has erupted and so damage in the formative stages is less likely. Instruments should not be inserted between a deciduous tooth and its developing permanent successor, and levering against the latter must be avoided. A dangerous consequence of closed extraction of a deciduous tooth is the accidental elevation of the permanent tooth or tooth bud. Rotational forces should not be employed with extraction forceps, because this will often result in deciduous tooth root fracture (Legendre, 1994).

If open extraction is deemed necessary, one or two releasing incisions are made, ensuring that they diverge and do not lie over the deciduous tooth root (Figure 12.21). A flap

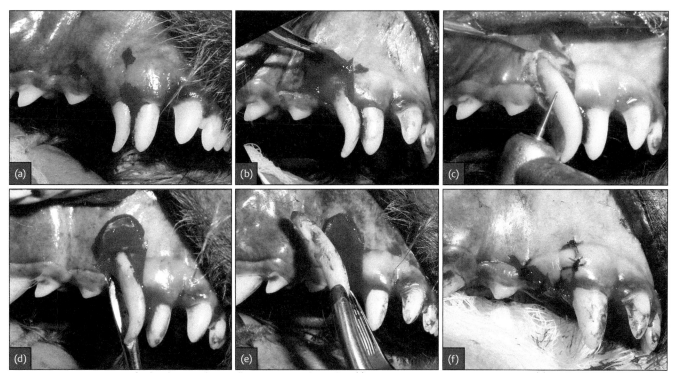

12.21 Open extraction of a deciduous right maxillary canine tooth in a dog. (a) Diverging releasing incisions are made. (b) A mucoperiosteal flap is raised. (c) Alveolectomy is performed. (d) The tooth is elevated and (e) extracted. (f) The wound is sutured closed.
(© Dr Alexander M. Reiter)

is raised, alveolar bone carefully removed, the tooth extracted and the flap sutured closed. A radiograph is taken if any doubt exists that the entire root was extracted. Removal of a fractured root tip must be achieved, as it could affect eruption of the permanent successor (Reiter, 2007).

Maxillary canine tooth

This large, single-rooted tooth is, unless severely affected by periodontitis, difficult to extract using closed extraction techniques. Its root courses in a dorsal and caudal direction with its apex projected above the mesial root of the maxillary second premolar tooth. Various flap designs with one or two releasing incisions have been described (Fitch, 2003; Tsugawa *et al.*, 2012) (Operative Technique 12.1).

During extraction, the apex of the root must not be tipped nasally, as this would perforate the thin plate of bone separating the alveolus from the nasal cavity, producing an acute oronasal communication. The elevator must also never be angled palatally between the canine tooth and the alveolar bone. If fracture of the bony plate occurs and results in perforation, haemorrhage or emergence of flushing solution may be noted from the ipsilateral nostril. An acute oronasal communication is treated by suturing the mucoperiosteal flap over the alveolus, as one would routinely close the flap raised for the extraction procedure (Smith, 1998; Reiter and Smith, 2005).

Mandibular canine tooth

Unless the periodontal tissues are severely compromised, this tooth is difficult to extract using closed extraction techniques. Various flap designs with one or two releasing incisions have been described (Smith, 2001; Volker and Luskin, 2012) (Operative Technique 12.2). A lingual approach for open extraction of the mandibular canine has also been reported (Smith, 1996). The mandibular canine root contributes considerably to the strength of the rostral mandible, which may be weakened after extraction. Bone grafting materials may be placed into the alveolus prior to closing the extraction site.

Maxillary fourth premolar tooth

This three-rooted tooth has one large distal and two smaller mesial roots (mesiobuccal and mesiopalatal). Various flap designs with one or two releasing incisions have been described (Carmichael, 2002; Reiter, 2007) (Operative Technique 12.3). When making the rostral releasing incision, the infraorbital neurovascular bundle emerging at the infraorbital foramen is to be avoided (particularly in brachycephalic breeds). When making the caudal releasing incision, the duct openings of the parotid and zygomatic salivary glands are to be avoided (Emily and Penman, 1994).

Maxillary first and second molar teeth (in the dog)

These three-rooted teeth have one large palatal and two buccal roots (mesiobuccal and distobuccal) (Vall, 2012). They can often be extracted using the closed extraction technique. Excessive force must be avoided, as it can result in iatrogenic trauma to the eye and periorbital tissues due to their proximity to the ventral floor of the orbit. If crown-root segments resist elevation or root fractures have occurred, an open extraction approach must be considered.

1. The gingival attachment around the teeth is incised.
2. When making a flap, care must be taken to avoid injury to the ducts of the parotid and zygomatic salivary glands. This can be accomplished by making a releasing incision that starts in the buccal mucosa dorsal to the salivary duct openings and curves forward towards the mesiobuccal line angle of the tooth, rostral to the salivary duct openings (Figure 12.22).
3. After raising a mucoperiosteal flap, sectioning into single-rooted crown-root segments is performed. First, the palatal crown-root segment is separated from the rest of the tooth by cutting in the fissure created by the two buccal cusps and the palatine cusp. Then, the mesiobuccal and distobuccal crown-root segments are separated by cutting through the fissure formed by the two buccal cusps.

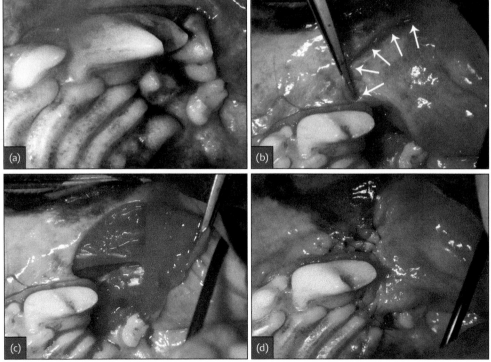

12.22 Open extraction of the left maxillary first molar tooth in a dog. (a, b) An incision is made from the buccal tissues dorsally, curving mesially in alveolar mucosa and gingiva, to the mesiobuccal line angle of the tooth (arrowed), creating a caudally pedunculated flap. (c, d) The flap is elevated, undermined, rotated and then sutured in place to completely close the extraction site without tension.
(© Dr Margherita Gracis)

4. Alveolectomy and crown-root segment elevation is then performed. The palatal crown-root segment can often be elevated and extracted without further alveolar bone removal.
5. Any sharp bony spicules are removed, the alveoli are debrided and lavaged, and the flap is replaced and sutured in a tension-free fashion.

Especially when only the first molar tooth is extracted, tension-free closure may not always be easily achieved. In select cases, and only if an oro-orbital fistula is not present, the flap may be placed to cover exclusively the buccal alveoli, using one or two bridge sutures from the flap margin to the palatal mucosa over the alveolus of the palatal root, which may be left open to heal by second intention. Alternatively, avoiding injury to the ducts of the parotid and zygomatic salivary glands, the skillful veterinary dentist may make a caudal releasing incision and/or free further mucosa to fully close the extraction site(s). When both molar teeth are extracted, an envelope flap may be sufficient to close the extraction site without tension (Ritchie, 2018). Damage to the salivary ducts can lead to sialocele formation, which in a few cases may require zygomatic and/or parotid sialoadenectomy.

Mandibular first molar tooth

This is a two-rooted tooth. In the dog, the mesial root is slightly larger than the distal root. In the cat, the mesial root is much larger and stronger, compared with the short and delicate distal root. Various flap designs with one or two releasing incisions have been described (Marretta, 2002; Smith, 2008a; O'Morrow, 2010) (Operative Technique 12.4).

In small-breed dogs, the apical portion of the roots of mandibular first molar teeth may reach into the ventral mandibular cortex (Reiter, 2007). Injury to the inferior alveolar vessels can result in haemorrhage that may significantly impair visualization of the surgical field. Injury to the inferior alveolar nerve may also cause neuralgia or altered sensation of lower jaw tissues. The extraction procedure is greatly complicated when root fragments are accidentally intruded into the mandibular canal.

Tooth extraction in cats

Tooth extraction in cats is performed in a similar fashion to dogs (Reiter, 2012), but the following points should be borne in mind:

* The cat's head is smaller, and its bones are more fragile than that of the dog
* The teeth of cats are more delicate, narrower and smaller than those of a dog of similar bodyweight; they become even more brittle when affected by resorption
* The furcation point of the mandibular first molar tooth in the cat is further distal than that of the dog's mandibular first molar tooth.

Feline teeth tend to fracture if extraction forceps are applied with force, and root fragments remaining in the alveolar sockets are a common complication, especially when the teeth are brittle due to tooth resorption (Reiter and Mendoza, 2002). Single-rooted crown-root segments after sectioning are more likely to fracture during leverage unless the force is applied very gradually. Traditional dental elevators are often too large for convenient use in cats, and smaller luxators, elevators and root tip elevators and forceps should be used (Lommer, 2012b; Reiter and

Soltero-Rivera, 2014). It is imperative for successful extraction that root fragments are not retained, particularly in the presence of stomatitis.

Multiple extractions in one quadrant

When extracting multiple teeth in sequence, it is important to consider which of the involved teeth is likely to be the most difficult to extract and use adjacent teeth to aid its extraction. The crown of one tooth may serve as a lever fulcrum for the dental elevator in extraction of an adjacent tooth. In dogs with severe generalized periodontitis and in cats with stomatitis and tooth resorption, several teeth and even the entire quadrant may be included in a single mucoperiosteal flap (Smith, 1998; Blazejewski et al., 2006; Smith, 2008b). When performed properly, this technique is faster and less traumatic than prolonged use of luxators, elevators or forceps in a closed extraction technique. Releasing incisions are made with the local neurovascular supply and effective closure in mind (Operative Techniques 12.5 and 12.6). In the case of full-mouth extraction, a single, large envelope flap (i.e. one without releasing incisions) may be utilized in each dental arch, going from the last molar tooth on one side to the last molar tooth on the other side.

Fractured and retained roots

Extraction of the entire tooth and its root(s) is recommended. Exceptions to this rule include retained roots identified on radiographs that are completely buried under intact and healthy gingiva and show no signs of endodontic or periapical disease. However, retained roots with intraoral or extraoral communication (sinus tracts through gingiva, alveolar mucosa or skin) or associated with periodontal, endodontic or periapical disease must be removed. Roots fractured during the extraction procedure or remaining after mandibulectomies and maxillectomies must also be removed to prevent infection and inflammation of the bone (Reiter and Mendoza, 2002).

Narrow-bladed luxators and elevators are worked circumferentially around the root. A trough can be cut adjacent to the root fragment to allow insertion of even finer instruments. Special root tip (apical) elevators and root tip forceps are used to elevate and remove very small root fragments. An oversized endodontic file can be used to retrieve the root fragment by threading the file into the root canal; with the aid of a root tip elevator, the root may then be luxated, elevated and retrieved by pulling on the endodontic file (Reiter, 2007; Beckman and Smith, 2011). If a root fragment cannot be removed in a closed fashion, a mucoperiosteal flap is raised and alveolar bone removed to outline the root fragment and facilitate its elevation and extraction. A radiograph should be taken to verify complete removal of the root. Retrieval of root remnants from the mandibular canal, infraorbital canal or nasal cavity after accidental repulsion into these spaces must be carefully planned to avoid significant haemorrhage (Woodward, 2006; Reiter and Soltero-Rivera, 2014).

Every reasonable effort must be made to retrieve fractured roots, but the risks associated with prolonged anaesthesia and increased removal of alveolar bone, especially in a weak mandible, must be weighed against the potential danger posed by a retained root. If the risk of complications from anaesthesia and tissue damage is greater than the advantage gained by extraction, leaving a periodontally and endodontically sound root fragment in place after thorough lavage and closure of the surgical site may be an acceptable (though not ideal) treatment plan. Fractured and retained roots should be noted on the dental record/chart (Moore and Niemiec, 2014). Diligent monitoring for clinical signs associated with infection is required, supported by follow-up radiographic examination. The owner should be informed about the presence of fractured or retained roots, as they are usually the first to recognize a change in their pet's behaviour that may be a result of pain and discomfort.

The practice of blindly pulverizing ('atomizing') fractured or retained roots using high-speed equipment is contrary to all principles of oral surgery and must be frowned upon and strongly discouraged (Reiter, 2007). This amateurish technique can create considerable iatrogenic trauma, such as:

- Incomplete removal of the tooth root
- Overheating of hard and soft tissues, leading to bone necrosis and delayed healing

- Injury to inferior alveolar and infraorbital neurovascular bundles
- Possible repulsion of root fragments into the nasal cavity, the infraorbital canal or the mandibular canal
- Transection of salivary gland ducts in sublingual tissues
- Submucosal and subcutaneous emphysema
- Emphysema and air embolism.

Retrieval of root fragments using this technique may result in more damage than leaving them in place. Roots are either removed *in toto*, or allowed to remain buried if judged to be harmless (Kertesz, 1993) – the latter being decided on radiographic evaluation.

In small-breed dogs the apices of some of the mandibular teeth may reach into the ventral mandibular cortex, beyond the mandibular canal. If an intraoral approach towards these root fragments is not possible or complicated by haemorrhage, then an extraoral approach may be used to retrieve them (Figures 12.23 and 12.24).

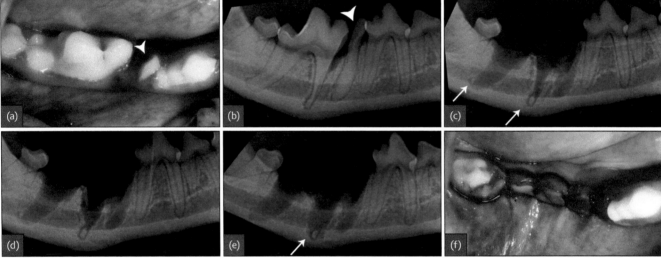

12.23 Vertical fracture of the mesial crown-root segment of the right mandibular first molar tooth in a 2-year-old Shi-Tzu dog following healing of a mandibular fracture at the same site. (a) Intraoral occlusal view and (b) lateral intraoral radiograph revealing the fractured piece of the tooth (arrowheads). (c) Root fragments (arrowed) remained deep in the alveoli following tooth extraction. (d, e) The fragment of the distal root was retrieved after further removal of alveolar bone, but visualization and extraction of the fragment of the mesial root (arrowed) was not possible due to significant haemorrhage from the inferior alveolar vessels. (f) Following haemostasis, the extraction site was sutured closed.
(© Dr Margherita Gracis)

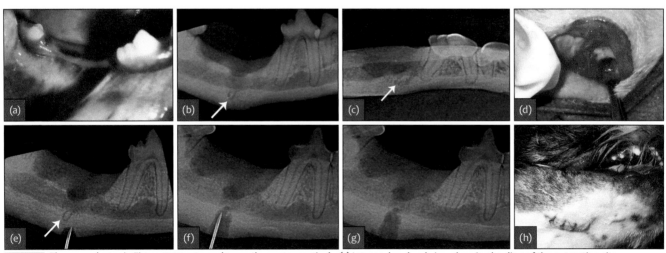

12.24 The same dog as in Figure 12.23 returned 2 months postoperatively. (a) Intraoral occlusal view showing healing of the extraction site. (b) Lateral and (c) occlusal intraoral radiographs, revealing the location of the fragment of the mesial root (arrowed) to be on the ventrobuccal aspect of the mandibular canal. (d) A full-thickness cutaneous incision was made over the ventral border of the mandible, and a small ostectomy was performed. (e) A radiograph was obtained with a radiopaque indicator in place to confirm the location of the fragment (arrowed). (f) Additional bone was removed to reach the root fragment, which was gently elevated. (g) A radiograph was obtained to confirm proper extraction. (h) The extraction site was sutured closed.
(© Dr Margherita Gracis)

Unerupted and intruded teeth

Unerupted or intruded teeth in animals with a permanent dentition should be extracted. A consequence of leaving an unerupted tooth in place is the formation of a dentigerous (tooth-containing) cyst, whose epithelial lining may in some cases undergo neoplastic metaplasia (Stapleton and Clarke, 1999; Taney and Smith, 2006; Edstrom et al., 2013).

1. A mucoperiosteal flap is raised.
2. Alveolar bone is removed over the tooth and its root(s), and the tooth is elevated and extracted. A multi-rooted tooth may be sectioned for a stepwise removal of crown-root segments. In the case of a dentigerous cyst, the epithelial lining of the cyst must be removed completely and submitted for histopathological examination.
3. The flap is replaced and sutured.

A clinically missing permanent maxillary tooth may have been intruded into the nasal cavity as a result of previous trauma. Patients can present with chronic rhinitis and epistaxis with owners unaware of the intruded tooth. Radiographic identification and evaluation of the tooth position is required. Surgical removal of such teeth may be accompanied by severe haemorrhage from the inflamed and infected nasal mucosa. Haemostasis can usually be achieved following curettage of the highly vascular granulation tissue that surrounded the intruded tooth, copious lavage with a refrigerated rinsing solution, temporary (a few minutes) packing of the wound with gauze, and final irrigation with a mixture of 0.25 ml phenylephrine 1% and 50 ml lidocaine 2% (0.05–0.1 ml/kg in cats; 0.1–0.2 ml/kg in dogs) before the site is sutured closed.

Crown amputation with intentional retention of resorbing root tissue

Ankylosed teeth and those with roots undergoing replacement resorption are commonly encountered in cats and sometimes in dogs as well. They cannot be easily elevated and extracted, even when open extraction principles are applied. An alternative to complete extraction of such teeth and roots (and only after radiographic confirmation of dentoalveolar ankylosis and root replacement resorption) is crown amputation with intentional retention of resorbing root tissue (DuPont, 2002).

The procedure begins by incising the gingival attachment around the tooth. A mucoperiosteal flap with or without releasing incisions is made. The crown is severed from the remainder of the tooth with a round or fissure bur attached to a high-speed handpiece under water irrigation. The resorbing root is further reduced with a round diamond bur to about 1–2 mm below the level of the alveolar margin. This allows a blood clot to form over the remaining root tissue into which alveolar bone can grow during healing. The flap is sutured without tension over the wound, and a postoperative radiograph is obtained serving as reference for future follow-ups (Reiter and Soltero-Rivera, 2014) (Operative Technique 12.7).

This technique is not recommended if closed or open extractions could be accomplished and is contraindicated for mobile teeth and those with periodontitis, endodontic disease and periapical pathology. Clients must be informed about the risks involved with this procedure (e.g. infection), and periodic monitoring of the surgical site must be performed by means of clinical and radiographic examinations (Reiter and Mendoza, 2002).

Complications of tooth extraction

Fractured roots

Fractured roots are a result of dental or mandibular/maxillofacial trauma, improper extraction technique or pre-existing root pathology (endodontic and periapical disease, dentoalveolar ankylosis and root replacement resorption). If the tooth being extracted has an inflamed, infected or necrotic pulp or is affected by periapical disease, every part of it must be removed to prevent further infection and avoid delay of healing. Crown sectioning must be complete and leverage forces applied for elevation of crown-root segments need to be directed as parallel to the roots as feasible and as far apical as possible, to prevent root fracture (Reiter, 2007).

The use of extraction forceps applied too far coronally on a tooth or crown-root segment, or applied with too much force, is also likely to result in root fracture. An audible crack can often be heard. A sharp-edged defect is visible and palpable at the end of the extracted root. Dental radiography is an invaluable tool in determining the position and size of the retained root fragment, aiding in its complete removal. If a root fragment cannot be retrieved and is left in place, a note is made in the dental record and the client informed about the complication (Lommer, 2012c). The surgical site should be evaluated periodically by means of clinical and radiographic follow-up examinations.

Root intrusion into the nasal cavity, infraorbital or mandibular canal is a serious complication (Taylor et al., 2004). Retrieval of root fragments from these spaces is difficult. Access through soft tissue and bone away from the extraction site may be required, and the operator should be prepared for possible haemorrhage to occur. Referral of these cases to an experienced veterinary dentist is desirable.

Haemorrhage

Bleeding can usually be controlled by means of digital pressure with a gauze swab. Cotton-tipped applicators and suction using fine tips greatly assist in cases where bleeding impairs visualization and removal of a tooth or root fragment. Severe bleeding is rare and likely to be due to injury of vessels in the mandibular or infraorbital canal or the mucosa of the nasal cavity. Packing a small amount of bone wax into an alveolus is usually sufficient to stop excessive bleeding. Bone wax should not be left in place, but removed after haemostasis is achieved. Application of cold compresses made from shredded ice wrapped in a gauze sponge can reduce blood flow sufficiently to allow a clot to form and, at the same time, retard postoperative swelling after flap surgery (Reiter, 2007).

In rare cases of excessive alveolar haemorrhage, the alveolus may be packed with cellulose meshes, gelatin powder/sheets, polysaccharide powder or collagen powder/sheets to aid in haemostasis. The gingiva must be sutured over the packs without tension. Vasoconstrictors are not recommended and should generally not be used in patients with cardiac problems, thyroid disorders or when halothane is used for inhalant anaesthesia.

Trauma to adjacent teeth, permanent tooth buds and soft tissues

Leverage against adjacent teeth must be avoided to prevent unwanted elevation and crown fractures of teeth not to be extracted. Complications of deciduous tooth extraction include damage to the underlying tooth buds of permanent successors. Instruments must not be inserted between a deciduous tooth and its developing permanent successor. Slight leverage against the latter could result in accidental elevation of the permanent tooth (Reiter, 2007).

Minor lacerations of adjacent gingiva commonly occur during the extraction procedure. More severe lacerations of soft tissues result from excessive elevation technique and slippage of sharp instruments. Gingival and alveolar mucosal defects thus created must be sutured appropriately. The use of a diamond disc for sectioning teeth is not recommended.

Sublingual oedema and salivary mucocele

Overzealous pharyngeal packing, tongue manipulation, excessive elevation of the alveolar mucosa on the lingual aspects of the mandibles and other iatrogenic trauma can result in oedematous swelling of the sublingual tissues. The sublingual oedema may be severe enough that breathing could be compromised during recovery from anaesthesia, and such patients may benefit from a single injection of intravenous dexamethasone (Reiter, 2007).

Excessive force and lack of instrument control can also cause injury to the ducts of mandibular, sublingual, parotid or zygomatic salivary glands, causing extravasation of saliva into submucosal and subcutaneous tissues and occasionally also the orbit (Adams et al., 2011). If breathing and masticatory function are not significantly compromised, postponing surgical treatment is feasible, as the salivary mucocele (sialocele) often resolves on its own in a few weeks. If it does not resolve, resection of the affected salivary gland–duct complex is preferred over marsupialization.

Trauma to the orbit and adjacent structures

Iatrogenic trauma to the orbit may occur during extraction of caudal maxillary teeth (Duke et al., 2014; Guerreiro et al., 2014). The cause of such trauma is related to the thin alveolar bone and proximity of the tooth roots to the ventral floor of the orbit. Orbital structures may be perforated by a pointed instrument, particularly in patients with severe periodontitis (Adams et al., 2011). Panophthalmitis may result. If antimicrobial and anti-inflammatory treatment fails, enucleation may need to be performed (Smith, 1998; Smith et al., 2003). Flushing of alveoli using a needle on a syringe may result in injection of non-sterile or tissue-damaging agents into the globe and is to be discouraged. Iatrogenic nasolacrimal duct obstruction following tooth extraction in a cat has also been described (Paiva et al., 2013). Frontal bone perforation and severe brain damage has been reported in the dog following improper extraction of maxillary molar teeth (Smith et al., 2003; Troxel, 2015).

Reduced alveolar bone height

Gingival connective tissue and periodontal ligament fibres attach the tooth to the jaw bone (Discepoli et al., 2013). Alveolectomy performed during an extraction procedure results in some loss of alveolar bone. There is also continued resorption of alveolar bone following tooth extraction, manifesting as apical recession of the alveolar margin (Blanco et al., 2011). Attempts to prevent or reduce continued loss of alveolar bone in edentulous sites of the mouth in cats and dogs by means of bone grafting showed mixed results (Araújo and Lindhe, 2005; Da Silva et al., 2012, 2013).

Fracture of the alveolus or jaw

A fractured alveolus occurs when excessive force is used during extraction, or when the bone overlying the root(s) has not been adequately removed. Unstable small bone fragments are removed before the extraction site is closed. Owners of animals with severe periodontal disease should be warned about an increased possibility of jaw fracture. The mandible may be prone to fracture during relatively routine pre- and intraoperative manoeuvres (when opening the mouth for examination or intubation, after placing a mouth prop, and during tooth extraction). Iatrogenic jaw fracture is most commonly associated with extraction of the mandibular canine (dogs and cats) or first molar teeth (small-breed dogs) and usually occurs when closed extraction techniques are used in areas weakened by severe bone loss (Reiter, 2007). This emphasizes the importance of preoperative dental radiography. A diseased and fractured mandible may never heal. Treatment includes extraction of diseased teeth in fracture lines, debridement of extraction sites and suturing of soft tissue to cover exposed bone, followed by orthopaedic repair.

Oronasal, oroantral and oro-orbital communications

Causes of oronasal, oroantral and oro-orbital communications involving the maxillary alveoli include severe periodontitis, periapical disease and iatrogenic trauma (Smith, 2000). In cats, such communications secondary to disease are rare because the thickness of the bone palatal to the roots of maxillary teeth is significant, and fistulas open relatively more frequently on the skin surface. A chronic oronasal or oroantral fistula results in rhinitis, sneezing, ipsilateral nasal discharge and difficulty in eating and drinking, and a defect may be seen in the upper dental arch, with oral epithelium confluent with nasal epithelium (Reiter, 2007).

If the nasal cavity, maxillary recess or orbit has been penetrated during the extraction process (acute communication), a tension-free flap must be raised to close the extraction site. In dogs, history of a chronic oronasal fistula typically reveals that a maxillary canine tooth has been lost or was previously extracted. Periodontitis results in resorption of the thin alveolar bone separating the root and nasal cavity. A deep periodontal pocket may be present on the palatal aspect of a maxillary canine tooth, causing communication between the oral and nasal cavities even though the tooth is still in place. The maxillary recess is located medial to the maxillary fourth premolar tooth, with some variations based on skull type and morphology. When the tooth is affected by severe periodontal disease, often the thin bone separating the alveoli from the recess is resorbed, and purulent material may collect into this space.

If an oronasal or oroantral communication is diagnosed, flushing of the ispilateral nasal cavity and surgical area should be performed prior to surgical closure to ensure removal of all debris. An absorbing pack should be placed in the pharynx during nasal flushing.

Orbital cellulitis and abscess formation may develop following dental disease of caudal maxillary teeth. Diagnosis of an oro-orbital communication following extraction of the molar teeth requires gentle retropulsion of the ipsilateral ocular globe while directly looking into the emptied alveoli. If the alveolar walls are not intact, the periapical soft tissues and blood contained in the alveolus will be seen moving according to the pressure applied over the ocular globe. If this is the case, the extraction site should definitely be sutured closed.

A single-layer labial-/buccal-based flap procedure is usually sufficient to repair a chronic oronasal, oroantral or oro-orbital fistula. Epithelium lining the fistula is resected, and apically diverging incisions are created into the alveolar and labial/buccal mucosa using a No. 15 scalpel blade. A full-thickness mucoperiosteal flap is raised with a periosteal elevator. The periosteum is incised at the base of the flap (as described earlier in this chapter to improve flap advancement). The flap is mobilized by blunt submucosal dissection using Metzenbaum scissors, advanced to cover the defect, and sutured to hard palate mucosa without tension in a simple interrupted pattern. Alternatively, a two-layer labial and buccal-based flap technique may be used; the first flap is overlapped and provides an epithelial surface for the nasal cavity and a connective tissue surface facing the oral cavity; the second flap is transposed and designed to cover the connective tissue surface of the first flap and also provides an epithelial surface for the oral cavity (Reiter, 2007).

Trauma from opposing teeth

Occlusal trauma may occur, particularly in cats, following the extraction of a maxillary canine tooth. Normally this tooth and supporting structures (gingiva and bone) keep the upper lip out of the way of the mandibular canine tooth when the cat closes its mouth. After extraction of the maxillary canine tooth the upper lip is not held out of the path of the opposing mandibular canine tooth, with the result that it may be pinched, punctured or lacerated (Reiter, 2007). Reducing the pointed tip of the mandibular canine tooth by 1 mm (taking care to avoid pulp exposure) is usually sufficient to solve the problem; exposed dentine should be treated with a layer of unfilled resin to reduce postoperative sensitivity. If the problem is ongoing, the mandibular canine tooth may be extracted; an alternative is crown reduction and vital pulp therapy or root canal therapy (Reiter, 2012).

Tongue hanging out of mouth

The rostral mandibular teeth serve as a basket to contain the tongue when it is at rest. When a mandibular canine tooth is extracted in dogs, the tongue may occasionally hang to the ipsilateral side when the mouth is open during panting (Reiter, 2007; Tsugawa et al., 2012). Commissuroplasty can be performed in cases of excessive drooling and lip dermatitis, though this procedure is most commonly indicated after partial or complete mandibulectomy procedures or pathological mandibular fractures.

Emphysema and air embolism

Emphysema sometimes occurs after use of air-driven high-speed equipment. This usually resolves spontaneously within days. It may also result from blowing air or air/water spray into submucosal tissues, particularly after deep submucosal dissection of large mucoperiosteal flaps. Emphysema can be effectively reduced or prevented with gentle digital pressure applied to the sutured flap for a few minutes to evacuate air bubbles and provide a seal between soft tissue and bone. Blowing air or air/water spray into alveolar sockets or on to bleeding tissues is contraindicated and risks causing air emboli (Gunew et al., 2008).

Local and systemic infection

Wound dehiscence is usually a result of tension on suture lines (Smith, 2008a). The extraction site is treated by means of resuturing, or left to granulate and epithelialize (healing by second intention). Infection and necrosis of alveolar bone occasionally occurs, particularly if the extraction procedure was excessively traumatic, caused loss of vascular supply to a segment of alveolar bone, or resulted in retained roots (Moore and Niemiec, 2014). Excessive heat generated during alveolectomy or alveoloplasty may also result in bone necrosis. Treatment consists of removal of sequestered bone, curettage until healthy bleeding bone is reached and a blood clot formed, and closure of the site with a healthy soft tissue flap. The rare condition of alveolitis (dry socket) in cats and dogs (more common in humans) is best prevented by allowing a blood clot to form in the debrided and lavaged alveolus after extraction and before suturing of the extraction site (Van Cauwelaert de Wyels, 1998). An extraction site that seems to be non-healing for 7 days or longer following surgery should be considered for biopsy to rule out the possibility of neoplasia.

Temporary bacteraemia has been described in cats and dogs during and after ultrasonic teeth cleaning and tooth extraction. It is not an indication for the perioperative use of systemic antibiotics in the otherwise healthy patient (Harvey, 1990). Systemic infection as a direct result of tooth extraction is anecdotally reported (Reiter et al., 2004; Westermeyer et al., 2013).

References and further reading

Adams P, Halfacree ZJ, Lamb CR et al. (2011) Zygomatic salivary mucocoele in a Lhasa Apso following maxillary tooth extraction. Veterinary Record **168**, 458–460

Anderson DM (2012) Surgical hemostasis. In: Veterinary Surgery: Small Animal, 1st edn, ed. KM Tobias and SA Johnston, pp. 214–220. Elsevier, St Louis

Araújo MG and Lindhe J (2005) Dimensional ridge alterations following tooth extraction. An experimental study in the dog. Journal of Clinical Periodontology **32**, 212–218

Beckman B and Smith MM (2011) Alternative extraction techniques in the dog and cat. Journal of Veterinary Dentistry **28**, 134–138

Blanco J, Mareque S, Liñares A et al. (2011) Vertical and horizontal ridge alterations after tooth extraction in the dog: flap versus flapless surgery. Clinical Oral Implants Research **22**, 1255–1258

Blazejewski S, Lewis JR and Reiter AM (2006) Mucoperiosteal flap for extraction of multiple teeth in the maxillary quadrant of the cat. Journal of Veterinary Dentistry **23**, 200–205

Boutoille F and Hennet P (2011) Maxillary osteomyelitis in two Scottish terrier dogs with chronic ulcerative paradental stomatitis. Journal of Veterinary Dentistry **28**, 96–100

Carmichael DT (2002) Surgical extraction of the maxillary fourth premolar tooth in the dog. Journal of Veterinary Dentistry **19**, 231–233

Clark WT, Kane L, Arnold PK et al. (2002) Clinical skills and knowledge used by veterinary graduates during their first year in small animal practice. Australian Veterinary Journal **80**, 37–40

Da Silva AM, Astolphi RD, Perri SH et al. (2013) Filling of extraction sockets of feline maxillary canine teeth with autogenous bone or bioactive glass. Acta Cirúrgica Brasileira **28**, 856–862

Da Silva AM, Souza WM, Souza NT et al. (2012) Filling of extraction sockets with autogenous bone in cats. Acta Cirúrgica Brasileira **27**, 82–87

DeBowes LJ (2005) Simple and surgical exodontia. Veterinary Clinics of North America Small Animal Practice **35**, 963–984

Discepoli N, Vignoletti F, Laino L et al. (2013) Early healing of the alveolar process after tooth extraction: an experimental study in the beagle dog. Journal of Clinical Periodontology **40**, 638–644

Duke FD, Snyder CJ, Bentley E et al. (2014) Ocular trauma originating from within the oral cavity: clinical relevance and histologic findings in 10 cases (2003–2013). Journal of Veterinary Dentistry **31**, 245–248

DuPont GA (2002) Crown amputation with intentional root retention for dental resorptive lesions in cats. Journal of Veterinary Dentistry **19**, 107–110

Edstrom EJ, Smith MM and Taney K (2013) Extraction of the impacted mandibular canine tooth in the dog. Journal of Veterinary Dentistry **30**, 56–61

Emily P and Penman S (1994) Extraction and oronasal fistula closure. In: Handbook of Small Animal Dentistry, 2nd edn, ed. P Emily and S Penman, pp. 95–105. Pergamon Press, Oxford

Fitch PF (2003) Surgical extraction of the maxillary canine tooth. Journal of Veterinary Dentistry **20**, 55–58

Gengler B (2013) Exodontics: extraction of teeth in the dog and cat. *Veterinary Clinics of North America Small Animal Practice* **43**, 573–585

Gorrel C and Robinson J (1995) Periodontal therapy and extraction technique. In: *BSAVA Manual of Small Animal Dentistry, 2nd edn*, ed. DA Crossley and S Penman, pp. 139–149. BSAVA Publications, Cheltenham

Guerreiro CE, Appelboam H and Lowe RC (2014) Successful medical treatment for globe penetration following tooth extraction in a dog. *Veterinary Ophthalmology* **17**, 146–149

Gunew M, Marshall R, Lui M *et al.* (2008) Fatal venous air embolism in a cat undergoing dental extractions. *Journal of Small Animal Practice* **49**, 601–604

Harvey CE (1990) Basic techniques – extraction and antibiotic treatment. In: *BSAVA Manual of Small Animal Dentistry, 1st edn*, ed. CE Harvey and H Orr, pp. 29–35. BSAVA Publications, Cheltenham

Harvey CE and Emily PP (1993) Oral surgery. In: *Small Animal Dentistry, 1st edn*, ed. CE Harvey and PP Emily, pp. 312–377. Mosby-Year Book, Inc, St Louis

Hobson P (2005) Extraction of retained primary canine teeth in the dog. *Journal of Veterinary Dentistry* **22**, 132–137

Holmstrom SE (2000) Exodontics (extractions). In: *Veterinary Dentistry for the Technician and Office Staff, 1st edn*, ed. SE Holmstrom, pp. 205–222. WB Saunders, Philadelphia

Holmstrom SE, Frost P and Eisner ER (1998) Exodontics. In: *Veterinary Dental Techniques for the Small Animal Practitioner, 2nd edn*, ed. SE Holmstrom, P Frost and ER Eisner, pp. 215–254. WB Saunders, Philadelphia

Kertesz P (1993) Oral surgery: I. Extractions. In: *A Colour Atlas of Veterinary Dentistry and Oral Surgery, 1st edn*, ed. P Kertesz, pp. 149–164. Wolfe Publishing, Aylesbury

Legendre LF (1994) Dentistry on deciduous teeth: what, when, and how. *Canadian Veterinary Journal* **35**, 793–794

Lipscomb V and Reiter AM (2005) Surgical materials and instrumentation. In: *BSAVA Manual of Canine and Feline Head, Neck and Thoracic Surgery, 1st edn*, ed. DJ Brockman and DE Holt, pp. 16–24. BSAVA Publications, Gloucester

Lommer MJ (2012a) Principles of exodontics. In: *Oral and Maxillofacial Surgery in Dogs and Cats, 1st edn*, ed. FJM Verstraete and MJ Lommer, pp. 97–114. Elsevier, Edinburgh

Lommer MJ (2012b) Special considerations in feline exodontics. In: *Oral and Maxillofacial Surgery in Dogs and Cats, 1st edn*, ed. FJM Verstraete and MJ Lommer, pp. 141–152. Elsevier, Edinburgh

Lommer MJ (2012c) Complications of extractions. In: *Oral and Maxillofacial Surgery in Dogs and Cats, 1st edn*, ed. FJM Verstraete and MJ Lommer, pp. 153–159. Elsevier, Edinburgh

Lommer MJ, Tsugawa AJ and Verstraete FJM (2012) Extraction of multirooted teeth in dogs. In: *Oral and Maxillofacial Surgery in Dogs and Cats, 1st edn*, ed. FJM Verstraete and MJ Lommer, pp. 131–139. Elsevier, Edinburgh

Lommer MJ and Verstraete FJM (2012) Simple extraction of single-rooted teeth. In: *Oral and Maxillofacial Surgery in Dogs and Cats, 1st edn*, ed. FJM Verstraete and MJ Lommer, pp. 115–120. Elsevier, Edinburgh

MacGee S, Pinson DM and Shaiken L (2012) Bilateral dentigerous cysts in a dog. *Journal of Veterinary Dentistry* **29**, 242–249

Marretta SM (2002) Surgical extraction of the mandibular first molar tooth in the dog. *Journal of Veterinary Dentistry* **19**, 46–50

Moore JI and Niemiec B (2014) Evaluation of extraction sites for evidence of retained tooth roots and periapical pathology. *Journal of the American Animal Hospital Association* **50**, 77–82

Niemiec BA (2008) Extraction techniques. *Topics in Companion Animal Medicine* **23**, 97–105

O'Morrow C (2010) Extraction of a mandibular first molar tooth (409) in a dog. *Canadian Veterinary Journal* **51**, 416–420

Paiva SC, Froes TR, Lange RR *et al.* (2013) Iatrogenic nasolacrimal duct obstruction following tooth extraction in a cat. *Journal of Veterinary Dentistry* **30**, 90–94

Reiter AM (2007) Dental surgical procedures. In: *BSAVA Manual of Canine and Feline Dentistry, 3rd edn*, ed. C Tutt, J Deeprose and D Crossley, pp. 178–195. BSAVA Publications, Gloucester

Reiter AM (2012) Dental and oral diseases. In: *The Cat: Clinical Medicine and Management, 1st edn*, ed. SE Little, pp. 329–370. Saunders, St Louis

Reiter AM (2013) Equipment for oral surgery in small animals. *Veterinary Clinics of North America Small Animal Practice* **43**, 587–608

Reiter AM (2014) Open wide: Blindness in cats after the use of mouth gags (guest editorial). *Veterinary Journal* **201**, 5–6

Reiter AM, Brady CA and Harvey CE (2004) Local and systemic complications in a cat after poorly performed dental extractions. *Journal of Veterinary Dentistry* **21**, 215–221

Reiter AM, Lewis JR and Harvey CE (2012) Dentistry for the surgeon. In: *Veterinary Surgery: Small Animal, 1st edn*, ed. KM Tobias and SA Johnston, pp. 1037–1053. Elsevier, St. Louis

Reiter AM, Lewis JR, Rawlinson JE *et al.* (2005) Hemisection and partial retention of carnassial teeth in client-owned dogs. *Journal of Veterinary Dentistry* **22**, 216–226

Reiter AM and Mendoza K (2002) Feline odontoclastic resorptive lesions – an unsolved enigma in veterinary dentistry. *Veterinary Clinics of North America Small Animal Practice* **32**, 791–837

Reiter AM and Smith MM (2005) The oral cavity and oropharynx. In: *BSAVA Manual of Canine and Feline Head, Neck and Thoracic Surgery, 1st edn*, ed. DJ Brockman and DE Holt, pp. 25–43. BSAVA Publications, Gloucester

Reiter AM and Soltero-Rivera M (2014) Applied feline oral anatomy and tooth extraction techniques. An illustrated guide. *Journal of Feline Medicine and Surgery* **16**, 900–913

Ritchie C (2018) A modified technique for extraction site closure of the maxillary molars in a dog. *Journal of Veterinary Dentistry* **35**, 42–45

Scheels JL and Howard PE (1993) Principles of dental extraction. *Seminars of Veterinary Medicine and Surgery (Small Animal)* **8**, 146–154

Smith MM (1996) Lingual approach for surgical extraction of the mandibular canine tooth in dogs and cats. *Journal of the American Animal Hospital Association* **32**, 359–364

Smith MM (1998) Exodontics. *Veterinary Clinics of North America Small Animal Practice* **28**, 1297–1319

Smith MM (2000) Oronasal fistula repair. *Clinical Techniques in Small Animal Practice* **15**, 243–250

Smith MM (2001) Surgical extraction of the mandibular canine tooth in the dog. *Journal of Veterinary Dentistry* **18**, 48–49

Smith MM (2008a) The periosteal releasing incision. *Journal of Veterinary Dentistry* **25**, 65–68

Smith MM (2008b) Extraction of teeth in the mandibular quadrant of the cat. *Journal of Veterinary Dentistry* **25**, 69–74

Smith MM, Smith EM, La Croix N *et al.* (2003) Orbital penetration associated with tooth extraction. *Journal of Veterinary Dentistry* **20**, 8–17

Stapleton BL and Clarke LL (1999) Mandibular canine tooth impaction in a young dog–treatment and subsequent eruption: a case report. *Journal of Veterinary Dentistry* **16**, 105–108

Taney KG and Smith MM (2006) Surgical extraction of impacted teeth in a dog. *Journal of Veterinary Dentistry* **23**, 168–177

Taylor TN, Smith MM and Snyder L (2004) Nasal displacement of a tooth root in a dog. *Journal of Veterinary Dentistry* **21**, 222–225

Troxel M (2015) Iatrogenic traumatic brain injury during tooth extraction. *Journal of American Animal Hospital Association* **51**, 114–118

Tsugawa AJ, Lommer MJ and Verstraete FJM (2012) Extraction of canine teeth in dogs. In: *Oral and Maxillofacial Surgery in Dogs and Cats, 1st edn*, ed. FJM Verstraete and MJ Lommer, pp. 121–129. Elsevier, Edinburgh

Vall P (2012) Maxillary molar tooth extraction in the dog. *Journal of Veterinary Dentistry* **29**, 276–284

Van Cauwelaert de Wyels S (1998) Alveolar osteitis (dry socket) in a dog: a case report. *Journal of Veterinary Dentistry* **15**, 85–87

Volker MK and Luskin IR (2012) Surgical extraction of the mandibular canine tooth in the cat. *Journal of Veterinary Dentistry* **29**, 134–137

Westermeyer HD, Ward DA, Whittemore JC *et al.* (2013) *Actinomyces* endogenous endophthalmitis in a cat following multiple dental extractions. *Veterinary Ophthalmology* **16**, 459–463

Woodward TM (2006) Extraction of fractured tooth roots. *Journal of Veterinary Dentistry* **23**, 126–129

OPERATIVE TECHNIQUE 12.1

Maxillary canine tooth extraction in the dog

INDICATIONS

Periodontal disease; tooth injury (wear, fracture, displacement); endodontic and periapical disease; malocclusion; oral inflammation; tooth resorption; caries.

POSITIONING

Lateral recumbency.

ASSISTANT

Preferable.

ADDITIONAL EQUIPMENT

Scalpel; periosteal elevator; round burs; round diamond burs; lactated Ringer's solution (or saline); dental elevators; extraction forceps; tissue scissors; thumb forceps; suture material; needle holder; suture scissors; gauze.

SURGICAL TECHNIQUE

Approach

The mouth is rinsed with a 0.12% chlorhexidine solution, and dental scaling is performed. Preoperative radiographs are obtained to evaluate root development, confirm lack of complicating factors, and identify signs of endodontic or periodontal disease.

Surgical manipulations

1   Incise the gingival attachment around the tooth.

2   Make diverging mesial and distal releasing incisions starting apical to the mucogingival junction, into the alveolar mucosa down to the bone and extending them towards the gingival margin at the mesial and distal aspects of the tooth.

3   Use a sharp periosteal elevator to free the gingiva and alveolar mucosa from the underlying bone labially, and elevate the palatal gingiva as an envelope flap to expose the alveolar margin.

4   Use a round bur with water irrigation to reduce the level of the alveolar bone overlying the root as needed. Narrow grooves can also be burred at mesial and distal aspects of the root to allow for better elevator purchase.

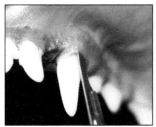 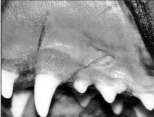 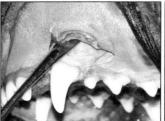 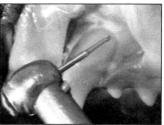

(© Dr Alexander M. Reiter)

5   Elevate and extract the tooth.

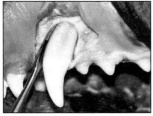 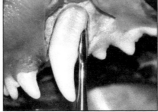 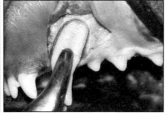 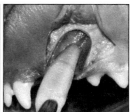

(© Dr Alexander M. Reiter)

→ **OPERATIVE TECHNIQUE 12.1 CONTINUED**

6 Incise the periosteum at the base of the flap with a scalpel blade, dissect its connective tissue with blunt tissue scissors, and ensure that the tension-free flap spans over the extraction site.

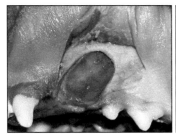 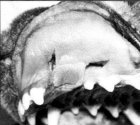 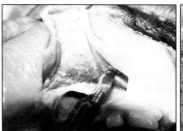 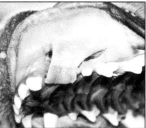

(© Dr Alexander M. Reiter)

7 Excise the flap margins, elevate the palatal gingiva, and proceed with debridement, smoothing of alveolar bone and lavage of the extraction site. Take a postoperative radiograph to confirm complete removal of dental tissue.

8 Appose the flap to the palatal gingiva by means of simple interrupted sutures. The corners of the flap are sutured first, and additional sutures are placed 2–3 mm apart and 1–2 mm from the flap edges.

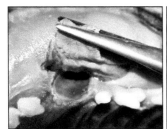 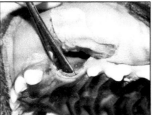 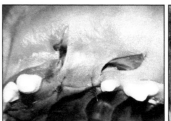 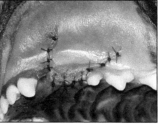

(© Dr Alexander M. Reiter)

PRACTICAL TIPS

- The distal releasing incision of the flap should preferably be created without cutting into the gingival sulcus of the first premolar tooth (or detachment of gingiva from this tooth)
- A triangular flap may also be used, utilizing a single releasing incision mesial to the canine tooth and extending the gingival horizontal incision to the first or second premolar tooth
- Stretching the alveolar mucosa dorsocaudally with a thumb will move the neurovascular bundle emerging from the infraorbital foramen away from where the distal releasing incision is made
- Avoid:
  - Injury to the neurovascular bundle at the infraorbital foramen
  - Creation of an acute oronasal fistula during alveolectomy or elevation of the tooth
  - Elevator purchase on the palatal aspect of the tooth, which could cause fracture of the thin bone separating the tooth from the nasal cavity and displacement of the apex into the nasal cavity

OPERATIVE TECHNIQUE 12.2

Mandibular canine tooth extraction in the dog

INDICATIONS

Periodontal disease; tooth injury (wear, fracture, displacement); endodontic and periapical disease; malocclusion; oral inflammation; tooth resorption; caries.

POSITIONING

Lateral recumbency.

ASSISTANT

Preferable.

ADDITIONAL EQUIPMENT

Scalpel; periosteal elevator; round burs; round diamond burs; lactated Ringer's solution (or saline); dental elevators; extraction forceps; tissue scissors; thumb forceps; suture material; needle holder; suture scissors; gauze.

SURGICAL TECHNIQUE

Approach

The mouth is rinsed with a 0.12% chlorhexidine solution, and dental scaling is performed. Preoperative radiographs are obtained to evaluate root development, confirm lack of complicating factors, and identify signs of endodontic or periodontal disease.

Surgical manipulations

1 Incise the gingival attachment around the tooth.

2 Make diverging mesial and distal releasing incisions starting apical to the mucogingival junction, into the alveolar mucosa down to the bone and extending them towards the gingival margin.

3 Use a sharp periosteal elevator to free the gingiva and alveolar mucosa from the underlying bone labially, and elevate the lingual gingiva as an envelope flap to expose the alveolar margin.

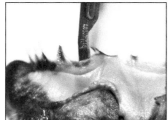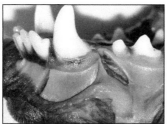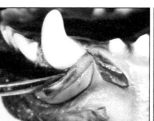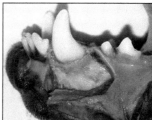

(© Dr Alexander M. Reiter)

4 Use a round bur with water irrigation to reduce the level of the alveolar bone overlying the root as needed. Narrow grooves can also be burred at mesial and distal aspects of the root to allow for better elevator purchase.

5 Elevate and extract the tooth.

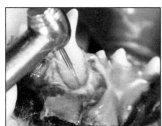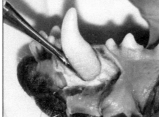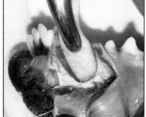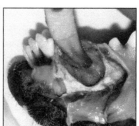

(© Dr Alexander M. Reiter)

→ **OPERATIVE TECHNIQUE 12.2 CONTINUED**

6   Incise the periosteum at the base of the flap with a scalpel blade, dissect its connective tissue with blunt tissue scissors, and ensure that the tension-free flap spans over the extraction site.

7   Excise the flap margins, elevate the lingual gingiva, and proceed with debridement, smoothing of alveolar bone and lavage of the extraction site. Take a postoperative radiograph to confirm complete removal of dental tissue.

8   Appose the flap to the lingual gingiva by means of simple interrupted sutures. The corners of the flap are sutured first, and additional sutures are placed 2–3 mm apart and 1–2 mm from the flap edges.

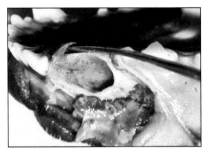 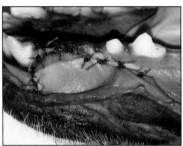

(© Dr Alexander M. Reiter)

PRACTICAL TIPS

- The distal releasing incision of the flap should preferably be created without cutting into the gingival sulcus of the first premolar tooth
- A triangular flap may also be used, utilizing a single releasing incision mesial to the tooth and extending the gingival horizontal incision distally to include the first or even the second premolar tooth. This will preserve the lateral frenulum of the lower lip, which is elevated and repositioned at the original position
- Avoid:
  - Injury to the neurovascular bundle at the middle mental foramen
  - Excessive elevator purchase between the mandibular canine and third incisor teeth, resulting in injury of the latter or fracture of the alveolus or mandible

OPERATIVE TECHNIQUE 12.3

Maxillary fourth premolar tooth extraction in the dog

INDICATIONS

Periodontal disease; tooth injury (wear, fracture, displacement); endodontic and periapical disease; malocclusion; oral inflammation; tooth resorption; caries.

POSITIONING

Lateral recumbency.

ASSISTANT

Preferable.

ADDITIONAL EQUIPMENT

Scalpel; periosteal elevator; round burs; round diamond burs; (cross-cut) fissure burs; lactated Ringer's solution (or saline); dental elevators; extraction forceps; tissue scissors; thumb forceps; suture material; needle holder; suture scissors; gauze.

→

→ **OPERATIVE TECHNIQUE 12.3 CONTINUED**

Approach

The mouth is rinsed with a 0.12% chlorhexidine solution, and dental scaling is performed. Preoperative radiographs are obtained to evaluate root development, confirm lack of complicating factors, and identify signs of endodontic or periodontal disease.

Surgical manipulations

1   Incise the gingival attachment around the tooth.

2   Make diverging mesial and distal releasing incisions starting apical to the mucogingival junction, into the alveolar mucosa down to the bone and extending them towards the gingival margin.

3   Use a sharp periosteal elevator to free the gingiva and alveolar mucosa from the underlying bone buccally, and slightly elevate the palatal gingiva to expose the alveolar margin.

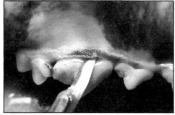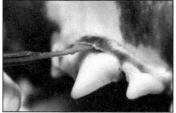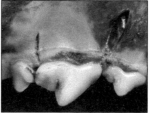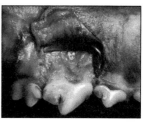

(© Dr Alexander M. Reiter)

4   Use a round bur with water irrigation to reduce the level of the alveolar bone overlying the mesiobuccal and distal roots as needed. Narrow grooves can also be burred at mesial and distal aspects of the roots to allow for better elevator purchase.

5   Section the tooth appropriately; separate the distal crown-root segment from the mesial portion of the tooth, and separate the mesiobuccal crown-root segment from the mesiopalatal crown-root segment.

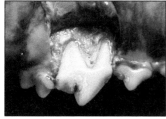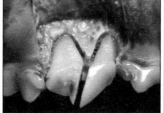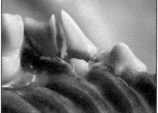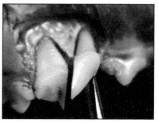

(© Dr Alexander M. Reiter)

6   Elevate and extract the mesiobuccal and distal crown-root segments, then reduce the septal bone overlying the mesiopalatal root, followed by elevation and extraction of the mesiopalatal crown-root segment.

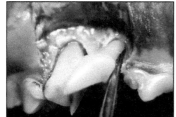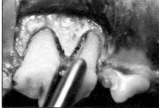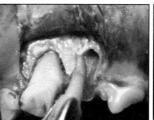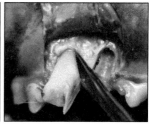

(© Dr Alexander M. Reiter)

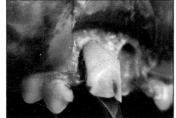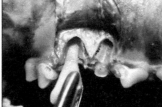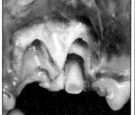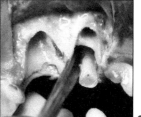

(© Dr Alexander M. Reiter)

→ **OPERATIVE TECHNIQUE 12.3 CONTINUED**

7 Incise the periosteum at the base of the flap with a scalpel blade, dissect its connective tissue with blunt tissue scissors, and ensure that the tension-free flap spans over the extraction site.

8 Excise the flap margins, elevate the palatal gingiva, and proceed with debridement, smoothing of alveolar bone and lavage of the extraction site. Take a postoperative radiograph to confirm complete removal of dental tissue.

9 Appose the flap to the palatal gingiva by means of simple interrupted sutures. The corners of the flap are sutured first, and additional sutures are placed 2–3 mm apart and 1–2 mm from the flap edges.

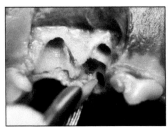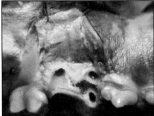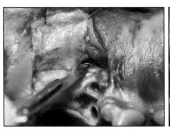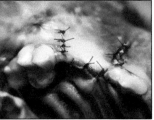

(© Dr Alexander M. Reiter)

PRACTICAL TIPS

- Slight elevation of the gingiva at the mesial aspect of the tooth will reveal the furcation between the mesiobuccal and mesiopalatal roots, facilitating proper sectioning between the mesiobuccal and mesiopalatal crown-root segments
- Slightly elevating the mucosa on the palatal aspect of the tooth will avoid injury to the palatal gingiva during sectioning between the distal and mesiobuccal crown-root segments
- Removal of dental tissue at the mesial and distal aspects of the tooth may improve elevator purchase in areas with limited interproximal space (i.e. between the maxillary third and fourth premolar teeth, and between the maxillary fourth premolar and first molar teeth)
- A triangular flap may also be used, utilizing a single releasing incision at the mesial aspect of the fourth premolar tooth, and extending the gingival horizontal incision distally to the first molar tooth
- Avoid:
  - Injury to the neurovascular bundle at the infraorbital foramen and the ducts of the parotid and zygomatic salivary glands during flap creation
  - Injury to the neurovascular bundle in the infraorbital canal during reduction of septal bone overlying the mesiopalatal root following extraction of the mesiobuccal crown-root segment
  - Injury to the mesiobuccal root of the maxillary first molar tooth during alveolectomy
  - Transportation of root tissue into the infraorbital canal, nasal cavity or maxillary recess
  - Creation of an oronasal or oroantral fistula during extraction of the mesiopalatal crown-root segment

---

OPERATIVE TECHNIQUE 12.4

Mandibular first molar tooth extraction in the dog

INDICATIONS

Periodontal disease; tooth injury (wear, fracture, displacement); endodontic and periapical disease; malocclusion; oral inflammation; tooth resorption; caries.

POSITIONING

Lateral recumbency.

ASSISTANT

Preferable.

→ OPERATIVE TECHNIQUE 12.4 CONTINUED

Scalpel; periosteal elevator; round burs; round diamond burs; (cross-cut) fissure burs; lactated Ringer's solution (or saline); dental elevators; extraction forceps; tissue scissors; thumb forceps; suture material; needle holder; suture scissors; gauze.

SURGICAL TECHNIQUE

Approach

The mouth is rinsed with a 0.12% chlorhexidine solution, and dental scaling is performed. Preoperative radiographs are obtained to evaluate root development, confirm lack of complicating factors, and identify signs of endodontic or periodontal disease.

Surgical manipulations

1 Incise the gingival attachment around the tooth.

2 Make diverging mesial and distal releasing incisions starting apical to the mucogingival junction, into the alveolar mucosa down to the bone and extending them towards the gingival margin.

3 Use a sharp periosteal elevator to free the gingiva and alveolar mucosa from the underlying bone buccally, and elevate the lingual gingiva as an envelope flap to expose the alveolar margin.

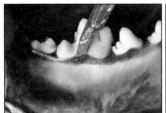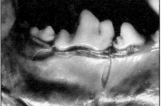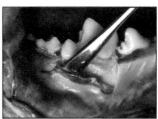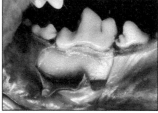

(© Dr Alexander M. Reiter)

4 Use a round bur with water irrigation to reduce the level of the alveolar bone overlying the mesial and distal roots as needed. Narrow grooves can also be burred at the mesial and distal aspects of the roots to allow for better elevator purchase.

5 Section the tooth appropriately.

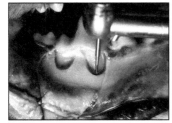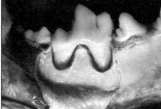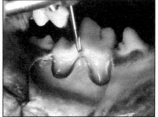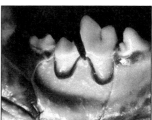

(© Dr Alexander M. Reiter)

6 Elevate and extract the mesial and distal crown-root segments.

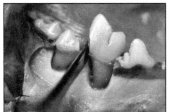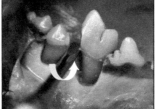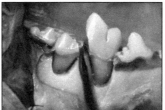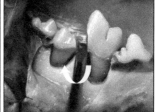

(© Dr Alexander M. Reiter)

→ **OPERATIVE TECHNIQUE 12.4 CONTINUED**

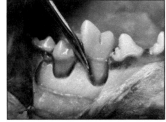
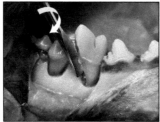
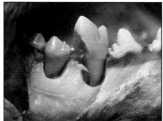
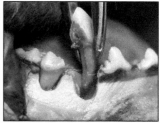

(© Dr Alexander M. Reiter)

7 Incise the periosteum at the base of the flap with a scalpel blade, dissect its connective tissue with blunt tissue scissors, and ensure that the tension-free flap spans over the extraction site.

8 Excise the flap margins, elevate the lingual gingiva, and proceed with debridement, smoothing of alveolar bone and lavage of the extraction site. Take a postoperative radiograph to confirm complete removal of dental tissue.

9 Appose the flap to the lingual gingiva by means of simple interrupted sutures. The corners of the flap are sutured first, and additional sutures are placed 2–3 mm apart and 1–2 mm from the flap edges.

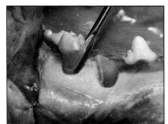
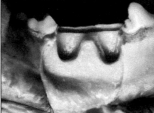
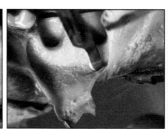
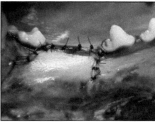

(© Dr Alexander M. Reiter)

PRACTICAL TIPS

- Creation of an envelope flap on the lingual aspect of the tooth will avoid injury to the lingual gingiva during sectioning between the mesial and distal crown-root segments
- An envelope flap may also be used, utilizing a single horizontal incision along the alveolar margin extending from the fourth premolar to the second premolar teeth
- Removal of dental tissue at the mesial and distal aspects of the tooth improves elevator purchase in areas with limited interproximal space (i.e. between the mandibular fourth premolar and first molar teeth and between the mandibular first molar and second molar teeth)
- Avoid:
  - Excessive flap elevation buccally and lingually
  - Injury to the neurovascular bundle in the mandibular canal during alveolectomy and elevation of crown-root segments
  - Transportation of root tissue into the mandibular canal
  - Excessive force during luxation and elevation of crown-root segments resulting in mandibular fracture

OPERATIVE TECHNIQUE 12.5

Extraction of the maxillary canine and cheek teeth in the cat

INDICATIONS

Tooth resorption; stomatitis; periodontal disease; tooth injury (wear, fracture, displacement); endodontic and periapical disease; malocclusion.

POSITIONING

Lateral recumbency.

ASSISTANT

Preferable.

ADDITIONAL EQUIPMENT

Scalpel; periosteal elevator; round burs; round diamond burs; (cross-cut) fissure burs; lactated Ringer's solution (or saline); dental elevators; extraction forceps; root tip elevators; root tip forceps; tissue scissors; thumb forceps; suture material; needle holder; suture scissors; gauze.

SURGICAL TECHNIQUE

Approach

The mouth is rinsed with a 0.12% chlorhexidine solution, and dental scaling is performed. Preoperative radiographs are obtained to evaluate root development, lack of complicating factors, and signs of endodontic or periodontal disease.

Surgical manipulations

1 Incise the gingival attachment around each tooth.

2 Make a horizontal incision along the alveolar margin from the mesiolabial aspect of the maxillary canine tooth to the distal aspect of the most caudal tooth to be extracted. Make a vertical releasing incision at the mesial aspect of the canine tooth starting apical to the mucogingival junction, into the alveolar mucosa down to the bone and extending it towards the gingival margin.

3 Use a sharp periosteal elevator to free the gingiva and alveolar mucosa from the underlying bone labially and buccally, and elevate the palatal gingiva as an envelope flap to expose the alveolar margin.

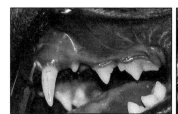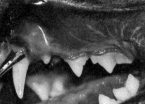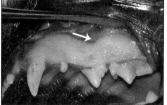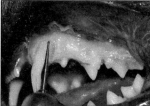

The arrow indicates the neurovascular bundle emerging at the infraorbital foramen.
(© Dr Alexander M. Reiter)

4 Use a round bur with water irrigation to reduce the level of the alveolar bone overlying the roots as needed. Narrow grooves can also be burred at mesial and distal aspects of the roots to allow for better elevator purchase.

→ **OPERATIVE TECHNIQUE 12.5 CONTINUED**

5 Section multi-rooted teeth; the maxillary first molar tooth may not need to be sectioned but may be extracted like a single-rooted tooth.

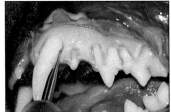 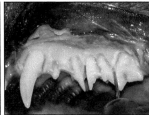 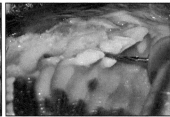 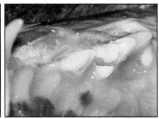

(© Dr Alexander M. Reiter)

6 Elevate and extract all teeth and crown-root segments.

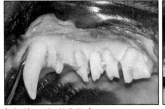 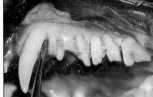 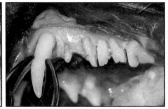 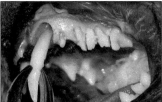

(© Dr Alexander M. Reiter)

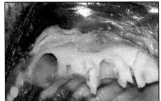 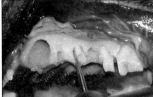 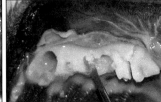 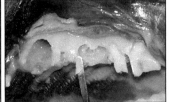

Fully extract any fractured roots by extending the labial/buccal alveolectomy using small elevators/luxators, as shown for the fractured mesial root of the left maxillary third premolar tooth.
(© Dr Alexander M. Reiter)

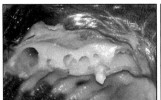 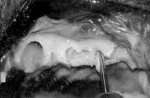 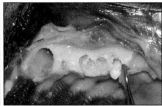 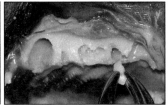

Reduce the septal bone overlying the mesiopalatal root (following extraction of the mesiobuccal crown-root segment) to facilitate its removal.
(© Dr Alexander M. Reiter)

7 Slightly elevate the palatal gingiva, and proceed with debridement, smoothing of alveolar bone with a large round diamond bur and lavage of the extraction sites.

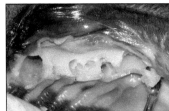 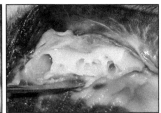 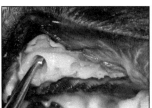 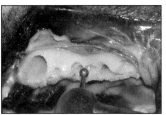

(© Dr Alexander M. Reiter)

8 Excise the flap margins, incise the periosteum at the base of the flap with a scalpel blade, dissect its connective tissue with blunt tissue scissors, and ensure that the tension-free flap spans over the extraction sites.

➜ OPERATIVE TECHNIQUE 12.5 CONTINUED

9 Appose the flap to the palatal gingiva by means of simple interrupted sutures. The corner of the flap is sutured first, and additional sutures are placed 2–3 mm apart and 1–2 mm from the flap edges.

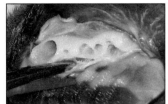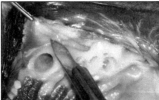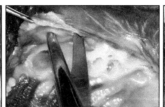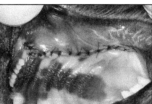

(© Dr Alexander M. Reiter)

PRACTICAL TIPS

- It is advisable to inspect and palpate the root apices and compare radiographs before and after extraction of teeth (prior to suturing of the flap) to confirm complete removal of dental tissue

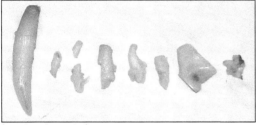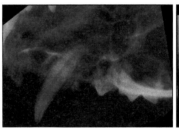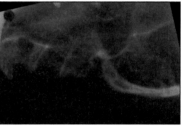

(© Dr Alexander M. Reiter)

- A large flap may be closed with a simple continuous suture pattern to minimize the number of knots in the mouth and reduce total anaesthesia time. However, the risk of wound dehiscence and postoperative complications should be considered when choosing this type of suturing technique
- It is wise for less experienced clinicians to extract one tooth at a time rather than to perform alveolectomy on multiple teeth, in case anaesthesia needs to be interrupted and the patient quickly awakened for medical reasons
- Avoid:
  - Excessive flap elevation labially/buccally and palatally as well as traumatic flap manipulation
  - Excessive bone removal
  - Injury to the neurovascular bundle at the infraorbital foramen or inside the infraorbital canal
  - Injury to the ducts of the parotid and zygomatic salivary glands
  - Transportation of dental tissue into the nasal cavity or infraorbital canal
  - Elevator purchase on the palatal aspect of the canine tooth, which could cause fracture of the thin bone separating the tooth from the nasal cavity and creation of an acute oronasal fistula or displacement of the apex into the nasal cavity

OPERATIVE TECHNIQUE 12.6

Extraction of the mandibular canine and cheek teeth in the cat

INDICATIONS

Tooth resorption; stomatitis; periodontal disease; tooth injury (wear, fracture, displacement); endodontic and periapical disease; malocclusion.

POSITIONING

Lateral recumbency.

ASSISTANT

Preferable.

ADDITIONAL EQUIPMENT

Scalpel; periosteal elevator; round burs; round diamond burs; (cross-cut) fissure burs; lactated Ringer's solution (or saline); dental elevators; extraction forceps; root tip elevators; root tip forceps; tissue scissors; thumb forceps; suture material; needle holder; suture scissors; gauze.

SURGICAL TECHNIQUE

Approach

The mouth is rinsed with a 0.12% chlorhexidine solution, and dental scaling is performed. Preoperative radiographs are obtained to evaluate root development, confirm lack of complicating factors, and identify signs of endodontic or periodontal disease.

Surgical manipulations

1 Incise the gingival attachment around each tooth.

2 Make a horizontal incision along the alveolar margin from the mesiolabial aspect of the mandibular canine tooth to the distal aspect of the most caudal tooth to be extracted. Make a vertical releasing incision at the mesial aspect of the canine tooth starting apical to the mucogingival junction, into the alveolar mucosa down to the bone and extending it towards the gingival margin.

3 Use a sharp periosteal elevator to free the attached gingiva and alveolar mucosa from the underlying bone labially and buccally, and elevate the lingual gingiva as an envelope flap to expose the alveolar margin.

4 Use a round bur with water irrigation to reduce the level of the alveolar bone overlying the roots as needed. Narrow grooves can also be burred at the mesial and distal aspects of the roots to allow for better elevator purchase.

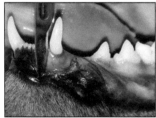 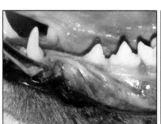 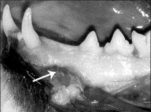 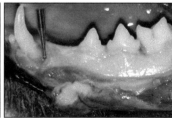

The arrow indicates the neurovascular bundle emerging from the middle mental foramen.
(© Dr Alexander M. Reiter)

5 Section multi-rooted teeth; pay particular attention to the mandibular first molar tooth, whose furcation separating mesial and distal roots is situated more caudally than the middle of the crown.

→ **OPERATIVE TECHNIQUE 12.6 CONTINUED**

6 Elevate and extract all teeth and crown-root segments.

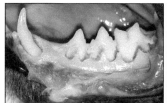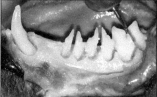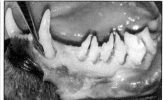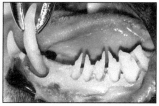

(© Dr Alexander M. Reiter)

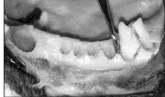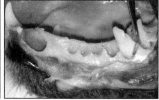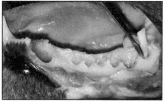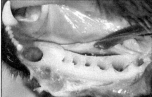

(© Dr Alexander M. Reiter)

7 Slightly elevate the lingual gingiva, and proceed with debridement, smoothing of alveolar bone with a large round diamond bur and lavage of the extraction sites.

8 Excise the flap margins, incise the periosteum at the base of the flap with a scalpel blade, dissect its connective tissue with blunt tissue scissors, and ensure that the tension-free flap spans over the extraction sites.

9 Appose the flap to the lingual gingiva by means of simple interrupted sutures. The corner of the flap is sutured first, and additional sutures are placed 2–3 mm apart and 1–2 mm from the flap edges.

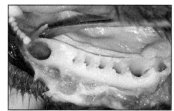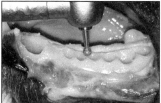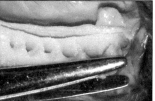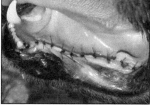

(© Dr Alexander M. Reiter)

PRACTICAL TIPS

- It is advisable to inspect and palpate the root apices and compare radiographs before and after extraction of teeth (prior to suturing of the flap) to confirm complete removal of dental tissue

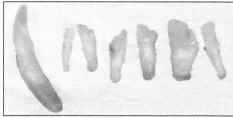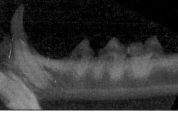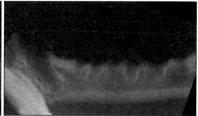

(© Dr Alexander M. Reiter)

- A large flap may be closed with a simple continuous suture pattern to minimize the number of knots in the mouth and reduce total anaesthesia time. However, the risk of wound dehiscence and postoperative complications should be considered when choosing this type of suturing technique
- It is wise for less experienced clinicians to extract one tooth at a time rather than to perform alveolectomy on multiple teeth, in case anaesthesia needs to be interrupted and the patient quickly awakened for medical reasons
- Avoid:
  - Excessive flap elevation labially/buccally and lingually
  - Excessive bone removal
  - Injury to the neurovascular bundles at the mental foramina or inside the mandibular canal
  - Transportation of dental tissue into the mandibular canal
  - Excessive force during luxation and elevation of crown-root segments, which could result in mandibular fracture

OPERATIVE TECHNIQUE 12.7

Crown amputation and intentional retention of resorbing root tissue in the cat

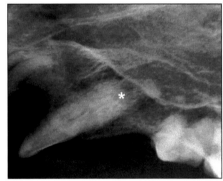

The asterisk (*) denotes the affected root of the left maxillary canine tooth.
(© Dr Alexander M. Reiter)

INDICATIONS

Presence of dentoalveolar ankylosis and root replacement resorption with simultaneous absence of tooth mobility, periodontitis, endodontic disease, periapical pathology and stomatitis.

POSITIONING

Lateral recumbency.

ASSISTANT

Preferable.

ADDITIONAL EQUIPMENT

Scalpel; periosteal elevator; (cross-cut) fissure burs; round diamond burs; lactated Ringer's solution (or saline); tissue scissors; thumb forceps; suture material; needle holder; suture scissors; gauze.

SURGICAL TECHNIQUE

Approach

The mouth is rinsed with a 0.12% chlorhexidine solution, and dental scaling is performed. Preoperative radiographs are obtained to evaluate root development, confirm lack of complicating factors, and identify signs of endodontic or periodontal disease.

Surgical manipulations

1 Incise the gingival attachment around the tooth.

2 Make a mucoperiosteal flap (including gingiva and alveolar mucosa) with or without releasing incisions.

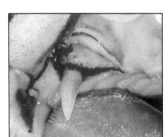

(© Dr Alexander M. Reiter)

3 Sever the clinical crown from the remainder of the tooth with a round (or cross-cut) fissure bur attached to a high-speed handpiece under water cooling.

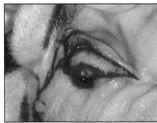

(© Dr Alexander M. Reiter)

4 Further reduce the resorbing root with a large round diamond bur to about 1–2 mm below the level of the alveolar margin.

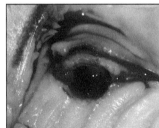

(© Dr Alexander M. Reiter)

5 Excise the flap margins, if necessary incise the periosteum at the base of the flap, dissect its connective tissue with blunt tissue scissors, ensuring that the flap spans over the extraction site in a tension-free fashion, and slightly elevate the palatal gingiva. Suture the flap over the wound.

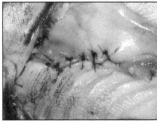

(© Dr Alexander M. Reiter)

→ **OPERATIVE TECHNIQUE 12.7 CONTINUED**

6 Obtain a postoperative radiograph.

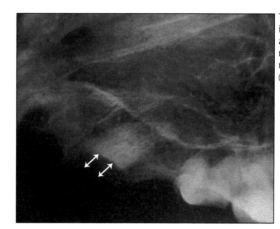

The double-headed arrows indicate the most coronal aspect of the cut root in relation to the alveolar margin.

(© Dr Alexander M. Reiter)

PRACTICAL TIPS

- This procedure should only be employed when closed or open extraction cannot be accomplished on teeth with radiographic confirmation of dentoalveolar ankylosis and root replacement resorption and absence of periodontitis, endodontic and periapical disease and stomatitis
- Reducing the resorbing root below the level of the alveolar margin allows a blood clot to form into which alveolar bone can grow above the remaining root tissue during healing

Chapter 13

Perioperative considerations in dentistry and oral surgery

Alexander M. Reiter and Ana Castejon-Gonzalez

This chapter provides information on topics not or only briefly covered in previous chapters. The topics include select intra- and postoperative considerations, the judicious use of antibiotics, the role of veterinary technicians/nurses and dental hygienists, safety in the workplace, equipment maintenance care and troubleshooting, considerations about dental scaling without anaesthesia, recommended home oral hygiene measures, suggested modalities of communication with clients and other professionals, and miscellaneous information about veterinary dental specialty colleges, veterinary dental organizations, and the scientific journals relevant to the specialty field.

Select intra- and postoperative considerations

Neurological deficits

There have been anecdotal reports and studies of cats developing blindness, and dogs and cats developing hearing loss and vestibular function compromise (particularly in geriatric patients), following dental procedures under general anaesthesia (Jurk et al., 2001; Stevens-Sparks and Strain, 2010). It has been suggested that the use of spring-loaded mouth gags represents a risk for the development of temporary or permanent post-anaesthesia blindness in cats. The role of the maxillary artery in supplying an extracranial network in cats was emphasized, which releases several arteries that pass through the orbital fissure into the cavernous sinus to form an intracranial arterial network from which cerebral arteries arise (Stiles et al., 2012).

Maximal mouth opening was shown to cause alterations in several indicators of maxillary artery blood flow in anaesthetized cats when evaluating electroretinograms (ERGs), brainstem auditory evoked responses (BAERs), magnetic resonance angiographies (MRAs) and dynamic computed tomography (CT) examinations (Barton-Lamb et al., 2013). The distance between the angular process of the mandible and the rostrolateral wall of the tympanic bulla in cats appeared to become shorter when the mouth was maximally opened, compressing the maxillary artery as it courses between these two bony structures and leading to reduced intracranial arterial supply, which was confirmed on CT (Scrivani et al., 2014). In a study of anaesthetized cats, ERGs and MRAs were performed with the mouth

closed, submaximally opened using plastic mouth gags of 20 mm, 30 mm and 42 mm, and maximally opened using a spring-loaded mouth gag. Submaximal mouth opening with a 42 mm plastic gag (the same length as a 1-inch needle cap) and maximal mouth opening with a spring-loaded gag produced alterations in ERG waveforms consistent with circulatory compromise, which was confirmed on magnetic resonance imaging (MRI) (Martin-Flores et al., 2014). A clinical case of global cerebral ischaemia with suspected subsequent respiratory arrest after repeated use of a spring-loaded mouth gag has also recently been described (Hartman et al., 2017).

The use of spring-loaded mouth gags should be discouraged, and caution should be exercised when wide mouth opening is necessary (Reiter, 2013) (Figure 13.1). The duration of maximal mandibular extension should be minimized to reduce the risk of masticatory muscle strain and injury to the temporomandibular joints, as well as to avoid decreased maxillary artery blood flow and cerebral ischaemia. Furthermore, the wider the mouth is opened, the tighter the lip and cheek become and the more difficult it will be to retract these tissues to accomplish dental and oral surgical procedures (Figure 13.2). Placing 30 mm or 20 mm plastic gags cut from needle caps (or commercially available gags as shown in Figure 9.2) between the maxillary and mandibular canine teeth enables adequate mouth opening for dental and oral sugical procedures in cats (Reiter, 2014).

Tracheal injury

Overinflation of the cuff can result in tracheal rupture in cats, and this complication has been reported mostly in association with dental procedures (Mitchell et al., 2000). Tracheal rupture occurred in cadaver cats when the endotracheal tube cuff was filled with more than 6 ml of air. Other suggested causes include iatrogenic trauma from endotracheal tube movement during oral manipulations and turning over of the patient without first detaching the hoses from the endotracheal tube. A clinically airtight seal can be obtained in cats by filling the cuff of a correctly sized endotracheal tube with 1.6 ± 0.7 ml of air (Hardie et al., 1999).

Signs associated with tracheal rupture include subcutaneous emphysema, coughing, gagging, dyspnoea, anorexia, fever, and pneumomediastinum (Mitchell et al., 2000). Tracheoscopy is the method of choice for documenting tracheal rupture. Longer tears can be found with the use of high-pressure, low-volume endotracheal tubes

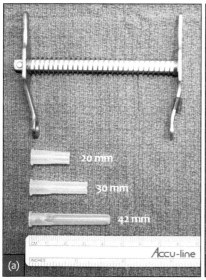

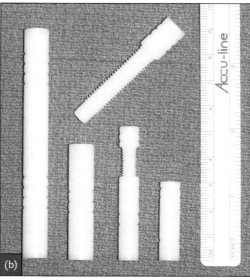

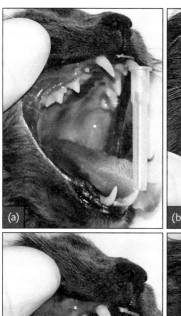

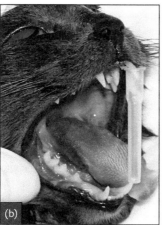

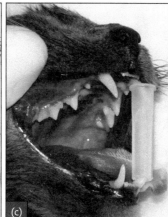

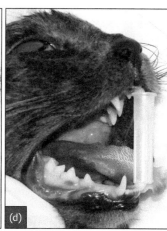

13.1 (a) Spring-loaded mouth gag advertised for use in cats and small dogs above needle caps cut to lengths of 20 mm and 30 mm, and a 42 mm needle cap. (b) Commercially available mouth props whose lengths can further be adjusted by unscrewing one part from another.
(© Dr Alexander M. Reiter)

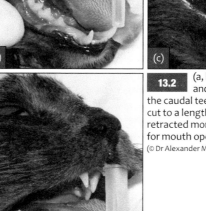

13.2 (a, b) When using a 42 mm needle cap for mouth opening, the lips and cheeks become very tight. This makes it difficult to fully access the caudal teeth and their supporting tissues. (c, d) When using a needle cap cut to a length of 30 mm for mouth opening, the lips and cheeks can be retracted more easily. (e, f) When using a needle cap cut to a length of 20 mm for mouth opening, the lips and cheeks can be readily retracted.
(© Dr Alexander M. Reiter)

(Hardie *et al.*, 1999). Most cats with tracheal rupture can be treated medically. Cats with worsening clinical signs such as severe dyspnoea (i.e. open-mouth breathing despite treatment with oxygen), suspected pneumothorax, or worsening subcutaneous emphysema should have surgery performed to correct the defect (Hardie *et al.*, 1999; Mitchell *et al.*, 2000).

Oral and oropharyngeal oedema

Swelling from oedema of oral tissues can be due to over-zealous pharyngeal packing, rough tongue manipulation, surgery in the sublingual region and excessive elevation of alveolar mucosa on the lingual aspect of the mandible, tonsillectomy and soft palate surgery (Reiter and Soltero-

Rivera, 2017). Breathing could be compromised during recovery from anaesthesia. Management ranges from a single injection of dexamethasone (0.1–0.2 mg/kg i.v.) during or at the end of the procedure to performing an emergency tracheostomy. The oedematous tongue can be wrapped with a gauze sponge soaked with a hypertonic solution prior to extubation.

Iatrogenic foreign body

Gauze sponges and other devices should be used for pharyngeal packing to avoid aspiration of fluids and debris during dental and oral surgical procedures (Figures 13.3 and 13.4). They should frequently be replaced during the procedure and be counted for safe and complete retrieval

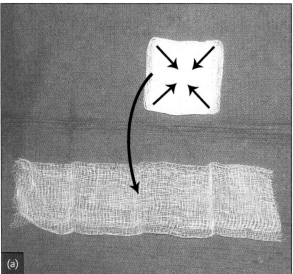

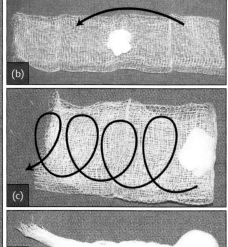

13.3 Pharyngeal packing for cats and small dogs using two small gauze sponges. (a) One sponge is opened. (b) The other sponge is wrapped to a ball and placed into the centre of the opened sponge. (c, d) The opened sponge is closed, and its ends are twisted. The bulkier part is placed into the pharynx, while the twisted, cord-like end is left to hang out from the side of the mouth.
(© Dr Alexander M. Reiter)

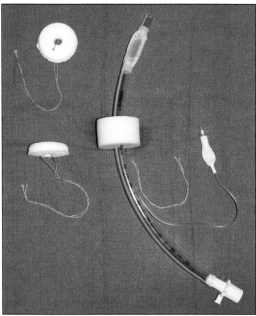

13.4 Polyvinyl alcohol (PVA) rings with loop string prior to hydration with water (left). Once it is hydrated with water, the expanding, soft, flexible and sponge-like ring is slid over the middle section of a cuffed endotracheal tube (right); after intubation, a finger is used to advance it along the tube into the pharynx. The disadvantage of these devices is that they cannot be replaced during a procedure when they become soaked with fluids.
(© Dr Alexander M. Reiter)

at the end of the procedure. Small sponges may sometimes also become displaced into the oesophagus. The throat of each patient should always be thoroughly inspected with the help of a laryngoscope prior to extubation to ensure that all foreign material has been removed (Reiter and Soltero-Rivera, 2017).

Tongue protrusion with an inability to reposition it into the oral cavity was described in an anaesthetized dog with limited mouth opening due to masticatory muscle myositis. Severe lingual and sublingual swelling resulted from venous congestion. Mandibular symphysiotomy was necessary to resolve venous congestion and to reposition the tongue into the oral cavity. It was recommended that the use of anaesthetic monitoring equipment on the tongue, such as a pulse oximeter probe, should be avoided in patients with

limited mouth opening (Nanai *et al.*, 2009). Excessive ventral pulling of the tongue in cats prior to intubation can cause puncture of the sublingual mucosa or underside of the tongue by pointed mandibular canine teeth (Reiter and Soltero-Rivera, 2017).

Ocular and orbital injury

Corneal damage can occur during prolonged anaesthetic episodes and has been reported with the use of sedatives, tranquilizers and/or analgesics. After 60 minutes under anaesthesia tear production, as measured using the Schirmer tear test (STT), decreases to 0. Corneal damage is more prevalent in animals with a small head and lagophthalmos (Park *et al.*, 2013). Eye lubricant (Figure 13.5) should therefore be frequently (i.e. at least every 20–30 minutes) applied during anaesthesia (Park *et al.*, 2013; Doering *et al.*, 2016). Administration of anticholinergics further decreases tear production (Doering *et al.*, 2016). If surgical drapes are not used to delimit the surgical area (e.g. the oral cavity), protecting the eyes is advised by

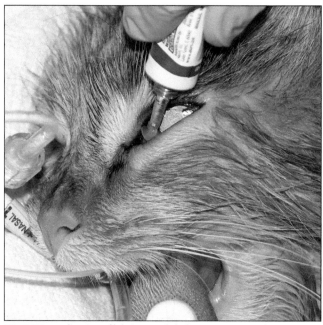

13.5 Application of lubricant ophthalmic ointment to the cornea.
(© Dr Alexander M. Reiter)

taping their eyelids closed when using the air/water syringe during dental scaling and polishing, during endodontic procedures where sodium hyplochlorite is used, or when handling sharp instruments around the maxilla. Post-operative opioids can also impair the animal's ability to blink, predisposing the eyes to desiccation and subsequent erosion or ulceration of their cornea.

Orbital penetration by dental elevators leading to ocular and brain trauma has been reported in dogs and cats associated with tooth extraction procedures (Smith *et al.*, 2003; Duke *et al.*, 2014; Guerreiro *et al.*, 2014; Troxel, 2015). Outcomes included recovery after antibiotic therapy, enucleation of the affected eye, and death from braincase fracture and brain abscessation. Early treatment and referral to a veterinary ophthalmologist are recommended. Awareness of the anatomical proximity of caudal maxillary tooth roots and the orbit, appropriate interpretation of dental radiographs, and proficiency in tooth extraction techniques will minimize the risk of these complications.

Injury to orbital structures (causing retrobulbar haematoma, transient vision loss, and glaucoma with permanent blindness) has also been reported in dogs and cats following maxillary nerve blocks (Alessio and Krieger, 2015; Perry *et al.*, 2015; Loughran *et al.*, 2016).

Trigeminocardiac reflex

Maxillofacial surgery in human patients represents a risk factor for the development of trigeminocardiac reflex. This reflex is elicited when a branch of the trigeminal nerve is stimulated, leading to increased vagal activity, bradycardia and asystole, and death. Sudden development of episodes of bradycardia and asystole secondary to trigeminocardiac reflex were reported in a puppy with limited mouth opening during cleft palate repair (Figure 13.6) (Vezina-Audette *et al.*, 2017). To allow access to the palate in that patient, the mandibular symphysis and intermandibular tissues were incised, the sublingual mucosa detached from the laterally deviated mandibles, and the tongue pulled caudoventrally. Trigeminocardiac reflex was thought to be a consequence of manipulation of branches of the trigeminal nerve (inferior alveolar nerve, lingual nerve, and major palatine nerve) during these procedures. The patient responded to glycopyrrolate and atropine injections that were administered periodically until completion of cleft palate repair (Vezina-Audette *et al.*, 2017).

Hypothermia and hyperthermia

Hypothermia is of particular concern when water is used to cool power instruments or rinse debris from the mouth. Steps should be taken to minimize the loss of body heat during anaesthesia. While thermally supported cats still experienced a drop in body temperature during dental procedures in one study, the drop was significantly greater in cats without thermal support (Hale and Anthony, 1997). Duration of pre-anaesthetic time, duration of anaesthesia, physical condition of the patient, reason for anaesthesia, anaesthetic risk, and dorsal or sternal recumbency of the patient during the procedure were found to be associated with postoperative hypothermia in cats and dogs (Redondo *et al.*, 2012a,b).

Hyperthermia is a concern in cats when opiates such as hydromorphone (with or without inhalation anaesthesia), ketamine, or both, are used. Opiates reset the threshold point controlled by the hypothalamus, causing a mild to

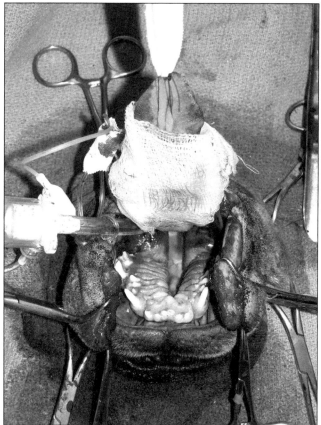

13.6 To allow access to the cleft palate in this puppy with limited mouth opening, the mandibular symphysis and intermandibular tissues were incised, the sublingual mucosa detached from the laterally deviated mandibles, and the tongue pulled caudoventrally, causing episodes of bradycardia and asystole secondary to trigeminocardiac reflex.
(© Dr Alexander M. Reiter)

moderate, and self-limiting, increase in body temperature (Posner *et al.*, 2010). Moreover, cats with concurrent tissue trauma may release pyrogenic cytokines that could eventually result in more severe hyperthermia. Cats with postoperative hyperthermia often respond favourably to intravenous fluid administration, removal of blankets in the cage, other cooling methods such as a fan and ice packs, and application of rubbing alcohol to footpads.

Intra- and postoperative bleeding

Severe oral bleeding can be due to injury of larger blood vessels, bleeding dyscrasias, lingual or palatal injury, oral inflammation, soft tissue trauma, oral neoplasia, or jaw fracture (Reiter and Soltero-Rivera, 2017). Inadvertent puncture of a larger vessel when regional nerve blocks are performed can sometimes cause haematoma formation with tissue swelling (Loughran *et al.*, 2016). Postoperative bleeding in retired racing Greyhounds appears not attributable to a primary or secondary haemostatic defect but could result from altered fibrinolysis (Lara-García *et al.*, 2008). Postoperative use of epsilon aminocaproic acid (EACA) has been shown to decrease postoperative bleeding in Greyhounds (Marin *et al.*, 2012).

Intravascular volume replacement is accomplished with crystalloids, colloids and/or blood products. Diffuse bleeding from nasal mucosa (e.g. after maxillectomy or palate surgery) can be stopped by wound irrigation with a mixture of 0.25 ml phenylephrine 1% and 50 ml lidocaine

2% (0.05–0.1 ml/kg in cats; 0.1–0.2 ml/kg in dogs). Other means of haemostasis include application of digital pressure, use of refrigerated rinsing solutions, astringents, bone wax, cellulose meshes, gelatin powder/sheets, poly-saccharide powder, collagen powder/sheets, thrombin in a gelatin matrix, fibrin sealants or cyanoacrylate tissue adhesives, and vessel ligation (Reiter, 2013). Bone wax (sterile beeswax) is particularly useful to control acute bleeding from alveoli during extraction of mandibular cheek teeth, but it should be removed after achieving haemostasis, as it may cause inflammation, granuloma formation, infection, and impaired osteogenesis if left *in situ* (Katz and Rootman, 1996; Wolvius and Van Der Wal, 2003; Katre *et al.*, 2010). A pressure bandage

(Figure 13.7) or temporary ligation of the carotid artery is rarely required for uncontrolled bleeding (Goodman and Goodman, 2016).

Emphysema and embolism

Emphysema sometimes occurs after use of air-driven equipment, or after blowing air or air/water spray into sub-mucosal tissues, particularly after deep dissection of large mucoperiosteal flaps. In the lower jaw, it is usually sub-cutaneous, as the air migrates to the intermandibular space and from there to the ventrolateral aspects of the face. Emphysema usually resolves within a few days. It can be reduced or prevented effectively with gentle digital

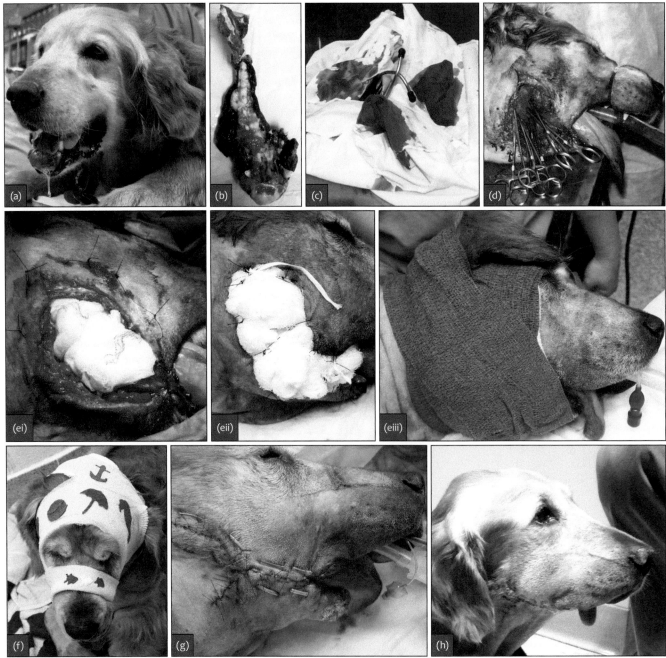

13.7 (a) A Golden Retriever dog with a malignant peripheral nerve sheath tumour had a (b) right total mandibulectomy and left partial mandibulectomy performed. Acute bleeding occurred on the morning of discharge (4 days after surgery); (c) the person walking the dog tried to control bleeding with a laboratory coat. (d) The dog was intubated, and repeated attempts at clamping bleeding vessels were unsuccessful. (e)(i–iii) A pressure bandage was applied after thoroughly rinsing the wound. (f, g) The wound was debrided daily, followed by application of new pressure bandages; the wound was closed 8 days after the initial surgery. (h) The dog returned 17 days after the initial surgery for suture removal.
(© Dr Alexander M. Reiter)

pressure applied to the sutured flap for a few minutes to evacuate air bubbles and provide an adhesive seal between soft tissue and bone (Reiter and Soltero-Rivera, 2017). Fatal air embolism was described in an anaesthetized cat that underwent tooth extraction. However, a definitive cause of death was not established because resuscitation attempts by external chest compression and positive pressure ventilation could have contributed to the post-mortem findings detected on radiography and autopsy (air in the vena cava, right atrium, auricle and ventricle, hepatic and renal veins) (Gunew *et al.*, 2008). Nonetheless, blowing air or air/water spray into an alveolar socket or root canal or on to denuded bone or bleeding tissue is strongly discouraged.

Vomiting and regurgitation

Vomiting and regurgitation may occur intra- or postoperatively, increasing the risk of aspiration especially in patients that have a decreased ability to open the mouth. Use of antiemetics perioperatively is indicated in patients with a history of vomiting or regurgitation and dogs receiving opioids (i.e. hydromorphone, morphine) (Hay Kraus, 2014; Davies *et al.*, 2015). Postoperative vomiting or regurgitation may compromise the healing of oral tissues and lead to wound dehiscence after repair of soft palate defects and is of particular concern following partial soft palate excision in brachycephalic airway obstruction syndrome (BOAS) patients. The use of antiemetics such as maropitant, metoclopramide and/or ondansetron should be considered for the perioperative care of these patients.

Muzzling

Muzzling can avoid excessive tension on intra- or extraoral suture lines during mouth opening, prevent the recurrence of temporomandibular joint luxation, provide definitive treatment of minimally displaced caudal mandibular fractures in adult pets and mandibular fractures in immature and young adult pets (Figure 13.8), support pathological mandibular body fractures in older pets, and represent temporary first-aid treatment of open-mouth jaw locking and mandibular fractures until definitive treatment is performed. Muzzling can also provide adjunct stabilization when used in conjunction with other treatment techniques (Reiter and Lewis, 2011; Somrak and Marretta, 2015). The use of custom-made tape muzzles or commercially available nylon muzzles allows some movement of the lower jaw while maintaining proper occlusal alignment and stabilization. Another advantage of nylon muzzles is that they can be laundered (Figure 13.9).

Tape muzzles were first described for the treatment of mandibular fractures in the early 1980s (Howard, 1981; Withrow, 1981). Fitting the trauma patient with an in-clinic fabricated adhesive tape muzzle is an easy, inexpensive, and non-invasive technique. To make a tape muzzle, first, a layer with the adhesive side of the tape outward is formed into a loop, encircling the upper and lower jaws. A second layer is added, with the adhesive side facing inward, directly on top of the first layer. The muzzle is applied snug enough for the dental interlock (interdigitation between maxillary and mandibular canine teeth) to be maintained, but loose enough to permit the tongue to protrude and allow lapping of water and a gruel diet. The gap

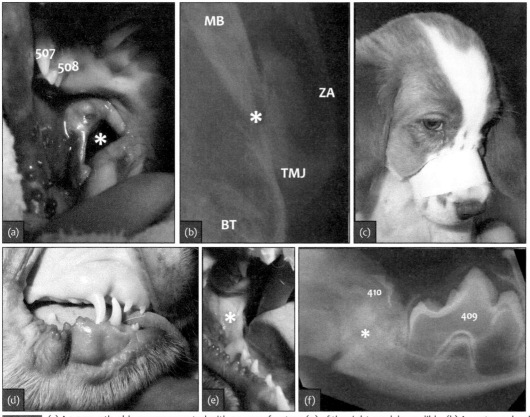

13.8 (a) A 2.5-month-old puppy presented with an open fracture (∗) of the right caudal mandible. (b) An extraoral radiograph was obtained, the fracture site was debrided, rinsed and sutured closed, and (c) a tape muzzle was placed. (d) The puppy returned 1 month later; there was good occlusion, the oral wound had healed (e) clinically and (f) radiographically (∗), and the tape muzzle was removed. 409 = permanent right mandibular first molar tooth; 410 = resorbing permanent right mandibular second molar tooth; 507 and 508 = deciduous right maxillary third and fourth premolar teeth; BT = bulla tympanica; MB = mandibular body; TMJ = temporomandibular joint; ZA = zygomatic arch.
(© Dr Alexander M. Reiter)

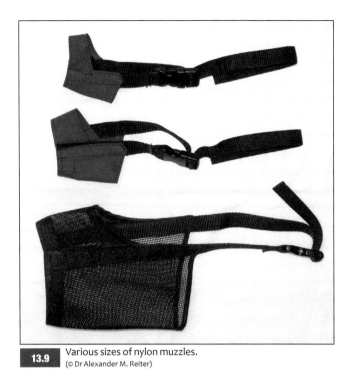

13.9 Various sizes of nylon muzzles.
(© Dr Alexander M. Reiter)

between the maxillary and mandibular incisors should be 8–15 mm in cats and small dogs and 20–25 mm in medium to large dogs. A loop ventral to the ears and around the neck is added (also adhesive side out for the first layer, then adhesive side in for the second layer), which may be tied like shoelaces (Figure 13.10a–c) to avoid over-tightening in growing patients and facilitate muzzle removal and replacement. Muzzling in cats and short-nosed dogs is possible by providing an additional middle layer running over the forehead (Figure 13.10d–f), which will effectively keep the muzzle in position (Reiter and Lewis, 2011).

It is best to discharge the patient with multiple identical tape muzzles (Figure 13.11), thus allowing change of a soiled muzzle every 2–3 days. Elizabethan collars prevent iatrogenic trauma to the eyes, face and paws of the patient during repeated attempts at removing the muzzle. Complications with muzzling include dermatitis from the muzzle becoming moist and soiled, swelling/congestion if too tight, incomplete stabilization of fractures resulting in non-union or malunion and subsequent malocclusion, delayed return to function by restricting jaw movement, heat prostration, dyspnoea in brachycephalic patients, and aspiration in the regurgitating/vomiting patient (Reiter and Lewis, 2011; Somrak and Marretta, 2015).

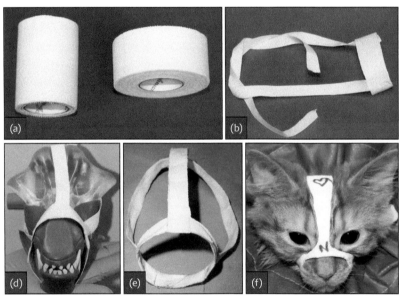

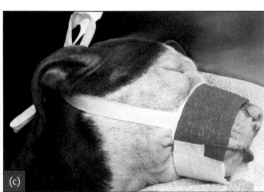

13.10 (a–c) The basic design of a tape muzzle consists of a loop encircling the upper and lower jaws connected to a loop running ventral to the ears and around the neck; the second loop may be tied like shoelaces. (d–f) A third loop running over the forehead and connecting the first and second loops often helps to effectively keep the muzzle in position in cats and short-nosed dogs.
(© Dr Alexander M. Reiter)

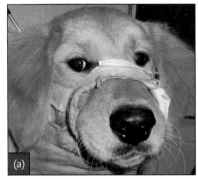
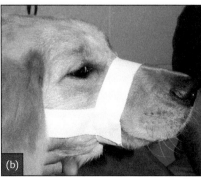

13.11 (a) Soiled tape muzzles should (b) be replaced daily or at least every 2–3 days.
(© Dr Alexander M. Reiter)

Nutritional support

Water is offered once the animal has recovered from anaesthesia. Generally, following oral surgery a soft diet is fed for about 2 weeks to prevent disturbance of wound healing. If pets were previously fed hard food, the kibble should be soaked in some water so that it can soften prior to feeding. This will avoid gastrointestinal upset from a sudden change of diet. It may take several days for a patient to adapt to the changed circumstances in the mouth before being willing to eat normally. Providing adequate nutritional support is imperative if the patient is not expected to eat within 2 to 3 days postoperatively. Partial or complete anorexia can occur in dogs and cats secondary to oral and maxillofacial trauma, intraoral pathology, and following oral and maxillofacial surgery or radiation therapy (Perea, 2008; Fink *et al.*, 2014). Feeding tube placement should be performed prior to maxillomandibular fixation or any procedure where wide mouth opening will be compromised.

Naso-oesophageal feeding tubes are for short-term nutritional support (less than 10 days), are easy to place, and do not require general anaesthesia. However, because of their small bore, they often get clogged by food or medications, unless an all-liquid diet is administered.

Oesophagostomy tubes are a better option when mid- to long-term nutritional support (about 2 months) is expected. Standard red rubber catheters, specific silicone or polyurethane feeding tubes can be used. Appropriate tube size will vary depending on the size of the patient. Size 12–14 Fr are recommended for cats and small dogs, while sizes 14–18 Fr can be used for larger dogs. Pet owners will be required to provide at-home feedings and tube care. The patient's nutrition plan can be individually customized based on its energy requirements using resting energy requirement formulas or via consultation with a veterinary nutritionist (Bexfield and Watson, 2010; Fink *et al.*, 2014). The use of balanced, commercially produced, liquid diets is preferable over the administration of regular soft diets diluted with water to avoid clogging of the tube and to meet nutritional requirements with a correct, non-excessive provision of water.

For placement of an oesophagostomy tube (Figures 13.12 and 13.13) the patient is positioned in right lateral recumbency. The left lateral neck, extending from the ramus of the mandible to the shoulder, is clipped and the skin aseptically prepared for surgery. Large, curved forceps are placed through the mouth and into the oesophagus. The tips of the forceps are pushed laterally (to make a small tent in the skin dorsal to the jugular vein)

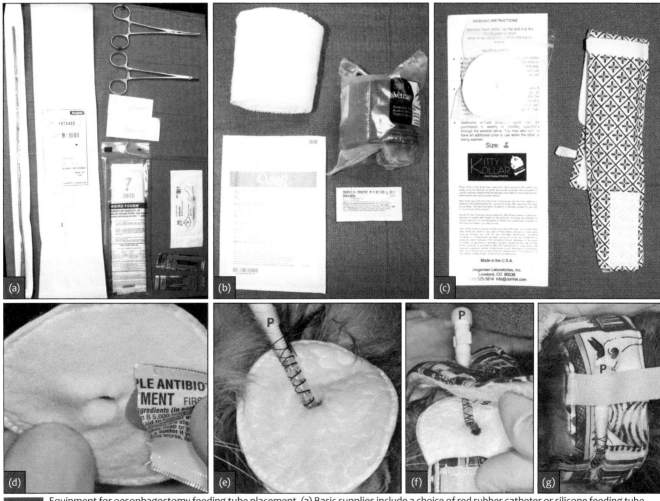

13.12 Equipment for oesophagostomy feeding tube placement. (a) Basic supplies include a choice of red rubber catheter or silicone feeding tube, scalpel blades, surgical gloves, large curved forceps, needle holder, nylon suture material, and a 'Christmas tree' adaptor with injection cap (for use with a red rubber catheter). (b) Neck wraps can be made by using non-adherent gauze pad, antibacterial ointment, cast padding, and a light layer of flexible self-adherent bandage material. (c–g) Washable fabric neck wraps of all sizes (e.g. Kitty Kollar®) are commercially available for cats and dogs. P = proximal aspect of the feeding tube.

(© Dr Alexander M. Reiter)

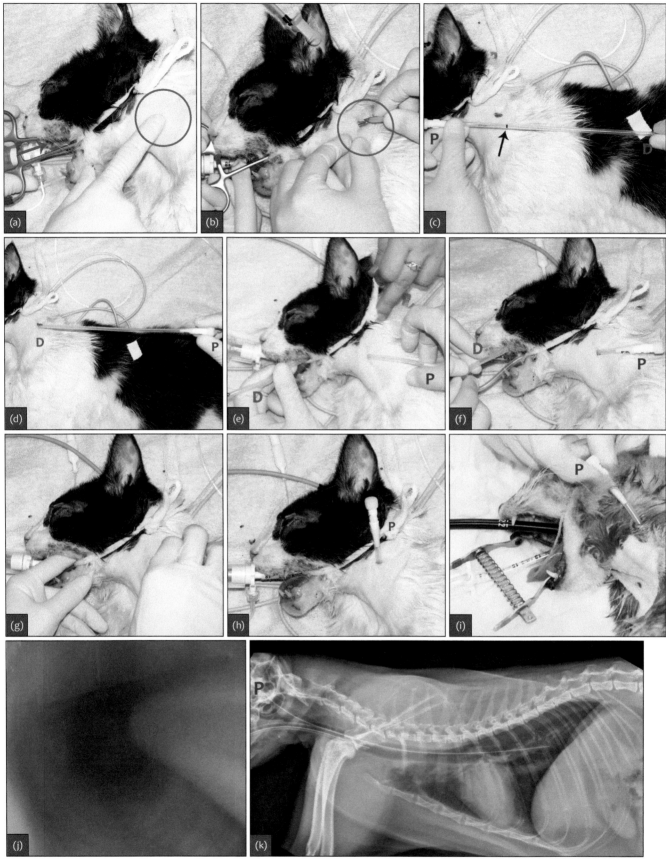

13.13 (a, b) Large, curved forceps are inserted into the oesophagus with the tips pushed laterally (dorsal to the jugular vein and ventral to the wing of the atlas); a full-thickness incision is made with a scalpel blade directly over the tips of the forceps through the aseptically prepared skin (circled), subcutaneous tissues, and into the oesophagus. (c, d) Measurement of the tube from the incision site to the eighth intercostal space (white tape on lateral chest); the tube is marked with a permanent marker (arrowed) before its distal end is grasped with the jaws of the forceps. (e, f) The distal tube end is pulled orally and out through the mouth and redirected back into the mouth. (g, h) The distal tube end is pushed down into the oesophagus with the operator's fingers, at which point the proximal tube end flips from pointing caudally to pointing rostrally. Proper tube placement is confirmed either (i, j) via endoscopy or (k) a lateral thoracic radiograph. D = distal end of the feeding tube; P = proximal end of the feeding tube. (continues) ▶
(© Dr Alexander M. Reiter)

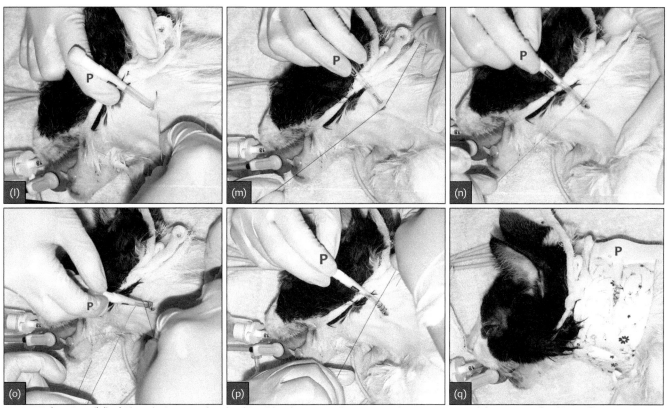

13.13 (continued) (l–q) The tube is secured to the skin with nylon sutures in a purse-string pattern around the stoma and a Chinese finger-trap pattern along its proximal end, followed by placement of a neck wrap (see Figure 13.12). P = proximal end of the feeding tube.
(© Dr Alexander M. Reiter)

and ventral to the wing of the atlas. A scalpel blade is used to make a small incision directly over the protruded tips of the forceps through the skin and subcutaneous tissues, and into the oesophagus. The tips of the forceps can now be pushed out through the incision (Fink *et al.*, 2014).

The tube should have been pre-measured and marked from the proposed insertion site to the seventh to ninth intercostal space to ensure that the end of the catheter is placed in the distal oesophagus and not across the lower oesophageal sphincter. The distal aspect of the feeding tube is placed into the jaws of the forceps, the forceps are locked, and the distal aspect of the tube is pulled orally and out through the mouth. The distal end of the tube is then redirected and pushed down into the oesophagus until the pre-marked area is at the level of the stoma. It is sealed with either a pre-existing injection port cover or a 'Christmas tree' adaptor and injection cap. The feeding tube placement should be checked with a lateral thoracic radiograph or via endoscopy to ensure proper placement in the distal oesophagus (Kahn, 2007; Fink *et al.*, 2014).

The oesophagostomy tube is secured in place with a purse-string suture in the skin surrounding the stoma followed by a Chinese finger-trap suture using 2 or 3 metric (3/0 or 2/0 USP) non-absorbable nylon suture material. A loose neck wrap can be placed using a non-adherent gauze pad, antibacterial ointment, cast padding, and a light layer of flexible self-adherent bandage material. The stoma should be monitored and cleansed daily using dilute chlorhexidine or povidone-iodine. An Elizabethan collar may be necessary to deter the animal from scratching at, and removing, the tube (Fink *et al.*, 2014).

The veterinary technician/nurse can maintain the tube, provide the feedings, and teach the client how to feed the patient at home. If the diet has been refrigerated, it can be warmed up in a bowl surrounded by warm water for 15–20 minutes. Microwaving should be done very carefully as it heats the food unevenly and can burn the oesophagus. Proper tube positioning should be verified by means of aspiration to achieve negative pressure. Then the tube is flushed with some water. If the animal tolerates the water without gagging or coughing, the administration of the calculated volume of diet can begin and be performed over the next 30 minutes. If the patient shows any signs of nausea, vomiting, regurgitation or discomfort, the administration of food should be stopped. Once the feeding has been completed, the tube is flushed again with some water, which will prevent the tube lumen from clogging. Then the tube is recapped. If the feeding tube is used to administer medications, one drug at a time should be given followed by flushing with water between administrations.

If there are no specific contraindications to oral feeding, patients with feeding tubes should also be offered food by mouth to see whether they will eat on their own. The patient's weight should be assessed daily, and electrolytes and other serum chemistry parameters should be monitored as needed. Once the patient is readily eating on its own, the feeding tube may no longer be required. Removal should be performed after 6–8 hours of fasting. The tube is flushed with water, the sutures are cut, the proximal tube end kinked (to avoid movement of any tube content within its lumen), and the tube removed in the awake patient. Oral feeding should be resumed a few hours after tube removal. The stoma will heal by second intention in a few days (Devitt and Seim, 1997; Levine *et al.*, 1997; Fink *et al.*, 2014).

Judicious use of antibiotics

Bacteraemia and endotoxaemia

Bacteraemia secondary to an oral condition occurs frequently in dogs and humans with periodontal disease during and after dental cleaning and tooth extraction (Black *et al.*, 1980; Limeres Posse *et al.*, 2016). The likelihood and severity of bacteraemia seems more related to the degree of periodontal disease than to the specific dental procedure performed, as there is not a significant difference between the number of positive blood cultures in dogs undergoing and dogs not undergoing dental procedures (Harari *et al.*, 1993).

In one study, bacteria were cultured from the blood (before anaesthesia, after intubation, 20 minutes after start of the dental procedure, and at 10-minute intervals until 10 minutes after completion of the dental procedure) and compared with those isolated from plaque in 20 dogs (Neives *et al.*, 1997). Up to 90% of the bacterial species isolated from the plaque were present in the blood, and bacteraemia was present in all dogs within 40 minutes from the start of the dental procedure (Neives *et al.*, 1997).

Bacteraemia may even occur in some dogs and humans after toothbrushing (Glass *et al.*, 1989; Hartzell *et al.*, 2005), and gentle mastication has been found to induce the release of bacterial endotoxins from oral origin into the bloodstream, especially when people have severe periodontal disease. This finding suggests that a diseased periodontium can be a source of chronic release of bacterial pro-inflammatory components into the bloodstream. However, bacteraemia is usually short-lived in healthy animals and humans, as the bacteria are eliminated by the host's immune system (Silver *et al.*, 1975). Therefore, it is not an indication for the perioperative use of systemic antibiotics in the otherwise healthy patient. Bacteraemia may be reduced by rinsing the oral cavity with diluted chlorhexidine prior to performing a professional dental cleaning or other oral procedure (Bowersock *et al.*, 2000).

A systemic inflammatory response was reported in one cat that presented with infected oral tissues after incomplete tooth extractions performed 10 days earlier (Reiter *et al.*, 2004). A second dental procedure was necessary to remove 22 tooth root remnants from this patient (Figure 13.14). Diabetic ketoacidosis and thromboembolism complicated the cat's recovery period and necessitated

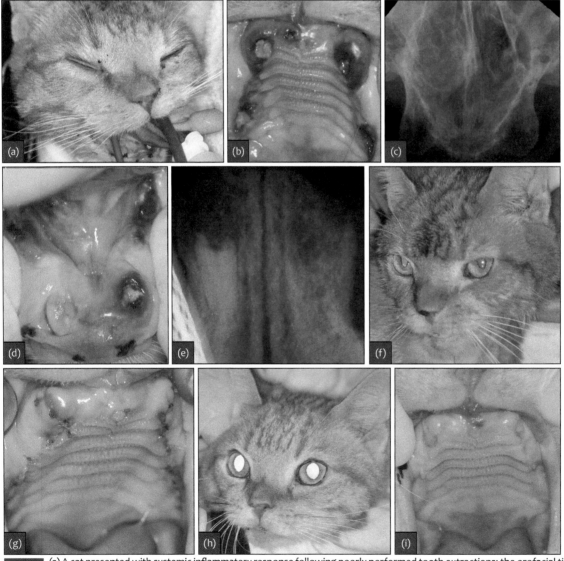

13.14 (a) A cat presented with systemic inflammatory response following poorly performed tooth extractions; the orofacial tissues were severely swollen. (b, c) Maxillary and (d, e) mandibular oral photographs and dental radiographs revealed numerous retained root remnants, gingivitis and purulent discharge from open alveoli. The cat returned (f, g) 3 and (h, i) 24 weeks following removal of root remnants and suturing of extraction sites, showing complete resolution of orofacial swelling and healing of extraction sites.

(© Dr Alexander M. Reiter, reproduced from Reiter *et al.* (2004), *Journal of Veterinary Dentistry*, with permission)

extended hospitalization. Postoperative examinations up to 52 weeks indicated continued improvement with moderate glycaemic control and chronic but stable renal failure. The cat died after further complications of diabetic ketoacidosis 20 months following root remnant extractions (Reiter *et al.*, 2004). In a prospective study, an attempt was made to assess whether periodontal disease can cause a systemic inflammatory response in otherwise healthy, adult client-owned dogs (Kouki *et al.*, 2013). There was a statistically significant relationship between the gingival bleeding index and the serum concentration of C-reactive protein, white blood cell count, and polymorphonuclear cell count. It was concluded that active periods of periodontal inflammation may be associated with laboratory values suggestive of systemic inflammatory response (Kouki *et al.*, 2013).

Bacterial resistance

Antibiotics make conditions favourable for overgrowth of some bacteria, including those that possess mechanisms of drug resistance. If a resistant organism is present, antibiotics will create 'selective pressure' favouring the growth of that organism (Radice *et al.*, 2006). A number of studies demonstrated that the development of bacterial resistance to antibiotics is correlated with the level of antibiotic use. Antibiotic resistance of nosocomial pathogens in veterinary hospitals is increased by the transfer of pets already colonized by resistant organisms from one location to another. Aged patients, those affected by chronic disease or immunosuppression may become more susceptible to bacterial infections, resulting in greater use of antibiotics (Radice *et al.*, 2006).

Worldwide spread of bacterial resistance to antibiotics is also due to the increased mobility of today's society. The number of pets has substantially increased in modern days, but their role in the dissemination of bacterial resistance has been given relatively little attention when compared with that of food animals, and a marked contrast is evident between the current policies on antibiotic usage in companion and food animals (Radice *et al.*, 2006). However, the practice of antibiotic overuse in cats and dogs has contributed to the worldwide development of bacteria resistant to antibiotics. Furthermore, the possible transfer of antibiotic-resistant bacteria from cats and dogs to humans has been acknowledged as a potential threat to public health (Booij-Vrieling *et al.*, 2010; Yamasaki *et al.*, 2012).

Reasons for antibiotic overuse

Numerous studies have determined that paediatricians prescribe antibiotics significantly more often to children if they perceive parents expect them, and significantly less often if they feel parents do not expect them (Watson *et al.*, 1999; Mangione-Smith *et al.*, 2001; Christakis *et al.*, 2005). The practice of antibiotic overuse in cats and dogs may also relate to inappropriate prescribing of drugs due to demand from the pet owner (client expectation), time pressure on the clinician (diagnostic uncertainty), legal considerations ('better be on the safe side'), and profitability aspects (selling medications). The best way to combat this situation is to educate the patient owners and veterinary surgeons (veterinarians) to decrease both demand and over-prescription. Unfortunately, there is a tendency to use antibiotics as part of the management of any animal with periodontal disease or other oral conditions, although there is no justification for this (Reiter and Soltero-Rivera, 2017).

Consequences of antibiotic overuse

In the mid-1990s, co-amoxiclav showed the highest *in vitro* susceptibility against all isolates (96%), all aerobes (94%) and all anaerobes (100%) sampled from subgingival areas in dogs, and enrofloxacin showed the highest *in vitro* susceptibility against Gram-negative aerobes (Harvey *et al.*, 1995a). A similar study performed in cats showed that co-amoxiclav had the highest *in vitro* susceptibility against all isolates (92%) and all anaerobes (99%, co-equal with clindamycin), and enrofloxacin had the highest *in vitro* susceptibility against all aerobes (90%) (Harvey *et al.*, 1995b).

By the mid-2000s, treatment of gingivitis with co-amoxiclav did not show clinical improvement of periodontal tissues in client-owned cats, but such improvement occurred in cats treated with clindamycin, doxycycline or spiramycin-metronidazole (Norris and Love, 2000). High resistance of anaerobic and aerobic bacteria to various antibiotics was found in dogs with periodontal disease, with anaerobic bacteria susceptible to co-amoxiclav, doxycycline, and erythromycin, and aerobic bacteria susceptible to co-amoxiclav, erythromycin, gentamicin, and sulfa-trimethoprim (Radice *et al.*, 2006).

In the mid-2010s, isolates from subgingival samples of dogs and cats with stage 2 and 3 periodontal disease revealed different resistance rates to ampicillin, amoxicillin and erythromycin between isolates, but similar high susceptibility to cefovecin (Khazandi *et al.*, 2014).

Select policy statements

The American Association of Endodontists issued the following statement on the overuse of antibiotics in 2012: 'The growing phenomenon of bacterial resistance, caused by the use and abuse of antibiotics and the simultaneous decline in research and development of new antimicrobial drugs, is now threatening to take us back to the pre-antibiotic era... The window of opportunity is rapidly closing' (American Association of Endodontists, 2012).

The American Dental Association stated the following in 2004: 'Any perceived potential benefit of antibiotic prophylaxis must be weighed against the known risks of antibiotic toxicity, allergy and the development, selection and transmission of microbial resistance.' Narrow-spectrum antibiotics (e.g. clindamycin, metronidazole, penicillin) should be used for simple infections, and broad-spectrum antibiotics (e.g. co-amoxiclav, cefalexin, azithromycin, erythromycin, and doxycycline) should be used for more complex infections (American Dental Association, 2004).

The American Veterinary Dental College (AVDC) released the following policy statement in 2005: 'The AVDC endorses the use of systemic antibiotics in veterinary dentistry for treatment of some infectious conditions of the oral cavity. Although culture and susceptibility testing is rarely performed on individual patients that have an infection extending from/to the oral cavity, the selection of an appropriate antibiotic should be based on published data regarding susceptibility testing of the spectra of known oral pathogens. Patients that are scheduled for an oral procedure may benefit from pre-treatment with an appropriate antibiotic to improve the health of infected oral tissues. Bacteraemia is a recognized sequela to dental scaling and other oral procedures. Healthy animals are able to overcome this bacteraemia without the use of systemic antibiotics. However, use of a systemically administered antibiotic is recommended to reduce bacteraemia for animals that are immunocompromised, have underlying systemic disease (such as clinically evident cardiac, hepatic, and renal diseases) and/or when severe oral infection is present. Antibiotics should never be considered to be a monotherapy for treatment of oral infections, and should not be used as preventive management of oral conditions' (American Veterinary Dental College, 2005).

Compulsory guidelines for prudent prescription patterns and use of antibiotics in small animals with periodontal disease or other oral conditions, which describe the minimum requirements to be followed by veterinary surgeons, are not available. Key elements of these guidelines should be the use of antibiotics on the basis of an exact (preferentially microbiological) diagnosis, choice of the most suitable antibiotic (antibacterial spectrum as narrow as possible, margin of safety as high as possible, and good tissue penetration if necessary), restricted use of antibiotics with last resort character, and adherence to label instructions (no underdosing or prolongation of dosing interval). Any deviation from the guideline recommendations should be justified and recorded (Radice et al., 2006).

Suggestions for antibiotic use

The clinician should distinguish between (1) the use of antibiotics for the treatment of specific oral infections (e.g. severe cellulitis, stomatitis, osteomyelitis, sialadenitis) in addition to surgical and other medicinal management of that disease and (2) the use of antibiotics to prevent or reduce bacteraemia or contamination during treatment of a select patient with a particular disease or condition (e.g. organ disease, endocrine pathology, immunodeficiency, implant carrier, simultaneous aseptic procedure elsewhere) (Lodi et al., 2012; Glenny et al., 2013; Ramasamy, 2014; Reiter and Soltero-Rivera, 2017).

Bacteraemia may occur during any periodontal procedure. Because this is usually short-lived in healthy animals, there is no need to place patients routinely on pre-, intra- or postoperative antibiotics. However, the prophylactic use of antibiotics is indicated in select patients with severe purulent infections (such as osteomyelitis), immunocompromising conditions (such as diabetes mellitus), and organ disease (such as renal disease). The drug of choice is intravenous ampicillin (22 mg/kg; when working in the mouth only) or cefazolin (20 mg/kg; when the skin outside the mouth is included in the surgery) given at induction (at least 20 minutes before bacteraemia is anticipated to happen) and repeated every 2 hours during the procedure (Reiter and Soltero-Rivera, 2017).

Systemic antibiotic treatment is not indicated for patients with periodontal disease except in very limited circumstances (Sarkiala and Harvey, 1993). The appropriate drug should ideally be used following culture and sensitivity testing, but the initial empirical use of known efficacious antibiotics may be acceptable in most instances for the treatment of polymicrobic odontogenic and oral infections. Systemic antibiotics can have a broader range of activity than topical antibiotics and can reach all periodontal tissues, but they only achieve a low local concentration at the diseased site. Antibiotics such as co-amoxiclav (13.75 mg/kg orally q12h in the US; 12.5 mg/kg orally q12h in Europe), clindamycin hydrochloride (11 mg/kg orally q12h) and, for severe osteomyelitis in dogs, metronidazole (30 mg/kg orally q24h for 10d, then 10 mg/kg orally q24h for 20d, in addition to radical surgical debridement) are the drugs of choice in cats and dogs (Nielsen et al., 2000; Jennings et al., 2015; Peralta et al., 2015; Reiter and Soltero-Rivera, 2017).

A doxycycline dosage of 2 mg/kg orally q24h appeared to be an appropriate sub-antimicrobial regimen for dogs with periodontitis (Kim et al., 2013). When using doxycycline at such low dosage, the medication's high affinity to hydroxyapatite and anti-inflammatory features are considered rather than its antibiotic effects. This dosage may be suitable for longer treatment in dogs without development of bacterial resistance (Kim et al., 2016).

Topical preparations of antibiotics are available for the treatment of deep periodontal pockets, delivering a very high local concentration of drug. Studies performed on Beagles to evaluate the efficacy of a subgingival delivery system for minocycline showed that when used as an adjunct to dental scaling and root planing, the minocycline periodontal formulation stimulated favourable clinical and antimicrobial responses (Hirasawa et al., 2000). This was represented by reduced total bacterial count, reduced periodontal probing depths and reduced bleeding on probing in the treated dogs. The clinical improvement was maintained for 13 weeks after the treatment was performed. Local application of 8.5–10% doxycycline or 2% clindamycin gel into cleaned periodontal pockets deeper than 4 mm also resulted in favourable clinical outcomes in dogs (Polson et al., 1996; Zetner and Rothmueller, 2002; Johnston et al., 2011).

Role of veterinary technicians/ nurses and dental hygienists

Definitions

The National Association of Veterinary Technicians in America (NAVTA) has a Committee on Veterinary Technician Specialties (CVTS) that governs technicians who excel at their professional discipline of special interest. The CVTS has specific guidelines for Veterinary Technician Specialists (VTS). The Academy of Veterinary Dental Technicians (AVDT; www.avdt.us) promotes the expansion of knowledge and education of veterinary dentistry among credentialled veterinary technicians of North America and grants the VTS (Dentistry) designation to qualified veterinary technicians that complete a credentials process and pass a specialty examination.

A registered veterinary dental hygienist is a licensed oral health professional who provides educational and therapeutic services to animal patients. Dental hygienists have advanced dental knowledge and clinical skills that enable them to perform oral health assessments and periodontal therapies. They also play an important role in the organization and efficient operation of many dentistry and oral surgery services in veterinary academic institutions.

Limitations imposed by law

Areas of responsibility of veterinary technicians/nurses and dental hygienists are summarized in Figure 13.15. Specialty-specific veterinary technicians/nurses and dental hygienists in good standing may perform dental and oral surgical procedures for which they have been qualified under the direct supervision of a veterinary surgeon. However, the supervising veterinary surgeon will be responsible for the diagnostic and treatment procedure performed on the patient.

As with all areas of veterinary medicine, there are limitations on what procedures a veterinary technician/nurse is allowed to perform. These limitations are imposed

- **Improving the client experience:** communicating with clients and referring veterinary surgeon as indicated by the responsible veterinary surgeon; triaging potentially urgent cases; providing home care instructions and demonstrating home oral hygiene; scheduling appointments and check-ups; performing follow-up examinations; and calling clients and referring veterinary surgeons about updates.
- **Performing diagnostic and treatment procedures:** performing physical examinations, oral examination, dental exploring and periodontal probing; charting and recording; taking and processing dental radiographs; performing dental scaling, root planing, gingival curettage, and dental polishing; placing medications into cleaned periodontal pockets; taking full-mouth impressions, obtaining a bite registration, and making stone models; fabricating tape muzzles; performing feeding tube care and wound management; demonstrating/providing home oral hygiene instructions; and removing sutures.
- **Performing sedation and anaesthesia:** premedicating and intubating patients; inducing and maintaining anaesthesia; administering local analgesia and regional nerve blocks; recovering patients from anaesthesia; and monitoring them postoperatively.
- **Assisting in the operating room:** preparing the operating room and table; providing instruments and supplies for specific dental and oral surgical procedures; and performing clinical research (obtaining measurements of periodontal attachment loss, gingival inflammation, plaque/calculus accumulation, etc.).
- **General nursing skills:** performing patient care (feeding, grooming, walking); obtaining blood and urine samples; submitting preoperative test requests; communicating with clinical laboratories; administering medications and fluids; placing catheters; providing perioperative care; and filing of dental and medical records.
- **Maintaining instruments and equipment:** performing routine maintenance and emergency repair of equipment; sharpening of instruments; being the primary contact for the manufacturer/supplier; ordering and maintaining inventory of all dental and oral surgical equipment, materials and supplies; and keeping the staff abreast of new products and techniques.
- **Teaching:** performing clinical teaching of other technicians/nurses, students, interns and residents; engaging in didactic and laboratory teaching during continuing education courses; and being role models with regards to safety in the workplace.

13.15 Areas of responsibility of veterinary technicians/nurses and veterinary dental hygienists (greatly dependent on country and state laws).

by law, but there are differences between the jurisdictions of different countries (or even states within a country). For the USA, the American Veterinary Medical Association (AVMA) has a Summary Report by State on the authority of veterinary technicians/nurses and other non-veterinarians to perform dental procedures (www.avma.org/Advocacy/StateAndLocal/Pages/sr-dental-procedures.aspx). The American Veterinary Dental College (AVDC) developed a position statement regarding veterinary dental healthcare providers as a means to safeguard the veterinary dental patient and to ensure the qualifications of persons performing veterinary dental procedures (www.avdc.org/Dental_Health_Care_Providers.pdf).

In the UK, practitioners are referred to the Royal College of Veterinary Surgeons (RCVS) Schedule 3 exemption (www.rcvs.org.uk/setting-standards/advice-and-guidance/code-of-professional-conduct-for-veterinary-surgeons/supporting-guidance/delegation-to-veterinary-nurses/). Veterinary surgeons, nurses/technicians and dental hygienists outside of the USA and UK should refer to their region's relevant legislation.

Safety in the workplace

Responsibilities and precautions

Employers and employees have responsibilities to one another to maintain a safe workplace. The employer has a responsibility to communicate the known hazards in the workplace, establish safety policies, and provide safety equipment to protect employees. Employees are responsible for learning about the known hazards in the workplace, implementing safety policies, and wearing the required personal protective equipment (Aller, 2005; Deeprose, 2007; Holmstrom and Holmstrom, 2013).

Safety is the most effective and least expensive insurance policy, and there are many precautions that can be taken. Primary and assisting clinicians should use instruments instead of fingers to retract tissue. Needles should not be recapped but disposed in a sharps container (Holmstrom and Holmstrom, 2013). The mouth should be rinsed with diluted chlorhexidine prior to performing dental or oral surgical procedures. Non-essential staff and pregnant women should leave the operating room during exposure of radiographs. Dosimeter badges

should be worn to recognize radiation overexposure. Disposable covers and barriers for objects, equipment and surfaces should be used to prevent patient cross-contamination and minimize clean-up time between patients (West-Hyde, 1995; Deeprose, 2007). Personnel should not store food, eat or drink in areas where patients are examined, treated or housed, biological specimens are handled, or medications are stored.

Personal protective equipment

The basic personal protective equipment needed for veterinary dentistry and oral surgery includes safety masks, protective eyewear, and gloves (Holmstrom and Holmstrom, 2013). They provide a barrier between the operator and the patient to reduce disease transmission from sources of infection. The concept of these precautions makes the assumption that any body fluid, non-intact skin, and mucus membrane from a patient contains an infectious agent, whether it actually does or not. One should err on the side of caution and prevent direct contact by wearing proper attire (West-Hyde, 1995; Aller, 2005).

Masks and protective eyewear are mandatory for anybody present in the dental operating room to avoid inhalation and corneal contamination by airborne microorganisms, and mechanical injury (Deeprose, 2007). This could consist of a surgical mask capable of high bacterial filtration and either goggles with solid side shields or a disposable face shield to protect mucus membranes of the mouth, nose and eyes from exposure to aerosols and splash risk (Figure 13.16). Respirator masks offer more protection than surgical masks (Holmstrom and Holmstrom, 2013). Appropriate eye protection is also mandatory for anybody in the dental operating room during surgical laser usage, and a laser plume evacuation system should be in place. Instrument-mounted or hand-held shields are needed when using light-curing units to block the blue light wavelengths that are harmful to the eye's retina (Figure 13.17). Operators should also wear a cap and gown over a scrub suit. Gloves (Figure 13.18) are needed to protect the operator as well as the patient from cross-contamination with bacteria (Deeprose, 2007). They also provide minimal protection from injury as a result of handling sharp instruments or pointed teeth. If a person near the operator gets injured, gloves can protect the operator from direct exposure to human blood. Powdered gloves must no

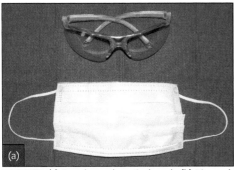
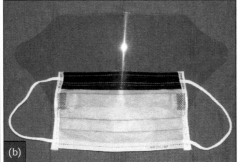
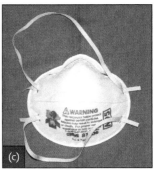

13.16 (a) Goggles and surgical mask. (b) Disposable face shield. (c) Respirator mask.
(© Dr Alexander M. Reiter)

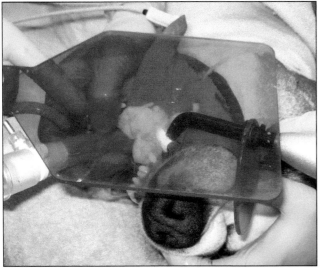

13.17 Instrument-mounted and hand-held shields are used for retinal protection during light-curing of a composite restoration at the right maxillary canine tooth of a dog.
(© Dr Alexander M. Reiter)

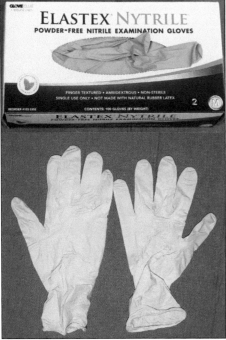

13.18 Powder-free nitrile gloves.
(© Dr Alexander M. Reiter)

longer be used due to documented health risks, and one should avoid latex gloves when there is concern about allergy (Aller, 2005).

Frequent hand washing is important in disease control, but hands could become dry, which may increase bacterial contamination. Using a good barrier type cream or lotion will prevent skin damage. Hands should be washed before donning gloves, after removing gloves, and between patients. Jewellery should not be worn for hand washing or during dental and oral surgical procedures, as it collects bacteria and tends to tear the gloves. Fingernails should be trimmed to <2 mm and cleaned to reduce accumulation of bacteria and prevent tears of gloves (Aller, 2005; Hardy *et al.*, 2017). If power scalers are used for a long period of time, it is possible for operators to sustain hearing loss. Some operators wear hearing protection while using power equipment (West-Hyde, 1995).

Animal bite protocol

During the initial consultation, opening the mouth should be reserved until the end of the physical examination. An oral examination should only be performed on cooperative patients to minimize the risk of being scratched or bitten. A bite wound should immediately be cleaned with soap and water, and a physician should be consulted. Protocols for a person bitten by a pet, for a patient presenting with a bite wound and uncertain rabies vaccination status, and for staff handling such a pet should be followed. If the animal is alive, a decision should be made whether the pet is a high-, moderate- or low-risk rabies suspect. The client should be informed if the pet has bitten a member of the staff. Follow-ups should be explained to the client based on the pet's rabies suspect risk category as well as the possible need for rabies testing if the animal dies or is euthanased. When applicable, the client is given the results of rabies testing from the laboratory, and the completion of the 10-day observation period of the animal is coordinated.

Ergonomics and musculoskeletal disorders

Ergonomics is the study of the interaction between people and their working environment, aiming at helping to improve efficiency, increase productivity, and reduce the number and severity of work-related musculoskeletal disorders (MSDs). It has also been defined as a scientific discipline devoted to the study and analysis of human work, especially as it is affected by anatomical, psychological, and other individual characteristics of people. Having good ergonomics provides an efficient, profitable, and pain-free work environment and increases the longevity of employment (West-Hyde, 1995; DeForge, 2002).

MSDs are impairments of body structures such as muscles, joints, tendons, ligaments, nerves, bones or an alteration of a localized blood circulation system caused or aggravated primarily by the performance of work and by the effects of the immediate work environment. They often result from inappropriate positioning, usually during repetitive use, and have been grouped as neck and shoulder disorders, back disorders, and hand and wrist disorders (Nemes et al., 2013; Sakzewski and Naser-ud-Din, 2014).

Two of the most commonly diagnosed MSDs in dental health care professionals are carpal tunnel syndrome (CTS) and thoracic outlet syndrome (TOS). CTS results from compression of the median nerve within the carpal tunnel, which is the passage for nerves, finger flexor tendons, and blood vessels. This can result in numbness and tingling of the thumb that may progress to a feeling of burning and pain in multiple digits. TOS is characterized by symptoms in the upper extremities, shoulder, chest, neck and head due to the pressure on the nerves and vessels at the thoracic outlet, which can lead to paraesthesia and pain of the hands upon elevation of the arms and/or weakness of the fourth and fifth digits. Dentists working in general private practice were more likely to report shoulder pain, while those working in periodontal practice were more likely to report forearm pain. Dental hygienists that use mostly hand instrumentation reported more neck pain, and those that scale most frequently with an ultrasonic unit would report more shoulder and back pain (Hayes et al., 2012).

Clinical signs, symptoms and consequences

Clinical signs of MSDs include decreased range of motion, loss of normal sensation, decreased grip strength, loss of normal movement, and loss of coordination (Aller, 2005). The symptoms often experienced are excessive fatigue in the shoulders and neck, tingling, burning or other pain in the arms, weak grip, cramping and stiffness of hands, numbness in fingers and hands, clumsiness and dropping of objects, and hypersensitivity in hands and fingers. The reported consequences of MSDs include inefficiency, decreased profitability, more sick days, change of career, and early retirement. MSDs account for 29.5% of reasons for early retirement among dentists that treat humans (Nemes et al., 2013; Gupta et al., 2014).

Risk factors

Poor operator positioning includes leaning forward abnormally and having feet not parallel to the floor, shoulders not squared or no lumbar support. These awkward positions are often assumed to coordinate the relative positions between people working together, to obtain optimal view of the field of interest within the patient's mouth, to provide a comfortable position for the patient, and to manoeuvre complex equipment and reach for instruments (DeForge, 2002; Gupta et al., 2014).

Tasks that require forceful exertions (e.g. tooth extraction) place higher loads on the muscles, tendons, ligaments and joints. Prolonged stresses can lead to MSDs when there is inadequate time for rest or recovery. Force requirements may increase with the use of an awkward posture, the use of narrow instrument handles that lessen grip capacity, and the use of the index finger and thumb to forcefully grip an object (DeForge, 2002; Gupta et al., 2014).

If motions are repeated frequently and for prolonged periods, fatigue and muscle-tendon strain can accumulate. Effects of repetitive motions from performing the same work activities are increased when awkward postures and forceful exertions are involved.

Repeated or continuous contact with hard or sharp objects, such as non-rounded table edges, and the use of narrow instrument handles or improper glove size may create pressure over an area of the fingers, hand or forearm that can inhibit nerve function and blood flow. Exposure to local vibration occurs when a specific part of the body comes in contact with a vibrating object, such as a power hand tool. Identified stressors include the psychological demands of performing a meticulous dental or oral surgical procedure under time pressure with little or no rest (DeForge, 2002; Gupta et al., 2014).

Prevention and treatment

The worker affected by MSDs should consult a physician, who may recommend a combination of diagnostic testing, exercise, massage, physical therapy, chiropractic work, medications, surgery, and limited patient schedule (Aller, 2005; Nemes et al., 2013). The operator needs to be aware of proper positioning, glove sizes, instrument design, modified pen grasp, chair design, tables, and loupes in order to prevent MSDs. Work is best done at a comfortable room temperature and low noise level. One should stand up every 20–25 minutes. It is equally important to exercise regularly to help maintain the core of the body. Exercise will also decrease pain, aid in proper movement/lubrication of the joints, increase blood flow and warm muscles, and decrease stress and injury (Aller, 2005; Holmstrom and Holmstrom, 2013).

The working environment should be arranged to the operator's needs for establishing good ergonomics (Figure 13.19). Proper body positioning should help to keep the patient and operator from harm (Aller, 2005; Deeprose, 2007). Ergonomics can help 'fit the job task to the employee' not 'fit the employee to the job task'. The feet of the operator should be flat on the floor, the thighs on a slight downward slant (or chair angled forward by 5–15 degrees), buttocks square in the chair, the spine central in chair (leaning forward slightly by 0–20 degrees), lumbar spine supported by a chair back, shoulders square (in a horizontal line), the arms in a neutral position (preferably supported by arm rests; upper arm abduction <20 degrees, forearm abduction <60 degrees), and the head flexed forward by 0–15 degrees (West-Hyde, 1995; DeForge, 2002; Holmstrom and Holmstrom, 2013).

The chair (Figure 13.20) strongly impacts posture and, therefore, musculoskeletal health (DeForge, 2002). The operator should position himself/herself first, and then the patient is positioned as needed. Adjustments will need to be done to the chair in between operators. There should be sufficient padding to support the operator's bodyweight. The chair should have a large seating area (thigh support), five caster stool, foot ring, and be adjustable for the height of the operating table. It may also have adjustable lumbar support and armrests, and a foot ring. To improve access and visibility to all areas of the mouth while maintaining the correct physical posture it is strongly recommended to use both a chair and an operating table that can be adjustable in height and inclination.

Improper glove size can contribute to hand and wrist constriction. Tight gloves impinge on the wrist causing repetitive impairment (i.e. vascular constriction, nerve compression, muscle fatigue and hand pain). Loose/baggy gloves can catch on inanimate objects causing injury. Gloves should be loose fitting across the palm and wrist region. The skin should not be red or blanch once the gloves are removed. Right- and left-fitted gloves are preferred over ambidextrous gloves (Aller, 2005; Holmstrom and Holmstrom, 2013).

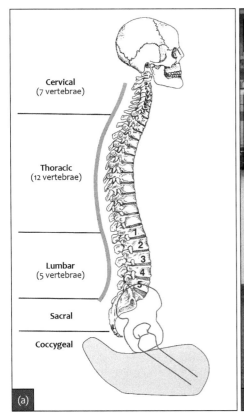

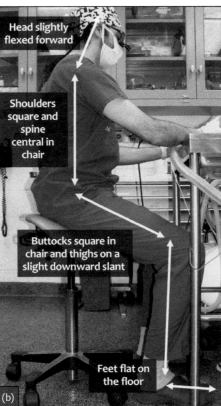

13.19 (a) Human spinal column in a saddle-sitting position, showing maintenance of normal spinal curvature even in a reach-forward activity. (b) Nearly perfect positioning of an operator.
(a, Reproduced with permission from Bambach Saddle Seat (Europe) Ltd.; b, © Dr Alexander M. Reiter)

Cervical (7 vertebrae)

Thoracic (12 vertebrae)

Lumbar (5 vertebrae)

Sacral

Coccygeal

Head slightly flexed forward

Shoulders square and spine central in chair

Buttocks square in chair and thighs on a slight downward slant

Feet flat on the floor

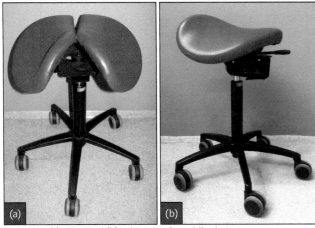

13.20 (a) Front and (b) side view of a saddle chair.
(© Dr Alexander M. Reiter)

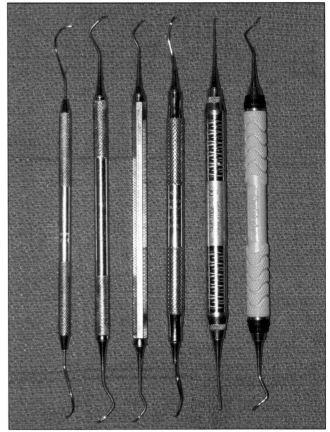

The instrument handle design is of utmost importance (Aller, 2005). Appropriate shape and pattern can provide traction and decrease a pinch grip. A lightweight (hollow) handle will improve tactile sensitivity and is less strenuous to use. A relatively larger diameter also decreases a pinch grip (a slender handle leads to cramping) (Figure 13.21). Instruments should be sharpened after each use, thus improving efficiency and reducing fatigue. The cord of a dental handpiece can be adjusted around an elbow so that its weight is not pulling on the operator's wrist. Similarly, the cord of an ultrasonic handpiece can be secured with the little finger or draped around the forearm (Figure 13.22) or over the neck.

13.21 Various instrument handle shapes; lightweight (hollow) and thicker handles with an appropriate pattern are preferred.
(© Dr Alexander M. Reiter)

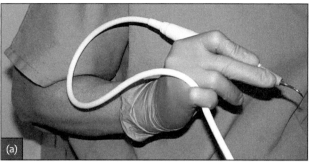
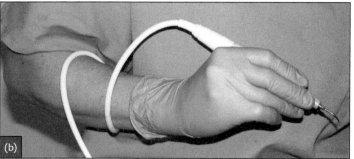

13.22 The cord of an ultrasonic handpiece can be (a) secured with the little finger or (b) draped around the forearm.
(© Dr Margherita Gracis)

The modified pen grasp should be utilized for holding most instruments and handpieces, facilitating tactile sensitivity and precise instrument control, and decreasing risk of tissue trauma (Aller, 2005). The index finger and thumb are placed on the instrument handle (to hold the instrument securely). The middle finger is rested lightly on the instrument shank (to support the instrument and guide its movement, which prevents it from slipping). The ring finger is placed on the tooth surface (giving strength to the working strokes and stability), and the little finger is placed against or next to the ring finger (but it does not really have a function).

Loupes and adequate illumination enhance proper positioning, reduce back and neck strain, and increase visibility (DeForge, 2002). There are several aspects to consider when purchasing loupes (Figure 13.23), including working distance (distance between the operator's eyes and the patient's mouth, which should be between 12 and 17 inches (30 and 45 cm)), declination angle (angle of the line of sight made with neutral eye position and the actual line of sight made by the declined eye chosen by the clinician; proper angle is neutral for all types of work), magnification (2.5–3.5x or 3.5–5x; lower magnification provides a wider view for general work; higher magnification gives a smaller view for greater detail), depth of field (difference between the nearest and farthest distances within which the object remains in sharp focus; should be large enough to allow the operator to move the head freely within a required working range), and weight and design of the frame (a lighter frame is more comfortable when wearing for a prolonged time; a larger frame allows for the magnification lens to sit lower) (Deeprose, 2007). The use of lightweight headlamps (that can be attached to the eye loupes) and quality surgical lamps is recommended to properly illuminate the surgical areas. Additional illumination may be provided by fibreoptics or LED self-generating dental handpieces.

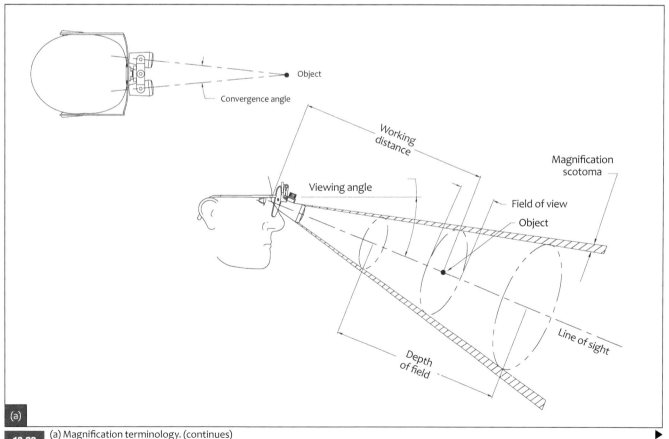

13.23 (a) Magnification terminology. (continues)
(Reproduced with permission from DP Medical Systems, Ltd)

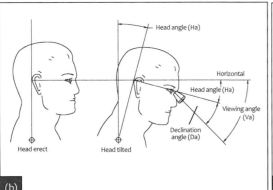

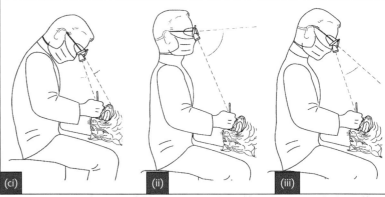

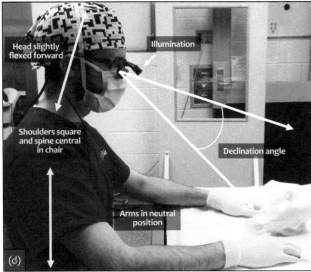

13.23 (continued) (b) Angle terminology. (c) Declination angle that is (i) too small, (ii) too large, and (iii) optimal. (d) Nearly perfect positioning of an operator in relation to the declination angle.
(b, c, Reproduced with permission from DP Medical Systems, Ltd.; d, © Dr Alexander M. Reiter)

Equipment maintenance care and troubleshooting

Sharpening of periodontal instruments

Sharp periodontal instruments are important to facilitate effective removal of dental deposits, reduce operator fatigue, and improve tactile sensitivity. Thorough periodontal debridement can only be accomplished with the use of sharp instruments (Angel, 2014). Each stroke of an instrument against the tooth will wear away the metal of the cutting edge, causing it to transform from a precise, sharp line at the junction of the face and lateral surfaces to a dull, rounded surface. Using a dull surface requires heavier lateral pressure against the tooth, reducing tactile sensitivity and creating hand fatigue. The dull surface will burnish the calculus, rather than causing it to be shaved off. Once burnished, this calculus is difficult to detect and remove (Lewis and Miller, 2010).

Instruments should be sharpened after cleaning and before sterilizing. This can be accomplished manually with sharpening stones or automated devices. Either way, it is critical to have a thorough understanding of the instrument design, including the cross-sectional shape and the line angles between surfaces, to enable a sharp cutting edge to be reestablished without creating changes in the instrument's original design. Two methods of manual sharpening can be used: stationary stone/moving instrument or moving stone/stationary instrument (Holmstrom, 2013a).

The latter method is described below. It requires the instrument to be held stationary while the stone is moved and provides a good view of the blade so that the angle can be precisely controlled.

Sharpening stones (Figure 13.24) may be flat or conical and include the synthetic, highly abrasive Carborundum (silicon carbide), the synthetic, medium abrasive India (aluminum oxide), and the natural, mildly abrasive Arkansas (aluminum oxide) (Holmstrom, 2013a). A wedge-shaped stone with rounded ends, giving two different

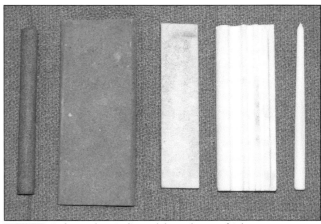

13.24 Carborundum, India, and three shapes of Arkansas stones (from left to right).
(© Dr Alexander M. Reiter)

diameters of curvature, is also available for use on instruments of different sizes (Robinson, 2007). More abrasive stones are used to sharpen very dull instruments, and less abrasive stones are utilized to produce a final, sharp cutting edge. A few drops of lubricant are required for most stones to keep metal particles from embedding into the stone and to reduce heat friction (Figure 13.25). The Carborundum stone can be lubricated with water or used dry. Arkansas and India stones are lubricated with an acid-free mineral oil (Robinson, 2007).

For sickle scalers and universal curettes, the instrument is held in the palm of one hand (palm grasp), positioned vertically with the face parallel to the floor, and the tip of the instrument is pointed toward the operator to sharpen the one cutting edge and away from the operator to sharpen the opposite cutting edge (Angel, 2014). Elbows should be braced against the side of the body for stability, and the procedure should be performed under good lighting. The stone is held with the fingertips of the other hand and should be placed against the lateral surface of the blade, forming an angle of approximately 110 degrees with the face of the blade (Figure 13.26). Area-specific (Gracey) curettes have one cutting edge that requires sharpening (Angel, 2014). If the instrument is held with the terminal shank vertically, the cutting edge is lower than the back of the blade. Thus, the instrument is held so that the face of the blade is horizontal, and then the cutting edge and toe are sharpened as for a universal curette.

Using light pressure, the stone is moved in short up-and-down strokes against the lateral surface of the instrument, beginning at the heel of the instrument and working towards the tip. When sharpening curettes, the stone is

also moved around the toe. At the point where sharpening allows the lateral surface to meet with the face, a black 'sludge' will appear on the face, consisting of stone oil, stone particles, and instrument particles (Holmstrom, 2013a). The procedure is finished with a few more light strokes, ending with a down stroke of the stone to remove particles that have been lifted from the metal. Instruments that have been over-sharpened and are excessively thin should be discarded.

Sharpened scalers and curettes can be tested on an acrylic stick (Angel, 2014). A syringe casing may also be used to check for sharpness. Sharp instruments will shave a thin slice from the surface. When held against light, dull instruments will reveal a reflective cutting edge, and more sharpening is required. A curette used for a long time and repeatedly sharpened may at some point acquire the shape of a scaler (the round toe becomes a pointed tip). Other instruments can also be sharpened with an appropriate stone. For example, periosteal elevators are sharpened on the flat face of the instrument using either a flat or a round sharpening stone (Angel, 2014).

Ultrasonic scaler

When using a magnetostrictive scaling unit with a metal stack transducer (other types of units may have slight variations according to manufacturer's instructions), the following steps should be performed prior to and after dental scaling:

- Plug the electrical cord to an outlet, set the water knob on high, power on lowest, step on the pedal and let water run through the handpiece (without insert) into the sink for a minimum of 2 minutes (every morning; repeat for 30 seconds in between patients)
- Hold the handpiece perpendicular to the floor while stepping on the pedal to completely fill the handpiece with water, which eliminates air bubbles that cause heat (repeat each time the insert is changed)
- Choose the tip design, remove the foot from the pedal, slide the insert into the handpiece until resistance is met at the rubber 'O' ring, and gently twist as the insert is completely seated
- Hold the handpiece parallel to the floor to adjust the power to low-medium and water to a spray so that the lowest power setting is used that will accomplish the task (activate the foot pedal before the tip of the insert is adapted to the tooth surface)

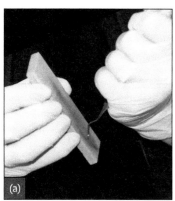
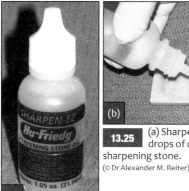

13.25 (a) Sharpening stone oil. (b) A few drops of oil are placed on an Arkansas sharpening stone.
(© Dr Alexander M. Reiter)

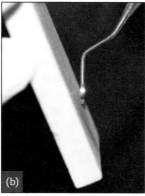
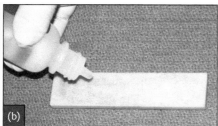
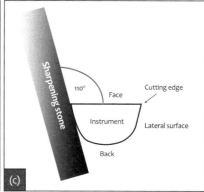
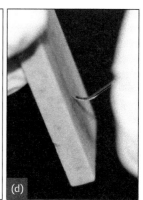

13.26 (a) The handle of a universal curette is held in the palm of one hand, with the terminal shank positioned vertically and the face of the working end parallel to the floor, and the sharpening stone is held with the fingertips of the other hand and placed against the lateral surface of the working end. (b) Close-up view. (c) Illustration showing that the sharpening stone and the face of the working end should form an angle of approximately 110 degrees. Using light pressure the stone is moved in short up-and-down strokes against the lateral surface of the working end. (d) When sharpening curettes, the stone is also moved around the toe.
(© Dr Alexander M. Reiter)

- Following ultrasonic scaling, wipe the unit, handpiece, and power cord with a non-immersion type disinfectant
- Observe the manufacturer's instructions for sterilizing the handpiece and inserts.

If the insert tip is not cavitating, adjust the phase, check the transducer, and inspect the tip for its shape and wear. The correct transducer should be purchased for the unit utilized (short (30 K) or long stack (25 K)). Inserts should be replaced if the transducer is bent or if the tip is bent or worn (Figure 13.27). An indicator guide (a card with printed tip outlines) should be used to determine the extent of tip bending and wear. If the tip is worn by 1 mm, there is 25% loss of efficiency. Inserts should be replaced when worn 2 mm (50% loss of efficiency). It is good practice to replace the inserts annually. If the handpiece and water get hot, the water pressure and flow should be checked and increased.

When using a piezoelectric scaling unit, all visible debris should be removed from the control unit, foot pedal, cables, handpieces and scaling tips using a hospital-grade surface disinfectant wipe. The disinfectant should be allowed to dry on the parts (preferably for 10 minutes). If using a disinfectant spray, it should not be sprayed directly on to the control unit or foot pedal. The handpiece and scaler tips can be steam-autoclaved according to the manufacturer's instructions. The tip should always be removed from the handpiece prior to sterilizing. When replacing the scaler tip to the end of the handpiece, over-tightening the connection with the tip wrench should be avoided, as this can cause the tip to jam.

The scaler tip should be routinely inspected for wear and shape, using the wear guide that accompanies the unit. The tips should be replaced when bent or shortened by use. Dropping the handpiece can cause fracture of the ceramic or crystal transducer located inside, resulting in a handpiece that will not vibrate. Once this breakage has

occurred, the entire handpiece must be sent to the manufacturer for repair. Water lines should be flushed for 2 minutes in the morning prior to use to remove any stagnant water left in the lines overnight. The scaling tip should be removed prior to flushing. It is also good practice to flush for 30 seconds between patients.

Microbial biofilms, consisting of colonies of bacteria, fungi and protozoa protected by a glycocalyx layer, form in narrow plastic tubing carrying water to ultrasonic scalers and handpieces and the air/water syringe of dental units (Figure 13.28). The primary source of microorganisms is the municipal water supply. The water filter needs to be changed if it gets clogged. Disinfectants can be introduced into the water supply to reduce the bacterial load. The manufacturer's advice on the type and strength of the disinfectant should be followed (Deeprose, 2007).

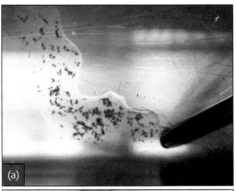

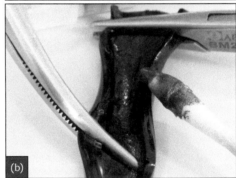

13.28 (a) Debris emerging from an ultrasonic handpiece. (b) Biofilm inside a cut plastic tube carrying water to an ultrasonic scaler.
(© Dr Alexander M. Reiter)

Dental unit

Regular machine maintenance and thorough cleaning and lubricating are essential to ensure trouble-free function. If there appears to be no power, one should check whether the dental unit is plugged in and switched on. The reset button may need to be used. If the oil tank of oil-lubricated air compressors is hot and there is a burning smell, one should check the oil level, listen for air leaks (hissing noise), determine if the handpieces and water bottle are tightly screwed to their connections, and check whether the regulator valve is stuck.

The pressure control knob allows water bottles to be depressurized before taking them off and being refilled with distilled or de-ionized water. If the water bottle cannot be unscrewed for refilling, the bottle should be filled slightly with air by pressurizing the unit, then the bottle can be unscrewed slowly (a hissing noise will be heard). A waterline cleanser/disinfectant should be used if there is mould growing in the bottle when distilled or de-ionized water is not being used.

13.27 (a) Intact metal stack transducer of an ultrasonic insert on top compared with one that is bent on the bottom. (b) An indicator guide is used to determine the extent of bending and wear of the tip of an ultrasonic insert.
(© Dr Alexander M. Reiter)

The compressor supplies the air needed to run the handpieces and to pressurize the water system. The silent-type compressor (requiring synthetic oil to prevent moisture from corroding sensitive disc valves) usually sits on the base of the dental unit. Its oil level can be checked at the site glass window while the unit is running. Oil recommended by the manufacturer needs to be added if the level is below half way (Robinson, 2007; Holmstrom, 2013a).

There are pressure gauges for the tank (largest gauge), the line (regulator), and handpieces. The maximum pressure for the silent-type compressor is 120 psi. It should be refilled with air when the pressure drops to 80 psi. One should check for air leaks. Maintenance care for the tank consists of at least weekly draining of condensation (reducing the pressure by turning off the compressor, draining the air pressure to almost zero by running a handpiece or air/water syringe, then slowly opening the valve to drain the condensation) (Holmstrom, 2013a).

The regulator pressure gauge (smaller of the two gauges) registers the pressure to the air lines. Pressure is adjusted to 80 psi by pulling up and rotating the knob on top of the unit. Additional gauges will monitor the pressure of the handpieces. These may be located on the front of the unit near the handpiece holders. To check for proper pressure, the handpiece is removed from the holder, the foot pedal is activated to full speed, and the lever on the gauge is observed. Adjustment knobs or screws (depending on the manufacturer) are located near each handpiece. The pressure should be 30–40 psi for the high-speed handpiece (depending on the manufacturer), 45 psi (35–50 psi) for the low-speed handpiece, and 40 psi (35–45 psi) for the sonic scaler. Occasionally, the air/water syringe will need maintenance and replacement parts, typically when the buttons do not retract when depressed or when water leaks on its own. Internal replacement parts can be purchased as a kit.

Handpieces

The low-speed handpiece must be lubricated at the end of each day. The lubricant is inserted into the smaller of the two larger holes (i.e. the air entry hole) (Figure 13.29), using a specified oil, and then the handpiece is operated forward and reverse (Robinson, 2007; Holmstrom, 2013a). The handpiece is disassembled, cleaned and oiled (mineral base with silicone) weekly. Overuse of oil can cause the handpiece to freeze. One drop or one spray is all that is required. A penetrating oil and water-displacing spray

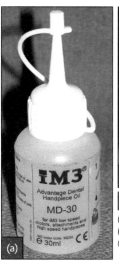
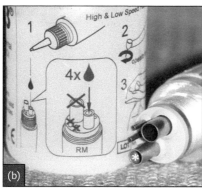

13.29 (a) Manufacturer lubricant for low- and high-speed handpieces. (b) The oil is inserted into the air entry hole (i.e. the smaller of the two larger holes (∗)).
(© Dr Alexander M. Reiter)

may be sprayed into the low-speed handpiece to remove residues, followed by the recommended lubricant. The handpiece should never be submerged into the ultrasonic instrument cleaner.

The high-speed handpiece (usually with a 4-hole Midwest connection to the supply hose) and sonic scalers should be lubricated daily with a spray-type cleaner and lubricant or another product recommended by the manufacturer (oil through the air entry hole) (Robinson, 2007; Holmstrom, 2013a). Maintenance of lube-free high-speed handpieces includes daily removal of the bur, blowing water/air into the chuck mechanism, drying with paper points until they come out clean, removing the turbine and cleaning inside the head (but no oiling) weekly. Cleaning of the inside of the head should be done prior to each sterilizing process.

The turbine is the internal portion of the high-speed handpiece. It can easily be damaged if the handpiece is used incorrectly. It is important to not run the handpiece without a bur, always ensure that burs are fully seated in the turbine (never having them extended to gain length, which results in greater lateral forces), not use bent or damaged burs, and always store handpieces with a bur or blank in place (Robinson, 2007). Turbines wear out over time and must be replaced periodically. This is often indicated by abnormal vibration, increased noise, failure of the turbine chuck to tighten around the bur, roughness felt when spinning the bur by hand, and intermittent stopping of the handpiece (Holmstrom, 2013a).

To change the turbine, a blank is placed in the handpiece. If the bur that is in the handpiece cannot be removed, caution should be exercised to keep from cutting the hands on the bur. Next, the small metal ring (wrench) supplied with the handpiece is placed on the cap of the handpiece. The handpiece cap is unscrewed and removed by rotating the wrench anti-clockwise. The turbine cartridge is removed from the handpiece head by pressing on the blank or bur. The new turbine cartridge is placed into the handpiece head. Finally, the new turbine cartridge is aligned with the pin side up. If the pin is not aligned with the slot, the turbine cartridge will not slide completely into the handpiece head (Holmstrom, 2013a).

If the bur in a high-speed handpiece stops spinning, one should check whether the compressor is on, evaluate the pressure setting of the handpiece, and check whether the cap of the handpiece is tightened. It is also possible that the operator has pressed too hard against the tooth, causing the bur to stall. The handpiece should be cleaned and lubricated if the bur slips out of the turbine and the handpiece run with a bur inserted for 30 seconds prior to use. If there is no water flow in the handpiece, one should check whether the compressor is on, the water flow pressure switch is on, and the water bottle is sufficiently full. The water flow knob at the handpiece should be inspected. One should check which line the handpiece is attached to, take it off, depress the foot pedal, and check if water is coming out. Mineral accumulations in the water line can be dislodged by passing a fine wire through the water intake hole and into the water exit hole of the handpiece. If water is leaking out of the back of the handpiece, one should ensure that the rubber gasket is in place. If the fibreoptic light does not work, the bulb should be evaluated by removing the handpiece and depressing the foot pedal to observe the presence of light. The connector sheath can be moved back to expose and replace the bulb.

If the bur in a low-speed handpiece does not spin, one should check whether the compressor is on, evaluate the pressure setting of the handpiece, ensure that the nose cone is pushed down tightly, check whether the chuck housing is locked or open, check the forward/reverse speed/direction ring, and determine whether there is too much or too little lubricant. If the prophy/contra angle does not spin, one should clean and lubricate it (single use for disposable prophy angles).

Sanitization, disinfection and sterilization

Sanitization refers to cleaning an object or area free from any dirt or dust. Disinfection is accomplished by application of a disinfectant to an inanimate object or an antiseptic to a living tissue. Sterilization refers to the removal of all living microorganisms and bacterial endospores from an object or instrument and is achieved by steam or chemical vapour under pressure, dry heat, and low-temperature sterilization processes (ethylene oxide gas, plasma sterilization) (Terpak and Verstraete, 2012; Reiter, 2013). Any instrument/equipment coming into contact with intact skin (e.g. X-ray head, blood pressure cuff, and stethoscope) should be sanitized. Any instrument/equipment coming into contact with intact mucus membranes but not penetrating them (e.g. dental mirror, dental handpiece) should at least be disinfected. Any instrument/equipment introduced into a patient's bloodstream, skin, and mucus membranes or otherwise sterile area (e.g. scalpel blade, hand curette, and dental bur) should be sterilized.

A designated processing area should be used to control quality and ensure safety during receiving, cleaning, disinfecting, sterilizing, packaging and storing of instruments and equipment. Dental water lines (including those of handpieces, ultrasonic scalers and air/water syringes) should be flushed daily for a minimum of 2 minutes prior to usage and for 30 seconds in between patients. Components permanently attached to air and water lines should be cleaned and disinfected. Dental handpieces and other devices that can be detached from air and water lines should be cleaned and sterilized. Instruments are soaked in hot water then scrubbed with detergent and rinsed (heavy-duty utility gloves should be worn), or they are laid in an ultrasonic cleaning bath, containing special solutions to enhance its cleaning activity (Holmstrom, 2013a). Selected instruments may be arranged into cassettes, which are then covered with steam-permeable wrappers and sealed with tape (Terpak and Verstraete, 2012; Reiter, 2013).

Packs should be loosely but evenly distributed within the sterilization chamber to allow circulation of heat and moisture. Steam in gravity displacement type sterilizers (15–30 minutes at 121.5°C) and high-speed prevacuum sterilizers (4–5 minutes at 132°C) tend to dull and rust carbon steel instrument cutting edges; thus, the use of a rust inhibitor is advised to prevent corrosion. Dry heat sterilizers (60 minutes at 160°C) can be used for delicate instruments that might be damaged or corroded by moist heat. Heat-sensitive objects such as powders, plastics, rubber and acrylic resin materials with low melting points may be treated with ethylene oxide gas or other low-temperature sterilization processes (Terpak and Verstraete, 2012; Reiter, 2013).

Dental scaling without anaesthesia

Fear *versus* risk of anaesthesia

Anaesthesia is essential for most diagnostic and treatment procedures performed in veterinary dentistry and oral surgery. Fear of general anaesthesia is a natural concern voiced by many pet owners. However, the risk of chronic oral infection and its systemic impact, for example, is far greater than the risk of a complication related to sedation or anaesthesia. Appropriately administered general anaesthesia carries an extremely low risk for the patient, as a result of a combination of pre-anaesthetic assessment of the patient (including blood tests and other tests as indicated), use of modern anaesthetic agents, regional nerve blocks (minimizing the depth of general anaesthesia required), and appropriate monitoring equipment. Many patients are awake and standing within 15–20 minutes of completion of the procedure and go home the same day. While no one can guarantee the outcome of anaesthesia, veterinary professionals are trained to provide safe anaesthesia and to minimize pain for pets.

Several studies have described the frequency of or risk factors for anaesthetic- and sedation-related death, which is referred to as death occurring within 48 hours of use of anaesthesia or sedation where surgical or pre-existing medical causes did not solely cause death. The overall risk of anaesthetic- and sedation-related death is approximately 0.1–0.2% in healthy and 0.5–4.8% in sick dogs and cats (Gaynor et al., 1999; Brodbelt, 2009; Bille et al., 2012). Factors associated with increased odds of anaesthetic- or sedation-related death are poor health status, increasing age, extremes of weight, increasing procedural urgency, duration and complexity, endotracheal intubation (in cats, possibly due to laryngeal trauma, spasm, or oedema), fluid therapy (possibly secondary to volume overload, especially in small-sized patients), and (in dogs) use of injectable agents for anaesthetic induction and halothane for maintenance or use of inhalant anaesthetics alone (compared with use of injectable agents for induction and isoflurane for maintenance). Pulse monitoring and use of pulse oximetry are associated with reduced odds in cats. Greater care with endotracheal intubation and fluid administration are recommended, and pulse and pulse oximetry monitoring should be routinely implemented. Greater patient care in the postoperative period could also reduce fatalities (Brodbelt et al., 2008).

Non-professional dental scaling

The term 'professional dental cleaning' refers to scaling and polishing of teeth with power/hand instrumentation performed by a trained veterinary health care provider under general anaesthesia. This is in contrast to 'non-professional dental scaling', which refers to tooth scraping procedures without polishing and performed on pets without anaesthesia, often done by individuals untrained in veterinary dental techniques. The latter, also known as 'anaesthesia-free dental cleaning' may be cosmetically pleasing to some owners. However, it provides a false sense of accomplishment by making parts of the crowns look good while neglecting the subgingival areas of the teeth where periodontal disease is active. The term 'cleaning' in this context is also misleading to pet owners who have the impression that after one of these procedures their pet's mouth is clean and healthy when in fact scratches are left in the tooth surface, making them more prone to immediate plaque accumulation.

The pet owner will often be told that it is just like a person going to the dentist, which is not the case. Human patients sit in the chair and open their mouths when requested, letting the trained professionals (dental hygienist or dentist) do their work. Because most people cooperate, dental scaling and polishing of human teeth can usually be completed successfully without restraint, sedation or anaesthesia. Nobody could expect an awake pet to patiently sit still during oral examination and treatment procedures that include exploring teeth and probing periodontal tissues with pointed instruments, obtaining dental radiographs with devices held in the mouth, and dental cleaning using sharp instruments.

For the untrained provider to access the mouth and perform scraping of teeth without anaesthesia, a pet must be physically restrained against its will. Anaesthesia-free dental cleaning performed by untrained individuals is inappropriate for several reasons, including incomplete oral examination (teeth further back in the mouth and surfaces of teeth facing the tongue and palate are not examined; dental radiography is not performed; large areas of painful disease are missed), significant safety concerns for the patient and operator (use of sharp instruments can injure the patient and may lead the pet to bite), insufficient cleaning of inaccessible tooth surfaces (a false sense of accomplishment is given when supragingival calculus has been removed but periodontal pockets filled with plaque, calculus and pus are not debrided), oral discomfort and serious pain (making the pet wary about home oral hygiene efforts, administration of medications, and awake oral examinations in the future), and accidental aspiration of debris without protection of the airways (which can result in dyspnoea, pneumonia and death) (Figure 13.30).

The American Veterinary Dental College (in 2004) and European Veterinary Dental College (in 2013) released position statements against the practice of non-professional dental scaling without anaesthesia. With some differences of regulations and laws between countries, only licensed veterinary professionals can practice veterinary medicine. Anyone providing dental services to animals other than a licensed veterinary surgeon, or a supervised and trained technician/nurse or dental hygienist, is practicing veterinary medicine without a license and is subject to criminal charges. Access to the gingival sulcus or periodontal pocket at all aspects of every tooth is impossible in a non-anaesthetized canine or feline patient. Removal of calculus on the visible surfaces of

the teeth has little effect on a pet's oral health, and the outcome is purely cosmetic.

Safe use of an anaesthetic or sedative in a dog or cat requires evaluation of the general health and size of the patient, to determine the appropriate drug and dose, and continual monitoring of the anaesthetized or sedated patient. Veterinary surgeons are trained in all of these procedures. Inhalation anaesthesia using a cuffed endotracheal tube provides three important advantages: cooperation of the patient with a procedure it does not understand; elimination of pain resulting from diagnostic and therapeutic procedures; and treatment of affected oral tissues during the procedure with protection of the upper airway and lungs from accidental aspiration of fluid, blood, debris, calculus, bacteria-rich aerosols, etc. Although anaesthesia will never be 100% risk-free, modern anaesthetic and patient evaluation techniques minimize the risks, and millions of dental cleaning procedures are safely performed each year in veterinary hospitals.

To minimize the need for professional dental scaling procedures and to maintain optimal oral health, daily home oral hygiene is recommended from an early age in dogs and cats. This, combined with periodic examinations of the patient by a veterinary surgeon and with professional dental cleaning under anaesthesia when indicated, will optimize life-long oral health for cats and dogs. When it comes to pet oral health, the risks of missed or untreated dental, periodontal, oral and maxillofacial pathology (including early signs of cancer) far outweigh the risk of anaesthesia. Non-professional dental scaling without anaesthesia appears like a cheap and quick fix. But pet owners should understand that they risk having greater expenses in the long term for problems that have gone unidentified and untreated for a number of years.

A very informative website created by the American Veterinary Dental College (and also translated into Italian) on the risks of anaesthesia-free dental procedures is available online (http://avdc.org/AFD/what-is-an-anesthesia-free-dental-cleaning/). It contains videos, printable oral health fact sheets and much information for both veterinary surgeons and pet owners.

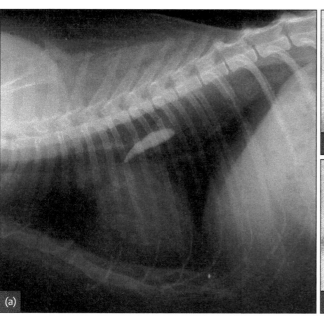

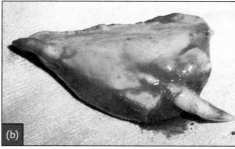

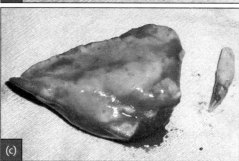

13.30 (a–c) Accidental aspiration of a maxillary canine tooth in a cat, requiring lobectomy for its removal.
(© Dr Alexander M. Reiter)

Home oral hygiene

Starting with clean teeth and healthy gums

Plaque control is a critical component in the maintenance of treatment success. When oral hygiene is less optimal and plaque is allowed to accumulate, it becomes thicker and more complex. Calculus forms when calcium carbonate and other calcium salts in salivary fluid crystallize on the tooth surface, mineralizing the plaque into a hard material. Following professional dental cleaning it takes 2–3 days for plaque to become sufficiently mineralized to form calculus that resists being readily wiped off by mastication or tooth brushing. Calcium salts are more likely to be deposited on plaque in an alkaline environment. Because the mouths of dogs and cats are slightly alkaline, they are more prone to deposition of calculus than humans (Harvey, 2005).

Professional dental cleaning followed by home oral hygiene is the gold standard for prevention of periodontal disease (DuPont, 1998; Gorrel, 2000). A painful mouth will make for a non-compliant pet and may cause the client to give up on tooth brushing and other home oral hygiene measures completely. Thus, it is often best to start with clean teeth and healthy gums (Figure 13.31). Educating the pet owner about home oral hygiene is an important role of the technician/nurse and dental hygienist. Tooth brushing techniques can be demonstrated and recommendations made for products that reduce plaque and calculus build-up, including the use of dental diets, dental chews, treats and toys, oral rinses, gels, toothpastes and drinking water additives (Hale, 2003). Decisions about what products to use can be facilitated by consulting the website of the Veterinary Oral Health Council (www.vohc.org). Performing home oral hygiene may allow for longer intervals between (and fewer surprises during) professional dental cleanings (Aller, 1993; Roudebush et al., 2005; Ray and Eubanks, 2009).

Professional dental cleaning in dogs followed by application of a sealant and weekly reapplication performed by a veterinary surgeon or technician/nurse provided significant improvement in plaque and calculus indices during an 8-week period (Gengler et al., 2005). Application of a barrier dental gel on to cleaned teeth and weekly reapplication by a technician/nurse showed significantly lower plaque scores in treated compared with untreated cats, but no significant differences were seen for calculus, gingivitis, or gingival bleeding (Bellows et al., 2012). In another study, a hydrophilic sealant containing polymers was applied following a professional dental cleaning in dogs to form a barrier film in the subgingival area and promote an aerobic environment in the gingival sulcus. After 30 days, plaque and calculus accumulation were significantly reduced at treated sites, but there was no significant difference for the gingival index score (Sitzman, 2013). Dental wax applied daily on to cleaned teeth on one side of the mouth by the dog owners for 30 days showed no significant difference in gingivitis or plaque accumulation scores when comparing treated and untreated sides. However, calculus accumulation scores were significantly lower for teeth receiving the dental wax (Smith and Smithson, 2014).

Tooth brushing

Tooth brushing has long been known to be imperative in maintaining oral health in pets (Richardson, 1965). Brushing should be initiated at a young age (e.g. at 8–12 weeks before any permanent teeth have erupted) to allow

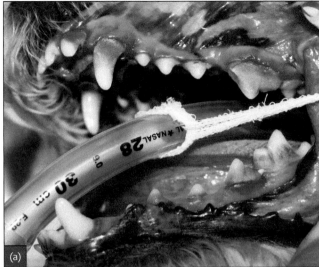

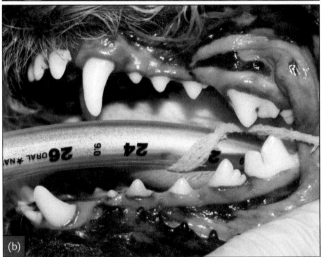

13.31 Showing owners (a) before and (b) after images of professional dental cleaning can be very inspiring and encourage them to start daily tooth brushing as part of a home oral hygiene regimen for their pets.
(© Dr Alexander M. Reiter)

the patient to become accustomed to daily home oral hygiene. The puppy or kitten should have gum massages with a finger to gain experience of having their mouths manipulated. Toothbrushing in cats may be more challenging than in dogs and will sometimes not go as easily as it is described (Ingham et al., 2002b).

One should start slowly and not force the issue, maybe let the pet lick the dentifrice from the finger, then off the toothbrush, gradually place the toothbrush into the pet's mouth, and add the brushing motions (Holmstrom, 2013b). It is not important that perfection is reached but that progress is made. Cooperation by the pet should be rewarded before tooth brushing is attempted again.

A survey of dog owners conducted 6 months following professional dental cleaning demonstrated that, despite the recommendation of daily tooth brushing, only 53% of the clients were still brushing several times a week, and 38% were no longer brushing at all (Miller and Harvey, 1994). This emphasizes the need for pet owners to be educated about home oral hygiene at each office visit.

Small pet-specific toothbrushes are available (Holmstrom, 2013b). Some cats and small dogs prefer finger brushes. Pet toothbrushes often are angled to assist in brushing the caudal teeth (Figure 13.32). It is important that the bristles of the toothbrush are soft. One can also

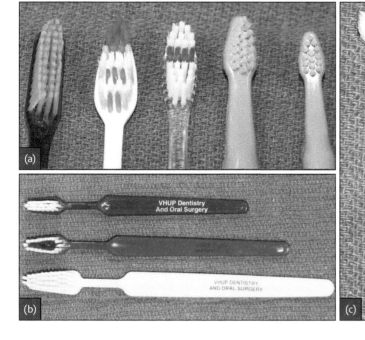

13.32 (a) Assortment of toothbrushes. (b) Brushes may be made with the hospital name on them. (c) Cat toothbrush with angled head and pointed bristles.
(© Dr Alexander M. Reiter)

use medicated wipes, gauze, and cotton-tipped applicators to remove plaque from the tooth surfaces. Single-use wipes are rubbed daily on the outside of the teeth to remove plaque. There are various pet dentifrices. Some of them are more abrasive to work on calculus, and others contain enzymes to reduce plaque (Lewis and Miller, 2010). Common flavours include malt, poultry, vanilla, mint, beef, and seafood. Some cats are very particular about new flavours. Human toothpaste must be avoided because it often contains foaming agents and fluorides that cause stomach upset and pose a health hazard when swallowed.

Many pets are reluctant to keep their mouth open, so it is best to brush while the mouth is closed with access to the teeth made by gently lifting of the lips and reflecting the cheeks (Lewis and Miller, 2010). The non-dominant hand should be placed in a C-shape around the muzzle of the pet so that the mouth is kept closed. The fingers of that same hand are used to raise the upper lip and retract the cheek backwards to make the teeth visible (Figure 13.33). The client should prioritize brushing in areas that collect the most plaque (usually the buccal surfaces of the caudal maxillary cheek teeth) in case the patient becomes uncooperative before the task is completed. It would be ideal if the pet allows mouth opening so that the lingual and palatal surfaces of the teeth also can be brushed (Ingham and Gorrel, 2001).

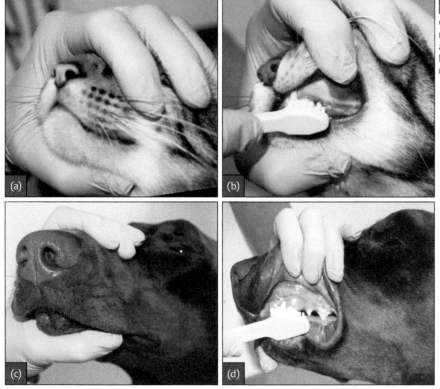

13.33 Toothbrushing in (a, b) a cat and (c, d) a dog. The non-dominant hand is placed in a C-shape around the muzzle of the pet so that the mouth is kept closed. The fingers of that same hand are used to raise the upper lip (and retract the cheek backwards) to make the teeth visible for brushing.
(© Dr Alexander M. Reiter)

The mechanical cleansing provided by daily tooth brushing is the most thorough method of plaque control for pets. The bristles may be rinsed in water only rather than covered with dentifrice because brushing becomes more difficult when the patient tries to eat the tasty paste (Lewis and Miller, 2010). When brushing with water is completed, the dentifrice can be applied to the gingiva and teeth as a treat and to provide enzymatic or antiseptic benefits. Offering a treat will create a positive reinforcement for the pet while creating a good habit. While dentifrice may be effective at a certain level, it is not more than the effect of brushing (Watanabe *et al.*, 2015; Watanabe *et al.*, 2016). Brushing with azithromycin-containing toothpaste was found to be useful in controlling ciclosporin-induced gingival enlargement in dogs (Rosenberg *et al.*, 2013).

The Bass technique directs the bristles at a 45-degree angle toward the gingival margin so that some of the bristles enter the gingival sulcus while other bristles are resting on the tooth adjacent to the gingival margin (Figure 13.34). Pressing lightly (too much pressure can irritate or damage the gingiva), very short back-and-forth strokes are made for 5-10 seconds before repositioning the toothbrush along the next group of teeth (Lewis and Miller, 2010). One should not spend more than a few seconds on each tooth in the mouth, making sure to prioritize brushing in areas that collect the heaviest debris (usually the buccal surfaces of the caudal cheek teeth). The modified Stillman technique is used in areas of periodontal surgery to minimize plaque accumulation while preventing trauma to the reattaching gingival tissue. The bristles are placed apical to the gingival margin with a gentle sweeping motion in the coronal direction against the gingiva and crown of the tooth without placement of bristles into the healing gingival sulcus (Lewis and Miller, 2010).

Numerous studies have indicated that daily tooth brushing is superior in maintaining periodontal health compared with brushing every other day (Corba *et al.*, 1986a; Corba *et al.*, 1986b; Tromp *et al.*, 1986b; Buckley *et al.*, 2011) and that brushing every other day is the minimum brushing frequency in dogs to maintain oral health (Tromp *et al.*, 1986a). One study showed that tooth brushing every other day did not maintain clinically healthy gingiva in dogs, and daily tooth brushing should be recommended to pet owners irrespective of dietary regimen.

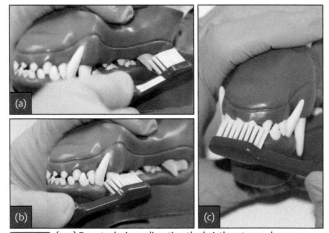

13.34 (a–c) Bass technique directing the bristles at a 45-degree angle toward the gingival margin. The client should prioritize brushing in areas that collect the most plaque (usually the buccal surfaces of the caudal maxillary cheek teeth) in case the patient becomes uncooperative before the task is completed.
(© Dr Alexander M. Reiter)

Providing a dental hygiene chew daily seemed to give an added health benefit when tooth brushing was less frequent (Gorrel and Rawlings, 1996b). A more recent study suggested that for brushing to significantly reduce plaque, calculus and gingivitis scores, it needs to be done daily or at least every other day (Harvey *et al.*, 2015).

Dental diets

The dental calculus scores were significantly higher in domestic cats eating commercially available canned and dry foods compared with feral cats consuming a diet consisting of small mammals, birds, reptiles and insects in Australia. However, there was no statistically significant difference in the prevalence of periodontal disease between these groups of cats (Clarke and Cameron, 1998). Thus, it may be inferred that a raw food diet consisting of meat and bones could play a protective role in the accumulation of calculus, but for reasons of food safety pets should generally not be fed raw meat or unpasteurized dairy products.

It is believed that feeding a soft diet that adheres to the tooth surfaces will contribute to plaque-induced periodontal disease (Watson, 1994). Cats fed on large kibbles with mechanical cleaning qualities had significantly less gingivitis and calculus compared with cats fed small kibbles (Vrieling *et al.*, 2005). Another study also reported that feeding a dry food diet had a positive influence on oral health, decreasing the occurrence of mandibular lymphadenopathy, accumulation of dental deposits, and development of periodontal disease in cats and dogs (Gawor *et al.*, 2006). There was also significantly improved oral health in cat and dogs when feeding a commercial dry diet compared with feeding a home-prepared diet (Buckley *et al.*, 2011).

Many commercial pet food manufacturers have considered the relationship of diets to the oral health of pets. Dental diets utilize the cleansing action of specially engineered dry kibble (mechanical action) and/or additives such as polyphosphates (chemical action) to prevent or retard plaque and calculus formation (Jensen *et al.*, 1995; Stookey *et al.*, 1995; Rawlings *et al.*, 1997; Logan *et al.*, 2002; Logan, 2006; Clarke *et al.*, 2010). Long fibres within a large kibble oriented in one direction help to keep the kibble from crumbling when a dog or cat bites into it. This design allows the kibble to mechanically scrape the sides of the teeth clean as they penetrate the kibble. An example of a chemical used to provide anti-calculus effects is polyphosphate, sequestering the calcium in plaque fluids to prevent mineralization of plaque and thus reduce calculus formation.

Dental chews, treats and toys

Dental chews, treats and toys are an important part of any pet oral health program. The daily addition of dental chews and treats was shown to reduce plaque and calculus accumulation, severity of gingivitis and oral malodour in dogs (Stookey *et al.*, 1995; Gorrel and Rawlings, 1996a; Gorrel and Bierer, 1999; Gorrel *et al.*, 1999; Hennet *et al.*, 2006; Stookey, 2009; Clarke *et al.*, 2011; Quest, 2013). Access to a flexible polymer chew toy was effective in significantly reducing calculus build-up in dogs (Duke, 1989). Providing a dental treat daily also seemed to give an added oral health benefit in dogs (Buckley *et al.*, 2011), in particular when tooth brushing was less frequent (Gorrel and Rawlings, 1996b).

Dental chews, treats and toys should not be too hard, as very hard materials can fracture teeth. Inappropriate dental chews, treats and toys include plastic bones made of hard nylon, cow hooves, antlers, rocks, large ice cubes, and wooden sticks. Meat bones (cooked and uncooked) are also too hard and do not mimic the effect of an animal tearing meat off a carcass. Tennis balls are very abrasive to teeth because they collect tiny particles of dirt and sand and will wear down the crowns and then cause pulp exposure. Acceptable toys include stuffed plush animals, flexible rubber bones, soft plastic balls, and ropes. They should be appropriate for the size of the pet, and caution should be exerted when the pet is left unobserved during play with toys. One can increase the pet's willingness to chew on toys by smearing appropriate and palatable food pastes or sauces on the product.

There was progressively less accumulation of calculus, less gingival inflammation and less alveolar bone loss in dogs that were given access to more types of chewing objects compared with dogs given access to fewer or no chewing objects. When the effects of individual chewing materials were analyzed, access to rawhides overall had the greatest apparent periodontal protective effect, and this effect was more apparent in dogs fed dry food only compared with those fed other than dry food only (Harvey et al., 1996). Rawhide has an excellent tooth cleansing action and is effective in significantly reducing plaque and calculus accumulation in dogs (Lage et al., 1990; Hennet, 2001). However, the size and shape of the product must be correctly matched with the chewing habits of the dog. Rawhide should be taken away following 20–30 minutes of gnawing to decrease the likelihood of gastrointestinal or choking problems from ingestion of a large piece.

The inclusion of chlorhexidine or polyphosphate further improved the efficacy of the product (Stookey et al., 1996). Dogs fed a dental treat once daily had significantly less gingivitis, plaque, and calculus compared with dogs that were fed an identical diet but received no dental treat. The inclusion of an antimicrobial agent such as 0.2% chlorhexidine resulted in significantly less plaque accumulation but did not further improve the efficacy of the product (Rawlings et al., 1998; Brown and McGenity, 2005). Thus, the abrasiveness of the dental treat rather than the antimicrobial activity of chlorhexidine may be the decisive factor in maintaining oral health in dogs.

There is less information available documenting the oral health benefits of dental chews, treats and toys in cats. One study demonstrated that the daily addition of a dental treat to the dry diet resulted in significantly less plaque and calculus accumulation on tooth surfaces. It was concluded that daily feeding of the dental treat helped maintain oral hygiene in cats; however, the authors also stressed that regular professional dental cleaning is still indicated (Gorrel et al., 1998; Ingham et al., 2002a).

Oral rinses, gels, and toothpastes

Oral rinses, gels and toothpastes can be applied to a toothbrush or directly to the teeth and gums as an adjunct preventive measure. Chlorhexidine is the most effective anti-plaque agent (Robinson, 1995). It binds to the oral tissues and tooth surfaces, and is gradually released into the oral cavity. A gel containing 0.12% chlorhexidine gluconate and other ingredients, including 0.15% sodium hexametaphosphate, 0.10% cetylpyridinium chloride, 0.61% zinc gluconate, and a fine abrasive (titanium dioxide), and applied to the teeth and gums in

dogs twice daily for one week resulted in significantly decreased plaque accumulation compared with control dogs (Hennet, 2002).

Dogs treated thrice daily with 0.2% chlorhexidine were found to have significantly less plaque, gingivitis, loss of attachment, and gingival recession than dogs treated similarly with water over a 5-year period (Tepe et al., 1983). The rinse is applied by squirting a small amount inside the cheek on each side of the mouth. The gel is smeared on to the side of the teeth and gums or applied as dentifrice on a toothbrush or finger brush. Chlorhexidine was also found to be effective for plaque control in dogs in the form of a bioadhesive tablet (Gruet et al., 1995).

Chlorhexidine is safe for pets and rarely causes problems, although it may have a bitter taste if palatability enhancers suitable for pets are not included. Except for the formation of a brownish discoloration at the tooth surfaces, no side effects were observed in dogs that had a 0.2 or 0.5% chlorhexidine rinse or gel applied to their mouths daily (Hull and Davies, 1972; Hamp et al., 1973). In one long-term study, however, plaque bacteria from chlorhexidine-treated dogs displayed reduced sensitivity to the drug after 18 months of daily treatment (Hamp and Emilson, 1973).

Some cats object to the taste of chlorhexidine. The clinical and microbiological effects of zinc ascorbate on oral health in cats were evaluated during a 42-day study period. Cats receiving zinc ascorbate gel applied to their teeth and gums showed a significant decrease in plaque, gingivitis, and anaerobic periodontal pathogens compared with control cats. Halitosis and calculus scores were not significantly different between treated and untreated cats (Clarke, 2001).

Plaque, calculus and gingivitis scores were significantly reduced in dogs whose mouths were rinsed every other day for 2 weeks with a solution containing *Lippia sidoides* essential oil compared with control dogs (Girao et al., 2003). Significant reductions in both plaque and gingivitis were observed in small-, medium- and large-breed dogs compared with control dogs when teeth were brushed daily during a 4-week period with an anti-plaque gel, containing purified water, organic pomegranate, organic blueberry, papain (papaya extract), and yucca extract, cinnamon extract, clove extract, chlorophyll, riboflavin (vitamin B2), ascorbic acid (vitamin C), zinc gluconate and glycerin (Milella et al., 2014). In an *in vitro* study, a non-toxic emulsion of free fatty acids (medium chain triglycerides) had significantly improved activity compared with a xylitol-containing formulation and similar activity compared with 0.12% chlorhexidine against canine and feline periodontopathogens (Laverty et al., 2015). Another study evaluated the antimicrobial activity of beta-caryophyllene against plaque bacteria in the dog *in vitro* and *in vivo*. The results showed that beta-caryophyllene was effective against plaque bacteria and resulted in significantly reduced plaque accumulation compared with untreated dogs and dogs treated with 0.12% chlorhexidine (Pieri et al., 2016).

Drinking water additives

Some plaque or calculus-retarding agents can be added to the drinking water. One study evaluated the effect of a drinking water additive in cats. Following a 56-day test period, the addition of xylitol to the drinking water was effective in reducing plaque and calculus accumulation (Clarke, 2006).

Communication

Clients and referring veterinary surgeons

Clients often educate themselves through the internet, searching for information about their pets' problems. Carefully designed websites containing information about diagnosis and treatment of commonly encountered oral diseases in cats and dogs play an important role in client education. Some websites allow clients to submit inquiries with questions about their pets or make appointments for initial consultations. Pertinent information about their pets' medical history and presenting complaint can already be uploaded at that time. It should be understood that both pets and their owners must be 'treated'. Pets are often considered family members, and each pet–owner relationship is unique. One should know how to interpret this relationship in order to use the right approach to the client and provide the appropriate care for the pet in each individual situation. Politeness, kindness, honesty, sincerity, reliability and taking time will be rewarded by clients returning for future appointments.

A complete general history must be obtained prior to performing a general and oral examination (see Chapter 3). The name and contact information of the referring veterinary surgeon should be obtained. Clients should provide a contact phone number under which they can be reached at any time. The client is asked to sign a general informed consent form that outlines a diagnostic and treatment plan, provides a range of estimated costs, and permits sedation/anaesthesia to move forward with the procedures suggested. Upon admission of a pet, the referring veterinary surgeon should be notified and kept updated; copies of medical records may need to be sent from the referring veterinary surgeon to have all information available. Pet owners should be informed about pre-anaesthetic test results, whether any other diagnostic tests will need to be performed, and when their pets will undergo anaesthesia. A communication log should always be completed after speaking with the client or referring veterinary surgeon's office, also detailing updates about cost estimates given so that other staff are aware about all circumstances relating the client and pet.

Many patients are sent home on the day of treatment once they have recovered from anaesthesia. If a patient remains hospitalized, clients appreciate being kept informed about their pets' continued care. Discharge instructions should contain sufficiently detailed information for patients that underwent diagnostic and treatment procedures and a brief summary for patients presented for check-ups. A large amount of information can be gleaned from past discharges of pets that have had similar procedures, which lends to the creation of templates that can be used for commonly encountered situations and then are individualized as needed. Copies of discharge instructions sent to referring veterinary surgeons may be accompanied by more personal letters. Maintaining good communication with referring veterinary surgeons is paramount. Cards can be sent to remind clients about annual check-ups, and newsletters about home oral hygiene and other topics may be emailed to maintain strong client relationships.

Dental laboratory technicians

Communication with a dental laboratory is needed for the fabrication of prosthodontic crowns (partial and full metal crowns), orthodontic appliances (indirect inclined planes and expansion screw devices), and prosthetic appliances (palatal obturators). Prosthodontic crowns are primarily utilized to restore and protect fractured or weakened teeth of dogs that put their dentition at risk of trauma (Fink and Reiter, 2015). Orthodontic appliances are needed to move maloccluding teeth into a position that provides a pain-free and functional occlusion. Prosthetic appliances are used to overcome functional or cosmetic deficiencies. It is important to provide the dental laboratory with as much information as needed about pertinent patient history and management, the area of the mouth to be treated, and the appliance that should be fabricated.

For prosthodontic crowns, this should include the tooth to be treated, whether it should receive a partial or full crown, endodontic and periodontal surgery previously performed on that tooth, and the type and location of the margin made (e.g. chamfer and supragingival). Instructions should be given about the preferred material for the prosthodontic crown and the thickness of the material at the prepared crown's tip and sides (Figure 13.35). The inside of the prosthodontic crown should be sandblasted, its outside surface polished, and the tip rounded. For orthodontic and prosthetic appliances, there will likely be additional information (e.g. whether it should be permanent or removable). Full-mouth impressions (or stone models), bite registrations, including detailed impressions of prepared teeth (Figure 13.36), photographs of the tooth/teeth/area of the mouth to be treated, and drawings of what is expected from the dental laboratory should be submitted (Fink and Reiter, 2015).

Pathologists

Close collaboration between clinicians and pathologists is desirable and beneficial to the patients. Detailed information about signalment, medical history and clinical signs of the patient, including history, clinical (location, size, colour, consistency, etc.) and radiographic or tomographic features (presence or lack of bone involvement) of the lesion of interest, tentative clinical diagnosis, thorough description of the bioptic specimen (e.g. description about the depth of sampling), and possibly even clinical images should be

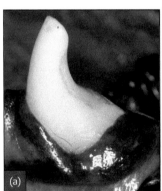
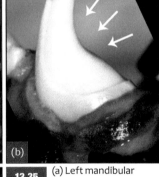

13.35 (a) Left mandibular canine tooth of a dog with severe abrasion on its distal crown surface. The tooth was prepared for receiving a partial ('three-quarter') crown. (b) The dental laboratory technician was instructed to not follow the contour of the prepared crown but to make the prosthodontic crown thicker in the area of severe abrasion (arrowed). (c) The cemented prosthodontic crown was fabricated as instructed.
(© Dr Alexander M. Reiter)

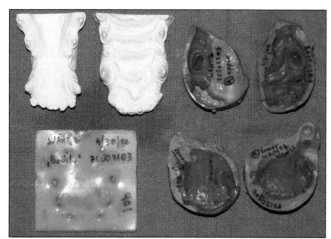

13.36 Items to be sent to the dental laboratory for prosthodontic crown fabrication: stone models (left top), bite registration (left bottom), and impressions of prepared canine teeth.
(© Dr Alexander M. Reiter)

shared with pathologists so that interpretation of cyto- and histopathological findings can be improved (Sapierzynski *et al.*, 2017). If the results do not fit the clinical picture, the clinician should contact the pathologist and discuss the case. Further important details may arise that could help in reaching a definitive diagnosis. It is also important that clinicians and pathologists agree on the utilized nomenclature and classification of pathology such as benign and malignant neoplasia.

Miscellaneous

American Veterinary Dental College and European Veterinary Dental College

A Diplomate has earned a veterinary degree from an accredited veterinary college/school, which was followed by a structured internship or its equivalent of varied clinical practice, completion of a specific training programme in dentistry and oral surgery, and passing the entry examination of the American Veterinary Dental College (AVDC; www.avdc.org) or European Veterinary Dental College (EVDC; www.evdc.org), the clinical specialist organizations accredited by the American Board of Veterinary Specialties (ABVS) and European Board of Veterinary Specialties (EBVS), respectively. Diplomates meet the highest standards for certification of knowledge and skills in veterinary dentistry and oral surgery.

Foundation for Veterinary Dentistry and European Veterinary Dental Society

The Foundation for Veterinary Dentistry (FVD; www.veterinarydentistry.org) emerged from the American Veterinary Dental Society (AVDS), which was founded in 1976 for the purpose of creating a forum for advancing the knowledge, education, and awareness of veterinary dentistry among veterinary surgeons, students, and the public. Membership in the FVD is open to any veterinary surgeon, dentist, hygienist, technician/nurse, or individual with an interest in veterinary dentistry. The FVD organizes together with the AVDC the annual Veterinary Dental Forum (VDF; www.veterinarydentalforum.org), which is the largest continuing education conference in veterinary dentistry in North America.

The European Veterinary Dental Society (EVDS; www.evds.org) is a non-profit educational organization that was founded in 1992. The aims of the society are to educate and train European veterinary surgeons in animal dentistry and promote clinical dental research, which will benefit animals and people. The EVDS is a UK registered charity (registration number 1128783) and is run by unpaid members elected by its membership. The EVDS organizes together with the EVDC the annual European Veterinary Dental Forum (EVDF; www.evdf.org), which is the largest continuing education conference in veterinary dentistry in Europe.

Journal of Veterinary Dentistry

As the journal of record in its field, the *Journal of Veterinary Dentistry* (JOVD; http://journals.sagepub.com/home/jov) is written for veterinary dental scientists, veterinary surgeons, dentists, and veterinary/dental technicians/nurses who are engaged in veterinary dental practice. The JOVD provides a continuing education forum that can serve as a reference source in the veterinary office. It publishes articles that provide practical and scientifically sound information covering not only the medical and surgical aspects of veterinary dentistry but also specific categories including anatomy, restorations, crowns, endodontics, orthodontics, periodontics, laboratory animal dentistry, and dental and oral biology as they relate to clinical practice. FVD or EVDS membership includes a subscription to the JOVD.

Frontiers in Veterinary Science

Frontiers in Veterinary Science is a global, peer-reviewed, indexed, open access journal that bridges animal and human health, brings a comparative approach to medical and surgical challenges, and advances innovative biotechnology and therapy. It includes numerous specialty sections. Its section *Veterinary Dentistry and Oromaxillofacial Surgery* (www.frontiersin.org/journals/veterinary-science/sections/veterinary-dentistry-and-oromaxillofacial-surgery) is devoted to the publication of high-quality research that contributes to the body of knowledge and/or the evidence-based practice in veterinary dentistry (oral anatomy, developmental and acquired conditions, oral medicine, oral pathology, periodontology, endodontics, prosthodontics, orthodontics, and other tooth-related and oral cavity diseases) and oromaxillofacial surgery (tooth extraction, tumour surgery, palatal defect repair, maxillofacial fracture management, and temporomandibular joint and salivary gland pathology).

Veterinary Oral Health Council

The Veterinary Oral Health Council (VOHC; www.vohc.org) is an entity of the American Veterinary Dental College (AVDC; www.avdc.org) and awards a seal of acceptance to products that successfully meet pre-set criteria for efficacy or effectiveness in mechanically and/or chemically controlling plaque and/or calculus deposition in dogs and cats. It is not a regulatory agency, and submission of results of clinical trials to the VOHC on behalf of a product is voluntary. Furthermore, it does not determine safety of a product but requires assurance by the company that a product is safe and meets all applicable regulatory requirements. The VOHC was founded in 1997, and the first seal of acceptance was awarded in 1998. Use of the VOHC outside the USA began in Canada, followed by Europe and Japan. It is now recognized worldwide.

References and further reading

Alessio TL and Krieger EM (2015) Transient unilateral vision loss in a dog following inadvertent intravitreal injection of bupivacaine during a dental procedure. *Journal of the American Veterinary Medical Association* **246**, 990–993

Aller S (1993) Dental home care and preventive strategies. *Seminars in Veterinary Medicine and Surgery Small Animals* **8**, 204–212

Aller MS (2005) Personal safety and ergonomics in the dental operatory. *Journal of Veterinary Dentistry* **22**, 124–130

American Dental Association (2004) Combating antibiotic resistance. *Journal of the American Dental Association* **135**, 484–487

American Association of Endodontists (2012) *Use and abuse of antibiotics.* Available at: https://www.aae.org/specialty/wp-content/uploads/sites/2/2017/07/ecfewinter12final.pdf

American Veterinary Dental College (2005) *Policy statement: The use of antibiotics in veterinary dentistry*; https://www.avdc.org/Antibiotic_Use_April_2005.pdf

Angel M (2014) Sharpening periodontal instruments. *Journal of Veterinary Dentistry* **31**, 58–64

Barton-Lamb AL, Martin-Flores M, Scrivani PV *et al.* (2013) Evaluation of maxillary arterial blood flow in anesthetized cats with the mouth closed and open. *Veterinary Journal* **196**, 325–331

Bellows J, Carithers DS and Gross SJ (2012) Efficacy of a barrier gel for reducing the development of plaque, calculus, and gingivitis in cats. *Journal of Veterinary Dentistry* **29**, 89–94

Bexfield N and Watson P (2010) How to place an oesophagostomy tube. *Journal of Small Animal Practice* **51**, 12–16

Bille C, Auvigne V, Libermann S *et al.* (2012) Risk of anaesthetic mortality in dogs and cats: an observational cohort study of 3546 cases. *Veterinary Anaesthesia and Analgesia* **39**, 59–68

Black AP, Crichlow AM and Saunders JR (1980) Bacteremia during ultrasonic teeth cleaning and extraction in the dog. *Journal of the American Animal Hospital Association* **16**, 611–616

Booij-Vrieling HE, van der Reijden WA, Houwers DJ *et al.* (2010) Comparison of periodontal pathogens between cats and their owners. *Veterinary Microbiology* **144**, 147–152

Bowersock TL, Wu CC, Inskeep GA and Chester ST (2000) Prevention of bacteremia in dogs undergoing dental scaling by prior administration of oral clindamycin or chlorhexidine oral rinse. *Journal of Veterinary Dentistry* **17**, 11–16

Brodbelt D (2009) Perioperative mortality in small animal anaesthesia. *Veterinary Journal* **182**, 152–161

Brodbelt DC, Pfeiffer DU, Young LE and Wood JL (2008) Results of the confidential enquiry into perioperative small animal fatalities regarding risk factors for anesthetic-related death in dogs. *Journal of the American Veterinary Medical Association* **233**, 1096–1104

Brown WY and McGenity P (2005) Effective periodontal disease control using dental hygiene chews. *Journal of Veterinary Dentistry* **22**, 16–19

Buckley C, Colyer A, Skrzywanek M *et al.* (2011) The impact of home-prepared diets and home oral hygiene on oral health in cats and dogs. *British Journal of Nutrition* **106**, S124–S127

Christakis DA, Wright JA, Taylor JA and Zimmerman FJ (2005) Association between parental satisfaction and antibiotic prescription for children with cough and cold symptoms. *Pediatric Infectious Disease Journal* **24**, 774–777

Clarke DE (2001) Clinical and microbiological effects of oral zinc ascorbate gel in cats. *Journal of Veterinary Dentistry* **18**, 177–183

Clarke DE (2006) Drinking water additive decreases plaque and calculus accumulation in cats. *Journal of Veterinary Dentistry* **23**, 79–82

Clarke DE and Cameron A (1998) Relationship between diet, dental calculus and periodontal disease in domestic and feral cats in Australia. *Australian Veterinary Journal* **76**, 690–693

Clarke DE, Kelman M and Perkins N (2011) Effectiveness of a vegetable dental chew on periodontal disease parameters in toy breed dogs. *Journal of Veterinary Dentistry* **28**, 230–235

Clarke DE, Servet E, Hendriks W *et al.* (2010) Effect of kibble size, shape, and additives on plaque in cats. *Journal of Veterinary Dentistry* **27**, 84–89

Corba NH, Jansen J and Fidler V (1986a) Artificial periodontal defects and frequency of tooth brushing in Beagle dogs (I). Clinical findings after creation of the defects. *Journal of Clinical Periodontology* **13**, 158–163

Corba NH, Jansen J and Pilot T (1986b) Artificial periodontal defects and frequency of tooth brushing in Beagle dogs (II). Clinical findings after a period of healing. *Journal of Clinical Periodontology* **13**, 186–189

Davies JA, Fransson BA, Davies AM *et al.* (2015) Incidence of and risk factors for postoperative regurgitation and vomiting in dogs: 244 cases (2000–2012). *Journal of the American Veterinary Medical Association* **246**, 327–335

Deeprose J (2007) Operator safety and health considerations. In: *BSAVA Manual of Canine and Feline Dentistry, 3rd edn*, ed. C Tutt, J Deeprose and D Crossley, pp. 56–66. BSAVA Publications, Gloucester

DeForge DH (2002) Physical ergonomics in veterinary dentistry. *Journal of Veterinary Dentistry* **19**, 196–200

Devitt CM and Seim HB (1997) Clinical evaluation of tube esophagostomy in small animals. *Journal of the American Animal Hospital Association* **33**, 55–60

Doering CJ, Lukasik VM and Merideth RE (2016) Effects of intramuscular injection of glycopyrrolate on Schirmer tear test I results in dogs. *Journal of the American Veterinary Medical Association* **248**, 1262–1266

Duke A (1989) How a chewing device affects calculus build-up in dogs. *Veterinary Medicine* **84**, 1110–1114

Duke FD, Snyder CJ, Bentley E and Dubielzig RR (2014) Ocular trauma originating from within the oral cavity: Clinical relevance and histologic findings in 10 cases (2003–2013). *Journal of Veterinary Dentistry* **31**, 245–248

DuPont GA (1998) Prevention of periodontal disease. *Veterinary Clinics of North America Small Animal Practice* **28**, 1129–1145

Fink L, Jennings M and Reiter AM (2014) Esophagostomy feeding tube placement in the dog and cat. *Journal of Veterinary Dentistry* **31**, 133–138

Fink L and Reiter AM (2015) Assessment of 68 prosthodontic crowns in 41 pet and working dogs (2000–2012). *Journal of Veterinary Dentistry* **32**, 148–154

Gawor JP, Reiter AM, Jodkowska K *et al.* (2006) Influence of diet on oral health in cats and dogs. *Journal of Nutrition* **136**, 2021S–2023S

Gaynor JS, Dunlop CI, Wagner AE *et al.* (1999) Complications and mortality associated with anesthesia in dogs and cats. *Journal of the American Veterinary Medical Association* **35**, 13–17

Geerts SO, Nys M, De MP *et al.* (2002) Systemic release of endotoxins induced by gentle mastication: association with periodontitis severity. *Journal of Periodontology* **73**, 73–78

Gengler WR, Kunkle BN, Romano D and Larsen D (2005) Evaluation of a barrier dental sealant in dogs. *Journal of Veterinary Dentistry* **22**, 157–159

Girao VC, Nunes-Pinheiro DC, Morais SM, Segueira JL and Gioso MA (2003) A clinical trial of the effect of a mouth-rinse prepared with *Lippia sidoides* Cham essential oil in dogs with mild gingival disease. *Preventive Veterinary Medicine* **30**, 95–102

Glass RT, Martin ME and Peters LJ (1989) Transmission of disease in dogs by toothbrushing. *Quintessence International* **20**, 819–824

Glenny AM, Oliver R, Roberts GJ and Worthington HV (2013) Antibiotics for the prophylaxis of bacterial endocarditis in dentistry. *Cochrane Database of Systemic Reviews* 10:CD003813. doi: 10.1002/14651858.CD003813.pub4

Goodman AE and Goodman AR (2016) Common carotid artery ligation to minimize blood loss during oral and maxillofacial surgery. *Journal of Veterinary Dentistry* **33**, 195–200

Gorrel C (2000) Home care: products and techniques. *Clinical Techniques in Small Animal Practice* **15**, 226–231

Gorrel C and Bierer TL (1999) Long-term effects of a dental hygiene chew on the periodontal health of dogs. *Journal of Veterinary Dentistry* **16**, 109–113

Gorrel C, Inskeep G and Inskeep T (1998) Benefits of a 'dental hygiene chew' on the periodontal health of cats. *Journal of Veterinary Dentistry* **15**, 135–138

Gorrel C and Rawlings JM (1996a) The role of a 'dental hygiene chew' in maintaining periodontal health in dogs. *Journal of Veterinary Dentistry* **13**, 31–34

Gorrel C and Rawlings JM (1996b) The role of tooth-brushing and diet in the maintenance of periodontal health in dogs. *Journal of Veterinary Dentistry* **13**, 139–143

Gorrel C, Warrick J and Bierer TL (1999) Effect of a new dental hygiene chew on periodontal health in dogs. *Journal of Veterinary Dentistry* **16**, 77–81

Gruet P, Gaillard C, Boisramé B *et al.* (1995) Use of an oral antiseptic bioadhesive tablet in dogs. *Journal of Veterinary Dentistry* **12**, 87–91

Guerreiro CE, Appelboam H and Lowe RC (2014) Successful medical treatment for globe penetration following tooth extraction in a dog. *Veterinary Ophthalmology* **17**, 146–149

Gunew M, Marshall R, Lui M and Astley C (2008) Fatal venous air embolism in a cat undergoing dental extractions. *Journal of Small Animal Practice* **49**, 601–604

Gupta A, Bhat M, Mohammed T, Bansal N and Gupta G (2014) Ergonomics in dentistry. *International Journal of Clinical Pediatric Dentistry* **7**, 30–34

Hale FA (2003) The owner-animal-environment triad in the treatment of canine periodontal disease. *Journal of Veterinary Dentistry* **20**, 118–122

Hale FA and Anthony JMG (1997) Prevention of hypothermia in cats during routine oral hygiene procedures. *Canadian Veterinary Journal* **38**, 297–299

Hamp SE and Emilson CG (1973) Some effects of chlorhexidine on the plaque flora of the Beagle dog. *Journal of Periodontal Research* **12**, 28–35

Hamp SE, Lindhe J and Löe H (1973) Long-term effects of chlorhexidine on developing gingivitis in the Beagle dog. *Journal of Periodontal Research* **8**, 63–70

Hardie EM, Spodnick GJ, Gilson SD *et al.* (1999) Tracheal rupture in cats: 16 cases (1983-1998). *Journal of the American Veterinary Medical Association* **214**, 508–512

Harari L, Besser TE, Gustafson SB and Meinkoth K (1993) Bacterial isolates from blood cultures of dogs undergoing dentistry. *Veterinary Surgery* **22**, 27–30

Hardy JM, Owen TJ, Martinez SA, Jones LP and Davis MA (2017) The effect of nail characteristics on surface bacterial counts of surgical personnel before and after scrubbing. *Veterinary Surgery* **46**, 952–961

Hartman EA, McCarthy RJ and Labato MA (2017) Global cerebral ischemia with subsequent respiratory arrest in a cat after repeated use of a spring-loaded mouth gag. *Journal of Feline Medicine and Surgery Open Reports* **3**:2055116917739126. doi: 10.1177/2055116917739126

Hartzell JD, Torres D, Kim P and Wortmann G (2005) Incidence of bacteremia after routine tooth brushing. *American Journal of Medical Sciences* **329**, 178–180

Harvey C, Serfilippi L and Barnvos D (2015) Effect of frequency of brushing teeth on plaque and calculus accumulation, and gingivitis in dogs. *Journal of Veterinary Dentistry* **32**, 16–21

Harvey CE (2005) Management of periodontal disease: understanding the options. *Veterinary Clinics of North America Small Animal Practice* **31**, 819–836

Harvey CE, Shofer FS and Laster L (1996) Correlation of diet, other chewing activities and periodontal disease in North American client-owned dogs. *Journal of Veterinary Dentistry* **13**, 101–105

Harvey CE, Thornsberry C, Miller BR and Shofer FS (1995a) Antimicrobial susceptibility of subgingival bacterial flora in dogs with gingivitis. *Journal of Veterinary Dentistry* **12**, 151–155

Harvey CE, Thornsberry C, Miller BR and Shofer FS (1995b) Antimicrobial susceptibility of subgingival bacterial flora in cats with gingivitis. *Journal of Veterinary Dentistry* **12**, 157–160

Hay Kraus BL (2014) Effect of dosing interval on efficacy of maropitant for prevention of hydromorphone induced vomiting and signs of nausea in dogs. *Journal of the American Veterinary Medical Association* **245**, 1015–1020

Hayes MJ, Taylor JA and Smith DR (2012) Predictors of work-related musculoskeletal disorders among dental hygienists. *International Journal of Dental Hygiene* **10**, 265–269

Hennet P (2001) Effectiveness of an enzymatic rawhide dental chew to reduce plaque in beagle dogs. *Journal of Veterinary Dentistry* **18**, 61–64

Hennet P (2002) Effectiveness of a dental gel to reduce plaque in Beagle dogs. *Journal of Veterinary Dentistry* **19**, 11–14

Hennet P, Servet E and Venet C (2006) Effectiveness of an oral hygiene chew to reduce dental deposits in small breed dogs. *Journal of Veterinary Dentistry* **23**, 6–12

Hirasawa M, Hayashi K and Takada K (2000) Measurement of peptidase activity and evaluation of effectiveness of administration of minocycline for treatment of dogs with periodontitis. *American Journal of Veterinary Research* **61**, 1349–1352

Holmstrom SE (2013a) Dental instruments and equipment. In: *Veterinary Dentistry – A Team Approach, 2nd edn*, ed. SE Holmstrom, pp. 78–116. Elsevier, St Louis

Holmstrom SE (2013b) Home-care instructions and products. In: *Veterinary Dentistry – A Team Approach, 2nd edn*, ed. SE Holmstrom, pp. 194–215. Elsevier, St Louis

Holmstrom LA and Holmstrom SE (2013) Personal safety and ergonomics. In: *Veterinary Dentistry – A Team Approach, 2nd edn*, ed. SE Holmstrom, pp. 117–134. Elsevier, St Louis

Howard PE (1981) Tape muzzle for mandibular fractures. *Veterinary Medicine for the Small Animal Clinician* **76**, 517–519

Hull PS and Davies RM (1972) The effect of a chlorhexidine gel on tooth deposits in Beagle dogs. *Journal of Small Animal Practice* **13**, 207–212

Ingham KE and Gorrel C (2001) Effect of long-term intermittent periodontal care on canine periodontal disease. *Journal of Small Animal Practice* **42**, 67–70

Ingham KE, Gorrel C and Bierer TL (2002a) Effect of a dental chew on dental substrates and gingivitis in cats. *Journal of Veterinary Dentistry* **19**, 201–204

Ingham KE, Gorrel C, Blackburn JM and Farnsworth W (2002b) The effect of tooth brushing on periodontal disease in cats. *Journal of Nutrition* **132**, 1740S–1741S

Jennings MW, Lewis JR, Soltero-Rivera MM, Brown DC and Reiter AM (2015) Effect of tooth extraction on stomatitis in cats: 95 cases (2000–2013). *Journal of the American Veterinary Medical Association* **246**, 654–660

Jensen L, Logan EL, Finney O *et al.* (1995) Reduction in accumulation of plaque, stain and calculus in dogs by dietary means. *Journal of Veterinary Dentistry* **12**, 161–163

Johnston TP, Mondal P, Pal D *et al.* (2011) Canine periodontal disease control using a clindamycin hydrochloride gel. *Journal of Veterinary Dentistry* **28**, 224–229

Jurk IR, Thibodeau MS, Whitney K, Gilger BC and Davidson MD (2001) Acute vision loss after general anesthesia in a cat. *Veterinary Ophthalmology* **4**, 155–158

Kahn SA (2007) Placement of canine and feline esophagostomy feeding tubes. *Laboratory Animals* **36**, 25–26

Katre C, Triantafyllou A, Shaw RJ and Brown JS (2010) Inferior alveolar nerve damage caused by bone wax in third molar surgery. *International Journal of Oral and Maxillofacial Surgery* **39**, 511–513

Katz SE and Rootman J (1996) Adverse effects of bone wax in surgery of the orbit. *Ophthalmic Plastic and Reconstructive Surgery* **12**, 121–126

Khazandi M, Bird PS, Owens J *et al.* (2014) *In vitro* efficacy of cefovecin against anaerobic bacteria isolated from subgingival plaque of dogs and cats with periodontal disease. *Anaerobe* **28**, 104–108

Kim SE, Hwang SY, Jeong M *et al.* (2016) Clinical and microbiological effects of a subantimicrobial dose of oral doxycycline on periodontitis in dogs. *Veterinary Journal* **208**, 55–59

Kim SE, Kim S, Jeong M *et al.* (2013) Experimental determination of a subantimicrobial dosage of doxycycline hyclate for treatment of periodontitis in Beagles. *American Journal of Veterinary Research* **74**, 130–135

Kouki MI, Papadimitriou SA, Kazakos GM, Savas I and Bitchava D (2013) Periodontal disease as a potential factor for systemic inflammatory response in the dog. *Journal of Veterinary Dentistry* **30**, 26–29

Lage A, Lausen N, Tracy R and Allred E (1990) Effect of chewing rawhide and cereal biscuit on removal of dental calculus in dogs. *Journal of the American Veterinary Medical Association* **197**, 213–219

Lara-García A, Couto CG, Iazbik MC and Brooks MB (2008) Postoperative bleeding in retired racing Greyhounds. *Journal of Veterinary Internal Medicine* **22**, 525–533

Laverty G, Gilmore BF, Jones DS *et al.* (2015) Antimicrobial efficacy of an innovative emulsion of medium chain triglycerides against canine and feline periodontopathogens. *Journal of Small Animal Practice* **56**, 253–263

Levine PB, Smallwood LJ and Buback JL (1997) Esophagostomy tubes as a method of nutritional management in cats: a retrospective study. *Journal of the American Animal Hospital Association* **33**, 405–410

Lewis JR and Miller BR (2010) Dentistry and oral surgery. In: *McCurnin's Clinical Textbook for Veterinary Technicians, 7th edn*, ed. JM Bassert and DM McCurnin, pp. 1093–1148. Saunders, St Louis

Limeres Posse J, Álvarez Fernández M, Fernández Feijoo J *et al.* (2016) Intravenous amoxicillin/clavulanate for the prevention of bacteraemia following dental procedures: a randomized clinical trial. *Journal of Antimicrobial Chemotherapy* **71**, 2022–2030

Lodi G, Figini L, Sardella A *et al.* (2012) Antibiotics to prevent complications following tooth extractions. *Cochrane Database of Systematic Reviews* 11:CD003811. doi: 10.1002/14651858.CD003811.pub2

Logan EI (2006) Dietary influences on periodontal health in dogs and cats. *Veterinary Clinical of North America Small Animal Practice* **36**, 1385–1401

Logan EI, Finney O and Hefferren JJ (2002) Effects of a dental food on plaque accumulation and gingival health in dogs. *Journal of Veterinary Dentistry* **19**, 15–18

Loughran CM, Raisis AL, Haitjema G and Chester Z (2016) Unilateral retrobulbar hematoma following maxillary nerve block in a dog. *Journal of Veterinary Emergency and Critical Care* **26**, 815–818

Mangione-Smith R, McGlynn EA, Elliott MN *et al.* (2001) Parent expectations for antibiotics, physician-parent communication, and satisfaction. *Archives of Pediatrics and Adolescent Medicine* **155**, 800–806

Marin LM, Iazbik MC, Zaldivar-Lopez S *et al.* (2012) Epsilon aminocaproic acid for the prevention of delayed postoperative bleeding in retired racing Greyhounds undergoing gonadectomy. *Veterinary Surgery* **41**, 594–603

Martin-Flores M, Scrivani PV, Loew E *et al.* (2014) Maximal and submaximal mouth opening with mouth gags in cats: Implications for maxillary artery blood flow. *Veterinary Journal* **200**, 60–64

Milella L, Beckman B and Kane JS (2014) Evaluation of an anti-plaque gel for daily toothbrushing. *Journal of Veterinary Dentistry* **31**, 160–167

Miller BR and Harvey CE (1994) Compliance with oral hygiene recommendations following periodontal treatment in client-owned dogs. *Journal of Veterinary Dentistry* **11**, 18–19

Mitchell SL, McCarthy R, Rudloff E *et al.* (2000) Tracheal rupture associated with intubation in cats: 20 cases (1996–1998). *Journal of the American Veterinary Medical Association* **216**, 1592–1595

Nanai B, Phillips L, Christiansen J and Shelton GD (2009) Life threatening complication associated with anesthesia in a dog with masticatory muscle myositis. *Veterinary Surgery* **38**, 645–649

Nemes D, Amaricai E, Tanase D *et al.* (2013) Physical therapy *versus* medical treatment of musculoskeletal disorders in dentistry: a randomized prospective study. *Annals of Agricultural and Environmental Medicine* **20**, 301–306

Nielsen D, Walser C, Kodan G *et al.* (2000) Effects of treatment with clindamycin hydrochloride on progression of canine periodontal disease after ultrasonic scaling. *Veterinary Therapy* **1**, 150–158

Nieves MA, Hartwig P, Kinyon JM and Riedesel DH (1997) Bacterial isolates from plaque and from blood during and after routine dental procedures in dogs. *Veterinary Surgery* **26**, 26–32

Norris JM and Love DN (2000) *In vitro* antimicrobial susceptibilities of three *Porphyromonas* spp., and *in vivo* responses in the oral cavity of cats to selected antimicrobial agents. *Australian Veterinary Journal* **78**, 533–537

Park Y-W, Son W-G, Jeong M-B *et al.* (2013) Evaluation of risk factors for development of corneal ulcer after nonocular surgery in dogs: 14 cases (2009–2011). *Journal of the American Veterinary Medical Association* **242**, 1544–1548

Peralta S, Arzi B, Nemec A, Lommer MJ and Verstraete FJM (2015) Non-radiation-related osteonecrosis of the jaws in dogs: 14 cases (1996–2014). *Frontiers in Veterinary Science* **2**, 1–7

Perea SC (2008) Critical care nutrition for feline patients. *Topics in Companion Animal Medicine* **23**, 207–215

Perry R, Moore D and Scurrell E (2015) Globe penetration in a cat following maxillary nerve block for dental surgery. *Journal of Feline Medicine and Surgery* **17**, 66–72

Pieri FA, Souza MC, Vermelho LL *et al.* (2016) Use of β-caryophyllene to combat bacterial dental plaque formation in dogs. *BMC Veterinary Research* **12**, 216; https://doi.org/10.1186/s12917-016-0842-1

Polson AM, Southard GL, Dunn RL *et al.* (1996) Periodontal pocket treatment in beagle dogs using subgingival doxycycline from a biodegradable system. I. Initial clinical responses. *Journal of Periodontology* **67**, 1176–1184

Posner LP, Pavuk AA, Rokshar JL, Carter JE and Levine JF (2010) Effects of opioids and anesthetic drugs on body temperature in cats. *Veterinary Anesthesia and Analgesia* **37**, 35–43

Quest BW (2013) Oral health benefits of a daily dental chew in dogs. *Journal of Veterinary Dentistry* **30**, 84–87

Radice M, Martino PA and Reiter AM (2006) Evaluation of subgingival bacteria in the dog and their susceptibility to commonly used antibiotics. *Journal of Veterinary Dentistry* **23**, 219–224

Ramasamy A (2014) A review of use of antibiotics in dentistry and recommendations for rational antibiotic usage by dentists. *International Arabic Journal of Antimicrobial Agents* **4**, 1–15

Rawlings JM, Gorrel C and Markwell PJ (1997) Effect of two dietary regimens on gingivitis in the dog. *Journal of Small Animal Practice* **38**, 147–151

Rawlings JM, Gorrel C and Markwell PJ (1998) Effect on canine oral health of adding chlorhexidine to a dental hygiene chew. *Journal of Veterinary Dentistry* **15**, 129–134

Ray JD and Eubanks DL (2009) Dental homecare: teaching your clients to care for their pet's teeth. *Journal of Veterinary Dentistry* **26**, 57–60

Redondo JI, Suesta P, Gil L *et al.* (2012a) Retrospective study of the prevalence of postanaesthetic hypothermia in cats. *Veterinary Record* **170**, 206

Redondo JI, Suesta P, Serra I *et al.* (2012b). Retrospective study of the prevalence of postanaesthetic hypothermia in dogs. *Veterinary Record* **171**, 374

Reiter AM (2013) Oral surgical equipment for small animals. *Veterinary Clinics of North America Small Animal Practice* **43**, 587–608

Reiter AM (2014) Open wide: Blindness in cats after the use of mouth gags. *Veterinary Journal* **201**, 5–6

Reiter AM, Brady CA and Harvey CE (2004) Local and systemic complications in a cat after poorly performed dental extractions. *Journal of Veterinary Dentistry* **21**, 215–221

Reiter AM and Lewis JR (2011) Trauma-associated musculoskeletal injuries of the head. In: *Manual of Trauma Management in the Dog and Cat*, ed. K Drobatz, MW Beal and RS Syring, pp. 255–278. Wiley-Blackwell, Ames

Reiter AM and Soltero-Rivera MM (2017) Oral and salivary gland disorders. In: *Textbook of Veterinary Internal Medicine, 8th edn*, ed. SJ Ettinger, EC Feldman and E Cote, pp. 1469–1476. Saunders, Philadelphia

Richardson RL (1965) Effect of administering antibiotics, removing the major salivary glands, and toothbrushing on dental calculi formation in the cat. *Archives of Oral Biology* **10**, 245–253

Robinson JG (1995) Chlorhexidine gluconate – the solution for dental problems. *Journal of Veterinary Dentistry* **12**, 290–31

Robinson J (2007) Dental instrumentation and equipment. In: *BSAVA Manual of Canine and Feline Dentistry, 3rd edn*, ed. C Tutt, J Deeprose and D Crossley, pp. 67–76. BSAVA Publications, Gloucester

Rosenberg A, Rosenkrantz W, Griffin C, Angus J and Keys D (2013) Evaluation of azithromycin in systemic and toothpaste forms for the treatment of ciclosporin-associated gingival overgrowth in dogs. *Veterinary Dermatology* **24**, 337–345

Roudebush P, Logan E and Hale FA (2005) Evidence-based veterinary dentistry: a systematic review of homecare for prevention of periodontal disease in dogs and cats. *Journal of Veterinary Dentistry* **22**, 6–15

Sakzewski L and Naser-ud-Din S (2014) Work-related musculoskeletal disorders in dentist sand orthodontists: a review of the literature. *Work* **48**, 37–45

Sapierzynski R, Czopowicz M and Ostrzeszewicz M (2017) Factors affecting the diagnostic utility of canine and feline cytological samples. *Journal of Small Animal Practice* **58**, 73–78

Sarkiala E and Harvey C (1993) Systemic antimicrobials in the treatment of periodontitis in dogs. *Seminars in Veterinary Medicine and Surgery* **8**, 197–203

Scrivani PV, Martin-Flores M, Van Hatten R and Bezuidenhout AJ (2014) Structural and functional changes relevant to maxillary arterial blood flow observed during computed tomography and nonselective digital subtraction angiography in cats with the mouth closed and opened. *Veterinary Radiology and Ultrasound* **55**, 263–271

Silver JG, Martin L and McBride BC (1975) Recovery and clearance of oral microorganisms following experimental bacteremias in dogs. *Archives of Oral Biology* **20**, 675–679

Sitzman C (2013) Evaluation of a hydrophilic gingival dental sealant in beagle dogs. *Journal of Veterinary Dentistry* **30**, 150–155

Smith MM, Smith EM, La Croix N and Mould J (2003) Orbital penetration associated with tooth extraction. *Journal of Veterinary Dentistry* **20**, 8–17

Smith MM and Smithson CW (2014) Dental wax decreases calculus accumulation in small dogs. *Journal of Veterinary Dentistry* **31**, 26–29

Somrak AJ and Marretta SM (2015) Management of temporomandibular joint luxation in a cat using a custom-made tape muzzle. *Journal of Veterinary Dentistry* **32**, 239–246

Stevens-Sparks CK and Strain GM (2010) Post-anaesthesia deafness in dogs and cats following dental and ear cleaning procedures. *Veterinary Anaesthesia and Analgesia* **37**, 347–351

Stiles J, Weil AB, Packer RA and Lantz GC (2012) Post-anesthetic cortical blindness in cats: Twenty cases. *Veterinary Journal* **193**, 367–373

Stookey GK (2009) Soft rawhide reduces calculus formation in dogs. *Journal of Veterinary Dentistry* **26**, 82–85

Stookey GK, Warrick JM and Miller LL (1995) Effect of sodium hexametaphosphate on dental calculus formation in dogs. *American Journal of Veterinary Research* **56**, 913–918

Stookey GK, Warrick JM, Miller LL and Katz B (1996) Hexametaphosphate-coated snack biscuits significantly reduce calculus formation in dogs. *Journal of Veterinary Dentistry* **13**, 27–30

Tepe JH, Leonard GJ, Singer RE *et al.* (1983) The long term effect of chlorhexidine on plaque, gingivitis, sulcus depth, gingival recession and loss of attachment in beagle dogs. *Journal of Periodontal Research* **18**, 452–458

Terpak CH and Verstraete FJM (2012) Instrumentation, patient positioning and aseptic technique. In: *Oral and Maxillofacial Surgery in Dogs and Cats*, ed. FJM Verstraete and MJ Lommer, pp. 55–68. Saunders, Philadelphia

Tromp JA, Jansen J and Pilot T (1986a) Gingival health and frequency of tooth brushing in the beagle dog model. Clinical findings. *Journal of Clinical Periodontology* **13**, 164–168

Tromp JA, van Rijn LJ and Jansen J (1986b) Experimental gingivitis and frequency of tooth brushing in the beagle dog model. Clinical findings. *Journal of Clinical Periodontology* **13**, 190–194

Troxel M (2015) Iatrogenic traumatic brain injury during tooth extraction. *Journal of the American Animal Hospital Association* **51**, 114–118

Vezina-Audette R, Benedicenti L, Castejon-Gonzalez A *et al.* (2017) Recurrent asystole and severe bradycardia during surgical repair of a congenital cleft palate in a dog. *Journal of the American Veterinary Medical Association* **250**, 1104–1106

Vrieling HE, Theyse LRF, Winkelhoff van AJ *et al.* (2005) Effectiveness of feeding large kibbles with mechanical cleaning properties in cats with gingivitis. *Tijdschrift voor Diergeneeskunde* **130**, 136–140

Watanabe K, Hayashi K, Kijima S, Nonaka C and Yamazoe K (2015) Tooth brushing inhibits oral bacteria in dogs. *Journal of Veterinary Medical Science* **77**, 1323–1325

Watanabe K, Kijima S, Nonaka C, Matsukawa Y and Yamazoe K (2016) Inhibitory effect for proliferation of oral bacteria in dogs by tooth brushing and application of toothpaste. *Journal of Veterinary Medical Sciences* **78**, 1205–1208

Watson AD (1994) Diet and periodontal disease in dogs and cats. *Australian Veterinary Journal* **71**, 313–318

Watson RL, Dowell SF, Jayaraman M *et al.* (1999) Antimicrobial use for pediatric upper respiratory infections: reported practice, actual practice, and parent beliefs. *Pediatrics* **104**, 1251–1257

West-Hyde L (1995) Occupational hazards in small animal dentistry. In: *BSAVA Manual of Small Animal Dentistry, 2nd edn*, ed. DA Crossley and S Penman, pp. 50–66. BSAVA Publications, Gloucester

Withrow SJ (1981) Taping of the mandible in treatment of mandibular fractures. *Journal of the American Animal Hospital Association* **17**, 27–31

Wolvius EB and van der Wal KG (2003) Bone wax as a cause of a foreign body granuloma in a cranial defect: a case report. *International Journal of Oral and Maxillofacial Surgery* **32**, 656–658

Yamasaki Y, Nomura R, Nakano N *et al.* (2012) Distribution of periodontopathic bacterial species in dogs and their owners. *Archives of Oral Biology* **57**, 1183–1188

Zetner K and Rothmueller G (2002) Treatment of periodontal pockets with doxycycline in beagles. *Veterinary Therapeutics* **3**, 441–452

Index

Page numbers in *italics* refer to figures
Page numbers in **bold** refer to Operative Techniques

carnivore 6
deciduous and permanent tooth differences 13–14
defence mechanisms/repair 31–2
dental formula/eruption schedule 14–15
dental occlusion 25–6
Modified Triadan System 15, *16*
odontogenesis/tooth development 6–7, 15
periodontium *17–18*, 20–1
physiology of dental tissues 31–2
radiographic anatomy 25
sensory perception 32
surgical anatomy 27–31
tooth eruption 7–12
tooth exfoliation 12–13
tooth morphology 21–4
(*see also* Deciduous dentition; Permanent dentition;
Tooth abnormalities; *and specific tooth types*)
Dentoalveolar ankylosis 62, 97, *98*
Deracoxib *130*
Desflurane 128
Developmental disorders
brachycephalic obstructive airway syndrome 265–7
calvarial hyperostosis 265
craniomandibular osteopathy 71, 115, 265
fibrous osteodystrophy 265, *266*
lip and palate defects 109, 260–4
periostitis ossificans 265, *266*
temporomandibular joint dysplasia 73, 264
tight lower lip 267–8
tongue anomalies 268
(*see also* Malocclusions; Open-mouth jaw locking;
Tooth abnormalities)
Dexmedetomidine 126, 128, *131*
Diagnostic imaging *see* Imaging
Diazepam 126–7, *131*
Dietary measures
feline chronic stomatitis 179
home oral hygiene 364
intra/postoperative 345–7
Digital radiographic systems 51, 52, *53*
Dilaceration 94, 257
Diphyodont dentition 6, 12
Direct inclined planes 251, *252*, **275–7**
Direct pulp capping *196*, *198*, 199
Disarming dogs, ethical principles 5
Disclosing solutions 37
Disease *see* Pathological conditions
Disinfection 360
Dobutamine *128*
Dolichocephalic head conformation 245
Domestic Shorthaired cat
endotracheal intubation *122*
feline chronic stomatitis *172*, *173*
palatal fracture repair *223*
oral eosinophilic granuloma *185*, 186
squamous cell carcinoma *280*, *285*
Dopamine, use in anaesthesia *128*
Dorsal marginal mandibulectomy **298–300**
Dorsoventral (DV) radiographic views 54
Doxycycline gel 156, **166**
Drinking water additives, home oral hygiene 365
Drug interactions, evaluation for anaesthesia 120
Dysplasia, temporomandibular joint 73, 264

Ear trimming, ethical principles 2
Ectodermal dysplasia 258
Education, client 287
(*see also* Clients, communication)
Elderly patients, evaluation for anaesthesia 120
Electrical burns, oral trauma surgery 217, *218*
Elevators 308–9, *310*, 312, *314*, 341
Embedded teeth 95, 258–9
Embolism 312, 318, 321, 342–3
Embryonic development of teeth 6–7
Emphysema, iatrogenic injury 321, 342–3
Enamel 6, 7, 14
anatomy 16–19
comparison of dental tissues *19*
deciduous and permanent tooth differences 14
fractures/infraction 100, *101*
hypomineralization 98–9, 254–5
hypoplasia 98, 99, 254–5
odontogenesis 6–7
pearls 7, 94, 258
radiographic anatomy *18*, 25
radiology 60, *61*, 62–3, 70
Endodontics
ethical principles 4
radiology 66, 67, *68*
techniques
contraindications 197
terminology/definitions *196*
traumatic injury 196–206
treatment algorithm *198*
Endodontics 102, 137
ethical principles 4
radiology 66, 67, *68*
Endotoxaemia, antibiotic use 348–9
Endotracheal tubes 121–4, 305, 338–9
Eosinophilic granuloma complex 114, 176, 185, 186
Epitheliotropic T-cell lymphoma (ETCL) 183, 184–5
Equipment
anaesthesia *121*, *125*, *132*
dental examination 36–7
exodontics 307–11
maintenance/care 356–60
oral and maxillofacial tumours 287
oral trauma surgery 208
orthodontics 248–9, **271**
periodontics 137–52
radiography 49–51, 52, 54
sanitization, disinfection and sterilization 360
(*see also* Instruments)
Ergonomics, for practitioners 197, 352–3
Eruption of teeth *see* Tooth eruption
Erythema multiforme (EM) 115, 176, 182–3
Ethics of treatment 1–3
endodontics 4
exodontics 5
orthodontics 3, 250
periodontics 3–4
prosthodontics 4
Ethylenediamine tetra-acetic acid (EDTA) solution 203
Etodolac *130*
Etomidate 127, *131*
European Domestic Shorthair *see* Domestic
Shorthaired Cat
European Veterinary Dental College (EVDC) 3, 48, 361, 367
European Veterinary Dental Society (EVDS) 367

Harmful practices, ethical principles 2, 4
Head conformation, and malocclusion 245
Head radiography 49, 54–8, 71
Health and welfare, ethics 1–2, 3, 4, 5
 (*see also* Safety)
Healthcare products 4, 46–7
Hearing loss, iatrogenic 338
Heart function, anaesthesia 119–20, 121
Heat injury, iatrogenic 138, 140, 154
Hedstrom files, root canal therapy *202, 203*
High-speed handpieces 140, 307, 359–60
Histiocytosis 188
Histology
 masticatory muscle myositis 191
 osteonecrosis/osteomyelitis 188
 tumours 285–6
Histopathology
 chronic stomatitis 176, 182
 erythema multiforme 183
 tumours 287
History-taking 33
Hoes, periodontal surgical instruments 146
Holding dental instruments *354,* 355, *355*
 (*see also* Modified pen grasp technique)
Home oral hygiene 362–5
 information for owners **166**
 periodontal disease 91
Husky, root canal therapy *201*
Hydromorphone *131*
Hygiene 91, 137, 153
 (*see also* Home oral hygiene)
Hypercementosis 103, *104*
Hypersalivation/hypersialism 113–14
Hypodontia 49, 63, 94, 256, 258
Hypothermia/hyperthermia, intraoperative 124–5, 341

Iatrogenic injury
 accidental aspiration 339, 343–4, 361
 emphysema and embolism 321, 342–3
 exodontics 319–21
 foreign bodies 339–40
 local/regional anaesthesia 132, *133,* 134
 mouth gags 36, 125, 338, *339*
 ocular/orbital 340–1
 oral and oropharyngeal oedema 339
 pulp 138, 140, 154
 tracheal 338–9
 trigeminocardiac reflex 341
Idiopathic osteomyelitis 188
Imaging 49
 foreign bodies 81, *82*
 jaw/temporomandibular joints 70–8
 neuromuscular conditions 79
 palatine tonsils/tongue 78
 radiological interpretation 60–2
 regional lymph nodes 77–8
 salivary glands 79–81
 techniques **83–8**
 teeth/periodontal tissues 63–9
 (*see also specific modalities*)
Immunological abnormalities, chronic stomatitis 172–80
Immunosuppressive drugs, feline chronic stomatitis 178
Immunotherapy, tumours 292

Impacted teeth 95, 259, 260, 304
Implants, ethical principles 4
Impression trays/materials 248, **271–5**
Incisivomaxillary canal, surgical anatomy 28, 29
Incisor teeth 16, 21–2
 exodontics 306, 311–12
 imaging techniques **83–5, 86–8**
 occlusion/orthocclusion 245
 surgical anatomy *30,* 31
Inclined planes, orthodontics 251, *252,* **275–7**
Indirect pulp capping *196,* 197–9
Inductive fibroameloblastoma 110, *279,* 283
Infections
 iatrogenic 304, 321
 immunological responses 91, 92
 malodour 37
 osteomyelitis 93
  (*see also* Inflammatory conditions; and *specific diseases*)
Inferior alveolar nerve block 135
Inflammatory conditions
 canine chronic stomatitis 180–2
 effects of tooth wear 100
 feline chronic stomatitis 172–80
 jaws/masticatory muscles/salivary glands 188–94
 nodular lesions of oral mucosa 185–8
 periapical abscess 103
 radiography 70–1
 soft tissue and bone inflammation 92–3
 systemic effects 91, 137
 tooth resorption 65–6, 97–8
 ulcerative lesions of oral mucosa 172–85
 (*see also* Infections)
Information, client 287
 (*see also* Clients, communication)
Informed consent 1, 2, 3, 4, 5, 304, 305
Infraorbital artery, surgical anatomy 28, 29, 32
Infraorbital canal 32
Infraorbital foramen, 32
Infraorbital nerve block 133–4
Inhaled anaesthetic agents 128
Injectable anaesthetic agents 128
Instruments 137–150
 air/water syringes 141, 156, **164, 166**
 burs 141, **167,** 199, 249, 307, 359–60
  12-fluted 148, 158, **170, 171**
  friction-grip (FG) 307
  tungsten carbide 141
 chisels 146
 elevators 148, 153, **167,** 308–9, *310,* 312, 314, 341
  Molt No. 9 148
 explorers 36–7, *43,* 44, 142, **164**
  11/12 ODU 142
  Orban 147, 148
  shepherd's hook 36, 142
 files 146
  Hedstrom *202, 203*
 forceps
  calculus-removing forceps 144, **164**
  pocket-marking 148, **170**
  root tip *307, 308, 310,* 317, **331, 334**
  thumb 149, **167,** 308
 gingival knives 147–8, **170**
  Kirkland 147, *148*
  Orban 147, *148*

Macrodontia 94, 256
Macroglossia 268
Magnetic resonance imaging (MRI) 59–60
    foreign bodies 81
    inflammation and infection 70
    lymph nodes 77
    neuromuscular conditions 79
    palatine tonsils 78
    salivary glands 79–81
    temporomandibular joint 72
    tumours 76–7, 285
Magnetostrictive scalers 137, *138*, 357–8
Major palatine artery, surgical anatomy 29
Major palatine nerve blocks 134
Malignant melanoma (MM) 111, 279–80
Malignant peripheral nerve sheath tumour (MPNST) 111, *112*, 279, 281
Malocclusions 95–6, 246
    classification 246–7
    ethical principles 3
    exodontics 304
    oral examination 41
    radiography *63*, 70
    terminology 246
        (*see also* Occlusion; Orthodontics)
Malodour, extraoral examination 37
    (*see also* Halitosis)
Maltese Dog
    tooth extraction *28*
    vital pulp therapy *200*
Mandible (lower jaw)
    fractures 31, 105–6, 137
    operative techniques **298–303**
    radiology 56–7, 60
Mandibular teeth
    exodontics 306, 316, 317, *318*, **325–6, 328–30, 334–5**
    imaging techniques **84–5, 88**
    linguoversion 251, 252
    occlusion/malocclusions 96, 246, 247
    radiology *61–8*, 69
    surgical anatomy *29, 30*, 31
    vascular supply 32
Mandibular canal *27, 28*, 31, 60
Mandibulectomy 113, 290–1, **298–303**
Marginal Line Calculus Index 47
Masks, personal protective equipment 351
Masseter muscle, surgical anatomy 28
Mast cell tumours (MCTs) 113, 279, 282
Mast cells, feline chronic stomatitis 176
Masticatory muscle myositis (MMM) 79, 94, 190–2
Mastiff, tight lower lip *268*
Mastocytoma 113, 279, 282
Maxilla (upper jaw)
    fractures 106
    operative technique **294–7**
    radiology 56, 60
Maxillary nerve blocks 134
Maxillary teeth
    exodontics 306, 316, **323–4, 326–8, 331–3**
    imaging techniques **83–7**
    malocclusions 247
    mesioversion 252–3, **277–8**
    radiology 60–1, *64–8*, 69
    surgical anatomy 27, 28, 29, *30*
    vascular supply 32

Maxillectomy 113, 289–90, **294–7**
Maxillofacial tumours 109–13, 279
Mayo scissors *149*, 150
Medetomidine 126, *131*
Medical records 33, *34–5*
    anaesthesia 119, *120*
    feline chronic stomatitis 179–80
Medium head conformation 245
Meloxicam *130*
Membranes, guided tissue regeneration 152
Mental foramina, surgical anatomy 31
Mental nerve blocks 135
Mepivacaine 132, *133*
Mesaticephalic head conformation 245
Mesenchymal stem cell therapy 178–9
Mesioversion, maxillary canine tooth 252–3, **277–8**
Mesocephalic head conformation 245
Metabolic conditions, radiography 70–1
Metastases, radiology 77–8
Methadone 130, *131*
Metzenbaum scissors 149
Michigan-O periodontal probes 37, 142, *143*
Microbiome, oral 175
    (*see also* Bacteriology)
Microdontia 94, 256
Microglossia 268
Micromotor units 141
Midazolam 126–7, *131*
Middle mental nerve block 135
Miller surgical curettes 146
Mineral trioxide aggregate (MTA) 199, 200, **229**
Miniature Pinscher, canine chronic stomatitis *181*
Miniature Schnauzer, malignant melanoma *279*
Minimum alveolar concentration (MAC) 128, 132
Mirrors, dental 36, 144, *154*, **164**
Missing teeth (hypodontia) 49, 63, 94, 256
Mixing spatulas, orthodontics 248
Modified pen grasp technique 140, 142, *143*, 144, 153, 355
Modified split U-flap 223–4
Modified Triadan System 12, *13*, 15, *16*, 33
Modified Widman flap procedure 156, 167
Molar teeth 23–4, *30*
    anatomy *17–18*, 31
    exodontics 176–8, 306–7, 313, 316–17, *318*, **328–35**
    imaging techniques **84, 85, 87–8**
    radiology 49, *60, 62, 63*
Molt No. 9 periosteal elevator 148
Morphine *128*, 131
Morphology of teeth 21–4
Mouth gags 36, 125, *197*, 223, 305, 338, *339*
Mouth opening/closing, extraoral examination 39
Mucogingival junction (MGJ) *17–18*, 20, *42*, **167**
Mucoperiosteal flaps 148, 156–7, 159, 161, **167**
Mucositis, radiation therapy 184
Mucus membrane pemphigoid (MMP) 183
Multilobular bone tumours 77, 111, *112*, 279, 281–2
Multi-rooted teeth, exodontics 312–13, 314
Musculoskeletal disorders (MDS)
    practitioner 352–5, *356*
    radiology 79
Muzzling, intra/postoperative 209, *210*, 343–4
Myoblastoma 111, *279*, 283

Surgical solutions...

BSAVA Manual of Canine and Feline
Abdominal Surgery
Second edition

Editors: John M. Williams, Jacqui D. Niles

This fully revised and updated edition provides a practical surgical reference that is easy to read and follow. Includes step-by-step Operative Techniques.

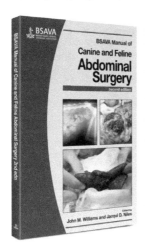

BSAVA Member Price
£61.75
Price to non-members: £95.00

BSAVA Manual of Canine and Feline
Head, Neck and Thoracic Surgery
Second edition

Editors: Daniel J. Brockman, David E. Holt, Gert ter Haar

This manual provides a practical, up-to-date approach to the head, neck and thoracic surgery in dogs and cats. Includes step-by-step Operative Techniques.

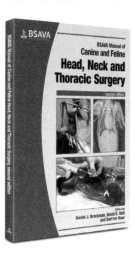

BSAVA Member Price
£58.50
Price to non-members: £90.00

BSAVA Manual of Canine and Feline
Fracture Repair and Management
Second edition

Editors: Toby J. Gemmill, Dylan N. Clements

This manual covers principles of fracture management, repair and management of specific fractures and the treatment and prevention of complications. Includes step-by-step Operative Techniques.

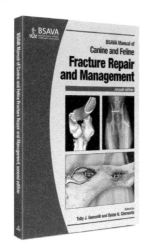

BSAVA Member Price
£61.75
Price to non-members: £95.00

BSAVA Manual of Canine and Feline
Musculoskeletal Disorders
Second edition

Editors: Gareth Arthurs, Gordon Brown, Rob Pettitt

This second edition presents a logically arranged and readily accessible source of practical information for the management of musculoskeletal disorders. Includes step-by-step Operative Techniques.

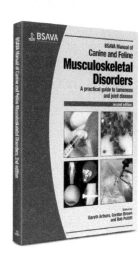

BSAVA Member Price
£61.75
Price to non-members: £95.00

WHERE TO BUY
Order print books at **www.bsava.com/store**
or call **01452 726700**
Order online versions at **www.bsavalibrary.com**

BSAVA Publications
COMMUNICATING VETERINARY KNOWLEDGE

BSAVA reserves the right to alter prices where necessary without prior notice.

BSAVA Manuals

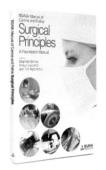 BSAVA Manual of Canine and Feline Surgical Principles: A Foundation Manual

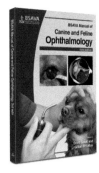 BSAVA Manual of Canine and Feline Ophthalmology, third edition

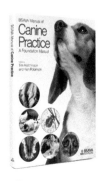 BSAVA Manual of Canine Practice: A Foundation Manual

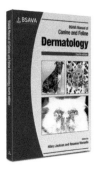 BSAVA Manual of Canine and Feline Musculoskeletal Disorders

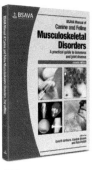 BSAVA Manual of Canine and Feline Dermatology

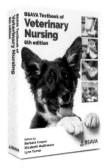 BSAVA Textbook of Veterinary Nursing, 6th edition

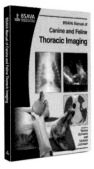 BSAVA Manual of Canine and Feline Emergency and Critical Care

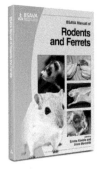 BSAVA Manual of Canine and Feline Shelter Medicine

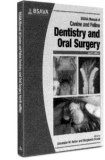 BSAVA Manual of Canine and Feline Anaesthesia and Analgesia

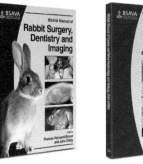 BSAVA Manual of Wildlife Casualties

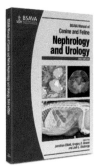 BSAVA Manual of Canine and Feline Haematology and Transfusion Medicine

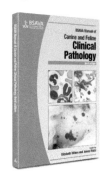 BSAVA Manual of Exotic Pets

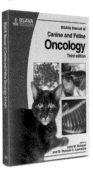 BSAVA Manual of Canine and Feline Oncology, Third edition

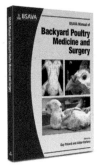 BSAVA Manual of Backyard Poultry Medicine and Surgery

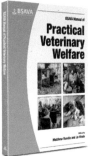 BSAVA Manual of Practical Veterinary Welfare

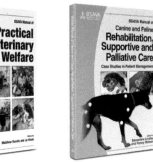 BSAVA Manual of Canine and Feline Rehabilitation, Supportive and Palliative Care

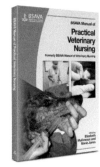 BSAVA Manual of Practical Veterinary Nursing

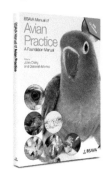 BSAVA Manual of Avian Practice: A Foundation Manual

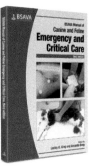 BSAVA Manual of Canine and Feline Thoracic Imaging

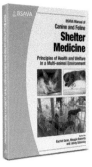 BSAVA Manual of Rodents and Ferrets

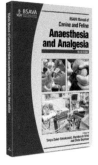 BSAVA Manual of Canine and Feline Dentistry and Oral Surgery

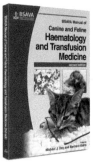 BSAVA Manual of Rabbit Surgery, Dentistry and Imaging

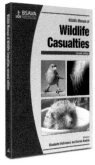 BSAVA Manual of Canine and Feline Nephrology and Urology

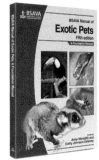 BSAVA Manual of Canine and Feline Clinical Pathology

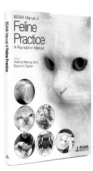 BSAVA Manual of Feline Practice: A Foundation Manual

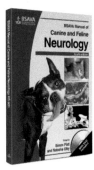 BSAVA Manual of Canine and Feline Neurology

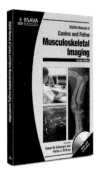 BSAVA Manual of Canine and Feline Musculoskeletal Imaging

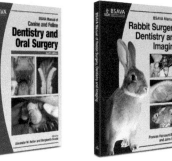 BSAVA Manual of Canine and Feline Head, Neck and Thoracic Surgery

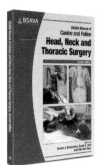 BSAVA Manual of Canine and Feline Behavioural Medicine, Second edition

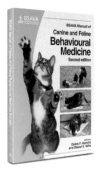 BSAVA Manual of Canine and Feline Radiography and Radiology: A Foundation Manual

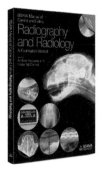

Tel: 01452 726700   Fax: 01452 726701
Email: administration@bsava.com   Web: www.bsava.com